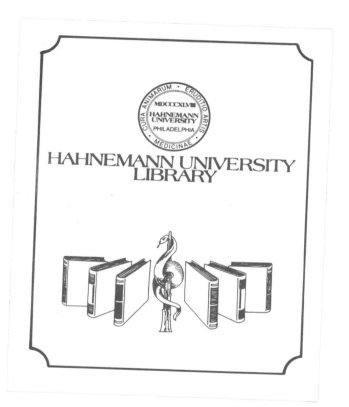

Orthopedic Pathophysiology in Diagnosis and Treatment

Orthopedic Pathophysiology in Diagnosis and Treatment

Jonathan Cohen, M.D.

Professor, Department of Orthopedic Surgery, Tufts University School of Medicine; Consultant, Orthopedic Surgery and Pathology, Children's Hospital Medical Center; Consultant, Orthopedic Surgery, Franciscan Children's Hospital; Deputy Editor, Journal of Bone and Joint Surgery, Boston, Massachusetts

Michael Bonfiglio, M.D.

Professor Emeritus, Department of Orthopaedic Surgery, University of Iowa College of Medicine and University of Iowa Hospitals and Clinics; formerly Chief, Section of Orthopaedic Surgery, Veterans Administration Medical Center, Iowa City, Iowa

Crawford J. Campbell, M.D.

Formerly Chairman, Division of Orthopaedic Surgery, Albany Medical College of Union University, Albany, New York; formerly Lecturer, Department of Orthopedic Surgery, Harvard Medical School and Massachusetts General Hospital, Boston, Massachusetts

■■■ **Churchill Livingstone**
■■■ New York, Edinburgh, London, Melbourne

Library of Congress Cataloging-in-Publication Data

Cohen, Jonathan, date
    Orthopedic pathophysiology in diagnosis and treatment/Jonathan
Cohen, Michael Bonfiglio, Crawford J. Campbell.
      p.   cm.
    Includes bibliographical references.
    ISBN 0-443-08070-4
    1. Orthopedics.   2. Physiology, Pathological.   I. Bonfiglio,
Michael, date.   II. Campbell, Crawford J.   III. Title.
    [DNLM: 1. Arthritis.   2. Bone Diseases   3. Connective Tissue
Diseases.   4. Fractures.   5. Muscular Diseases.   WE 140 C678o]
RD732.C64   1990
617.3—dc20
DNLM/DLC   89-22215
for Library of Congress   CIP

Distributed in the United Kingdom by Churchill Livingstone, Robert Stevenson House, 1–3 Baxter's Place, Leith Walk, Edinburgh EH1 3AF, and by associated companies, branches, and representatives throughout the world.

Accurate indications, adverse reactions, and dosage schedules for drugs are provided in this book, but it is possible that they may change. The reader is urged to review the package information data of the manufacturers of the medications mentioned.

The Publishers have made every effort to trace the copyright holders for borrowed material. If they have inadvertently overlooked any, they will be pleased to make the necessary arrangements at the first opportunity.

Acquisitions Editor: *Robert A. Hurley*
Production Supervisor: *Sharon Tuder*

Production services provided by Bermedica Production

Printed in the United States of America

First published in 1990

To the giants on whose shoulders we stand, especially Dr. Howard Hatcher.

Preface

More than fifty years ago Codman took the brash step of prefacing his book on the shoulder, a medical classic, with an embarrassingly frank account of his personal life. He believed that the book's readers should know the author's character. The authors of this book are not so brash, but we will, nonetheless, set forth our credentials briefly.

All three of us have been active orthopedic surgeons for three decades in practice and in academic environments. All three of us have had special, early education in bone pathology, two in the Chicago school (Phemister and Hatcher) and one in Boston (Wolbach and Farber). All of us have seen the subject of the pathology of bone carried forward by pathologists with special interest in skeletal disease: Jaffe, Lichtenstein, Dahlin, Spjut, Dorfman, Fechner, and Ackerman. We all have taken active roles in education in local hospitals and also at the national level, with particular attention to musculoskeletal pathology. We have been active in the pathology committee of the American Academy of Orthopedic Surgeons and the discipline of pathology as incorporated in the examination of the American Board of Orthopaedic Surgery. Our writings on bone lesions speak for themselves.

The idea for this book derived its impetus years ago during the meetings of the Pathology Committee of the American Academy of Orthopedic Surgery and during Oral Examinations in Pathology of the American Board of Orthopedic Surgery, spurred by the late Mary Sherman.

When the three of us planned to write the book we shared the responsibility of organizing and writing the text. Two of us (M.B. & C.J.C.) assumed the preparation of cases and illustrations and the third (J.C.) the responsibility of editing the final text; but the death of C.J.C. in 1983 shifted the three functions to the two survivors. We are confident that Dr. Campbell's ideas and philosophy, particularly on controversial subjects, coincide with the ideas and explanations incorporated in this book. All three of us were well aware that the available books on bone pathology did not meet some of the needs of clinicians and students. With few exceptions, they treat bone tumors and tumorlike lesions, to the exclusion of other processes. Those lesions have also been well described from the point of view of pathologists and radiologists, notably in books by Jaffe, Lichtenstein, and Aegerter and Kirkpatrick, Spjut, Dorfman, Fechner, Ackerman, and Schajowicz.

Our intent was to write a book that surveyed the principal musculoskeletal lesions encountered in practice. We wanted to emphasize those pathological and pathophysiological features important to the clinician, that is, the features important for diagnosis and treatment. By diagnosis we mean not only classifying the lesion adequately, but also defining those morphological features of its biological behavior that have important implications with regard to the patient's symptoms and signs and that influence the sequence of diagnostic studies. Ideally as the stages of interaction between doctor and patient progress, the range of diagnostic possibilities should narrow until a definitive diagnosis is reached. Then, all choices in treatment can be reviewed. By treatment we mean characterizing the morphological elements of the lesion as they influence choice and planning of a treatment regimen. One can then administer the clinical treatment that seems most promising.

We also believe that the exact consequences of each maneuver of treatment on all the tissues involved should be examined in conjunction with the diagnostic maneuver. This subject might be called the pathophysiology of therapy. It was our credo, from the outset, that one has to appreciate the possible morphology of the lesion and the operation of a reparative process. If the surgeon is to optimize his or her use of all the factors promoting repair and minimize the influence of factors hampering repair, he or she must understand what changes are occurring in the tissues, both those in and around the lesion and those of the repair process itself. The morphology, to a major degree, reflects those pathological and physiological changes.

In examining board candidates on "interpretive skills" (formerly "pathology"), we noted that the thought processes critical in diagnosis and treatment were not often emphasized in resident education. The chapter on interpretive skills derives its title from that portion of the board examination in which we participated for many years. However, its contents primarily are an outgrowth of regular conferences on correlative pathology that each of us has conducted in his academic programs.

We earnestly hope our efforts will achieve the objectives we have set forth, and we hope our work here will stimulate every reader to think effectively about the lesions that are the basis of orthopedic surgery, and the therapy that is its *raison d'etre.*

Jonathan Cohen, M.D.
Michael Bonfiglio, M.D.

Acknowledgments

No book can be completed without the support and effort of many people.

At Iowa City the support of our colleagues Carroll Larson, Reginald Cooper, and John Kasik, who provided office space and departmental resources, is particularly appreciated, but none of the words would reach the goal of publication without the dedicated work of our secretaries, Pamela Smith, Myrtle Meeker, Jeanette Marsh, Kathy Cady, Cheryl Reyhons, Nancy Grubb, Jan Freel, Lori Schneider, and Laura Cole.

For the illustrations and photomicrographs we are grateful in particular to Louis Facto at the Iowa City Veterans Hospital Medical Media Production and Linda Rohret at the same service, and at the Audio Visual Center of the University of Iowa College of Medicine to Steve Thalken, Ed Heffron, and Larry Perkins, and to Jerry Maynard, Fred Ohlerking, and John Busse at the Orthopaedic Pathology Laboratory, Department of Orthopaedic Surgery, University of Iowa.

Our wives, Louise Cohen, Ruth Bonfiglio, and Catherine Campbell, encouraged and cajoled us (with reason) from beginning to end. To them no words can express our appreciation.

Contents

Interpretive Skills

The traditional sequence of medical interactions between patient and physician, applicable to orthopedics as elsewhere, is, first, registration of the chief complaint followed by the medical history and then elicitation of physical findings. What follows is variable, including perhaps obtaining appropriate laboratory data, e.g., radiographs. The plan of treatment or of further investigation, if needed, is then mapped out.

The emphasis throughout this book is on how the pathologic characteristics of a lesion affect its treatment. To allow us to focus on those characteristics, we must devote less attention to other aspects of orthopedic lesions, which are covered by and large in standard texts. We choose to begin the book with a chapter on interpretive skills, discussing the processes by which a surgeon accumulates the evidence needed for treating a patient with a specific lesion. It then seems appropriate to review the interpretive skills that have to be applied at all of the steps in the sequence of service to a patient.

OVERVIEW

History

Starting with the medical history, it should be realized that all of the data gathered during history-taking are later used for the inductive and deductive reasoning processes that go on in the mind of the orthopedic surgeon as he or she elicits other findings, whether during the physical examination or when studying laboratory data. It has often been said that the importance of the skill of eliciting the history of an illness or injury cannot be overemphasized. However, the facts in such matters do not lend themselves easily to description or quantitation, or even to verification, and only too often the data that one calls facts depend for their reliability on uncertain and variable traits of patients and the physician, as well as the circumstances of the history-taking.

History-taking is a highly individualized process, and the best history-takers are those who have developed two tools essential to the task. One is a sensitivity to the patient at hand, and the other is knowledge of the several techniques that meet the wide variety of situations one encounters. To elicit the important "facts" one must always deal appropriately with an informant whose state of mind, articulateness, purposes, and even character have been assessed on the spot. History-taking with an intelligent, educated, and calm informant is worlds away from history-taking when a patient is unintelligent, inarticulate, unobservant, or terrified to the point of distorting symptoms or sequences of events. Once the history-taker has assessed the informant's state of mind and reliability — a process that may occur within seconds of the primary encounter — then the approach should be chosen which is designed to meet the special elements noted while assessing the patient.

In the context of most specialty practice, at least in the United States, selection of patients for referral to specialists (triage) is done by primary care physicians (generalists), internists, pediatricians, and so on. Most often these physicians refer the patient to the orthopedic surgeon with a more or less extensive work-up (except for emergencies). Even when the work-up has been extensive and its main features relayed to the consultant, the burden of history-taking and triage is not lifted from the shoulders of the orthopedic surgeon. Often the effort for history-taking does not begin where the referring physician left off. Rather, it may start exactly where the triage physician started—at the beginning—with the added obstacles (1) of discounting a history that may be irrelevant, superficial, imperfect, or even downright misleading, and (2) dealing with a patient whose apprehension has been considerably augmented by the prospect of what lies ahead.

In orthopedic conditions, however inclusive or exclusive the term, there usually are symptoms of pain of one kind or another, a disturbance in motor function, or a deformity. Usually there is a combination of these complaints. Compared to the symptoms that occur in patients by and large, this list is short; nevertheless, the orthopedist must keep in mind that, except for deformity, each of the symptoms may well relate to a nonorthopedic condition. Conversely, what seem to be symptoms irrelevant to orthopedics may well have their origins in lesions properly termed "orthopedic." The job of triage of patients who belong under the care of not only primary physicians but also orthopedic surgeon-physicians and those who do not is a primary responsibility of the orthopedic surgeon. This physician must develop the skill of eliciting and interpreting any symptoms whatsoever so that the interpretation leads logically to step-by-step collection of whatever data are needed for diagnosis and treatment.

Skills in the handling of therapeutic problems and establishing good relations with patients often begin with elicitation of the history. Perhaps only experience can teach interpretive skills in this area, particularly in regard to the interpretation of pain, perhaps the most subjective of all symptoms. Given the wide range of patients' perception of and accommodation to pain, the surgeon's skill in interpreting the importance of a patient's pain can well be the cornerstone of the diagnostic sequence of fact finding as well as of the therapeutic regimen. Many special systems have been devised to evaluate the pain component of particular conditions, especially for the assessment of each such condition relative to operative indications and postoperative end results. All of the systems apply to special situations (e.g., total hip or knee replacement arthroplasty) and are not relevant to ordinary, everyday conditions of practice.

Limitations of space forbid elaborate consideration of how one should elicit the facts from a patient and then develop interpretive skills in relating those facts to one's knowledge of anatomy and pathophysiology. The solution to the anatomical problem is to associate each symptom with the structure that probably is maximally involved. The pathophysiological problem is resolved by establishing a list, in descending order of probability, of the process that may be under way. Solving these two problems often may be extraordinarily difficult even on the restricted subject of pain. Some typical patterns are easily recognized and need not be described; but even the seasoned practitioner, reviewing failures and mistakes, may well realize that often misinterpretation of symptoms was responsible for this first wrong step along the path to misdiagnosis. The failure to obtain adequate information from the patient heads the list of inadequacies in clinical competence, as determined by a study conducted for the National Board of Medical Examiners. It may come as a shock to a busy practitioner to be told that as his or her practice grows the history-taking procedures, because they are time-consuming, tend to become more sketchy; and despite growing expertise, omissions and mistakes tend to multiply. The following two cases demonstrate the role played by patterns of pain in diagnosis as related to orthopedic problems.

Case 1-1 An 8-year-old boy had complained daily of pain in his back for 2 months. Although the pain is not disabling, even in regard to participation in sports, it is becoming more severe and is now interfering with sleep. He takes aspirin for the pain, sometimes as often as three times a day. Other than the pain in the back, he has had no complaints and is in good health.

This pattern of pain, so distinctive for osteoid osteoma, must be considered with one fact particularly in mind, i.e., the patient's age. Children, especially teenage boys, rarely have pain in the back, except for the transient after-effects of injury. Elicitation of a history of injury in this case would merely cloud the diagnostic problem. The question now arises: Are there any historical details that might be helpful? There are, and they illustrate an important principle: A single diagnostic entity should never be so uppermost in the doctor's thoughts as to prevent entertainment of other possibilities. With the pain pattern as given, localization of the pain would be helpful, as would any symptoms of radiation of pain or sensory disturbance. Elicitation of these historical elements should not be conducted in a manner that, however methodical, could be characterized as an elaborate checklist. It should follow the sequence dictated by the particular circumstances. Each item of information should lead to questions related to it, i.e., questions that would support the most probable diagnosis or, more importantly, support other diagnoses. In this case, other possibilities are spondylolysis, a tumor of bone or of the spinal canal or paraspinal structures, herniated intervertebral disc, or an infection.

Each possibility evokes a series of questions, but here a practical consideration — efficient use of medical time — enters the equation, and another principle applies as well: The medical history need not be elicited as an entity separated from other steps leading to a diagnosis. In case 1-1, for instance, physical findings may well allow the physician to minimize the questioning. However, the physician's desire to save time should not suggest that in a case such as this one an x-ray examination is undoubtedly needed, so why not have it done right away? This route is a pernicious one because it invalidates the important precepts already discussed with reference to symptoms. In addition, it violates another principle; that is, the kind of x-ray examination performed should be tailored to the information available. Not enough information is yet at hand in case 1-1 to specify what radiographic views should be requested.

Physical Examination

At this point it would not be amiss for the physician to perform a physical examination. Suppose the physical examination is done (not perfunctorily) and the following positive physical findings are recorded: mild scoliosis (Fig. 1-1A) that is predominantly lumbar (Fig. 1-1B), considerable paraspinal muscle spasm in the lumbar region, limited straight-leg raising (Fig. 1-1C), and a normal neurological examination (reflexes, sensation, strength). These findings obviously support a diagnosis of osteoid osteoma.[2] They should provoke the physician to conduct a more intensive examination of the lumbar spine with regard to finding minimal tenderness in any one particular spot or perhaps slight swelling or deformity in a particular region of the lumbar spine. It should be mentioned that, in contrast to the repetitive nature of the questioning of the patient for historical details, repeated examinations are not as easily come by, and therefore the physical examination should be conducted in as detailed and complete a way as possible when the opportunity is provided. It certainly is not inappropriate to re-check physical findings from time to time, but in general different parts of the physical examination should not be separated in time or each part performed without reference to other parts.

Whereas one positive physical finding should stimulate the examiner to try to elicit other associated findings, there should be some general, personally individualized pattern to the examiner's examination that allows for departure from the ordinary sequence of tests while ensuring that there would be no important omissions. Lumbar scoliosis in the case under consideration and the spasm of the paraspinal muscles should not erase from the examiner's thoughts the possibility that a rectal examination may be of value if the details of the history or subsequent findings by radiograph, for example, so indicate. The mental checklist implied here differs from routine checklists in that it focuses the examiner's attention on the adequacy of the examination and is designed to avoid the pro forma routine of a checklist that, when repeated too often, blurs the problem-solving process by making slavish the adherence to a routine for routine's sake.

After the physical examination has been completed, it is obvious that an x-ray examination is in order; let us assume that the views obtained from it are pertinent to the problem as presented. Let us also assume that the x-ray examination shows no findings that are diagnostic. Suppose a scoliosis is present, for instance, but no localized osseous lesion can be seen (Fig. 1-1D). An important fact that relates to localization of osteoid osteoma in the spine should then be recalled by the physician in

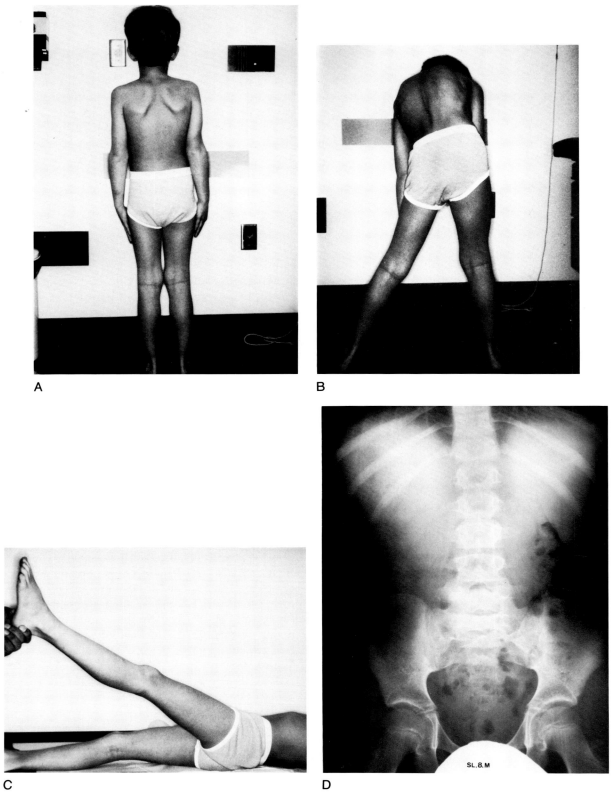

A

B

C

D

Fig. 1-1. Case 1-1. **(A)** Mild scoliosis to the left. **(B)** The forward bending position shows a paraspinal muscle spasm in the lumbar region. **(C)** Limited straight-leg raising is present on the left. **(D)** Radiograph of the lumbosacral spine with mild left scoliosis. *(Figure continues.)*

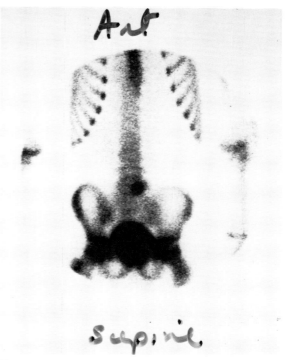

Fig. 1-1 *(Continued)*. (**E**) Supine bone scan. Positive left L5 lamina and pedicle. (**F**) AP radiograph of the lumbar spine of an 8-year-old boy shows an aneurysmal bone cyst (arrow) of the L4 transverse process. (**G**) Oblique view reveals an osteoblastoma or chondromyxoid fibroma (arrow) of the pedicle.

E

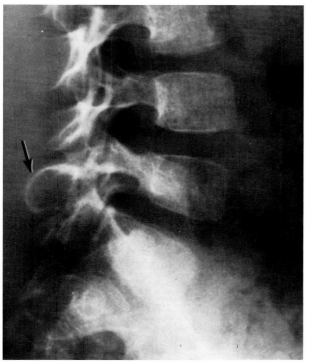

F

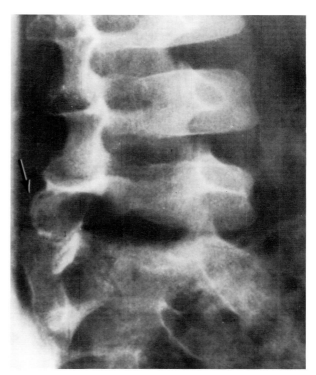

G

charge, otherwise the diagnosis will be delayed, often for weeks or months: That fact is that osteoid osteoma in the spine sometimes is so difficult to recognize from the radiographic examination that it is even missed on several such examinations, often over a period of many months. The physician knowledgeable about the subject, given no radiological findings of osteoid osteoma, should think in terms of a bone scan for the diagnosis because it is the most sensitive way to make the diagnosis in the absence of positive radiographic findings (Fig. 1-1E).[1]

The point is, in this case, that the pattern of pain is so distinctive and the findings are so supportive of a diagnosis of osteoid osteoma that the physician should pursue that diagnosis even if negative radiographs are obtained. Of course, if the radiographic findings are indicative of another of the lesions mentioned above (Fig. 1-1F,G), or even if the lesion is a small facet fracture in the healing stage, the diagnosis is then followed by the treatment appropriate to the entity.

Case 1-2 Another example of how elicitation of a medical history is governed by the principle that each bit of information elicited should fit into a rational pattern of problem-solving is as follows: Supposing that 1 week after an injury to the knee a female college student seeks consultation because of continuing pain and swelling. Given the wide spectrum of traumatic lesions that occur at the knee and the nontraumatic lesions first brought to one's attention when there is an injury, the delineation of what would be the best approach to the specific problem varies widely with the circumstances. One approach might be chosen if the young woman enters the consulting room on crutches, whereas another would be appropriate if she enters limping, and a third if she enters walking without a limp. One approach may be appropriate to a sports medicine clinic in the college and another to the private practitioner's office. Previous familiarity of the surgeon with injuries of the knee in the young woman, or elicitation of such a history, also might dictate a variation in the approach, as do the details of the specific injury or the evaluation of the degree of swelling. Each one of the half-dozen items just mentioned may be evident within seconds or minutes of the patient's encounter with the physician. If the problem-solving is to be an effi-

cient process, the physician must take into account not only all of the facts in retrospect (as in a statistical regression analysis) but also those possibly in prospect. For instance, recurrent subluxation of the patella is a common lesion in young women, whereas strain of the medial collateral ligament, the most common injury of the knee in young men, is uncommon in young women except for those who indulge in the more violent athletic activities. Relatively common lesions should be sought first. It is much more effective if the surgeon has a mental list of suspected lesions, in order of priority, rather than "ruling out" first one condition, however uncommon or common, and then another, as if a diagnosis is best reached by exclusion. When conditions permit and an accurate and firm diagnosis is not easily come by, the best practical course may be to administer appropriate conservative therapy as for a diagnosis that the surgeon knows is a provisional diagnosis, contingent on the course of the symptoms. The patient, when apprised of the way in which matters are being carried forward, may then be encouraged to become more precise as to symptoms and to cooperate better with therapy.

Returning to case 1-2, the young woman with knee pain, let us assume for the sake of the example that the patient has not been seen before, is being cared for in an office setting, and walks in with only a mild limp. Assume further that routine questioning about the pain yields the following historical items: Onset: 1 week earlier she sustained a valgus injury during a basketball game; location of pain: medial mostly but also circumpatellar; character of pain: sharp in episodes, perhaps several times per day especially during certain activities such as going down the stairs and playing basketball. Several specific series of questions about the course of a specific episode of pain should then be pursued. One is the typical chronological pattern characterizing subluxation of the patella, another the plica shelf syndrome, another the fat pad syndrome (all common lesions in the young athletic woman). The history-taker may not have in mind a list of all the lesions that might make a young woman present with pain and swelling in the knee, but he or she should surely know the most common ones and should try to establish as quickly as possible if one fits the case. The history here might be rather short (on a provisional basis) because, as with the previous example, more history can be elicited during and after the physical examination.

As to the examination, assume for the sake of the example that the examination reveals no abnormality at the hip, only minor swelling at the knee, indefinite tenderness at the joint line medially, a full range of motion except for the limited flexion attributable to the swelling, and only moderate atrophy of the quadriceps musculature. Before doing the specific physical tests that pertain to the knee (most of them dependent on knowledge of the pathological anatomy of the specific lesion of the knee under test) the examiner should not be so intent on performing the examination that the implications of the positive findings are not contemplated. The positive findings form the *objective* evidence in the case, and they must be much more strongly supportive of the diagnosis than the subjective findings, i.e., those elicited by history-taking. In the presence of swelling, the examiner should be asking whether the swelling represents synovial fluid, blood, or perhaps hypertrophic synovial membrane. It should be wondered if the amount of swelling is consonant with the details of the history (e.g., timing, character of the injury) and if the degree of swelling now present is on the wane, whether in previous episodes the patient has had less or more swelling, and what the course of the swelling was during those other episodes.

Specific Tests

Coming now to the specific tests applicable to the knee, any physician, including one who specializes in sports medicine or sees large numbers of patients with injuries to the knee, should defer a routine of specific tests that, for example, begins with the McMurray test for torn meniscus, the Lachman test for anteroposterior laxity, and rotary instability tests according to the techniques of Slocum, Losee, or MacIntosh until the knee is gently examined. The examiner should be aware that subluxation of the patella may be the diagnosis and thus should instead begin with observing how the patella tracks up and down during flexion and extension of the knee in gait; it should also be observed whether the course of tracking is straight or crooked when the patient is sitting or supine. The sideways mobility

and tenderness of the patella and the ligamentous attachments should be tested and the extent of valgus present in both knees assessed. Meanwhile, the examiner can be formulating questions with regard to findings that may have just become apparent. For example, if the tracking of the patella appears abnormal, the question could be asked if when an episode of pain is experienced there is an accompanying feeling of something out of place in the knee, with perhaps a clicking sound when the displaced structure falls into place. This finding is pathognomonic of a subluxation of the patella as well as of displacement and reduction of a meniscus.

Assume now, in the example, that all of the evidence indicates a diagnosis of recurrent subluxation of the patella. If the situation is clear and not evocative of a need for immediate measures to further pursue the diagnosis or for immediate rigorous therapy, the therapeutic program, e.g., quadriceps exercises, may be formulated. However, the case should not be left incomplete with regard to the physical examination in particular. Other signs that might be important with regard to the nature of the pathological lesion should be carefully elicited. Crepitation on one of the posterior facets of the patella should be an important element of the record, so it becomes clear if the patient also has the chondromalacia that so commonly results from recurrent subluxations. The normal contralateral knee should be examined not only as a control on the findings particularly of chondromalacia but also for recording abnormalities of other types because in cases of subluxation of the patella the condition is often bilateral. The severity of the physical findings and the details of the history of the case then become important factors in the decision of whether to have radiographic documentation, particularly of hypoplasia of the lateral condyle of the femur or sclerosis of the subchondral bone of the patella — important findings in the particular case. Radiographs are not needed routinely — only if some doubt exists about the diagnosis or if other diagnoses are entertained, e.g., osteochondritis dissecans or chondromalacia.

For each of the two cases we described the possible thought processes of the physician as the information that becomes available is digested during the course of the first encounter with the patient. It is evident that these thought processes are difficult to illustrate because in the evolution of each specific pattern there are changes that occur as the bits of information come into view. The most important point is that the examiner's mind must be working in two directions: One involves elicitation of information bit by bit, and the other is concerned with conceptual appreciation of the lesions that may be present.

To consider the possible lesions, whether they are many or few, the surgeon first must know the lesions that are expected to evoke the specific symptoms and physical findings presented by the patient. Only then can the value of a single bit of information be considered. In some situations a single bit of information can categorically eliminate from consideration one or more lesions; or, conversely, a single bit of information can be diagnostic (i.e., it is *pathognomonic*).

In the cases described, there would be no single bit of information in the history and physical findings of the 8-year-old boy (case 1-1) that categorically rules in or out any one of the diagnoses mentioned, although specific bits of information might support or fail to support individual diagnoses to a varying degree. In contrast, with reference to the college girl (case 1-2), a physical finding of tenderness at the attachment of the medial collateral ligament or painful crepitation when the patella is rubbed along the femoral groove may be pathognomonic, respectively, of (1) a tear or sprain of the medial collateral ligament or (2) chondromalacia of the patella.

One of the most common errors in the second direction of thinking is for the examiner to jump prematurely into thinking that a single lesion is the only one that is likely and that other lesions have been reliably ruled out. Too often this error is made either because only one or at most a few lesions have been considered in any important way or because the examiner fails to give due importance to the *provisional* nature of the diagnostic process until the evidence becomes adequately supportive. The supportive evidence is strongly dependent on a conceptualization of the nature of the pathologic lesion in an anatomic or physiologic sense.

It has already been emphasized that a sequential series of interviews and examinations may well be the best way to build the structure of evidence for the diagnosis. The next part of that structure, after the history and physical findings have been elicited, depends on the decision as to what should be the next step. In some cases the history and physical findings so strongly indicate a specific diagnosis that there is no need for a next step; i.e., no radiological or laboratory tests need be pursued. Perhaps then a therapeutic test of sorts would be the most effective way to solve the patient's problem. However, when the lesion is a serious one and would not be likely to spontaneously recede with rest or other short-term conservative measures, the diagnosis must be clarified further by the appropriate radiographic and laboratory studies.

PHYSICAL EXAMINATION

Every specialist, during training, was drilled (or should have been) about how thorough the physical examination should be, especially in regard to his or her particular field of interest. Yet it is surprising that the goal of eliciting positive diagnostic physical findings so often eludes the practitioner. Perhaps this phenomenon can be attributed to the outstanding advances that have been made in the laboratory during recent years. In fact, laboratory findings may be becoming the staff on which many practitioners lean, somewhat to the exclusion of physical findings.

In so-called orthopedic cases, the referring generalist (or internist or primary physician) nearly always displays uncertainty about musculoskeletal findings on examination. He or she may readily acknowledge a lack of competence concerning physical findings that can be elicited only if the physician has a good working knowledge of anatomy. With the recent deemphasis of the study of gross anatomy, particularly of the musculoskeletal system, in medical schools, there is an extra burden on orthopedic surgeons to apply anatomical expertise to the physical examination. In the two cases that follow, it becomes evident that the need for interpretive skill in eliciting physical findings is just as great as that needed for eliciting a history. It is also evident that, as with history-taking, one positive physical finding prompts a search for other confirmatory or contravening findings. At every step the examiner should have a goal (the diagnosis) in mind. Check-lists that presuppose a sequence of items adding up to a diagnosis just do not fit the usual clinical situations because each item may have variable reliability or specificity.

Consider case 1-1, the 8-year-old boy with back pain. Perhaps the first step in the physical examination of the patient would be a look at his back, at which time he would be asked to localize as well as possible the site of his pain. Before that initial step in the examination is reached, however, a perceptive examiner watches the undressing process. It might reveal, for instance, distress while assuming the positions needed to unlace one's shoes — an observation that should suggest to the examiner spasm of the muscles of the back (from osteoid osteoma?) or hamstring tightness, often seen with disc herniation, spondylolysis, or spondylolisthesis. Before the examiner begins to cover the requisite list of observations on gait, stance, mobility of joints, strength of muscles, and so on, the pattern of positive physical findings that relate to the back may be sketched out. This list might include straight-leg raising, side bending, forward bending, and even a cursory neurological examination, depending on the nature of the positive physical findings elicited. The gait–stance–mobility sequence then is a list that serves not only to confirm the pattern of the physical findings but also to ensure that there are no inadvertent omissions. The neurological check on reflexes and sensation and a glance at the feet to identify cavus or other deformity might be enough to rule out a diagnosis of spinal tumor, diastematomyelia, or other rare lesion. The essence of the procedure, however, is to fix one's mind on the one, two, or three most likely possibilities and strive to build the evidence for them step by step.

Suppose in case 1-1 that the definite physical findings are spasm in the paraspinal lumbar musculature on one side, mild scoliosis with concavity toward the opposite side, limited straight-leg raising, and no neurological deficit. It then becomes apparent what radiological examinations would be appropriate; considerations of availability and practicality might dictate that these tests be done together or in sequence, but at the very least the routine films would be examined soon after the physical examination was performed. The word

"performed" is used instead of "completed" to emphasize a point referred to earlier in regard to elicitation of the history. The radiographic findings may well be such that the examiner wants to review some findings that either were not elicited or were equivocal. Suppose, for instance, that the locus of osteoid osteoma was not seen but there was some erosion of a pedicle. The previous, rather perfunctory elicitation of neurologic deficits would now be supplemented by a more elaborate examination. The strength of each muscle would be checked — with areas of hypesthesia or anesthesia sought more diligently so that a spinal tumor would not be missed. In other situations, e.g., where an intervertebral disc proves radiologically to be narrow or a lytic lesion arouses suspicion of infection, laboratory tests might be ordered on the spot or hospitalization recommended for further investigation (e.g., spinal tap, myelogram, biopsy).

Note that at each step of the inductive reasoning process (from the part to the whole) the pathophysiology of each lesion provisionally diagnosed must be kept in mind. In case 1-1, for instance, an erosive process close to the zygoapophyseal joint might irritate the joint, as might an osteoid osteoma. Irritation of the zygoapophyseal joint would explain the scoliosis and the limited straight-leg raising. Does the narrowing of the intervertebral disc mean that infection or tumor or even eosinophilic granuloma has broached the annulus? If so, is it possible to arrive at a more definite diagnosis without biopsy?

Case 1-2, the college girl with a traumatized swollen knee, also can provide insights into the development of interpretive skills as they pertain to the physical examination. Let us select for convenience the history of a fresh week-old injury without preceding chronic trouble. The other physical findings that might be elicited would differ so much, depending on if there is marked swelling and discomfort, that the interpretation of each finding must be governed by those elements.

It may seem like heresy to suggest that physical findings might well be elicited before a detailed history is recorded or that the two might be explored concomitantly. Yet it would be only natural for the examiner, seeing the young woman limping into the examining room with an obviously swollen knee, to seat the patient on the examining table and immediately look at the knee while asking the obvious questions. Of course the circumstances of the injury require detailed documentation.

Frequently the examiner focuses on those details that pertain to a biomechanical explanation of the damage. For example, what ligament(s) might be torn by a twisting, forceful, internal rotational movement of the femur on the tibia with the knee in flexion or perhaps after a blow to the medial surface of the knee while it was flexed? The danger here is that the examiner may gloss over important details of the history that have pathophysiological significance. If the injury was incurred during athletics, was the patient able to continue playing; and if not, was she able to limp off the field? Do the circumstances of the injury resemble those that might be present if the patella was dislocated either with spontaneous reduction or manual reduction? When was the swelling first noted? If it was minutes after the injury, it would bespeak hemorrhage from a vessel(s) of moderate size. If it was noted only the next day, the vessels involved might have been small ones. Were crutches used right away? Was the patient able to sleep that night, and if not did her knee throb? What was the course of the swelling and pain during the 7-day interval, and what was the therapy? Here the examiner would be considering if it was likely that the volume of hemorrhage in the joint was increasing, if it was resorbing, or if the swelling represents exudate rather than hemorrhage.

In addition to the acute symptoms, the patient would also be closely questioned about previous injuries or symptoms that might be related to the injured knee in particular but also to other joints. Much of such questioning can be taking place as the knee is being examined.

If at the initial consultation the knee is so markedly swollen and painful that all motion is interdicted, it may be possible to elicit only those two physical findings, both indicative of a large amount of fluid or blood in the joint. However, the swelling should reveal the anatomical limits of the knee, ballooning of the suprapatellar pouch, and the parapatellar fat pads as well as the posterior recess. Discoloration indicative of hemorrhage usually is absent because the intraarticular blood is relatively distant from the skin surface and separated from it by capsule, fat, and so on. Given these physical findings, the examiner can be certain that the injury has caused intraarticular hemorrhage and can then be thinking of what structures could have been torn within the joint to cause the bleeding. Correlations of the history and the findings at this juncture might be helpful: Was the injury forceful enough to avulse a ligament's attachment to bone or even to fracture the bone? If so, perhaps the best next step would be radiography even though exposures might be limited because of the flexed position of the knee. If the injury was such that one might visualize the possibility of posterior dislocation of the fibula, the vascular status of the leg should be ascertained as well as the possible presence of a neurological deficit.

If for the purpose of developing the theme of interpretive skills the extensive swelling in the patient with obvious severe discomfort and the physical findings of a tender, tense joint are interpreted as evidence of hemorrhage under pressure in the joint, the lesions that are possible include some that could be diagnosed radiologically (e.g., avulsion of the tibial spine, plateau fracture, patellar fracture). Moreover, if the historical details fit any of these lesions a radiological examination with the views that might reveal any of those lesions would be the next step (Fig. 1-2A,B). In all likelihood a radiographic study would be desirable in any case; but in some instances it can be deferred for a few days — if the swelling was not extensive and if the discomfort was also somewhat less than implied above.

At this point in the discussion of case 1-2, the options available for further pursuit of diagnostic measures would be considered by the physician. Probably the most conservative of all of these measures is a short period of immobilization to see if it would alleviate the symptoms and swelling. Some physicians would consider removing the hemorrhagic fluid, partly to reduce the pain in the joint and partly to facilitate the radiological examination either by allowing the flexion contracture to be eliminated or, with an obviously severe injury, by allowing valgus stress views to be obtained under cover of a local anesthetic instilled into the joint. If there is a hemarthrosis, one would expect that the fluid would reaccumulate; a hemarthrosis that is not massive, however, is a strong contraindication to aspiration. The possibility of introducing infection into a joint with exudate is an added argument against such a course of action.

The introduction of arthroscopy has provided

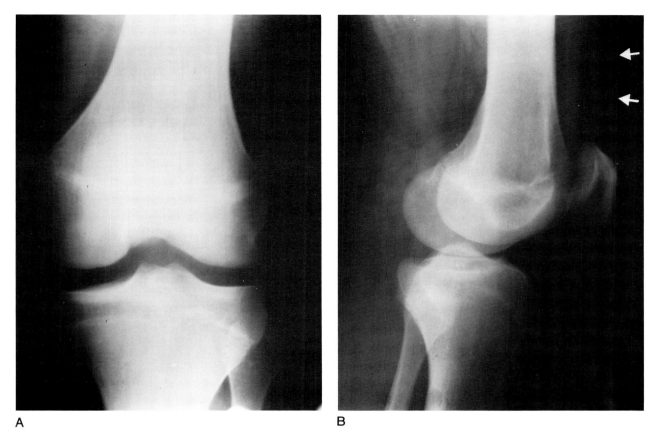

A   B

Fig. 1-2. Case 1-2. **(A)** AP radiograph of the left knee. **(B)** Lateral radiograph shows displacement of the suprapatellar fat pad by fluid (arrows).

the means to arrive at an early diagnosis. In some cases arthroscopy is important, i.e., in cases where a severe injury to ligaments is likely. It is easier to suture the torn ligaments in these patients at an early stage than after a delay of a week or more. Such injuries are uncommon, however, particularly in women, and in the case under discussion such a measure would probably not be useful.

RADIOGRAPHY

Interpretive skills pertain to all phases of diagnosis. After the history and physical examination are concluded, often the most severe test of the examiner's interpretive skills relates to the interpretation of radiographs. Traumatic lesions occupy a large fraction of the practice of orthopedic surgery, and be-

cause they pose such different radiographic problems from those associated with nontraumatic conditions there should be a different emphasis in their interpretation. This point becomes evident when we analyze the radiographs of the two cases already considered from the clinical standpoint.

The surgeon involved in either traumatic or nontraumatic cases undoubtedly views the films while keeping in mind the salient features of the patient's history and physical examination. This process is in some contrast to the approach to films by radiologists, who nearly always are not aware of much of the data in the case. For that reason, radiologists tend to start their study of a film or set of films with a surveying routine. During that survey, in cases in which a pronounced abnormality is detected, the abnormality usually relates to the clinical problem under investigation. The radiologist generally is concerned with the possibility that other, less prominent abnormalities — some related to the "primary" lesion, others serendipitous, and still others irrelevant — may be detected on the film. A surveying routine is followed so there is no inadvertent neglect of any abnormality that may be displayed.

The surveying routine varies with the personal preference of the radiologist. Because teaching ways to develop interpretive skills in regard to radiographs of orthopedic patients tends to be allocated in residency programs to radiologists, these specialists generally teach what they practice — that surveying the films is the first order of business. What medical student has not been at a radiology conference or on rounds where the radiologist or orthopedic surgeon throws a film on the view box and either says nothing whatsoever or asks "What do you see?" implying in either case that the picture tells all. Not uncommonly, the teaching radiologist, in order to emphasize the value of the surveying routine, presents films on which, in addition to the prominent abnormality there are findings that overshadow the abnormality that is of primary interest to the clinician. In contrast, the clinician, with a knowledge of the patient's complaints and physical findings, cannot possibly view the films in that context. He or she naturally focuses on the probable area of abnormality as indicated by the clinical data. The clinician's education in this area has presupposed that the clinical data are in hand as the films are viewed.

It should not be inferred that, for the clinician's purposes, the radiologist's review of the films is not essential except as a means of confirming a diagnosis and uncovering findings that, although present, are not particularly helpful so far as treatment of an orthopedic lesion is concerned. Medicolegal considerations require that an attempt at rigorous reporting of all abnormalities be made, regardless of whether they pertain to the patient's trouble. Institutional requirements of hospitals particularly are such that the report must be complete and be rendered by a certified radiologist. Although these considerations are important for all concerned, for the clinician they constitute distractions from the paramount purpose of the radiograph — pursuit of the diagnosis and then institution of treatment.

The circumstances of viewing the radiographs also play an important role in the disparity of attitudes between radiologist and clinician. When the clinician views the radiographs, more often than not historical and clinical details of the case have just become known, especially when the case is a traumatic one. Whatever the role of the radiologist in viewing and reporting the findings of radiographs and in teaching interpretive skills of radiology, situations abound where the clinician must render his or her own interpretation of the radiographs, without help, and therefore must have the requisite interpretive skills relevant to these responsibilities. Such skills include not only interpretation of the important features of a lesion but also, importantly, judgment as to whether the radiographs that have been obtained are adequate for the purpose and display the findings that are being sought. The last point is important because often the first misstep leading to misdiagnosis or mistakes in treatment can be traced to acceptance of radiographs that were not adequate for either technical or other reasons. Under these circumstances the clinician may be judged inadequate in terms of radiologic interpretive skills, and the radiologist, viewing the films perhaps the next day with the patient unavailable, cannot remedy the situation.

To develop interpretive skills in radiography of orthopedic cases, therefore, the orthopedic surgeon must approach the task keeping in mind the integration of the radiograph with the clinical data. The method of viewing the radiographs should, however, also be integrated (as was the history-taking and physical examination) with a concomitant appreciation of possible pathological lesions as each bit of information is recorded. On the one hand, the radiographic characteristics of the lesion should be registered as basic stepping stones to a radiographic differential diagnosis; on the other hand, each feature of the radiograph should be placed in the context of the pathological process that is most likely responsible for the abnormal finding.

The first step when viewing the films is registering the appropriate observations, i.e., the existence of specific abnormal shadows. An example is the existence of a remodeling change in the contour of a bone or an area of radiolucency in a bone. With recognition of a radiolucency, the borders of that area may be characterized — and if they are irregular, the lesion may be termed lytic. Immediately after that kind of abnormality is recognized, the interpretation of its significance along pathological lines is pursued, as radiographs reflect gross pathological change. In the first example, any change involving remodeling of the gross contours of bone must be thought of as an extraordinary, chronic change; therefore such acute lesions as infection and malignant tumor might well be discounted as improbable. In contrast, the irregular edge of the lytic lesion implies acute destruction of bone, and that in itself means that the process at hand probably is acute, e.g., an infection or malignant tumor. A lytic zone in itself should always bring to the viewer the idea that some nonbony tissue is present within the bony borders, and the question whether the tissue is fat, fluid, pus, tumor, cartilage, or fibrous tissue should arise immediately.

Sometimes a single finding provokes a train of thought that includes so many possibilities the clinician cannot review them all in a short time and come to any worthwhile conclusion. In such instances, perhaps the best course is to keep under consideration the most common lesions that fit the radiographic picture and the most probable interpretation of the abnormality of that single finding while additional supplemental characteristics are sought on the radiograph. Such features might be sets of observations, e.g., the size, contour, and exact localization of the lesion.

In recent years the computerization of information has led to approaches, in processes such as we are describing, in which each bit of information is programmed according to its presence or absence — and even according to the probability of its presence or absence — in all conceivable situations. Until an enormous amount of data can be accumulated, with computerization in mind, the computer approach to interpretation of radiographs cannot be practical. Instead, the clinician's mind must act, to a degree, like the computer by asking such questions as the following: If the lesion is 1 cm in diameter, what lesions tend to fall within that measurement? If the lesion is 10 cm in diameter, what lesions tend to be that large? Analogous questions are raised in the clinician's mind with regard to the exact location of the abnormality and so on.

We have indicated a few of the radiographic features that characterize orthopedic lesions. There are many other features of radiographs that should be part of the observational processes of each clinician who views the films (e.g., the presence of a periosteal reaction). Strangely enough, some of the textbooks devoted to the radiology of skeletal disorders do not address the observational information bits that are essential to recognition of patterns of abnormality. Three texts that do address this problem are those of Ferguson[3], Murray and Jacobson[4] and Eideken and Hodes[5], and there may be others. In addition to the observational bits that have already been mentioned (e.g., radiolucent area, destructive border) others may be mentioned to indicate the scope of the list: the presence of a soft tissue mass, the contour and density of that mass, the presence of stippling within a bony lesion or a permeative character, and the contour of the lesion, either intraosseous or extraosseous.

Once the clinician has examined and interpreted the radiographs in a particular case, the need for further investigative methods must be explored and the tests decided upon, a decision that rests strongly on two elements. One is the confidence the clinician has in the diagnosis (or provisional diagnosis) formulated, and the other is his or her conception of the need for more information with regard to the treatment intended. Often the history, physical findings, and ordinary radiographs lead to a diagnosis so strongly supported by the data that no other diagnosis need be entertained. If the treatment for the patient is standard and does not require special data obtainable only by additional means, it is obvious that further delineation of radiographic features of the lesion or other laboratory results are not needed.

In academic centers particularly, there is a tendency to use excessive investigative measures for spurious reasons. Sometimes there is a tendency to order tomograms, computed tomograms or arteriograms, and other specialized radiographic tests; often they are obtained merely for the edification of the academic community and provide little help to the clinician treating the patient. If the judgment of the clinician in charge is that the diagnosis is a confident one and that no additional information is needed for treatment to be prescribed, good arguments can be advanced against further investigation. Aside from the economic costs and the additional exposure of patients to unnecessary radiation, obviously prime considerations, the unnecessary tests are to be deplored for another, less obvious but also important procedural reason. The resident and student should *not* be inculcated with a philosophy that completeness of work-up requires all "relevant" tests, e.g., bone scans and the like. If the student is exposed to that thinking, one inculcates the idea that the physician must rely on those procedures to arrive at difficult diagnoses. In such a process the student's problem-solving ability is neglected as are his or her clinical skills; and the main tools for problem-solving—observational and interpretive faculties—are left unsharpened.

Clinical Examples

In case 1-1, the boy with back pain, ordinary radiographs are ordered with the expectation of seeing in them the features of osteoid osteoma. With the knowledge that this lesion, in the spine particularly, may be difficult to recognize, arrangements have been made for the clinician to view the ordinary films and, if necessary, to obtain additional ones on the spot. In this case the films (Fig. 1-1) reveal the scoliosis that was detected clinically. Suppose that, in addition, an abnormality of the transverse process of a lumbar vertebra was noted and that the lesion is essentially a radiolucency. The clinician should at once pose several questions. Let us assume that the observer can categorically state that the lesion in question bears no resemblance to osteoid osteoma; i.e., a close look at the involved transverse process shows that, in addition to its size, the ballooned aspect of the bone, the radiolucent center, and the somewhat scalloped edges support a different diagnosis. Moreover, there seems to be in one sector an interruption in the continuity of the shell of the lesion.

The observer should now be considering what pathological processes might be at work to produce a lesion that is expansile, lytic, and provocative of the train of symptoms exhibited by this young boy. At this point, a seasoned practitioner might interrogate the boy further as to whether the onset of his more acute symptoms was occasioned by some traumatic episode, or if the nocturnal pain was the initial symptom becoming increasingly severe. The clinician may conclude that the history of accentuated nocturnal pain was elicited without reference to a minor traumatic episode. This practitioner might well put the diagnosis of aneurysmal bone cyst high on the list primarily because of the ballooning aspect of the lesion but also because of its location, so common with that entity, the age of the patient, and the absence of systemic symptoms. If the possibilities of a low grade infection or benign tumor such as fibroma or chondroma were also considered, it would indeed be realized that it is of little value to assign each one a relative probability.

The seasoned practitioner should realize that the best treatment for whatever this lesion represents is probably total excision of the involved bone. One basis for this conclusion is that proof that the lesion is an aneurysmal bone cyst or any of the other lesions mentioned depends on histological examination of the tissue. In that case, there is no need for better delineation of the anatomy of the lesion by tomography or computed tomography (Fig. 1-3), and there is no reason to obtain a bone scan to show if bone production in the lesion is an important element of it. If the possibility of an inflammatory lesion is even casually entertained, the determination of systemic indications of inflammation (e.g., leukocyte count, erythrocyte sedimentation rate) might be permitted on the grounds of their simplicity and innocuousness; but in truth, the results of those tests, even if they were strongly positive, would not change the clinician's objective of excising the lesion. Excision is preferred over any other operation (e.g., biopsy) because the bone involved is expendable and the likelihood of a cure, with excision, is maximal.

With reference to case 1-2, the college girl with the injury to the knee, mention has already been made of routine radiographs that might show a fracture of the tibial spine, patella, or tibial plateau. None of these lesions is likely, however, in a young woman who has endured pain and swelling in her knee for an entire week after an injury without having consulted a physician. A much more likely injury to evoke abnormal radiographic findings is osteochondritis dissecans, previously silent clinically, with an acute complicating detachment of the overlying articular cartilage. This lesion is rare compared with lesions already mentioned, which do not cause radiographic abnormalities other than effusion within the joint, the so-called internal derangements. Other, uncommon bony abnormalities may also be considered if their radiographic abnormalities are revealed (e.g., a tumor that has involved the joint, such as a giant cell tumor or chondromyxoid fibroma). Most of the time, the patient under consideration would not reveal specific radiographic findings other than those associated with effusion of the joint (Fig. 1-2), and the course of this patient's care would be as indicated above —a trial of conservative therapy. The possibilities of further radiographic investigation at the moment would not be in order, nor would extensive laboratory tests be considered worthwhile. However, if after a period of conservative therapy there is persistence of the findings, both physical and radiographic, the persistent symptoms and signs might be a good indication for further investigation, repetition of the ordinary radiographs, special tests, and arthroscopy.

LABORATORY EXAMINATIONS

Most patients seen in consultation by orthopedic surgeons have had a work-up by a generalist, internist, or pediatrician; and usually a series of routine laboratory tests, and perhaps some special tests as well, have been done. In contrast, in orthopedic work-ups, routine laboratory testing generally cannot be applied. For some patients, however, the orthopedist must see to it that the routine has been adhered to strictly. For instance, patients with back pain should never be allowed to proceed under treatment or observation without urinalysis and, in the case of older individuals, without laboratory testing for such lesions as multiple myeloma, leukemia, or prostatic disease. Patients with rheumatoid arthritis ordinarily should be cared for by both rheumatologist and orthopedic surgeon, the former being the one most responsible for laboratory testing.

Interpretative skills of the orthopedic surgeon in regard to laboratory tests therefore should reflect a knowledge of what tests can be helpful in the specific instances where a diagnosis is being pursued and where the symptoms, signs, and perhaps radiographs introduce a variety of possibilities best elucidated (or perhaps capable of some elucidation) by appropriate laboratory testing. Orthopedic surgeons rarely are called on to develop a fine expertise in laboratory testing, as would be expected for internists and pediatricians. Orthopedists should be familiar with standard tests, however, and under appropriate conditions order such tests, perhaps confirmed by repetition; under conditions of abnormal findings unrelated to their specialty, they should seek the collaboration of appropriate specialists for systemic treatment of the patient.

PATHOLOGY

In contrast to other texts on orthopedic surgery, the pathological features of the orthopedic patients' lesions are emphasized in this book. The treating orthopedic surgeon should be aware of the special properties of the specific lesion under consideration. Thus he or she must have a firm, working knowledge of the normal microanatomy of the musculoskeletal tissues and of their more common pathological alterations. In recent years the teaching of microanatomy, both normal and pathological, has become sketchy in medical schools because of a shift of emphasis to three other areas: the newer basic sciences (molecular biology and chemistry, electron microscopy), behavioral sciences, and socioeconomic subjects. As a result, classical histology and pathology have lost ground, and their integration into clinical work has suffered.

For the education of an orthopedic surgeon in residency, therefore, special emphasis on the classical subjects is needed, and the emphasis must be on the function and dysfunction of the musculoskeletal tissues. The special application of this subject to the orthopedic field may be illustrated by just one example, The microscopic elements of bone—cancellous and cortical—have patterns that bear an intimate relation to load-bearing. They relate as well to physiological processes such as remodeling in response to changes in metabolism (e.g., renal disease or disuse).

Fractures (i.e., destruction by overload of the bony substance) must be understood in relation to the microscopic features of the substance fractured—its biomechanics, including its mechanical properties. The physiology of repair of a fracture must be understood as based on the extent and pattern of microanatomical disruption; any operation on bone requires that the surgeon have that same body of knowledge of microanatomy. The same principle applies to injuries to ligaments, for example, or operations on tendons. Understanding microanatomy, however, does not require that the orthopedic surgeon have the degree of technical expertise of a pathologist in terms of interpreting the histology of tumors. It is not appropriate for orthopedic surgeons to be able to recognize and characterize all cells seen in every lesion, nor is it appropriate for him or her to be able to form a diagnosis based on cellular patterns and special stains. Nevertheless, the orthopedist should be aware of the basic principles in these matters, so that use of the pathologist's expertise and facilities is maximal in regard to care of the patient.

If the surgeon does develop interpretive skills in microanatomy and pathology, one consequence is that treatment, including operations on the musculoskeletal tissues, can be planned more appropriately. If the surgeon understands what the lesion looks like histologically, he will undoubtedly be more proficient when he does a biopsy in providing the pathologist with diagnostic tissue than if he had little or no concept of what the microscope might reveal. If the clinician well versed in pathology were draining the focus of an infection, he or she would not be satisfied with merely obtaining material (pus and tissue) that would reveal the organism. It would be anticipated that removal of the sequestrated bone, detected grossly, and judicious provision for drainage of foci of an infection adjacent to the abscess (that might be loculated) might also be of benefit. Eliminating the pabulum on which the bacteria feed and multiply thus constitutes a sound therapeutic principle to be applied to the patient's lesion. However, the limits imposed on the excision of devitalized bone or suppurative exudate are delineated according to additional pathophysiological knowledge. Gross recognition of what constitutes devitalized tissue or exudate limits the extent of the excision. Maximal preservation of blood supply to the remaining viable tissue and minimal extension of the operative trauma to noninvolved tissue also limits the operative manipulations. Thus when treating osteomyelitis, knowledge of the

pathological process may well allow the surgeon to maximize the benefit of the operation, thereby causing less dependence on the efficacy of antibiotics. This treatment choice is especially valuable if later, when the bacteriological studies are complete, it is found that the organisms in question are not especially sensitive to the usual antibiotics or that the organisms are unusual. In that event the new knowledge may require additional investigative and therapeutic maneuvers, but the appropriate operation has already been completed.

The knowledge of microanatomy emphasized above is not considered applicable only to surgical treatment, in all of its aspects mentioned. Although there will be additional reference to measures appropriate for biopsy of tumors (see Ch. 9) or for surgical maneuvers for fractures (see Ch. 5) or infections (see Ch. 2), the surgeon should use a knowledge of pathophysiology at all stages of conservative treatment as well as for operative treatment and diagnosis. Conservative treatment of a fracture can be used as an example of how markedly treatment can vary depending on how certain questions are answered according to their pathophysiological implications. These questions include the following.

How much displacement has there been? This question, interpreted pathophysiologically, implies that the more displacement that occurs, the more hemorrhage and other interposing elements may exist between the bony fragments. It also implies that the more displacement there is, the more the soft tissues in the neighborhood have been damaged, perhaps to the point of necrosis. It implies further that with progressively more displacement, there is more periosteum that has been stripped from the bony fragments and more bone devitalized by ischemia.

What kind of bone has been fractured? This question implies that a segment of cancellous bone such as might be found in the metaphysis, being wholly cancellous, would therefore be more likely to heal rapidly compared with a fracture that occurs through thick, cortical bone.

Answers to the question of *how long the fractured extremity might have to be immobilized* strongly depends on the nature of the fractured segment. Cancellous bone that is impacted would require, for repair, the elaboration of cancellous trabeculae across a narrow gap—surely a process that requires perhaps 3 to 4 weeks until sturdy consolidation is achieved. A thin wall of compact bone might require several more weeks for reconstruction. A thick, compact bony tube might require several or many months.

What is the relation of the fracture to the adjoining articulation? The answer here presupposes the pathophysiological principle that the immobilization of a joint by conservative means over a long period constitutes a greater hazard—permanent loss of motion to the articulation—than would a short period of immobilization.

PLANNING THE OPERATION

To conclude this chapter let us consider planning for the operations on the two cases described. In case 1-1, the boy who had a lesion of the transverse process of the vertebra (Fig. 1-1F,G), excision of the lesion is the ideal treatment. Based on the surgeon's expectations concerning the gross findings at operation, are there any unusual preparations that need be made for that procedure? The answer is "few," because the operative approach is straightforward and without danger to the large nerves, blood vessels, or viscera; moreover, the surgeon's confidence that the lesion is benign is nearly 100 percent. Knowing, however, that there have been cases in which removal of aneurysmal cysts have been complicated by excessive hemorrhage from the lesion, and on the off chance that the lesion might be something else, perhaps a hemangioma, the surgeon would have prepared for the possible complications of hemorrhage with blood for transfusion as needed.

The plan, then, would be first to expose the entire posterior aspect of the involved transverse process extraperiosteally to determine if the periosteum has been broached by lesional tissue. It is expected that the specimen would include the fracture revealed by the radiograph. This may not be apparent grossly, but microscopically it would be evident as would the expected repair reaction. Having decided that the transverse process is expendable, no preparations would be needed for re-

construction of the excised tissue. Then, after the lesion has been fully excised in one piece, a radiograph of the block of tissue would be obtained and the tissue processed for histological study. If it could be cut across without fragmentation or distortion, the procedure in the operating room might allow the surgeon to assess immediately the character of the internal nonosseous tissue; however, if the bony margin were too hard or brittle for easy section (i.e., if it required sawing), sectioning would best be avoided, and the entire block of tissue would be processed in the pathology laboratory by fixation en masse, decalcification, and then sectioning. If the block could be sectioned easily with a scalpel and the internal tissue revealed the typical mottled multicystic hemorrhagic surface found in an aneurysmal cyst, or the smooth gray glistening and chondroid texture typical of chondromyxoid fibroma, the immediate knowledge of the provisional diagnosis might well be helpful to both the surgeon and the patient's parents.

With case 1-2, let us suppose that the young woman has had persistence of the swelling in the knee, mild though it is, despite a 2-week period of symptomatic therapy, i.e., immobilization and non-weight-bearing. Let us suppose further that the radiographs, on repetition, reveal no abnormalities other than slight effusion in the joint. The lesions of the knee joint in young women that may occur have been well described by Smillie, who stated that subluxation of the patella was the most common such lesion. If our patient has slightly accentuated genu valgum, and if motion of the patella from side to side can be elicited manually with symptoms of pain and tenderness during that examination, the probability of that diagnosis is high. In that case, interpretation of the pathological sequence is that the initial trauma was an accentuation of the habitual slight or recurrent subluxation, with moderate trauma to the synovial membrane and subsequent traumatic synovitis.

The other lesions introduced by Smillie as common in the type of patient described include lesions of the anterior portion of the meniscus (not only tears but also compression injuries and subluxations) and traumatic necrosis of the fat pad. These lesions are not such that they would require immediate investigation by arthroscopy. If other lesions such as tears of the anterior cruciate ligament or the so-called plica shelf syndrome were contemplated, arthroscopy might be of value, particularly for the latter because during the procedure the plica could be divided.

For all of these lesions the microscopic pathology would have to be more or less speculation based on the gross findings and the chronology of the symptoms. If the signs and symptoms are not sufficiently severe to justify an arthroscopic examination, at this point in the patient's care a regimen of quadriceps exercises with gradually increasing activity, under appropriate activity and medical observation, might well be the therapy of choice, with arthroscopy deferred until the symptoms and signs warrant. Should the patient improve during the subsequent weeks, the actual pathological lesion may remain in doubt, but provisionally one of the commoner lesions would be selected for diagnosis, probably subluxation of the patella. If during subsequent weeks the more acute symptoms recur, the course of investigation would include arthroscopy and then possibly arthrotomy.

REFERENCES

1. Gore DR, Mueller HA: Osteoid osteoma of the spine with localization aided by ^{99m}Tc polyphosphate bone scan. Clin Orthop 113:132, 1975
2. Keim HA, Reina EG: Osteoid osteoma as a cause of scoliosis. J Bone Joint Surg [Am] 57:163, 1973
3. Ferguson AB: Roentgen Diagnosis of the Extremities and Spine. Paul B. Hoeber, New York, 1943
4. Murray RD, Jacobson HG: The Radiology of Skeletal Disorders. Churchill Livingstone, New York, 1977
5. Eideken J, Hodes PJ: Roentgen Diagnosis of Diseases of Bone. Williams & Wilkins, Baltimore, 1967

2

Inflammation and Infection

Inflammation is an important cause of disease as well as a component of many other diseases in orthopedic patients. The spectrum of the diseases in which inflammation plays an important role, if not the primary one, is wide. That role often is so important that the success of treatment of a patient depends entirely on successful treatment of the inflammation. Two examples are pertinent: The first is an obvious one where the inflammation is caused by a primary infection with microorganisms, as in osteomyelitis or suppurative arthritis. The second, also obvious, is a developing infection in an open fracture or at an operative site. In either example the *infection*, i.e., the invasion by microorganisms, must be treated not merely because of its obvious local consequences but because of its obvious threat to the life of the patient. The likelihood that the organisms will invade further is the risky element in both circumstances.

In contrast, there are situations where the role of the inflammation is secondary to an underlying disease process, in which case the inflammation may not require aggressive treatment. An example is the patient who has a necrotic tumor with inflammation at the margins. In such a patient treatment of the inflammation is entirely irrelevant to the primary lesion even though the signs of inflammation may be more obvious than those of the primary lesion. Treatment of the inflammation may moderate the symptoms, but it does not have an important curative effect on the tumor.

The inclusion of the large number of lesions of varying etiology in this chapter highlights the contrast between the diversity of the lesions and the similarity of the inflammation whatever its cause. From the point of view of pathophysiology, the inflammatory sequences and histologic components of all the conditions are similar, so we must infer that similar fundamental processes are at work whenever there is inflammation. Examination of pathologic specimens from many lesions, even fractures, reveals similar findings of inflammation. It may be acute or chronic, and it may exist in addition to the tissue changes of the primary lesion. Only rarely (i.e., only with primary infections) are the pathological characteristics of a specimen specific or nearly specific for the inflammatory disease process in question. Even in those instances the specificity rests on the histological demonstration of the pathogenic organism(s).

In the broadest sense, inflammation is undoubtedly the most common of all pathological processes. Undoubtedly, infections are among the most frequent primary lesions, but inflammation also accompanies many other pathological processes of frequent occurrence, including those caused by trauma, some metabolic diseases (e.g., gout), and even neoplasia. Specific lesions, e.g., primary infections with microorganisms such as tuberculosis or syphilis, consist of identifiable (e.g., specific) changes—the tubercle and the gumma—in which the causative organism can be demonstrated (and then identified by bacteriological manipulations). However, some inflammations, on the basis of histological patterns, can be considered nearly specific. An example is rheumatoid arthritis. The inflammation here is not absolutely specific because it can, albeit rarely, be seen with nonrheumatoid lesions. The cause of the inflammation of rheumatoid arthritis is not a microorganism that can be specified, despite innumerable efforts to identify responsible organisms.

A more important justification for including the many conditions discussed in this chapter is the implication that inflammation is diagnosable as such. It is. The presence of inflammation should be recognized, and in most situations its severity easy to assess, by its classic signs and symptoms. This statement is obviously true for acute inflammation in superficial locations but less so where the process is deep-seated. Chronic forms of inflammation may not be easy to recognize. If there is acute inflammation affecting a considerable volume of tissue, the laboratory findings usually include evidence indicative of that inflammation (e.g., leukocytosis). However, even if the laboratory findings are pathognomonic of acute inflammation, an underlying disease process may exist as well. Pursuing this train of thought, treatment directed at the (secondary) inflammation per se is similar to that for a primary inflammation, but missing the underlying disease process is a grievous error. Of course, treatment of the inflammation, as well as the underlying lesion, is helpful for many patients in whom inflammation is superimposed on other tissue changes due to an underlying disease.

The most important point here is that *infection is only one of the causes of inflammation.* Because infections are so common, especially if one includes minor, superficial ones, the physician may understandably think of infection first when signs of inflammation are encountered. He or she always must be on guard, however, not to neglect the other possibilities. There are several important reasons why lowering one's guard has become a common error. One is the overwhelming promotion by the pharmaceutical industry of a host of drugs that are easily available and are effective antibiotic agents. The tendency to use those agents in modern therapy has overshadowed older, tried-and-true measures of therapy that, though nonspecific, are often neglected. One need only reflect on the content of postgraduate lectures on the treatment of infection to make the point. "Supportive treatment" of the patient rarely includes the classical therapeutic agents such as hot packs and immobilization of the infected part. The lectures may even pass over the systemic supports — rest, diet, and sedation — so that the "meat" of the lecture can be presented. The "meat" then includes the various classes of antibiotic drugs, their mode of action, relation to the changing nature of the bacterial flora, dosage, monitoring by laboratory analysis, and so on. Few specialists in infectious disease nowadays mention immobilization or elevation of an extremity, hot packs, or incision and drainage — the classical modalities of treatment for infection based on pathophysiological principles. The practitioner may be lured into routines that do not include identification of organisms and use of *the* antibiotic that is most appropriate. Those steps may be bypassed as time-consuming, with the argument that the use of a "broad-spectrum" antibiotic is more expedient.

At referral centers, patients are often seen in whom an inadequate, ill-conceived therapeutic regimen of antibiotic therapy has been pursued: A provisional diagnosis of infection was made, and antibiotics were prescribed that were sometimes changed serially after several days on the presumption that if the first or second drug did not work it was because the bacterial organism was resistant. The delay and the inadequacies in diagnosis of such cases are often portrayed as lapses either because the physician did not think of doing the sophisticated bacteriological testing that was needed to identify an infectious organism or even of doing other laboratory tests to identify other inflammatory lesions. The calamity is that the thinking *did not* proceed along the lines necessary for understanding the lesion of this particular patient. Pathophysiology did not even come to mind.

The usual study of inflammation in clinical courses for medical students emphasizes relatively superficial, local inflammations (infections); the quartet of tumor, rubor, calor, and dolor bear witness to that emphasis. In many if not most orthopedic patients who have acute inflammation, regardless of whether infectious, the affected structures may be deep-seated — so deep, in fact, that the first two members of the quartet, swelling and redness, may escape notice. The associated edema and increased blood flow may be confined to the deeper tissues as well and thus cannot be detected superficially. The other two members of the quartet, pain and local heat, usually are evident with either superficial or deep involvement, but their contribution to the body of evidence that leads to a diagnosis of inflammation is not an important one because pain can be caused by many lesions and local heat may be imperceptible.

It is much more important for the surgeon to diagnose inflammation based on the evidence inherent in a good physical examination that elicits findings other than the four cardinal signs just mentioned; under present programs of instruction in medical schools, the findings of the physical examination are not given enough emphasis. A common reason for misdiagnosis or delay in diagnosis of inflammatory lesions is that the emphasis has now focused on laboratory testing. To a great extent, the dwindling emphasis on the elicitation of physical findings follows that in other classic subjects — mainly anatomy and pathology. The effect of this changing educational emphasis on the treatment of orthopedic patients has been a major cause for misdiagnosis and delay in diagnosis in general; in particular, of an inflammatory lesion.

Most orthopedic patients arrive for treatment by the surgeon on referral from generalists or other specialists. Often there has not been an adequate attempt, by a physical examination, to determine the anatomical localization of the inflammation or whatever other lesion is present, particularly if the extremities are involved. Because an examination of the extremities requires good working knowledge of anatomy, most physicians are not comfortable in the pursuit of an anatomic localization of a lesion. Application of pathophysiological principles in diagnosis, then, can be only rough at best; therefore when a patient is referred to an orthopedic surgeon for diagnosis, use of the surgeon's anatomical and pathophysiological knowledge may be the single most important element in the initiation of the proper diagnosis and treatment of the patient.

ACUTE INFLAMMATION

Acute inflammation, whether elicited by an infection with pyogenic bacterial organisms or an acute irritant such as a splinter, needs no detailed description with regard to its basic components, the exudation of fluids from the blood, the thrombosis and other vascular changes, and the local accumulation of millions of inflammatory cells in the affected tissue. These three phenomena can easily be appreciated in histological preparations even in the early stages of the infectious process.

An acute, severe suppurative process, if superficial, usually poses little diagnostic problem to clinicians, although mapping its extent and its involvement of anatomical structures may be difficult. However, a full understanding of the lesion must include an accurate evaluation of its chronology as well as its extent and cause. Chronologically, the onset of swelling in an inflamed superficial part can generally be detected within a few hours, either by the patient's direct observation of redness and swelling if the inflammation is superficial or by the symptoms of pain. When a deep structure is infected, pinpointing the onset of the inflammatory processes may be impossible, but even then the onset can be approximated within a day or two, providing the process is one of severe inflammation (suppuration) and not an inflammation caused by an attenuated organism or an irritant (in which case the inflammation is less severe). The onset of swelling therefore may be thought of as indicative of the onset of the suppuration. It represents essentially the exudative process, but that may develop much more rapidly than either the cellular or the vascular components of the inflammation, so that even during the first hours of the development of a lesion measures (e.g., drugs such as kinin blockers) that may be appropriately used, directed at halting or even reversing the exudation, might not be appropriate for either the vascular or the cellular phenomena. In reciprocal fashion, a measure aimed at ameliorating the cellular component of the suppuration (e.g., steroids) might be ineffective or even harmful in terms of its effects on the exudative or vascular components. Once the inflammation passes from the acute stage, i.e., after 2 to 4 weeks, the exudative and vascular phenomena, with which therapy will have been primarily concerned, play lesser roles in the process. The center stage, in regard to attacking the inflammation, is then occupied by necrosis, immune phenomena, and cellular responses such as fibrosis and, in bone, resorption and new bone formation. The cases presented below portray some of the variations in the inflammatory process and correlate pathophysiology with therapy.

Case 2-1   A patient had severe cellulitis of the forearm of 2 days' duration caused by trauma to a furuncle. The diagnosis is simple. There would be obvious reddened, brawny tissues that are tender and that center around the furuncle. The pain on contraction of neighboring muscles might indicate extension of the suppuration to muscle. The short duration of the process might imply that direct involvement of the underlying bones would not be likely, although that possibility and the possibility of a hematogenous (retrograde) extension should not be dismissed. However, the physician downgrades these possibilities. Their important implications for therapy can be put aside because most infections of bone occur by introduction of bacteria from the general circulation; they rarely stem from direct propagation of an infection of the soft tissues into bone (except when there has been extensive open trauma). The pathological process here would include massive exudation, diffuse cellular infiltration of the subcutaneous and muscular tissues with many polymorphonuclear leukocytes, and concomitant microthrombosis of vessels. More extensive thrombosis, perhaps of larger vessels, would not be likely because of the short duration of the process; nor would necrosis of much tissue be a likely possibility because of the extensive collateral circulation and the absence of confining tissues surrounding and partially strangulating the inflamed part.

The physicians' interpretation of the case, as presented, would surely admit of no other provisional diagnosis than an acute suppurative bacterial infection. That remote possibilities could be entertained *at this stage of the patient's illness* may be kept in the back of one's mind, but it should not stimulate a move for *any* further investigation. The important fact to bear in mind is that a furuncle is, possibly without exception, a suppurative bacterial infection of a hair follicle. The prima facie temporal and anatomical association between that lesion and the cellulitis should be reason enough to postpone all laboratory studies (white blood cell count for leukocytosis, urinalysis for glucose, and radiograph for involvement of bone). These tests should be done only if the history of how the lesion developed or of the patient's medical status suggests that

the case, as presented, is not simple. For example, the patient may be under treatment for a systemic disease that compromises immunological mechanisms, he may have diabetes predisposing him to infection, or the involved forearm may have had previous trouble. In the absence of these possibilities or others that may be elicited by questioning, one laboratory test — identification of the bacterial organism — would be worthwhile. A smear of the pus from the furuncle might reveal cocci (most likely staphylococci), and the antibiotic therapy, begun immediately, might target that class of organism. However, because the inflammation is in its most acute, early stage, therapy should include an attack on the vascular and exudative aspects of the inflammation.

The most obvious measure to reduce the exudation is elevation of the part, but that measure is expected to have little or no direct effect on either the cellular or the vascular components of the inflammation. One other mechanical measure designed to reduce exudation, i.e., active massage as produced by muscular contraction, is inadvisable here because of the tendency of the muscle contractions to spread the invading organisms. Chemical means for reducing the exudation, perhaps by use of fibrolysins or steroids, might also be entertained. These measures also would not be expected to affect the cellular or vascular components of the inflammation in any substantial way, and their use as primary therapy can be criticized in view of possible side effects. Only when measures that are potentially less harmful have failed (elevation, hot wet applications, rest) do these drugs have a place.

The measures just described might be employed to ameliorate the cellular components of the infection, and their use is predicated on the surgeon's concept of the cellular configuration of the affected tissue. One other situation also might be entertained. If the surgeon views the process as a diffuse one, without significant (gross) accumulation of pus, i.e., no abscess formation, it could readily be concluded that removal of an accumulation of fluids by incision and drainage would not be effective; however, hot wet packs, designed to promote blood flow, therefore help resorb the exudate. Under circumstances where it is thought that there is indeed such an accumulation, as diagnosed by the presence of a fluctuant mass in the forearm, an incision might well be helpful. If the cellular infiltrate is diffuse and not constituted as pus, any incision removes little of that infiltrate and tends to spread the infection to all parts traumatized by the surgical procedure.

The one measure that alone might be considered effective with respect to the vascular components (vasodilatation, stasis) of the inflammation is the application of moist heat. It not only increases the vascular flow to the part but may thereby halt or retard the progression of the thrombosis.

It has already been mentioned that one therapeutic weapon that must be considered simultaneously but not exclusively is the administration of antibiotic drugs. The surgeon's attention to the bacteriologic cause of the infection may take several forms. As mentioned for the furuncle, bacteriologic study beginning with a smear and Gram stain is appropriate, and the antibiotic that might be appropriate to the morphology of the organism identified might then be begun immediately if no contraindication exists. However, subsequent cultures and studies of the sensitivity of the organism to antibiotics might decree that a different antibiotic be used, and then the change should be effected as soon as possible.

Consider now some of the possible findings that would alter the diagnostic and therapeutic prescriptions described above. If there were physical findings indicative of a severe systemic involvement, e.g., a high fever, "toxemia," or "toxic shock," or if the swelling, redness, and tenderness in the forearm were severe enough to raise the suspicion that the infection predated the 2-day history or was caused by an organism of high virulence, the other measures mentioned might well be instituted, and still others might be pursued. Blood cultures would be appropriate, as would admission to the hospital so the antibiotic could be given intravenously and the patient monitored for developments.

Perhaps some justification is needed for the course of action advocated when the above findings do not obtain, i.e., reliance on a history (as brief as noted above) and physical examination, and dispensing with laboratory tests, even radiographs. A provisional diagnosis, entertained for a day or two while appropriate therapy is in progress, allows a determination to be made about the severity of the infection and how amenable it is to the elements of treatment, i.e., rest, heat, and antibiotics. The laboratory tests can be done later if the physical findings do not abate and especially if they worsen.

The emphasis on entertaining a provisional diagnosis "for a day or two" introduces a principle in therapy that is considered in more detail as it relates to fractures (see Ch. 3). The principle is to apply a step-by-step approach to a diagnostic as well as a therapeutic regimen, rather than a rigid unified program, instituted as by reflex. In the "day or two" during which a number of diagnostic measures are undertaken and completed, therapy of an interim character is applied that is appropriate to the situation and with minimal risks, but not necessarily including one or more of the therapeutic agents that, after the "day or two" are evidently appropriate. The results of the diagnostic measures may well alter the therapeutic program and so may changes in the course of the lesion during the "day or two."

One of the other lessons relative to case 2-1 follows from the precept that the pathological process should be addressed on its merits early in the therapeutic process. The choice of antibiotic therapy should not be considered as the first, sole, or most important element in treatment of the patient. The diagnosis of infection finds such strong support in the history and physical findings that the interim trial of therapy takes priority over any elaborate testing maneuvers. One example from a rapidly growing "armamentarium" of possible diagnostic tests is the bone scan, purportedly used to "rule out" involvement of the bone. Its use would probably do no good — it would only delay the beginning of treatment and conceivably might even be harmful for this reason. A positive test is not conclusive evidence of involvement of the bone, as too many false-positives are encountered. With the scan positive, one might well conclude that intravenous antibiotics should be administered. There would follow a rather long period of hospitalization and an even longer period of therapy, both of which are unnecessary, harmful, and expensive. This situation is but one example of ways that adherence to rigid routines of diagnosis that do not depend strongly on assessment of pathophysiological processes can harm a patient, and it is done on the pious pretext of a complete evaluation. From the foregoing, one should not infer that the treating physician must be miserly when ordering tests. Tests that are appropriate and can convey important information, positive or negative, should be ordered, e.g., a series of blood cultures if the fever is high or if there is a history of repeated infections.

Infections less severe than that just described manifest lesser low-grade local manifestations by slower, less obvious encroachment on adjacent tissues and slower development of the cardinal signs. They do not necessarily manifest proportionately less severe systemic indications of infection, however. In fact, severe cellulitis, as just described but affecting only a few square centimeters of surface, may not evoke any systemic signs or symptoms such as fever and malaise or it may evoke severe symptoms (if, for instance, there is septicemia). Even more importantly, the laboratory evidence of infection—leukocytosis, "shift to the left" in the hemogram, and elevation of the erythrocyte sedimentation rate (ESR)—should not, under those circumstances, be considered quantitative evidence of the severity of the local infection. When serial tests are done, they may serve only roughly as indications of how the localized lesion is progressing or regressing. Those tests may be of value to the surgeon's evaluation of the patient's immune response and assessment of the virulence of the infection organism, but the physical signs of progression or regression of the infection take precedence over laboratory tests so far as the local and antibiotic treatment are concerned.

Suppurative infections therefore can manifest a spectrum of severity, ranging from mild to fulminant. To complicate the surgeon's evaluation of any one lesion, the pathological changes in the tissues rarely are homogeneous, and it is to be expected that the tissues at the periphery of the infection, because they have been affected for a much shorter time than the tissues at the center, show different patterns. The cellular patterns reveal these differences: As the most acute, fulminating phase of the infection gradually subsides and the infection becomes more chronic, the millions of polymorphonuclear leukocytes show necrosis and liquefaction (pus formation); then, as they are being resorbed, the phagocytic cells (histiocytes) and the cells implementing the immune reaction of the tissue (lymphocytes and plasma cells) gradually become predominant. Somewhat later, but overlapping in time, fibrocytes appear, and there is neocapillary formation, concomitant with recanalization of thrombosed vessels. These changes begin at the periphery of the lesion and gradually progress toward the center, so that pus at the center is "walled off" and lends itself to drainage by surgical incision.

Portrayal of the acute pathological changes of inflammation, as caused by infection, includes little recently acquired knowledge. In fact, the entire description, as given, could fit in textbooks of several decades past. A conscientious pursuit and portrayal of newer information involves so many substances and processes that mention of only a few serves to give an idea of the complexity of inflammation, in its broadest sense.

Edema and exudation depend largely on vasodilation and capillary permeability, and those traits in turn may be regulated by substances such as histamine (secreted by mast cells), prostaglandins (cyclooxygenases, metabolic products of the injured cells), and various serotonins (probably derived from platelets). The cells that compose the major morphological elements seen during the acute phase of inflammation depend for their concentration in the inflamed area on some more recently studied substances—leukotrienes, for instance. Mention should also be made of the details of the clotting sequence and clot lysis because those two sequences affect not only hemorrhage (as well as hemostasis by thrombosis) but also the clotting of exudate and the removal of that exudate.

Many, if not most, of the more recent attempts at improving therapy for inflammation have as their cornerstone the idea of devising a synthetic substance that limits, or stops, the action of one of the natural substances mentioned above (e.g., histamine), the concept being that a certain physiologic process, once initiated, accelerates and gets out of hand. The synthetic substance then is supposed to act as an antimetabolite, neutralizing the excessive specific metabolite. In that way, it is hoped, the runaway process may be brought under control. Sometimes the synthetic substance is planned on the chemist's drawing board, but often a particular physiologically active substance is tested empirically. An example of the latter therapeutic trials is the use of corticosteroids, prescribed in a large variety of inflammatory processes with little understanding of the way it serves as an antimetabolite. The chances of error with that type of empirical therapy are exemplified by the cases of steroid therapy provided to patients who have a systemic disease for which the therapy is appropriate, but who also have an occult infection. That infection may then be sometimes aggravated to the point of disaster.

In general, one can assert that there is no single chemical substance administered systemically that is helpful for treatment of inflammation in the generic sense. This statement may seem startling, and it requires a serious assessment by each reader, not only as to whether it is true for every drug in use and in prospect (note that antibiotics are not included in this discussion) but also as to whether the concept of limiting a runaway physiological rogue is valid. The conservative view, at present, is that if there is a substance that might be useful in *all* inflammatory conditions — whether given systemically or in topical form — its benefits are minor if not disputable. Even if the particular drug has strong advocacy on a theoretical level, the empirical evidence for its usefulness often is shaky at best, and so too is the evidence for its safety. Two tentative conclusions are thus forced upon us: (1) Chemotherapy for inflammation per se is in trial status at present; and (2) the older, nonchemical therapy for inflammation need not, as a rule, include "antiinflammatory" drugs, except in the specific situations mentioned below (e.g., corticosteroids for rheumatoid arthritis). The all-too-common phenomenon of giving one drug for a valid purpose but then having to give another to treat the side effects should not enter into modern therapy of inflammation. A third conclusion is that, regretfully, the new knowledge accumulated on the pathophysiology of inflammation has so far affected therapy little *if at all*.

The acute infections just described involved superficial soft tissues only. The rapidity of the evolution of signs and symptoms during the spreading phase of the infection as well as during its containment and resolution under therapy — a matter of hours or a few days — depends in part on the character of those tissues. When the connective tissue is loose and permits swelling, dilution of the infecting organisms, and increased blood flow, rapid changes are the rule, and the surgeon must expect such changes in the appearance of the lesion or the affected part; thus it should be examined at least once a day. When the tissue is not loose, as exemplified by the tight compartments of fat in the heel or palm covered by thick skin, the progress of the infection may be accelerated by the restriction offered to swelling, thus impeding the defenses. The tight compartments also promote the process of necrosis of the impacted structures (e.g., fat cells, tendons) whose blood supply is easily compromised. Acute infections of the hand (see Fig. 2-6) are notorious for their tendency to fulminating progression, and severe sequelae may be the result if prompt treatment is not administered or if the treatment is inadequate. One may temporize for a few days with an infection of the thigh or forearm, or procrastinate on surgical measures while observing the results of conservative and antibiotic treatment; but with infections of the fingers, palm, and so on, time is of the essence. Early incision is needed because the dangers of disseminating infection, so prominently featured in the past as disadvantageous, are of lesser importance now, given the advantages of stemming the necrosis, identifying the causative organism(s), and administering the most effective antibiotic agent.

These principles apply with added force to all acute deep infections, not only osteomyelitis and pyogenic arthritis. The important feature common to the deep infections, as distinguished from the superficial ones, is that they tend to be in a more advanced stage of development when first recognized. It stems from the fact that the deeper the tissue that is infected, the less obvious are the symptoms and signs.

If a deep structure is recognized as infected acutely, and there has been a delay in diagnosis, as has already been mentioned, the infection usually has reached the stage of suppuration and abscess formation so that the need for urgent treatment by incision and drainage constitutes an *emergency,* perhaps on the first encounter of the patient with the physician. However, not all acute infections are suppurative, and the physician must differentiate between suppurative and nonsuppurative inflammation at an early stage.

Case 2-2 A 1-year-old girl is referred by a pediatrician for urgent consultation. The girl's symptoms 1 week prior to presentation were irritability during diapering and swelling of the right thigh. These symptoms had worsened, and 2 days before presentation the girl refused to stand or toddle as usual. There had been no fever or loss of appetite. The mother stated that the physician was concerned there might be an infection in one hip, and she brought along radiographs obtained the same day that had been reported negative by a radiologist. Under these circumstances, the crucial elements for diagnosis, and therefore for treatment, are the findings on physical examination of the hips. One's initial interpretation of those findings can be described by answering two questions. First, and more importantly, exactly where is the trouble? Second, what is the probable nature of the trouble? The pediatrician undoubtedly focuses concern on the hip joints; and because one must have absolute confidence in the findings as elicited, mention should be made of some difficulties that often arise in such situations. An irritable baby, who already has had at least two recent examinations may be recalcitrant to easy motion of any joint, particularly an inflamed hip. With much patience, as if playing with the child, both hips are flexed to 90° and jiggled through a small range of flexion and extension. Such a regimen, in this case, reveals no asymmetry and gradual easing of resistance. Similar jiggling in rotation is then attempted in flexion and extension. This examination reveals no asymmetry in flexion but when one tries to lay the lower extremities flat (i.e., in full extension of the hips) there is some resistance on the affected side. That is a signal to stop and return to the flexed position. Even a slightly forceful stretch of the involved leg makes the baby resist subsequent movement of the hip. So, with the hips now flexed, the test of rotation is further pursued.

Suppose first external and then internal rotations show that the hips rotate 45°, then 55°, and so on symmetrically and easily. The examiner then can make a first important interpretation, i.e., that the inflammation, if that is the trouble, is *not* in the hip joint. If it were, easy passive internal rotation would not be possible. The reason is that *any* inflammatory involvement of the joint (i.e., exudate in and irritation of the synovial membrane) thickens it, so that it cannot unfold and stretch easily. Moreover, because the small external rotators

of the hip are closely apposed to the membrane, they are the muscles that are first irritated by synovial inflammation; and they therefore are the first to show a limited stretch; i.e., there is limited internal rotation.

Having determined that the hip is not inflamed, one can now attempt to locate anatomically the inflamed structure. The resistance to extension is the clue to follow. In the context of the otherwise negative findings, including the absence of fever and trauma, and the acute onset, this positive indication of trouble anterior to the hip joint should stimulate one to consider the structures there. Among those structures, the lymph glands lying on the iliopsoas muscle should be accorded attention at this point in the diagnostic sequence because swelling of these glands is a common phenomenon in infants. If other glands (inguinal, axillary) are also swollen, the presumption is that the deep iliac glands are as well. The provisional diagnosis of lymphadenitis follows. Questions to pursue are as follows: Was the current problem preceded by a respiratory infection several weeks previously? Are the involved glands tender? Does the infant allow deep palpation?

With the provisional diagnosis (lymphadenitis), the question of what to do next is easily answered: Give the patient a few days of rest while the situation is monitored. Two items constitute unfinished business before the child is sent home, however. One is verification of the radiologist's interpretation of normal findings on the x-ray films. The other is communication with the pediatrician, who may have important information and who will be involved, at least in the observation of the patient and perhaps in treatment. The pediatrician's previous systemic findings, record of laboratory tests (a WBC count probably was done), and knowledge of previous infections may confirm the provisional diagnosis. If so, there is no need to perform elaborate tests to pursue other possible, although unlikely, diagnoses.

The phenomenon of swollen lymph glands in multiple sites in infants following a systemic or respiratory infection, although it is called lymphadenitis here, is not an inflammation analogous to inflammations of other tissues, as described above. Rather, it is a proliferative reaction of lymphoid follicles in response to the antigens elaborated by either the infecting organism or the inflamed tissues (e.g., respiratory epithelium). Because the inflammatory processes of exudation and vasodilatation are absent, and because they are the reasons an inflammation can develop so quickly but also subside quickly, one should not expect the proliferated tissue to subside in a day or so. However, the proliferated lymphoid tissue is not inflamed, and so the muscles on which it rests can accommodate to the increased pressure afforded by the enlarged mass of the nodes, provided that mass does not continue to increase. Therefore the girl's flexion contracture can be expected to resolve spontaneously within a few days. The condition is self-limited and is not likely to be influenced by any therapy other than rest.

It should be recognized that the confidence one has in the validity of the provisional diagnosis confers on the process of differential diagnosis a different time frame than is customary. During the day or two of rest therapy for the patient, the physician may do the mental exercise of differential diagnosis, which provides a plan for whatever new developments arise. Possible diagnoses to consider, although not likely under the conditions of presentation of this patient (case 2-2), are osteomyelitis of the femoral neck and suppurative arthritis of the hip. Advocacy of either diagnosis requires the presence of etiologic organisms of low virulence (or else there would be fever, leukocytosis, and more serious positive findings involving the hip joint because of the probability of involvement of the synovial membrane covering the femoral neck). The lack of evidence of this pathological extension permits, even dictates, a policy of deferring such examinations as a radioactive bone scan until there is more justification. Of course, the implication is that one is sufficiently confident of the validity of the provisional diagnosis and of the control one has of the observational environment that, should the inflammation not subside in a few days or should it intensify, the appropriate measures could be instituted in good time.

Mention should be made of other lesions that might be entertained as outside possibilities — to be kept in mind but not now pursued by diagnostic testing. *Toxic synovitis* of the hip can be entertained despite the absence of swelling of the joint that should be demonstrable radiologically. As a diagnosis it cannot be entirely dismissed on negative radiological grounds because of the absence of more severe limitation of motion of the hip, particularly on internal rotation. As a clinical entity, toxic synovitis presents a variable course, benign though the course may be, and the essential difficulty here is the lack of good evidence of exactly what this clinical entity represents histologically or immunologically. Innumerable observers have recorded its clinical characteristics, but the histology of the synovial membrane, allegedly inflamed, has not been studied, and no etiological agent has been implicated despite the widespread prevalence of the condition and much speculation as to its pathophysiology.

One other entity always should be kept in mind, i.e., *coxa plana* or *Legg-Calvé-Perthes* disease (see Ch. 7). That condition undoubtedly was considered by the pediatrician because it is a common cause of the type of motor disability of the hip in children that is under consideration. The physician should be aware, however, that this lesion is not common in those under the age of 2 years. The diagnosis is worthy of a place in the discussion but not in the active pursuit of a more definitive diagnosis for several reasons. One is that, along with osteomyelitis and septic arthritis, it is a common cause of permanent impairment. Another is that, as a chronic lesion, its first manifestation may well be similar to that depicted above; and in cases where it does develop, the physician may well search retrospectively for clinical or radiological findings that should have been recognized and were not.

CHRONIC INFLAMMATION

Although it is conventional to categorize inflammation as acute, subacute, and chronic, the division between any two stages is never sharp. One would find it difficult to construct definitions of delineations based on objective data, either clinical or histological. In the last stages of an acute inflammation, as mentioned, the polymorphonuclear leukocytes no longer are the overwhelmingly predominant cells. Concomitantly, there is less of an exudate of the fibrin-rich fluid. Yet with subacute inflammation and even with chronic inflammation there still is some exudate, and the inflamed tissue contains some polymorphonuclear leukocytes. The predominating feature of chronic inflammation is the constellation of elements that in varying amounts comprise granulation tissue, i.e., histiocytes, lymphocytes, new blood vessels, and scar. Perhaps the only way one can distinguish the scar of normal repair from the tissue of chronic inflammation is the continually increasing numbers, in paravascular and other focal loci, of lymphocytes, histiocytes, and plasma cells. They are always evident in an active inflammation. With both acute and chronic processes there is fibrogenesis of collagen, but in the scar of normal repair the foci of cells are few and small, without signs of active extension.

The convention is to arbitrarily designate as acute an inflammation that begins acutely and recedes within a 6-week period. If it persists somewhat actively after 6 weeks and has not receded by 3 months (the subacute interval), one may arbitrarily call the inflammation chronic. It should be realized that this temporal spectrum disregards some important variables. One is the volume of the inflamed tissue. If the volume initially inflamed acutely is large, it may not be possible for a chronic stage to be avoided, even if the stimulus for the inflammation can be effectively removed. If infectious organisms can be killed by the physiological defense mechanisms, with or without the aid of antibiotics, or if a large irritating foreign body can be extracted, the large volume of inflamed tissue most likely includes tissues devitalized by thrombosis of their vessels. The devitalized tissue, which must be resorbed, then, is a secondary irritant that stimulates inflammation. Different types of tissue vary in terms of the ease with which they can be resorbed—tendons and bone being much more chronic irritants than epithelial cells, muscle, or loose fibrous tissue. Thus the volume and the type of tissue affected by the inflammation are two factors affecting chronicity.

A third factor, just mentioned in passing above, is the persistence of the agent(s) causing the inflammation. If the antibiotic drug does not kill the organisms but, rather, decreases their rate of multiplication or their toxicity, or merely enhances somewhat the effectiveness of the host's cells (phagocytes) or antibodies for neutralizing the invaders or their toxins, the inflammation may become chronic. It may well be prolonged in regard to the acute cellular reactions, the histological criteria of chronicity, and the progressive spread of the organisms, even though they have been somewhat inhibited in their multiplication and toxicity (virulence).

There also are immunological phenomena that constitute still another factor influencing the transition of an acute infection to the subacute stage, the chronic stage (one end of the spectrum), or resolution, i.e., restitution of the tissue to its previous normal state (the other end of the spectrum). These phenomena are mediated by antibodies and are influenced by other substances (e.g., complement, prostaglandins). Their presence in the circulating blood is under active study, particularly as each relates to infection. These substances must be active locally in tissues as well as in the blood, acting either directly on the organisms or on the defensive cells of the host. The concept that the combat between organisms and tissues often does not end in decisive victory for either but, rather, persists as an armed truce, means that immune mechanisms have been mustered or developed sufficiently to contain the organisms but not destroy them. With this concept in mind, we can explain how an inflammation can be chronic but not progressive and how it can be transformed by a variety of mechanisms into a spreading lesion where for months or years it was not progressing. Conversely, a chronic inflammation treated so as to fortify the defenses may thereby be converted to an end-stage scar.

The summary just provided of the histological sequences in inflamed lesions serves as a common background to the specific infections now to be considered. Each of these infections is characterized according to the anatomical location as well as other special features (e.g., mode of entry of the organism, the usual organisms responsible for the infection). Examples of the various lesions are provided to emphasize the special diagnostic and therapeutic aspects of each as they relate to the histological sequences.

OSTEOMYELITIS

Infection of bone marrow is still encountered on occasion in orthopedic practice, although its incidence has declined markedly since the advent of antibiotics. The principles of inflammation as described above apply, but they are importantly influenced by the anatomical character of the bone affected. With the acute osteomyelitis of long bones of children, the bacteria settle in the metaphysis, having been carried there by the blood.[5,14,17] The likelihood that the portal of entry is hematogenous for that kind of infection should invite inquiry into the source of the organism. Any pediatric patient with an acute case should have repeated blood cultures performed routinely. If furuncles, a streptococcal sore throat, or a septicemia is the presumed source of the bacteria, smears and cultures of blood should be examined, preferably repeatedly if they are negative at first. In most cases early identification of the responsible organism is possible, and usually the appropriate antibiotic can then be prescribed,[3] as discussed below. When no extraosseous infection can be identified, one may postulate a hematogenous source as the result of organisms introduced not from an infection elsewhere but from portals that normally allow a few bacteria to enter the bloodstream (e.g., from the mouth during the act of chewing). If routine organisms (staphylococci, streptococci, pneumococci) are not retrieved, special cultures may allow identification of one of a host of other, rarer organisms and even for facultative pathogens.

The bacteria lodge ordinarily in a small thrombus in one of the vessels of the metaphysis (Fig. 2-1). The vessels in that region are end-vessels in the sense that a narrow sinusoid executes a hairpin turn

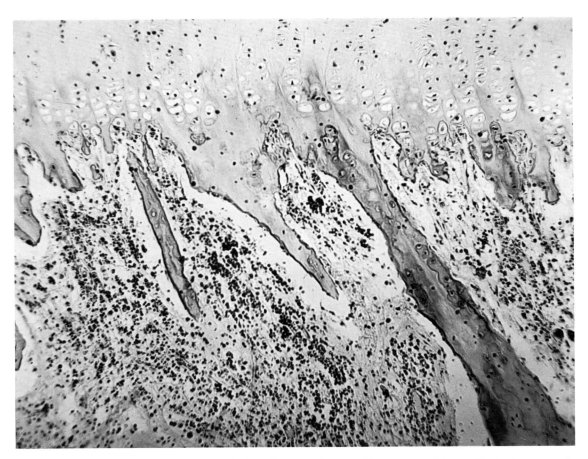

Fig. 2-1. A metaphysis near an epiphyseal plate showing clumps of bacteria within capillaries between the trabeculae of bone. Intertrabecular inflammatory exudate is present. ($\times$400)

as it reaches the epiphyseal cartilage, and the blood flow must be sluggish in that turn. Moreover, that part of the bone is most susceptible to minor injury. Even during the ordinary course of running, for instance, in which there is cyclic compression of the cartilage against its supporting bone, the microscopic vessels in that bone must, perhaps physiologically rather than pathologically, suffer microthrombosis. The concept that is offered is that one need not invoke a specific injury to explain a thrombosis. In recent years the idea has been advanced that this region of the bone is prone to microfractures, also as a physiological phenomenon.

As the infection then proceeds, there is exudation and cellular accumulation, as already described, but they occur within the narrow confines of the cancellous bone (Fig. 2-1). The structure there typically is similar to that of a rigid sponge, i.e., a mass of small cubicles, approximately 1 to 2 mm on a side, communicating with each other by pores on each side. Sinusoids pass from cubicle to cubicle, but most of the cubicles do not contain a sinusoid. When there is a sinusoid, it goes through the pores, coursing mostly in the axial directions. The source of the sinusoids is one of the metaphyseal arteries, and sinusoids drain ultimately into the metaphyseal veins. A unique feature of this tissue is the absence of lymphatics. Most of the marrow space in each cubicle is filled by interstitial fluid and hematopoietic cells.

Addition of exudate in any cubicle soon compromises the vessel in it if there is one, and the pores leading to other cubicles are then also obstructed. Unlike limiting membranes in soft, extraosseous tissues, the walls of the cubicles allow little swelling of the soft tissue in the cubicles; and as exudate presses into the interstitial tissue, cubicle after cubicle is compromised. In addition to the exudate, the tissue there also is affected by thrombosis owing to impedance to blood flow; necrosis is the result. The confluent mass of necrotic tissue makes an ideal medium for multiplication of organisms, there being no flow of blood to stay their progress. As more and more of the circulating bed is thrombosed, first the marrow cells die, and then more and more bony trabeculae become necrotic. The bony matrix, however, not only is more resistant to resorption than are the degeneration products of the cells but also is denatured by the lytic enzymes

released by the cells. After having been exposed to those enzymes, the matrix becomes even more resistant to resorption than bone substance rendered necrotic by avascularity. Depending then on the virulence of the bacteria and the immune mechanisms of the patient, the infection spreads.

In preantibiotic days the spread might traverse the thin layer of cortex in the metaphysis and spread underneath the periosteum so that in time the entire bone might be surrounded by the purulent exudate.[5] More often, however, some point in the periosteum would give way, and the abscess would be spontaneously decompressed into the soft tissues of the extremity.

How large a mass of bone that then might be affected varies. If the entire diaphysis is surrounded by pus, it will be entirely necrotic; but if only a small area of cortex is devascularized, it may well be gradually resorbed. Necrotic bone can undergo resorption only when there are viable cells because that process depends not only on secretion of enzymes from those cells but also on active phagocytosis. The cell to which that function is ordinarily assigned is the osteoclast. The controversies on how osteoclasts form and how they work need not be entered into here. Suffice it to say that, as the tide of battle swings from extension of the infection to its containment, the viable front of tissue allows resorption of the adjacent necrotic bone while it elaborates a lining membrane of fibrous tissue. When there is resorption of the interfacial elements of the necrotic trabeculae and the cortex, the remaining necrotic bone constitutes a sequestrum. The sequestrum might be just a wafer of cortex, the devascularized cancellous bone having been absorbed; alternatively, it may be a large piece of bone or many small pieces.

From the standpoint of diagnosis, one may well ask at what stage in the sequence of events just described would the patient first be likely to experience pain in the affected part and when would the other symptoms, signs, and laboratory tests provide evidence for staging the process and planning the therapy. These questions may best be discussed with reference to an actual case.

Case 2-3 A 4-year-old boy was first seen after pain of 5 days' duration that had become progressively more severe and localized to just below the knee on the shin. During the last day or two his knee would not extend fully, and the shin had become tender and slightly swollen. There was no history of injury or specific illness. During the history-taking that elicited the above items, it was noted that the boy seemed slightly flushed, lethargic, and feverish. The physician's suspicions included osteomyelitis as a possible diagnosis, even before the physical examination was done. The suspected osteomyelitis was presumed to be of at least 5 days' duration and was presumed to involve the tibial cortex, including perhaps some periosteum. The presumption was entertained because the absence of sensory nerves in the interstices of cancellous bone allows many pathological processes to intensify there without triggering pain fibers in afferent nerves. One therefore would expect that, should osteomyelitis be the diagnosis, there would already be extensive necrosis as well as suppuration in the tibial metaphysis. When the physical findings of localized brawniness of all tissues about the upper part of the tibia, marked tenderness there, and increased heat were elicited, the presumption of infection was strengthened; it was strengthened further when the boy was shown to be feverish. When the motion of the knee was found to be limited, not by evidence of fluid in the joint but, rather, because of muscle spasm, one began to suspect that the inflammation had reached the sites where muscles were attached to the tibia (not the attachments of the synovial membrane, because then one would expect a joint effusion to be evident).

It is obvious in this case that the work-up would have to include hematological tests (hemogram, ESR, and blood cultures). The immediate x-ray examination might be expected to verify the diagnosis; but because 5 days of infection of bone nearly always is not long enough to allow a sufficient amount of bone to be resorbed for the lysis to be discernible on the radiograph, one might expect to see the more subtle, earlier finding of diffuse swelling of the soft tissues (see Fig. 2-3A,B). That expectation should stimulate the physician to take two precautions with regard to the radiographs. One is to have films of the contralateral tibia for comparison with the affected one, a measure that best demonstrates the swelling. The second precaution is to have the exposure requested of the x-ray technician be one for contrasting soft tissue structures. When there is widespread edema and acute inflammation, many vessels of the area are congested, and they can be seen as streaks in the soft tissue but only if the radiograph has the appropriate exposure.

It is at this point in the case that the plan of therapy is worked out. As soon as the physical examination has been completed, a splint is applied to the extremity (removed only for radiography) and the child is transported to the hospital, with no weight-bearing on the involved extremity. While arrangements for hospitalization are made, as many of the delays inherent in the hospital "work-up" should be bypassed if possible. The findings on physical examination and radiography provide options as to how best to proceed. If, for instance, the boy's fever is not high, and he does not feel particularly sick, and if the radiograph shows only slight swelling, it is permissible to defer surgical measures. It is *not* permissible, however, to defer antibiotic treatment here (as in the case of cellulitis above) until the responsible organism is identified. The reason for the difference in the two cases is that in the cellulitis case the progression of the infection (in the soft tissues) is not nearly so dangerous as it is in bone, where it has been shown that a time interval of 2 hours (probably) to 6 hours (certainly) suffices to allow necrosis of the trabeculae. Such a delay would certainly extend the necrotic zone.

An antibiotic active against streptococci and most staphylococci (the most common organisms responsible for osteomyelitis in the boy's age group) must be given to achieve high serum levels as quickly as possible. Thus immediate intravenous therapy should be started, preceded only by blood cultures (to avoid possibly false-negative results owing to the efficacy of the antibiotic). That program would be started with the expectation that after a short time, e.g., 6 to 12 hours, the fever would abate and so would the pain.

If there were a point of maximal tenderness or other indication (swelling, radiologic evidence) of beginning localization of the suppuration, it would be worthwhile to aspirate that area. The aspirate might then be smeared for identification of organisms, either intracellular or extracellular. Of course the aspirate would be cultured.

One might proceed with incision and drainage if the proper indications are present. The arguments for such treatment are fortified when the fever is high, there is extensive swelling, or, worse, there is evidence of a longer duration of infection (signs of destruction of bone on the radiograph or of periosteal "reaction," i.e., deposition of a layer of subperiosteal bone). Arguments in favor of incision and drainage include the likelihood that there is pus under pressure underneath the periosteum and in the medullary canal; in such cases it would be helpful to drain the lesion so as to avoid subperiosteal dissection of the pus, devascularization of cortical bone, and sequestrum formation. Another argument is that one could identify the organism from any pus obtained and therefore start drug therapy with an antibiotic of known efficacy against that organism. Perhaps this favorable situation would pertain if a smear of the pus at the operating table revealed the characteristic coccal pattern. If the smear did not allow an organism to be identified and one relied on the culture, the time saved in plating the culture would be an advantage. Some physicians might argue that once the pus has reached the periosteum, it can be sampled by aspiration without surgical drainage. Advocacy of that procedure is based on the presumption that most if not all of the damage to cortical bone had already occurred, and the sequestration of that bone is inevitable anyhow. If the infection had reached that stage, the surgical procedure would not avoid any of the sequelae that would be likely. The surgically minded physician might argue that more pus would form after the aspiration, under pressure, and that pus should be drained. It could also be argued that surgical exposure of the infected metaphysis would promote further drainage of exudate, thereby limiting thrombosis and necrosis. It actually may help by removing some necrotic tissue that might be resorbed only with difficulty and over a protracted period of time.

Before further discussing therapy, some remarks about the diagnosis are appropriate. When ordinary radiographs leave little room for doubt that the right diagnosis is osteomyelitis, i.e., when the history (recent acute onset, localized pain) and physical findings (fever, tenderness, swelling) fit, one or two laboratory tests might be helpful. The ordinary hemogram serves as an indicator of the patient's resistance to infection and as a baseline for later determinations on how well the infection is being handled; the ESR also serves that purpose.

These tests are probably not needed for the diagnosis itself. No other tests are likely to be helpful and so should be considered only if there are important deviations from the information as presented above. Three instances can be mentioned: (1) If the child had been feeling poorly for some days or weeks before the onset of the pain; (2) if the radiograph indicated a more generalized process than osteomyelitis (e.g., leukemic infiltration); or (3) if the degree of bony destruction was not commensurate with a 5-day infection (e.g., a malignant tumor). Any important deviation would then override the urgency of the need for an immediate program of therapy starting with intravenous administration of an antibiotic; superseding that step are steps that would lead to a more proper provisional diagnosis.

Case 2-4 A 3-year-old boy was first seen 6 days after the onset of a fever with shaking and chills, and thereafter gradually increasing pain in the anterior aspect of the right thigh. During the illness, he had stayed in bed. Two weeks previously he had received an antibiotic for a skin infection on the abdomen. (He had a history of repeated furuncles.) When first seen, the boy's temperature was 39°C, and the outstanding physical findings were a flexion contracture and marked restriction of motion of the hip. The radiograph (Fig. 2-2A) revealed fluid in the hip, and a hemogram showed marked leukocytosis. Aspiration of the hip elicited a small amount of pus in which staphylococci were evident. Open drainage of the hip and neck of the femur was done, and appropriate antibiotics were administered with immediate beneficial effects — subsidence of the fever and the pain. Thereafter the boy was treated conservatively despite the development of extensive changes diagnostic of osteomyelitis (Fig. 2-2B). He had laboratory evidence of septicemia (with a complication of myocarditis) and therefore was hospitalized for several days. His antibiotic treatment was continued for three months. No additional physical signs of osteomyelitis were elicited, and over a period of 10 months the radiographs (Fig. 2-2C,D) showed resolution of the process. No sequestration was apparent.

Some of the data in this case, interpreted according to pathophysiologic principles, provide an instructive chronological pattern. The child likely

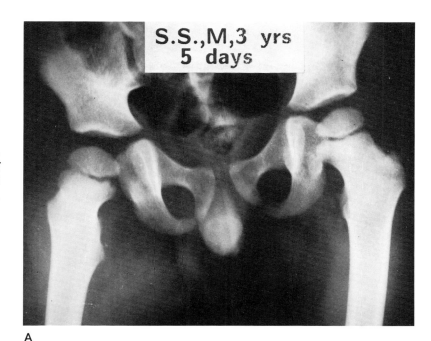

S.S.,M,3 yrs
5 days

Fig. 2-2. (A) Case 2-4. Soft tissue swelling of the right thigh with widening of the articular cartilage space is present 5 days after the onset of acute symptoms.

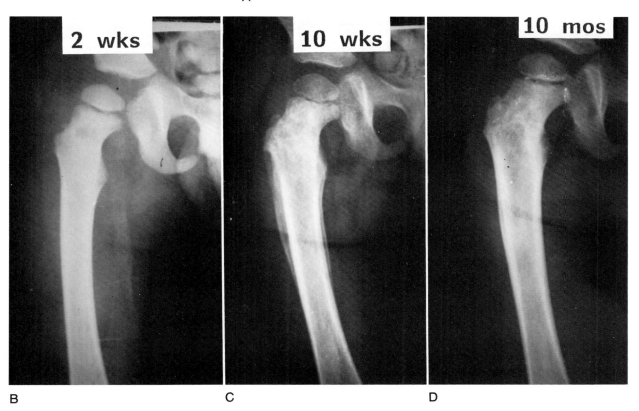

2 wks

10 wks

10 mos

A

B

C

D

Fig. 2-2. (B) At 2 weeks widening of the cartilage space and swelling of the joint capsule is evident with slight subluxation of the femoral head. (C) At 10 weeks the density of the proximal femur is increased and periosteal new bone is seen. The femoral head is not subluxated. (D) At 10 months the osteomyelitis and septic arthritis have resolved.

had a systemically lowered resistance (immunity) to staphylococci, and his abdominal furuncle probably was the hematogenous source for the infection at the hip. One could also speculate that minor, even unperceived, trauma was the episode responsible for localization of the lesion in the hip, and that the osteomyelitis in the femoral neck preceded, by a few days, the pyogenic arthritis.[5] According to this interpretation, the osteomyelitis might have elicited only minor (and unrecognized) signs prior to the onset of the chills, which then would be attributed to two mechanisms. One is the breakthrough of pus into the joint and the greatly increased absorption of toxic materials from the large synovial surface, and the other is the sudden influx of bacteria and toxins into the bloodstream.

Two other features of this case are noteworthy on chronological grounds. One is the fact that the hip joint developed almost normally during the 11 years of follow-up, and the other is that the osteomyelitis resolved spontaneously without permanent sequelae. Pus in a joint is a notorious destroyer of articular cartilage, so much so that an accepted precept is that any evidence raising a suspicion that there is fluid in a joint that may be pus should constitute a surgical emergency — to be met by aspiration of the fluid and then drainage of the joint.[11,12,14] Destruction of the cartilage begins within a matter of hours ordinarily, and therefore in the present case, where presumably the pus broke through into the joint a few days prior to aspiration, it seems remarkable that there was no evidence of destruction.

This happy but unusual end result should not be regarded as justification for a delay in the institution of drainage, even in "selected" cases. Rather, it should serve to emphasize that the results of treatment, however administered, are uncertain regarding the joint.[6,8–10,13]

The end result, as it pertains to the *infected bone,* which also was seen in this case, came about under a regimen of no further surgical treatment. Two pathophysiological principles contributed. One was that the infectious focus in the bone had already been decompressed by the breakthrough of the abscess into the hip joint and then by the surgical drainage of that joint. Pus under pressure remained in the bone (as noted when the surgical

window into the neck of the femur was made), and there was prompt subsidence of fever once the hip and bone were drained.

It is arguable if the bony focus should have been drained as well as the hip. As matters turned out, there was extensive involvement of the upper part of the femoral diaphysis and undoubtably extensive necrosis. Despite that fact, no protracted suppuration ensued with attendent formation of a cortical sequestrum. The reason for this fortunate circumstance is that in very young children, especially infants, the bony cortex is thin and much more porous than in older individuals, and therefore it can more easily be lysed and absorbed. The principle to be emphasized, then, is that septic necrosis of bone modified by antibiotic therapy is not inevitably followed by prolonged suppuration and formation of unabsorbable sequestra. If the bone is cancellous it is nearly always resorbed, and even extensive cortical areas are remodeled, especially in the young, and need not be removed prophylactically. Possibly in the present case more extensive surgical maneuvers for draining the infected focus of bone would have increased the quantity of necrotic bone.

Case 2-5 A 3-year-old boy presented with an obvious cellulitis on his right leg (Fig. 2-3A,B). He had a history of a second degree burn in the area, incurred 1 week before, and a blow to the shin 1 day before presentation, soon after which he developed a high fever, convulsions, and other symptoms and signs pathognomonic of septicemia. Immediate smears of the crust on his leg and a blood culture yielded staphylococci. Antibiotic treatment was begun. The cellulitis developed into an abscess by the eighth day of hospitalization, and it was drained; radiographic evidence of involvement of the bone did not become evident until 4 weeks later (Fig. 2-3C,D) at which time the medullary cavity of the tibia was incised and drained (Fig. 2-3E). At that time the boy had largely recovered from the septicemia and displayed no evidence of abscess formation in other locations. However, during the 4-week course of the acute illness his leukocyte count rarely rose above 13,000/mm³, and it was evident that there was profound systemic debilitation. These systemic conditions did not play a role in the therapy of the tibial infection, however, although in retrospect perhaps they should have.

The medullary cavity of the tibia was grossly purulent, and a large oblong segment of bone was removed that proved to be necrotic. After 3 months, during which time there was profuse drainage, the radiographs revealed a large cortical sequestrum; it was removed, after which drainage ceased and the wound healed. At that time and during the ensuing several years there was a severe, progressive valgus deformity (first noted at 20 months after the onset) (Fig. 2-3F,G) and shortening of the tibia, so that not only was a series of osteotomies required but also a leg length equalization procedure. An additional complication, an equinus deformity on the affected limb, also developed secondary to the extensive postinfectious scarring that occurred on the posterior structures of the calf, and that too required a surgical reconstruction.

The pathogenesis of the osteomyelitis of the tibia obviously can be attributed to spread of staphylococci from an infected area of skin that had a crust due to the preceding burn. The blow to that area probably was the immediate cause of the septicemia. There was hematogenous dissemination of the organism to the tibial location in all probability, and so the osteomyelitis did not result from direct invasion of organisms from the cellulitis. That lesion, however, served to mask the bony involvement by clinical signs as well as radiographically, and the result was involvement of tibial metaphysis. As revealed by the subsequent deformity, the infection must have encompassed nearly all of the lateral portion of the epiphyseal cartilage.[5]

It is only natural to ask if this unfortunate series of complications of the infection could have been mitigated, if not avoided, by therapy. The lapse of nearly a week at the onset of the infection before treatment was given to the boy at age 3 certainly meant that the entire metaphysis and most of the diaphysis had to be destroyed, if not by actual sepsis then by thrombosis of all the vessels. However, the epiphyseal cartilage was not rendered necrotic in toto, although its lateral segment must have been damaged, probably by thrombosis of the vessels (the epiphyseal vessels) that supply it. The pathophysiological sequence, if thrombosis occurred, would include either a slow-down or a stoppage of growth of that segment of epiphyseal cartilage so that a valgus deformity develops. When the damage is severe, there may be (and may have been in this case) premature closure of the epiphyseal cartilage laterally, in which event a bar of bone would or did form, spanning the cartilage and joining the epiphysis and metaphysis.

This pathophysiological sequence can be interrupted by interposition by any of several substances (fat, polymers), as suggested by Langenskiold, where the bar of bone otherwise would form (see Ch. 5). That was not done in the present case (which was treated before Langenskiold's work was published). In view of the severity of the deformity and its onset so soon after the infection had been cured, it would have been so treated early on if the boy was seen after Langenskiold's treatment was shown to be effective. It should be noted that the development of the knee was not compromised, other than by the secondary mechanical effects of the valgus deformity. This lack of damage to the articular cartilage is ascribable to its nutrition (from synovial fluid) having been maintained, because no thrombosis extended to the vessels of the synovial membrane.

Case 2-6 A 6-year-old boy had an insidious onset of pain in the back. After a few days it radiated to his left flank and became so severe that after 2 weeks he could climb stairs only by crawling. He was first seen at this point by a doctor who noted spasm of the spinal muscles, extreme tenderness in the lower part of the back, and markedly positive straight-leg raising tests bilaterally. He had a low fever. He was hospitalized, and blood tests showed an ESR of 87 mm/hour and leukocytosis. Radiographs of the back revealed no abnormality (Fig. 2-4A,B). After a week of bed rest, the physical signs and laboratory findings did not change, and the fever continued. A myelogram revealed no abnormality. After another week, new radiographs revealed thinning of the L3–L4 intervertebral disc (Fig. 2-4C,D), and a diagnosis of pyogenic vertebral osteomyelitis (previously designated "provisional") was then considered definitive despite the lack of tissue confirmation and identification of the causative organism. Antibiotic treatment and plaster cast immobilization relieved all the symptoms

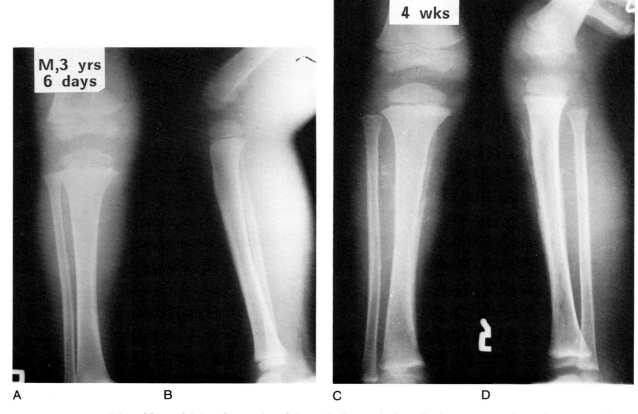

Fig. 2-3. AP (**A**) and lateral (**B**) radiographs of the right leg including the knee joint 6 days after onset of symptoms. Soft tissue swelling of the leg is present. The presumptive diagnosis is acute osteomyelitis in this 3-year-old boy, although the bone does not yet show any reaction. AP (**C**) and lateral (**D**) radiographs at 4 weeks show extensive alteration of the proximal part of the tibia including the diaphysis. There is periosteal new bone and increased density. *(Figure continues.)*

and signs. The hematological evidence of infection receded, and the radiographic course of the L4–L5 lesion was one of gradual sclerosis of the L4 bone adjacent to the disc, which maintained its narrowed thickness (Fig. 2-4E,F).

This case demonstrates an osteomyelitis of lesser severity than was seen in the previous two cases; but whether it is ascribable to the anatomy of the involved area or to low virulence of the organism is unknown. More often than not vertebral infections are not the acute, septic, abscess-forming processes described in cases 2-4 and 2-5.[1,16] When they occur in patients who abuse drugs or whose immunity is suppressed by steroids (two common circumstances in adults), the organisms involved

frequently are unusual ones, and often more than one species is cultured. However, as in the present case, the symptoms and signs are not severe enough to justify biopsy or aspiration. It must be presumed that the cancellous bone of the vertebra, which constitutes the primary focus of infection, can be decompressed by breaking through the end-plate and annulus fibrosis, as in the case illustrated, or through the thin cortices of the vertebral body anteriorly or laterally. When the abscess does become decompressed in that way, the presumption is that not enough pus is formed to be recognized as a paravertebral abscess or a psoas abscess, as occurs usually when the tubercle bacillus is the organism involved.

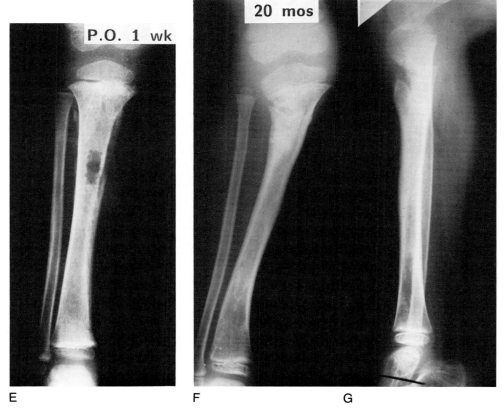

Fig. 2.3 *(Continued).* **(E)** AP view shows a surgical window in the metaphyseal diaphyseal region. Considerable periosteal new bone is present. **(F&G)** At 20 months a valgus deformity is seen on the AP radiograph **(F)**. Alteration of the lateral aspect of the proximal tibial epiphysis suggests a partial arrest **(G)**.

In recent years, probably because of the widespread and somewhat indiscriminate use of antibiotics, there have been cases of osteomyelitis in cancellous bone, not uncommonly caused by organisms of low virulence.[4] When long bones are involved the cases pursue a course similar to that described in Fig. 2-2 but differ in that the radiographic changes include lysis of the affected bone as well as sclerosis and periosteal reaction (sometimes in the onion-skin pattern), and these cases often raise differential diagnostic problems (e.g., tumor, eosinophilic granuloma).

Cases 2-1, 2-2, 2-4, 2-5, 2-6 and 2-7 can be used to point out that the various laboratory tests that are available should be applied with discrimination and sparingly; that is, every test done should have the justification that it will provide worthwhile information. The hematological tests are the simplest of all and are better indicators of the systemic severity of the infection and the patient's reactivity studied longitudinally than is the body temperature. Radiographs also done longitudinally have their own obvious justifications provided the intervals chosen are long enough to allow skeletal changes to be demonstrable.

With the current emphasis on the laboratory one may hear persuasive arguments for such techniques as bone scans with radioisotopes of several types or for computed tomography (to help determine the geometry of the lesion). Such arguments lose all force if the diagnosis is firm to start with. In addition to increasing medical costs, such tests nearly always impose unnecessary and harmful delays in treatment. Computed tomography or

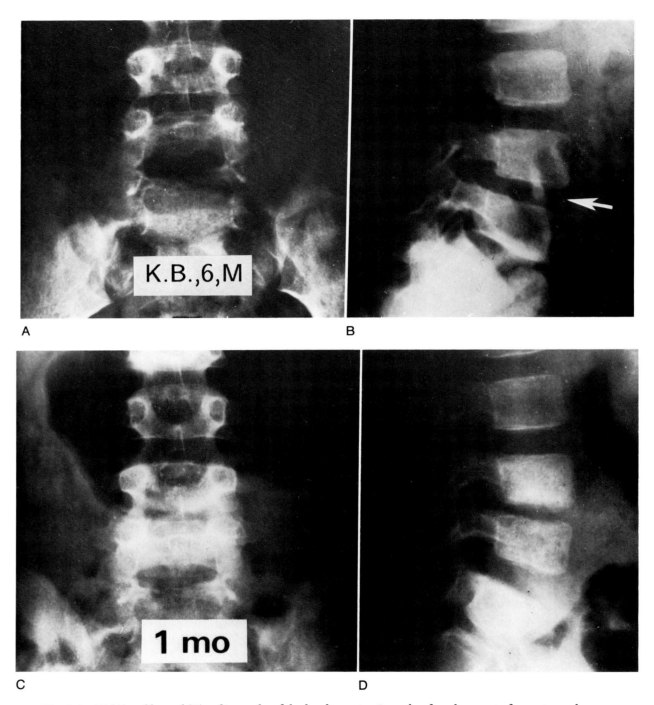

Fig. 2-4. AP (**A**) and lateral (**B**) radiographs of the lumbar spine 3 weeks after the onset of symptoms show no obvious abnormality at the level of tenderness. (**C&D**) Thinning of the L3–L4 intervertebral disc. *(Figure continues.)*

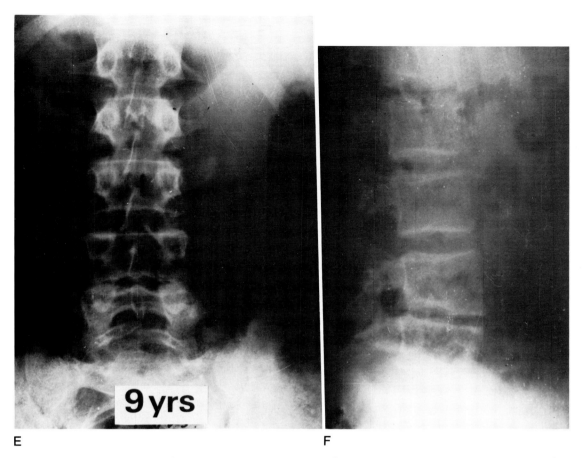

E   F

Fig. 2-4 *(Continued)*.   (E&F) There is persistent narrowing of the L3–L4 disc and increased density of the vertebral plates 9 years after the onset. (From Bonfiglio,[1] with permission.)

magnetic resonance imaging (but not both) on occasion is justified when the geometry of the lesion should be delineated. In the case illustrated (which dates back to a time before those tests were developed) either of those tests might have obviated the perceived need for a myelogram (to show if there was extension of the lesion into the spinal canal). Either of the tests would have been adequate to the purpose, avoiding the definite but small risk attending myelography and would involve comparable expense.

There may be some justification for aspiration (really aspiration biopsy) of the lesion of the disc and vertebra once it became evident radiographically but certainly not before, i.e., a blind aspiration is not justified in the absence of any radio-graphic indication as to the disc to be aspirated. The arguments for such a procedure are that there is a good chance that the organism will be retrieved and appropriate antibiotics could then be administered, that some measure of decompression can be accomplished, and that definitive diagnosis may be confirmed, i.e., that eosinophilic granuloma would be ruled out (or demonstrated). The arguments against its performance, which prevailed in this case, were that the short duration of symptoms and signs and the rapid changes on the radiographs were so characteristic of vertebral osteomyelitis; and that in such a typical case, in which there is little risk of rapid progression, a trial of conservative therapy would be best. If it failed, biopsy would then be in order.

Treatment

The three options to the first step in treatment have been alluded to. The physician should know the advantages and disadvantages of each as well as their indications and contraindications.

1. The patient whose onset of illness was only a few days before presentation, whose radiographs are negative or somewhat equivocal, and who might have had a sore throat or upper respiratory infection beforehand might well have a lesion that is small and caused by streptococci. In such a case it is permissible to start by administering, by injection, a high dose of antibiotic that is potent against streptococci (given their great susceptibility) and to have the child's fever and condition monitored in the hospital or even at home if conditions are optimal. Oral antibiotic therapy is continued for 1 or at most 2 days, provided no worsening of the child's condition becomes evident. Even then, should the fever persist drainage of the focus is indicated on the premise that the antibiotic is inappropriate and pus is collecting. The advantage of this therapeutic regimen, in addition to the obvious avoidance of surgery, is that a lesion of lesser magnitude than those described below deserves less radical therapy. However, the surgeon should not fall into the trap of minimizing therapy because the initial response is good. The affected extremity should be immobilized in a cast; the patient should not bear weight on the affected limb; and the prescribed antibiotic regimen should be continued for several weeks to ensure that any necrotic bone is absorbed while there still is antibiotic coverage. In this way the necrotic bone does not act as a focus for reactivation of the infection because all the organisms were not killed or because there is seeding of the focus from a bacteremia.

2. The regimen in which the bone is first aspirated and then the above treatment is followed might be appropriate when the radiographic findings are interpreted as being diagnostic of an accumulation of pus rather than merely edema. The hope of retrieving the causative organism must be balanced against the disadvantage of traumatizing the infected focus. Even if a large-bore needle is used, there always is a risk that it will be occluded by the tissue, and any pus that may be present will not be aspirated. Multiple punctures may be made when no aspirate is evident. Even though cultures prepared from the needle may eventually yield the organism, the surgeon will have little confidence in the success of the aspiration meanwhile, and the choice of antibiotic will reflect that uncertainty. Finally, aspiration is essentially a blind procedure; and when cortical and cancellous bone are the tissues to be perforated, there is a strong likelihood that the needle will not accomplish this perforation or, if it does, will push the pus further into the bone. In our opinion, the pros and cons of invasion of the lesion with a needle versus a scalpel strongly favor the scalpel because an incision allows drainage, if needed, and it allows gross observation of the affected area. Any necrotic cortical bone that is grossly identifiable but not evident on radiograph can be removed in part to obtain pus from an abscess that has not yet perforated the cortex. If a parent of the patient has an irrational prejudice against surgery, aspiration may be an acceptable option. In any case, the adjuvant measures, i.e., immobilization perhaps supplemented by hot wet applications and always accompanied by prolonged antibiotic therapy, are mandatory.

3. Most patients who have osteomyelitis that is acute need surgical treatment because often the lesion has progressed to the point of considerable suppuration and necrosis before the physician is consulted. If radiographs are to be relied on for a diagnosis, in an early case (e.g., one of less than 10 days' duration) one should be aware that usually there is no discernible abnormality in the bone. Even a slight periosteal reaction, i.e., deposition of a thin layer of bone superficial to the cortex and identifiable because there is a layer of radiolucent reactive tissue between it and the cortex, is not evident for the first 10 days or so. What the radiograph shows, in the early case, is extensive exudate and vascular congestion surrounding the bone — pathophysiological evidence of a segmental reaction to the pathogenic organisms. When such a picture obtains, especially if the site of presumed infection is not superficial and therefore no localizing signs exist, there is justification for a bone scan to help localize the lesion. Only a few days are required for a necrotic stage in the lesion to be reached. The radiographs do not allow one to diagnose *necrosis* until the bone adjoining the necrotic

focus is resorbed, which takes at least a week and usually longer. Therefore, unless the organism responsible for the infection is of low virulence, one may consider that a patient whose infection can be thought of as having aged a week or more has the indications for surgical therapy unless there are important mitigating circumstances.

During the 1980s there have been several modifications suggested for "improving on" the basic procedure of draining the pus and removing what can be identified as necrotic tissue, including sequestra. Although they can only be mentioned here (i.e., continuous suction, intermittent lavage with detergents or antibiotics), there is insufficient evidence, in our opinion, to show that any modification has a better chance to cure the infection or to cure it more rapidly than the basic surgical procedure itself. Of course that procedure must be done properly.

Some basic surgical principles must be kept in mind. One is that free drainage of the exudate is one of the primary objectives of the procedure. The more exudate (pus) that can be drained, the less there is to be resorbed and the shorter is the time required for repair. Whereas surgical teachings generally emphasize dependency and avoidance of "deadspace," it is more important in osteomyelitis patients to emphasize that the anatomical character of the cancellous bone with its cubicles whose intercommunications have been obstructed poses a dilemma to the surgeon. It cannot be recognized at the operating table which cubicles should be removed (they are too small to just be "opened"). Pus can be recognized, and if it is somewhat walled off the surgeon can be sure that the focus, which presumably contained exudate under pressure, has been drained.

Whether more should be done is the question; and if so, how much more? From the pathophysiological point of view, removing the tissue that has walled off the pus can be justified. The pus would not be under pressure unless the abscess wall, in this case including not only fibrous tissue but also some necrotic bone, retarded absorption of the exudate or was responsible for increasing its volume. Curetting the wall thus would be a proper surgical procedure. Further curettement would be improper because there would be no guide—by either actual observation or conceptualization of the pathology—to setting a limit. At that stage of the operative procedure, the same surgical principle as is discussed (see Ch. 3) for debridement of a wound obtains, i.e., that a step-by-step routine be adopted. It is proper to limit the removal of tissue and wait for clinical indications to guide one as to whether more should be removed. If one or more cubicles still contain exudate under pressure, once the principal focus has been attended to the patient will continue to be febrile and to have the expected leukocytosis and so on, whereas if the pressure in the affected cubicles diminishes (as the consequence of relief of pressures nearby, as well as the effectiveness of the antibiotic) the fever subsides and so does the leukocytosis.

Up to this point, cases have been described as if, with proper therapy addressed to several contingencies, all would turn out well, keeping the infection from developing into a chronic lesion. Other contingencies can exist, however, that affect the course of the lesion adversely.

One fascinating example of the natural history of osteomyelitis, as a chronic lesion, has appeared as two letters written by the physician-subject, whose disease in the tibia began when he was 8 years old and kept recurring. It recurred 30 times over a period of nearly 50 years despite antibiotic treatment. His second letter is so interesting that a quotation from the last paragraph seems apropos.[2]

> Erythromycin has been used since 1963 for threatened recurrences, and clindamycin, which is distributed well in bony tissue (with no side-effects for me), was used in 1975. The aim has been to stop recurrences altogether, but do these antibiotics actually abort the recurrence, or prevent an escape or extension of the infection? The short answer is that I do not have the courage to answer this question by submitting to random testing—no antibiotic versus antibiotic. But I think the appropriate antibiotic does abort the recurrence. However, it does not prevent subsequent flare-ups. It does seem, however, that, even if shamefaced, the organism returns to lurk behind an avascular wall. And it waits patiently too.

In this cited case and in case 2-5 the lesion started in the tibia, but its course depended largely on the precise location of the lesion. Case 2-5, as described, had the focus of infection (a small one) just

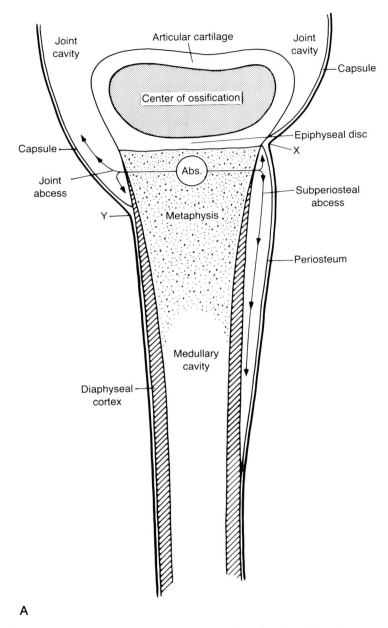

A

Fig. 2-5. (A) Proximal metaphysis and secondary center of ossification, depicting routes of escape of an abscess in osteomyelitis. *(Figure continues.)*

under the cortex, in the metaphysis. Suppose, however, the focus were somewhat larger and was located centrally, as in the physician's case (Fig. 2-5A). Six possible spontaneous avenues of escape of the pus are noted (Fig. 2-5B), the first of which might well have been the surgical drainage tract.

Each of the others would engender different consequences. Intracapsular evacuation of the abscess would mean a pyogenic arthritis, the effect of which was illustrated in case 2-4. Whereas the effect of relieving the pressure might well be some relief of the pain and fever, the development of an

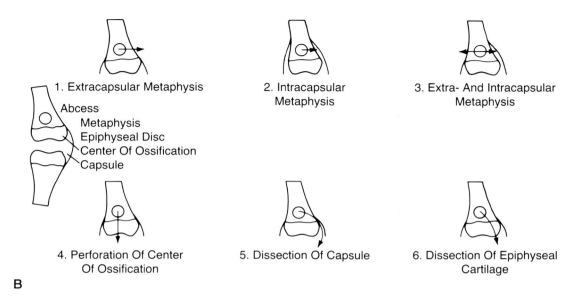

1. Extracapsular Metaphysis

2. Intracapsular Metaphysis

3. Extra- And Intracapsular Metaphysis

Abcess
Metaphysis
Epiphyseal Disc
Center Of Ossification
Capsule

4. Perforation Of Center Of Ossification

5. Dissection Of Capsule

6. Dissection Of Epiphyseal Cartilage

B

Fig. 2-5 *(Continued).* **(B)** Six possible escape routes of a metaphyseal abscess in acute hematogenous osteomyelitis. (From Hart,[5] with permission.)

effusion in the knee would be an ominous sign in terms of the future for that joint. Perforation of the epiphyseal cartilage either centrally or at the periphery would mean destruction of growth potential (case 2-5), and that complication would become evident only after several months, at least, or perhaps after a year or two. Nearly always the perforation is not exactly central in location, so that not only will there be some diminution in the ultimate length of the bone but also distortion of the joint's axes of rotation, i.e., a deformity that is progressive. The dissection of the capsule and the extracapsular involvement, seen in Figure 2-5B, are not without potential for inhibition of growth, because the inflammation of the soft tissue structures that contain the arteries and veins serving the epiphyseal as well as the articular cartilage may include thrombosis of those vessels. That situation, of course, might well be followed by necrosis and destruction of a variable extent of the cartilage.

Comment

Acute osteomyelitis similar to that in case 2-4 (Fig. 2-2) and case 2-5 (Fig. 2-3) was once common; now it is uncommon in developed countries. The cases reported herein have been considered at length to illustrate the pathophysiological principles of the lesion and its therapy. The variations on the theme are diverse and cumulatively constitute a common cause of morbidity. One variation is osteomyelitis caused by staphylococci of low virulence. Whether the ambient bacterial spectrum is changing and organisms of low virulence are more numerous is a matter for speculation, but certainly such organisms are being recovered from patients who have received steroids or antibiotic treatment for nonorthopedic conditions, and it is only natural to wonder if those drugs permit or even induce the development of strains of organisms that previously were uncommon or did not exist. Other variations on the theme are the infections caused by many different organisms, other than staphylococci and streptococci. Some of those arcane organisms are facultative pathogens. In addition, some of the individuals harboring those infections are "immunologically suppressed," e.g., those on prolonged steroid therapy or suffering from diseases that affect the leukocytes, complement, or antibody formation. A distinct group of patients who represent still another variation on the theme are drug addicts, whose obvious portal of entry of arcane organisms is by self-administered intravenous injections. For unknown reasons, their not-so-obvious infections often are located in the vertebrae.

Special circumstances attach to so many of these variations on the theme that we have had to select a few cases, primarily to illustrate the pathophysiological principles that are the subject of this book. Those principles are equally applicable to the diagnoses and treatment of infectious lesions caused by organisms that in the textbooks of previous decades were accorded separate chapters. Tuberculosis heads the list, but, depending how detailed the account, it might also include chapters on fungal infections, and chapters on other chronic bacterial infections, sometimes subdivided to several or many parts, e.g., one on brucellosis, one on leprosy, and so on. Despite the fact that histologically some of the organisms mentioned elicit cellular reactions that are typical for (or sometimes designated as "consistent with") those organisms (e.g., the tubercle bacillus, the spirochete of syphilis, or the mycobacterium of leprosy), none of those *reactions* is absolutely specific for the organism. To make the diagnosis specific, the organism must be retrieved and identified.

All of the organisms in question cause chronic inflammation; and the features of the chronic inflammation that are present in the lesions of the various infections are much more important from the point of view of therapy than in regard to the differences in histology. Not that it is unimportant for the organisms to be identified: it is important, but for reasons that essentially do not pertain to surgical treatment. They may pertain to epidemiological and socioeconomic considerations, but it should be emphasized that, in regard to therapy, they largely affect the choice of an antibiotic regimen, not the localized treatment directed at the lesion. Even if a particular organism that is retrieved from a chronic infection is absolutely refractory to every antibiotic, and such organisms are rare indeed, the principles of therapy for chronic infections already discussed (and further considered in Chapter 4) would apply.

Thus a consideration of organism-specific infections, one by one, as addressed to pathophysiology, obscures by repetition the essential principles. Those principles include considerations of anatomy that can be illustrated by the following case.

Case 2-7   A 40-year-old man was injured in a fight when his fist struck his opponent in the mouth. The injury was a transverse laceration 2 cm long over the metacarpophalangeal (MP) joint of the right ring finger. It was treated by intensive washing and débridement, loose suture, and application of a splint. One week later the wound and the entire hand became red and swollen; antibiotics were administered and were continued for 3 weeks. At that time, the wound was healed, but there was a painless fluctuant swelling over the MP joint, which could flex only 15°. Aspiration of the swollen joint yielded a sanguineous exudate that cultured *Staphylococcus epidermidis*. Radiographs showed loss of the joint space and subchondral bony resorption (Fig. 2-6A,B). When drainage and débridement of the joint was in process under general anesthesia, it was seen that the articular cartilage on both the phalanx and metacarpal had been resorbed, as had much of the metacarpal head. Neither flexor nor extensor tendon sheaths were exposed. Multiple organisms later were cultured from the débrided tissues. The wound was left open in the hope that, when healed, the joint would function as a pseudarthrosis. The outcome, however, was healing with little motion in the metacarpophalangeal joint or in the interphalangeal joints.

This case, although exhibiting the all-too-common error of handling wounds caused by human bites epitomized as initial poor handling of the wound, is not presented merely to emphasize that such wounds should not simply be washed, should not be sutured, and should not be expected to be protected from infection by a single antibiotic. Such a wound also should not be allowed to go unchecked for a week. Putting those errors to one side, it should be noted that only after débridement of the wound could it be determined that several organisms (and incidentally not the relatively benign one initially cultured) were responsible for the severe infection that not only destroyed all the cartilage of the joint within a period of 1 week but also spread to the neighboring tendon sheaths. Thus after the tendons were encased in scar, it was, for practical purposes, impossible to salvage any function for the finger. The anatomical features of the site of infection were the cardinal considerations.

The contrast between the complete failure of treatment for the infection of the *joint* specified in

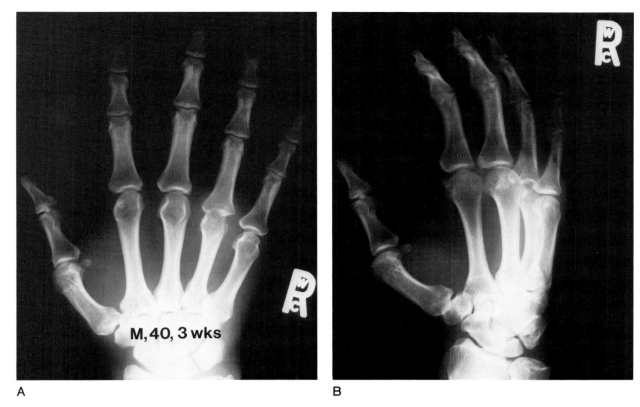

Fig. 2-6. AP (**A**) and oblique (**B**) radiographs of the hand show loss of articular cartilage space of the MP joint of the ring finger with reduced density of the subchondral cortex of the metacarpal head.

this case (as distinct from the tendons, for example) and the success of case 2-4 (Fig. 2-2) is emphasized, as is the need for extra precautions when treating infections in the hand where the motions of tendons and joints are so easily impaired. In case 2-4 the hip joint, secondarily exposed to pus from spontaneous decompression of osteomyelitis of the femoral neck, also was subjected to the destructive effects of enzymes from the exudate probably for several days (not 3 weeks as in this case). However, whether the fact that in young children the articular cartilage is several times as thick as in adults, whether the cartilage of the hip is several times as thick in a young child as is the finger joint in the adult, or whether during the first few years of life (some say until age 8) the articular cartilage retains potential for restitution, there was no residual loss of articular cartilage in case 2-3, whereas in the finger of the present patient the loss was complete.

The hand presents perhaps the most compelling instance in the body where anatomic complexity in a small volume of tissue — affects the course of an infection and the impairment as a result. However, the principles that govern its therapy are no different from those that apply to other sites — if each of the tissues is considered individually. The skin on the palm and the palmar surfaces of the fingers, like the skin of the sole of the foot, is thick and tightly bound to underlying structures by fibrous bands that convert the space between it and the bone underneath to tight, fat-filled compartments. Infection in such compartments acts in the same way as infection in the rigid compartments of cancellous bone. There is little tolerance for exudation. Swelling quickly leads to ischemia and necrosis in such a structure. The tendon sheaths tunneling between the skin and bone not only offer channels for rapid dissemination of infectious fluids but also expose the vessels of the tendons, at the vincula, to bacteria and their toxins. Thus thrombosis can occur easily, and as a consequence so can necrosis of the tendon fibers.

The pathophysiological sequences in bones and joints have already been discussed. Both these structures in the hand are not to be distinguished from similar tissues elsewhere in the body; however, their superficial location would make it easier to diagnose progressive involvement of individual structures were it not for two facts. (1) The structures are in such proximity that the signs of involvement — the four cardinal signs of inflammation (e.g., swelling) — are perceived as affecting a whole region rather than one structure. (2) The function of one structure often is so closely linked with that of another that when one is involved it often seems like the other is as well. The lack of precision in delineating the extent of the infection is one obstacle to precise surgical treatment: The surgeon cannot easily determine how far to go when evacuating pus and establishing good drainage. The other obstacle is that the objective with regard to reconstitution of the infected structures whose essential function is movement (articular cartilage, tendons in tendon sheaths) demands that there be a minimal amount of scar formed, and therefore motion of the structures should be instituted early, i.e., within a few days of the treatment. In contrast, the objective of reconstitution of infected bone, subcutaneous tissue, and fat is best achieved by immobilizing the part, elevation, and hot, moist applications. Resolution of this dilemma, however, can be achieved by putting the affected member (in this case the finger) through its range of motion once or twice daily and immobilizing it the rest of the day. However, in this case, although extension of scarring to the tendons might thus have been decreased somewhat, but not destruction of the metacarpophalangeal joint, the major problems associated with reconstruction of a functional finger remain. Because the ring finger is somewhat dispensable to ordinary function of the hand, especially if not normally mobile, and because its reconstruction might be suboptimal while taking many months of treatment, during which the patient could not use the hand, the best option for definitive treatment in this case would probably be a ray resection of the finger and metacarpal.

INFLAMMATION CAUSED BY VARIOUS AGENTS

One group of cases, mentioned in passing at the beginning of this chapter, deserves brief elaboration at this point because they exemplify another pathophysiological principle: that inflammation per se is a process caused by several etiological agents; and when more than one agent is at work, diagnosis (and treatment) may be difficult. Three kinds of cases illustrate the problem. One is the patient with active rheumatoid arthritis who develops sepsis – bacterial infection in an affected joint. Another is the patient with sickle cell disease, who has had a number of crises affecting one or more joints but who develops the sepsis (often due to enterococci or *Salmonella*) in one joint. A third is the patient who has Gaucher's disease and develops sepsis in a segment of bone (or a joint) that has been the site of previous symptoms. In these three cases, the secondary infection is superimposed on a primary inflammation that was due to obvious rheumatoid arthritis in the first case, and to necrosis of bone, possibly complicated by microfractures, in the other two cases.

The clinician may be unaware of the true state of affairs in regard to treatment of the infection because of a preoccupation with the primary disease and, with that preoccupation, may ignore the sepsis or its possibility. Once sepsis is suspected, it may not be easy to prove it exists, and the surgeon then faces the problem of how far to go diagnostically beyond the ordinary hematological tests. Is aspiration of the affected area indicated or contraindicated? Is delay indicated or contraindicated? Once sepsis is confirmed, therapy poses similar problems. Is total reliance on antibiotics indicated or contraindicated? Is delay of surgery indicated or contraindicated? One pathophysiological principle might be emphasized, however; that is, if surgical treatment (drainage, removal of necrotic tissue) is undertaken, its character depends on the ascertained abnormalities in those infected tissues, as conditioned by the primary disease, the anatomical site, and the septic process.

These cases, difficult as they are to diagnose and treat, do not compare in difficulty to another set of cases that now come under scrutiny, i.e., postoperative sepsis after prothesis placement in which metallic or other implanted devices are used. Whether the implant was for fixation of a fracture or a replacement prosthesis, the problem it poses to the surgeon, in addition to diagnosis and treatment of the sepsis, is that the purpose it was designed to serve must be reconsidered. Does the purpose retain priority over the new need for treatment of the sepsis? Must the surgeon who implanted the device and thought it the best answer to a therapeutic problem acknowledge failure, and even perhaps some culpability? What are the therapeutic options now?

These questions are far from simple, and the first element considered when arriving at answers is delineation of the tissues involved in the septic process. If within the first few postoperative days fever, leukocytosis, and purulent drainage from the operative wound are present and organisms are demonstrated in the exudate, that process, acute suppuration, can easily be conceptualized as the response of the bony tissues harboring the implant and is probably not localized to any one focus along its surface. This process is easily distinguished from one in which the fever, leukocytosis, and purulent drainage occurs somewhat later, perhaps after 2 to 3 weeks possibly preceded by evidence of a hematoma in the wound or sanguineous drainage. The sepsis is not as acute, yet it does not readily conform to the designations "subacute" or "chronic" either. Certainly there is acute inflammation, and perhaps bacteria are recoverable from the exudate; but the presumption is that the hemorrhage (hematoma, sanguineous exudate) played some role in allowing the infection to start. Thus the important question is if the implant played or is playing an important role. If the bacteria are less pathogenic than in the instance described as "acute suppuration" cannot be determined by bacteriological methods and can only be presumed on the basis of the patient's signs, systemic and localized.

At the other end of the spectrum of infection is the case in which symptoms and signs that raise suspicion first appear only months or years after surgery. The prosthesis that becomes loose is a good example of the diagnostic problem.

Given the broad spectrum of the process of sepsis, the surgeon's regimen of treatment must be tailored to the individual case, but it also must conserve whatever benefits are salvageable from the implantation operation. Although removal of the device (and necrotic tissue if there is any) and open drainage may well be an optimal procedure for septic foci, the result may also be unacceptable because of the loss of function that depended on the continuing presence of the implant, e.g., an intramedullary nail, another fracture fixation device, or a total joint prosthesis. When those devices are essential for continuing activities of the individual and when the sepsis is low grade, meaning that it is extending slowly or showing a steady state between active inflammation and scar formation so that there is no threat to the life of the patient, it may well be that the preferred course is to administer antibiotics in the hope of destroying all bacteria and thus alleviating the sepsis. Perhaps cure is not achieved, and a few bacteria survive, but a small degree of septic activity may be tolerated by the patient.

It is not so, however, when the sepsis is of high grade. In such an event, it not only spreads to adjoining tissues but may well invade the blood. Systemic involvement of other organs is then a likely consequence, and, accordingly, the patient's life is threatened. The hope that antibiotics alone can save the situation should not blind the surgeon to the risks. Removal of the implant and drainage of the infected area is mandatory to diminish those risks, and delay in so doing, for whatever reason, should be avoided. The surgeon should bear in mind that, in such a case, if treatment of the sepsis is successful there will be a second opportunity for reconstruction. Thus interim treatment of the patient, while the sepsis is addressed, includes measures to facilitate the deferred reconstruction procedure.

The wide spectrum of the pathophysiology of postoperative sepsis is superimposed on two other spectra in the situation. The first concerns the individual lesion for which the operation was performed. For instance, the spectrum of a fresh closed fracture treated electively by so-called closed intramedullary nailing might include the degree of comminution of the fracture, which in turn implies the extent of the trauma to the soft tissues, which indicates the amount of necrotic tissue available as a culture medium for the bacteria. This spectrum also includes the situation in an open, highly contaminated, but not comminuted, fracture. Analogous spectra would pertain to any other lesion, e.g., osteoarthritis, for which an operation might have been done.

The second spectrum, on which the sepsis is superimposed, concerns the role being played by the device at the time the sepsis develops. Here we mean the composite of chronological, anatomical, and functional variables that always are interacting and are the basis of the presepsis therapeutic rationale. For example, consider the chronology as it pertains to the closed, uncomminuted fracture, now immobilized with an intramedullary nail. Should the sepsis have developed within a few days, a few weeks, or a few months from the date of insertion of the nail, the pathophysiological implications would differ so greatly that they might be the overriding element in the conceptualization of a therapeutic regimen. Similar variability would be evident with regard to anatomy and function.

Having so many variables with which to contend, the surgeon's course of action, often described as "individualized treatment," may be developed through consideration of the options. These options represent the spectrum of treatment consonant with the three spectra described above, i.e., the spectrum of sepsis, the spectrum of the preoperative lesion, and the spectrum of the operative treatment after which the sepsis developed. The options obviously include antibiotic treatment, surgical drainage (with or without débridement), removal of the device, and substitution of another device.[7]

When to do what is the overriding question, and the surgeon should avoid the pressures of expedience so far as possible, thereby acting on principle, for best results. If the signs of sepsis are not fulminating, antibiotic treatment would best be delayed for a day or two during which time the responsible organism can be identified and appropriate drugs chosen. Expedience might dictate immediate administration of a broad-spectrum antibiotic as soon as sepsis is diagnosed; but even so, the septic exudate should be obtained for culture before the antibiotic is prescribed.

If immobilization of the fracture fragments in the example above is important to the composite treatment of the patient (e.g., if the patient had multiple injuries) and if other methods of immobilization introduced unacceptable risks or conditions of treatment (traction, external fixators), the best option in terms of removal of the intramedullary nail might be to defer it until the sepsis is under control or possibly until either callus forms at the fracture site or there is evidence of septic nonunion.

Thus the pathophysiological principles that govern the choice of treatment in each case might be envisaged at the onset of treatment, and the proper option(s) should be chosen, over time, with careful regard to the changes that are occurring in the tissues and the probabilities that are inherent in the particular case. There are many causes of inflammation other than pure bacterial infection, as we have mentioned at the beginning of the chapter, and it has been shown that inflammation can be superimposed on other essential noninflamed lesions.

OTHER CAUSES OF INFLAMMATION

There are some lesions in which inflammation can be attributed to one of three etiological agents other than bacteria (or fungi, or other infectious organisms). (Although those organisms include various parasites, it seems remarkable that viruses are missing from the list, unless one chooses to entertain that possibility for as yet unproved associations, e.g., varicella, Paget's disease.) We characterize the three etiological agents in question as: (1) mechanical trauma (other than fracture or that caused by an accident—in a single episode); (2) repetitive, cyclic trauma (several traumatic episodes); and (3) systemic causes. As will become evident, many patients have lesions that fall into more than one of the three categories; moreover, many of the lesions described can be secondarily infected, so that sepsis can be superimposed on the nonseptic, noninfectious inflammation.[15] Some of the lesions are so common they represent a sizable fraction of the ordinary practice of an orthopedic surgeon. That the discussions about them are brief or perhaps they are just mentioned therefore should not be considered an indication of their importance but, rather, a reflection of how suitable they are for illustrating pathophysiological principles.

Mechanical Causes of Inflammation

The common condition *hallux valgus,* or *bunion* (see Fig. 8-22), illustrates the principle that inflammation usually is the prime determinant to the patient of whether medical care (or surgery) is needed. Although the deformity may well be attributable in most cases to shoes that press the hallux into valgus, it is the pressure of the shoe over the metatarsophalangeal joint that elicits the pain. It is not only the skin that is irritated but also the deeper tissues, so that the inflammation, acute or chronic, or both, results in the development of a bursa (with bursitis) and even an osteophyte on the protruding metatarsal head. Treatment of the acute inflammation, i.e., relief of the pressure, hot applications, or even just avoiding the use of shoes, relieves the symptoms, although they recur unless the mechanical irritant is removed.

Another common lesion attributable to a mechanical mechanism is *paronychia.* Here the mechanics may be less obvious but instructive nevertheless. In most cases the hallux is involved and, as with bunions, pressure from a narrow shoe may be implicated, but here the pressure forces the soft tissue on either side of the nail up against the sharp border of the nail. Although daily application of the pressure by the shoes need not be prolonged over a period of years, as with bunions, the lesion may require a secondary irritative agent for development. The secondary agent may be a bacterial infection in the groove next to the nail; but even before the cause for inflammation is evident, the chronic inflammation from the pressure may affect the adjacent nail bed, so that the nail, instead of growing out smoothly, generates an irregular lateral (or medial) edge against which there is compression of the soft tissues. The resultant irritation then may well start a vicious cycle: the more the soft tissue swells, the greater the stimulus for more swelling. Ultimately, if there is enough swelling, the epithelium is eroded, and bacteria enter the scene. Here too, as with bunions, treatment of the inflammation (or infection) may be helpful, but the primary cause, the irregular border of the nail, must be addressed if there is to be a cure.

The *bursitis* that has been mentioned under the topic of bunions, is not to be equated with inflammation of any bursa whatsoever. Sometimes (e.g., with olecranon bursitis) the situation is comparable. Repetitive trauma is often demonstrable, as is secondary bacterial infection. In other situations, however, the pathological process may be inflammation secondary to a degenerative process, possibly one that triggers a minor traumatic lesion. Such a situation characterizes most cases of trochanteric bursitis, where the trauma (advanced as the best explanation but never demonstrated histologically to our knowledge) is a tear in the tendinous attachments of muscles on the base of the trochanter, the tear being the consequence of degenerative changes in the fibrous tissues.

The same mechanism may apply in the frequent involvement at the shoulder, interestingly presented more than a half-century ago by Codman. He used the terms subacromial bursitis, calcific tendinitis, and periarthritis and even illustrated gross changes in a few autopsy cases without, however, documenting those changes with the subject's clinical history or function or findings on physical examination in vivo. Unfortunately, up to the present, similar circumstances have been the rule with reference to studies on these ill-defined lesions of the shoulder, so there is a paucity of histological evidence as to their pathophysiology. There has been a profusion of speculation, however, and the most recent advocacy is one that uses impingement as a mechanism. The inflammation that may be evident (mostly as symptoms of pain and spasm, mildly and infrequently by redness or swelling, and rarely by gross microscopic findings in the structure allegedly inflamed) is postulated to be secondary to irritation of the rotator cuff by rubbing or pressure from the surface of the overlying acromion process. If the structure becomes roughened by periosteal deposition, demonstrable radiographically or grossly, it is considered supportive of the impingement concept, additional support being derived from a test in which pain is elicited either by manual compression of the supposedly involved surfaces or by their movement in a specific sector. However, the available clinical evidence comprises many cases with variable histories, variable physical findings, and variable responses to the many therapeutic approaches; thus one can select a group that supports whatever pathophysiological mechanism one dreams up. Therefore no attempt can successfully define principles unless it is accompanied by better histological and other evidence than has yet been made available. The so-called acute bursitis that elicits symptoms for a few days or weeks, and is apparently cured by an injection of corticosteroid into the subdeltoid bursa, cannot be a simple acute inflammation of the walls of the bursa—but what its histological basis might be is not yet known. The demonstrated complete tear in the rotator cuff that responds well to several weeks of rest and perhaps some physical therapy may well have a secondary inflammatory component alleviated by that regimen, but surely the tear cannot heal in that time. We must conclude that there are several lesions that for clinical purposes have been grouped under the heading "bursitis." At present the grouping is one of convenience and does not allow precise delineation of the structure(s) involved; moreover, it may not represent primary inflammatory conditions at all despite the "itis" suffix. This subject is discussed further in Chapter 6.

A final subgroup of inflammatory lesions arising from mechanical injury are those due to irritative substances. This group includes many cases in which the offending substance is of metabolic origin. The substance may normally be present in small amounts and therefore not a substance whose chemical properties are responsible for the irritation.

Gout is one of the disorders in this group; here urate crystals are present in large amounts in synovial membranes, subcutaneous tissues, or even bone. The idea that the urate crystals irritate by the physical action of their accumulated surfaces is inferred from the acute inflammatory zone that surrounds foci of crystals (see Fig. 8-15) and by the fact that washing synovial membranes free of the crystals (as by arthroscopic lavage of an affected joint) often provides instant relief of pain. Another example of a substance of metabolic origin is the calcium polyphosphate crystals of *pseudogout* or *chondrocalcinosis* (see Fig. 8-17). Here too lavage of an affected joint relieves the symptoms.

The more frequent exogenous substances that cause inflammatory lesions (not including embedded foreign bodies such as bullets or wood or glass splinters, which are more properly classified in the category of inflammations caused by single epi-sodes of trauma) include such substances as methylmethacrylate particles from prosthetic implantations, polyethylene particles, silicone particles (see Fig. 10-4), and metal particles (see Fig. 10-2), where there has been abrasive wear or deterioration of a porous surface.

All of these endogenous and exogenous substances that cause inflammation serve to emphasize the principle that any inflammation present must be regarded in conjunction with the associated circumstances (e.g., a systemic illness, a preceding operation), and the inflammation must always be differentiated from inflammation caused by infection or potentiated by a secondary infection.

Trauma-Induced Inflammation

Inflammation attributable to repetitive trauma includes such conditions as *DeQuervain's disease* (tenosynovitis of the common tendon sheath of the abductor and extensor pollicis longus) and similar involvement of other tendons, many of which do not have definite sheaths, so the condition is referred to as *tendinitis*. These conditions assume importance not only because they are encountered so frequently but because they often are occupational in origin and, even more often, are caused by sports activities of individuals strongly committed to their sport. Even though they pose few therapeutic problems because they usually respond well to rest and applications of heat, they do present a problem in pathophysiology. Little direct information exists on the histological abnormalities of, for example, achilles tendinitis, even when it is chronic and develops to a degree where there is a painful, hard protuberance at the insertion of the tendon in the os calcis. The same applies to "tennis elbow," and the various problems that occur in such athletes as baseball pitchers, football quarterbacks, hurdlers, and ballet dancers. Most of the lesions in question are best postulated as tears in the fibers of tendons, ligaments, or fascia—tears that involve so few fibers and with so little displacement of the torn ends that they cause no hemorrhage, only microscopic accumulation of exudate (see Fig. 6-5E). Such tears, repeated many times, would be expected at some point to generate painful stimuli when the structure is stressed but perhaps no stimuli when the structure is at rest. It is emphasized that the foregoing postulate is just that, and that therapy for these lesions rests on empiricism rather than principle. Nevertheless, when empiricism includes doctrinaire reports that fail to provide rigorous documentation of data and advocate therapeutic regimens that may include techniques that put the patient at substantial risk, e.g., invasive procedures, as with the use of steroid injections, the surgeon must view such empiricism with well deserved suspicion. In contrast, classical therapy for inflammation, i.e., resting the part, should never be ignored.

Systemic Causes of Local Muscle Skeletal Inflammation

The systemic causes of diverse lesions is a hodgepodge of inflammatory processes, some of which are attributable to immunological reactions or other mechanisms, often unknown. Some of these lesions are exceedingly common although obscure in their pathophysiology. A typical example is *fibrositis*, a focal inflammation in fibrous tissues, e.g., fascia, in a patient who has none of the findings of rheumatoid arthritis, and so on. These lesions may be called by various names, e.g., *fasciitis* when the focus seemingly is restricted to that type of structure (e.g., plantar fasciitis), or *myositis*, when intermuscular connective tissues are involved. The muscle itself is rarely the actual site of the inflammation. Sometimes not only are the intramuscular fibrous strands affected but also those at their surface; then the term *dermatomyositis* is used.

Other inflammatory lesions, seemingly the result of infectious agents but for which no agent has yet been isolated, may be included in this wastebasket of lesions — *eosinophilic granuloma*, for instance. A solitary or paucifocal eosinophilic granuloma, with its typical and diagnostic histological pattern, presents two features that support the proposition that some irritative agent is at work. One is the large number of histiocytes that are seen, indicating intensive phagocytosis of as yet unidentified material, possibly exogenous. The second is the presence of eosinophils, so often indicative of allergic reactions, again possibly to exogenous material (organisms?). It seems strange that so typical a histological pattern should be associated with a lesion so variable in its clinical manifestations as to be considered a mimic of other lesions (osteomyelitis with unusual infectious organisms, for example). It also is difficult to explain pathophysiologically why the same histological pattern should sometimes present in multifocal form and with such different clinical attributes in the disease called *Hand-Schüller-Christian's disease (histiocytosis X)* or in the infantile, largely visceral affection, *Letterer-Siwe's disease.*

The therapy for these lesions must take into account the well demonstrated fact that they often disappear spontaneously. When they do not elicit symptoms of importance, and are not progressive, or do not introduce risks (e.g., for fracture), a few weeks or months of observation is recommended; but here too empiricism dictates that the most rational and least risky therapy is to obtain a biopsy specimen to make or verify the diagnosis but, in so doing, to remove as much of the lesion as is convenient without necessitating a reconstructive procedure. Of course, biopsy should not be done for multiple lesions or for lesions in locations where extirpation of tissue is a hazard not to be undertaken lightly (e.g., a lesion in the vertebra). In such cases the chemotherapy that has proved effective (vinblastine) is the obvious choice once the case is diagnosed histologically.

Infantile cortical hyperostosis is another lesion that can best be put into the categorical wastebasket of systemic lesions because it is so often multifocal and so often accompanied by indications of systemic involvement (leukocytosis, fever). Histologically, the lesions are typical of subacute inflammation, but no organisms have yet been isolated from the paucifocal lesions. The disease is intriguing from the pathophysiological point of view in that no logical speculation has been forthcoming as to why special bones are affected (clavicle, mandible, and occasionally long bones of the extremities), why the disease typically runs its course regardless of the therapy used, why only infants are infected, and why in recent years the disease has practically disappeared, at least in developed countries.

REFERENCES

1. Bonfiglio M, Lange TA, Young MK: Vertebral osteomyelitis. Clin Orthop 96:234, 1973
2. Falkner F: Chronic osteomyelitis — personal paper. Lancet 415, 1976
3. Gillespie WJ, Mayo WM: The management of acute hematogenous osteomyelitis in the antibiotic era, a study of the outcome. J Bone Joint Surg [Br] 63:126, 1981
4. Hall BB, et al: Anaerobic septic arthritis and osteomyelitis. Orthop Clin North Am 15:505, 1984
5. Hart VL: Acute hematogenous osteomyelitis in children. JAMA 108:254, 1937
6. Jackson RW, Parsons CJ: Distension irrigation treatment of major joint sepsis. Clin Orthop 96:160, 1973
7. Jupiter J, Harris WH: Direct Implantation of Total Hip Replacements in Septic Hips in the Adult. AAOS Instructional Courses. CV Mosby, St. Louis, 1982
8. Kelly PJ: Bacterial arthritis in the adult. Orthop Clin North Am 6:973, 1975
9. Kelly PJ: Infections of Bone and Joints in Adult Patients. AAOS Instructional Courses. CV Mosby, St. Louis, 1977
10. Kelly PJ, et al: Bacterial (suppurative) arthritis in the adult. J Bone Joint Surg [Am] 52:1595, 1970
11. Morrey BF, et al: Suppurative arthritis of the hip in children. J Bone Joint Surg [Am] 58:389, 1976
12. Paterson DC: Acute suppurative arthritis of infancy and childhood. J Bone Joint Surg [Br] 52:474, 1970
13. Petty W: Infection of synovial joints. p. 10:75. In Evarts CMcC (ed): Surgery of The Musculoskeletal System, Churchill Livingstone, New York, 1983
14. Sherman MS: Acute and chronic osteomyelitis. Surg Clin North Am 29:117, 1949
15. Sherman MS: The non-specificity of synovial reactions. Bull Hosp Joint Dis 12:110, 1951
16. Stone DB, Bonfiglio M: Pyogenic vertebral osteomyelitis in the adult: a diagnostic pitfall for the internist. Arch Intern Med 112:491, 1963
17. Waldvogel FA, Mideroff G, Swartz MN: Osteomyelitis: a review of clinical features, therapeutic considerations and unusual aspects. N Engl J Med 282:198 and 316, 1970

3

Introduction to Fractures

The healing of fractures produced by low-energy injury is examined in this chapter. We begin with such relatively simple ones as compression fractures in cancellous bone and undisplaced or minimally displaced fractures of cortical bone. These low-energy fractures include many of the relatively common fractures, e.g., compression fracture of the spine, some diaphyseal fractures of long bones such as greenstick fractures in the forearm, fractures of the femoral shaft, and stress fractures (either cancellous or cortical). The cellular features of the stages of fracture healing are portrayed, and the dimensions and their variations are emphasized.

The characteristics of repair imposed by high-energy injury to bone and soft tissues are considerably different from those caused by low-energy injury and so are considered separately (see Ch. 4).

Injury, in the narrow and orthopedic sense of the word, means mechanical injury. There are other agents not ordinarily classified as traumatic, however — chemical, thermal, radiant, immunochemical — that injure tissues in somewhat similar fashion as regards the histologic sequence. Consideration of these agents, though, would divert us from the focus of the chapter, mechanical injury to bone. In any case, the severity of injury depends not so much on the actual agent as on three other factors: the degree of disruption of the continuity of tissues, the anatomy of the tissue disrupted, and the temporal pattern of application of the disrupting agent.

Extensive disruption may mean a large, jagged laceration of the skin and underlying muscles with a comminuted fracture of the underlying bone, or it may mean that a wide expanse of skin and other soft tissues, as well as the bone, has been devitalized by a blow from a blunt object, e.g., an automobile. Obviously, the *anatomy* of the disrupted tissue refers in part to nerves and vessels as well as bone, muscle, and skin, but just naming those structures does not bring into focus other anatomical aspects of the injured area, such as its capacity to permit extensive extravasation of blood (as in the pelvis) or the reverse (as in a compartment syndrome in the leg). The *temporal pattern* of the disrupting agent means not only its velocity, as in the diverse effects of gunshot wounds by different missiles (shotgun pellets, pistol bullets, shrapnel, high-velocity rifle bullets) but also the pattern of subsequent mechanical injuries, as during transport, attempts at immobilizing the part, and definitive treatment, including operative manipulations.

GRADATIONS OF INJURY

Mechanical injury to any bone always involves injury to the adjacent soft tissues. In some instances, fracture of a long bone may be accompanied by only a trivial degree of disruption of periosteum and muscle, as with a child's greenstick fracture or any stress fracture, but most fractures are accompanied by some degree of disruption of the periosteum and adjacent muscles. Cases where the degree of soft tissue injury is of major importance because it affects repair of the bony injury are discussed later in the chapter and in Chapter 6. In other situations, when injury to the soft tissue structures (e.g., nerves, vessels, tendons, ligaments) may be more important than the injury to the bone, the aspects of repair and impairment, including treatment peculiar to each structure, are considered separately (see Ch. 6).

The process of bone repair, although it is similar after most fractures, presents important differences in diverse clinical situations. It seems appropriate therefore to discuss first the general process and then some special situations. It is convenient to discuss the simplest aspects of fracture healing as it occurs first in cancellous and then in cortical bone, and we then quantitate several types of injury. This discussion is followed by consideration of specific associated clinical problems such as fracture into a joint, an epiphyseal injury, a slipped capital femoral epiphysis, an avulsion fracture, ununited fractures, radiation injury and pathological fracture (see Ch. 5) and reactions to implanted devices (metals and plastics) (see Ch. 10).

Aseptic necrosis occurs to some extent in every fracture. In some the extent is so great as to overshadow everything else (see Ch. 7), and in some anatomical sites a large fragment of bone is at high risk for this adverse sequence of events. Examples are the femoral head (especially after a dislocation of the hip or a subcapital fracture of the femoral neck), the humeral head (after a four-part fracture of the proximal end of the humerus), the body of the talus (after fracture of the talar neck or a subtalar dislocation), the proximal pole of the carpal scaphoid (after a scaphoid fracture or fracture dislocation), and the carpal lunate.

INTERPRETIVE SKILLS APPLIED TO INJURY

In chapter 1, where we described interpretive skills as they relate to diagnosis and treatment, we provided clinical examples that illustrated correlations of historical details, physical findings, radiographs, and so on. There are special aspects of these data that apply to fractures, particularly in the acute stages, that require elaboration here because, with fractures, the physiological changes caused by the lesion may assume more importance than the morphological changes when treatment is being planned. What is happening, i.e., *physiological changes* at the fracture site, from moment to moment dynamically overshadows the morphological alterations that are seen in histological preparations.[2-6,11-13,17,18,37] In the lesions previously considered (e.g., osteoid osteoma) the structural pathology was emphasized, but for fractures it is necessary to view the traumatic event and its sequela primarily in a temporal framework. That conception of the ongoing process is imperative if one is to understand the continuum of reaction and repair. There are four components that constitute the natural sequence of events following the injury, while there are additional circumstances that bear on the process and complicate the therapy. An important delay in, or even reversal of, the repair process may be caused by allowing complicating circumstances to endure or by administering ill-advised therapy when it runs counter to physiological principles.

CONTINUUM OF INJURY AND REPAIR

The continuum of tissue reactions in a fracture from the moment of injury to completion of the repair is an essential concept that should be recognized. We can distinguish, for the purpose of exposition, four components of the process: hemorrhage and necrosis, organization of the hematoma, fibroosseous callus formation, and remodeling. Each component may be followed independently, even though their overlaps in time and in localization must be recognized, and they may interact with one other.

A description of the chronology of the processes of healing divides the sequence into arbitrary stages. The stages that seem of practical relevance are the following. The first stage is one in which hemorrhage and necrosis predominate. This stage may last only a few minutes, or it may go on for days. Where there is a progressive vascular deficiency, the necrosis may progress for even a week or two. The second stage, organization of the hematoma, begins within a few days of the injury, but in focal areas within the injured part there may still be hemorrhage or necrosis weeks after the organization is well under way. The third stage, formation of fibroosseous callus, and the fourth stage, remodeling of the callus, are discussed in the individual examples below.

Changes that occur at the instant of injury are described for several illustrative injuries, followed by changes seen during the subsequent minutes (or hours), during the subsequent week, and finally during the repair sequences, which may go on for several weeks, months, or even years.

The wide range of clinical patterns and pathological manifestations must be appreciated. Fractures occur in numerous locations, and there are various types of fracture for each location. Despite these variations the pathophysiological processes in the repair process are surprisingly similar. That is true for the fracture due to mechanical trauma as well as for a repair process occurring in response to an infection, or after a surgical procedure or after nonmechanical injuries.

FRACTURES IN CANCELLOUS BONE

Acute Events

The range of physiological and histological responses in fractures is best depicted by examples. The first example is a compression fracture through the *cancellous bone* of a vertebra (see Fig. 3-1). The mechanism of injury typically is forcible flexion of the spine. In adults it may occur during an automobile accident as the body is jackknifed forward, or when an individual jumps from a height and lands on his feet (or buttocks). The force of the injury is transmitted to the most vulnerable vertebra, typically the first lumbar vertebra because of the relatively mobile segments below that level and the relatively immobile segments above it. In an old person with osteopenia (see Fig. 5-34) the same mechanism for a compression fracture obtains, but the energy required for fracture is much less and may be the result of minor trauma—as little as a sneeze or a stumbling movement. Whatever the patient's age, the amount of energy absorbed at the fracture site influences not only the degree of displacement of the fracture fragments (in this case the amount of compression, i.e., loss of vertebral height) but also the amount of bone and soft tissue that becomes necrotic immediately.

The energy having been absorbed by compression and displacement of bone, the next stage of the process, occurring mostly during the minutes immediately after fracture, consists predominantly of hemorrhage. That generally is proportional to the disruption of the vessels of the bone, bone marrow, and periosteum. The anatomical features of the vertebra may afford little opportunity for extensive hemorrhage from all three sets of vessels. It is not likely, in the osteopenic patient, that the periosteum of the vertebral body is torn by a compressive displacement. None of the vessels in question is large. Nevertheless, some hemorrhage infiltrates any available tissue plane, including the extradural layer of loose connective tissue. In distinct contrast, the compression fracture of a vertebra in a young patient initiated by a fall from a height might well include a tear not only of periosteum but also of the envelope of ligamentous tissue around the vertebral body, perhaps by a transitory displacement that therefore is not evident on radiographs. In either case, during the first few minutes after the fracture the process of thrombosis gradually tamps the many disrupted vessels and decreases the rate of hemorrhage. It should be evident that in the osteopenic case the total amount of hemorrhage is much less than in the case in which trauma was more severe. It also should be evident that any further mechanical motion at the fracture site starts new hemorrhagic outflow. Thus neither patient should be moved, except under compelling circumstances, except to be placed in a position of comfort that can be maintained on a stretcher during transport and subsequent treatment. Ideally, the position on the stretcher can be maintained for hours or days.

One of the mechanical effects of hemorrhage is interference with blood flow in the small vessels that have not undergone thrombosis. Recurrent hemorrhages plus the thrombosis are then responsible for whatever tissue necrosis occurs. Little energy needs to be absorbed, however, in these low-energy fractures other than that involved in the displacement. When repeated hemorrhages are provoked by moving fragments, they tend to increase the volume of tissue that becomes necrotic —beyond that already destroyed by the energy absorbed at the fracture site and that rendered ischemic by thrombosis. Another important poten-

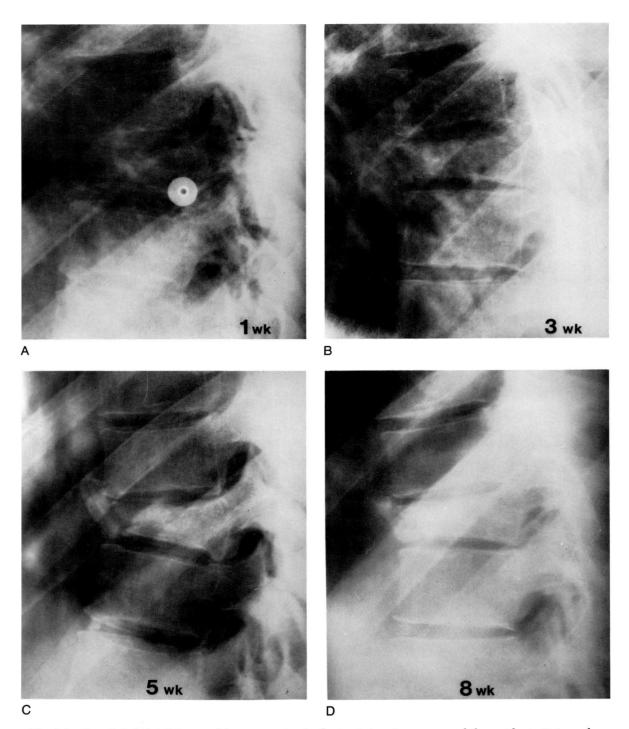

Fig. 3-1. Case 3-1. (**A**) A 34-year-old man sustained a flexion injury in an automobile accident. At 1 week a lateral radiograph shows a compression fracture of the body of T9 and wedging of the anterior aspect of the vertebral body. He was treated recumbent. (**B**) At 3 weeks, a lateral radiograph shows that the body has evidence of an increase in density anteriorly. The patient is now able to turn in bed. (**C**) At 5 weeks, the bony repair anteriorly reflects the extent of the original injury to the vertebral body. The callus is now stable enough to allow the patient to be up and walking with a body jacket of plaster or other material immobilizing the spine (or a thoracic spine orthosis). (**D**) At 8 weeks. *(Figure continues.)*

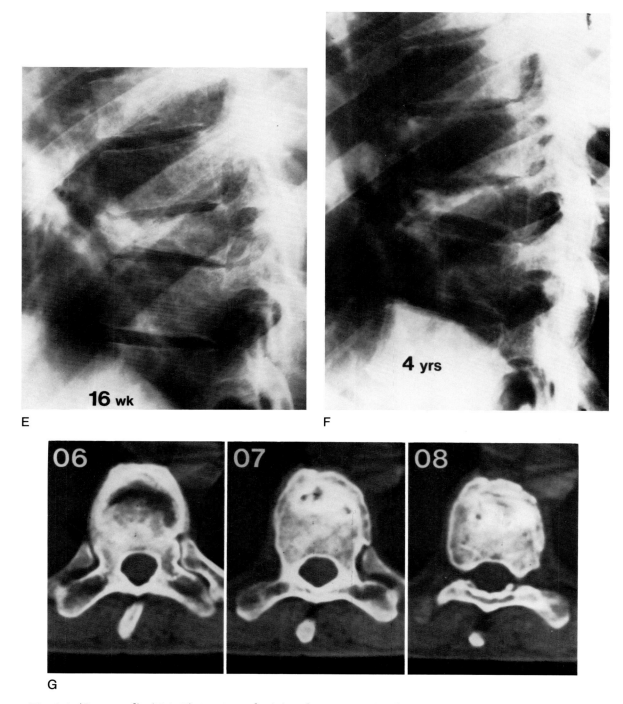

Fig. 3-1 *(Continued).* **(E & F)** At 16 weeks **(E)** and at 4 years **(F)** the vertebral body density indicates a healed fracture. **(G)** CT scans of T9 cut at 5-mm intervals show the cross-sectional anatomy of the bony repair at those levels.

tial mechanism for necrotizing bone is pressure on and obstruction of small vessels by the exudate from those vessels (including lymphatics) supplying the adjacent tissues. Such exudation invariably follows hemorrhage. One can readily conceive of dissection by hematoma of more and more of the torn edge of periosteum from the underlying bone, so that the blood supply and drainage by the periosteal circulation of the underlying bone is gradually reduced or even eliminated. With an impacted osteopenic vertebral fracture, however, if the periosteum is intact and the mechanical abutment of the cancellous fracture fragments is intrinsically stable, the amount of necrotized bone is negligible. However, the anatomical and clinical (diagnostic) implications of possible pressure of hemorrhage and exudate on the important structures close by (spinal cord and nerve roots) should be evident.

Intermediate Events

Once active hemorrhage and production of exudate cease (within a day or two of the injury if the part is undisturbed), the third stage, repair, can begin. Because even in the compressed vertebra, osteopenic or not, there are broad opposed surfaces of cancellous bone with relatively thin cortical fragments and minimal disruption of periosteum, the fracture fragments stabilize. The trabeculae of bone in one of the two main fragments of the vertebra have become impacted into the marrow spaces of the other fragment and vice versa so that the injured area is stable; in fact, it is so stable that a good deal of force might be needed to separate the fragments if that were desirable; it is not. As soon as the patient's pain is alleviated, i.e., after most of the muscle spasm has disappeared and the irritation from hemorrhage and exudation has subsided, the stable fracture site is capable of weight-bearing if excessive strain is avoided, even prior to repair of the impacted elements. The return to a functional state might well be accomplished within 2 to 3 weeks, much less time than is needed for repair of the fracture and much sooner than with a displaced cortical diaphyseal fracture of even a small bone, e.g., a digit.

Case 3-1   This case (Fig. 3-1) illustrates one end of

the spectrum of pathophysiological processes of fractures, i.e., prompt formation of a functional biomechanical state. In this extreme case, hemorrhage and exudation reach their maximum within days of the injury, at which time the products begin to be resorbed. The extravasated blood and fluids are quickly recycled, and the reconstructive phenomena begin to predominate, including resorption of any necrotic bone and deposition of a small amount of callus that not only replaces the necrotic bone but also welds the main fracture fragments together. It may take several weeks before the fracture can be considered "healed," and the process may then persist at a slower rate for many weeks thereafter.[5] The latter period of time would be the remodeling stage of the callus. It should be emphasized, however, that because of the mechanical stability of the fracture fragments *from the start* these weeks of repair do not have important implications for therapy, prognosis, or complications. All that is needed for such a fracture is protection against reinjury and rapid mobilization of the patient as soon as he or she is comfortable.

A compression vertebral fracture has several important properties that characterize it as the simplest type of *gross fracture* that occurs in cancellous bone. The word "gross" is inserted here to alert the reader to the implication that *microscopic fractures* occur frequently in osteopenic bone and may indeed be the essential factor in the slow shortening of the spine in the elderly (see Ch. 5). With a compression fracture, there first is minimal displacement of the fragments, shown in a quantitative way radiographically by the amount of the impaction. Despite the loss of the vertical height of the vertebra, a minimal volume of necrotic tissue must be resorbed. Such minimal volume represents the impacted trabeculae. The compressional apposition of the two broad surfaces of cancellous bone characteristic of the lesion, in addition to stabilizing the fragments, provides a large area of viable tissue on either side of the injury from which repair can be initiated. That repair tissue, consisting of (1) cells capable of elaborating fibrous, cartilaginous, and osseous matrix and (2) capillaries from which new capillaries can sprout, is what is called *callus*.[36,39] The minimal distance between the viable parts of those trabeculae on either side of the fracture line and the lack of micro-motion that would impede repair allows even a small amount of callus to bridge the gap. Lastly, there is an intact envelope of soft tissue surrounding the fracture fragments, so that the amount of hemorrhage is sharply restricted and the larger blood vessels needed to supply the capillaries for the repair stages are not injured.

As mentioned above, the end result with this fracture differs somewhat from that with most other fractures in that whatever repair and remodeling occur at a microscopic level in the callus they do not affect the final shape, i.e., the degree of compression of the injured vertebral body. The question has been raised if acceptance of the deformity of the vertebral body is proper, and if an attempt should be made, as with other fractures, to minimize deformity. A number of empirical observations have shown that it is important *not* to disturb the position of the fragments. Attempts to restore the height of the vertebral body by hyperextending the spine are ill-advised for several reasons. If a moderate force is used (e.g., by having the patient remain recumbent over a sandbag positioned at the fracture), the attempt is nearly always unsuccessful. If stronger forces are used and the fragments are disimpacted, the fracture gap is large; and even if the reduced position is maintained for some weeks, the gap does not fill with firm callus. Thus when the patient begins to stand, the original deformity reemerges, and healing is then slow for at least two reasons: The chronology of the reparative tissues (osteogenic cells, capillaries) has been interrupted, and the stability of interlocking trabeculae has been eliminated.

The consequences of the fracture, without compression of any neural structures, nevertheless include some mechanical derangements. One is alteration in the relations of the zygoapophyseal joints of the spine, not only in the segments of the region affected but, because of postural alterations, in other segments as well. Second, the shortening of some muscles and lengthening of others, although their effects may not cause *permanent* impairment of muscle function, constitute transient sequelae that affect the rehabilitation regimen, i.e., physical therapy. In individuals who are not elderly, the derangement of zygoapophyseal joints nearly always can be compensated for by adaptation of the spine's multiple segments, so that its posture as a unit is not much affected. In spines that are not flexible, however, the derangement may constitute an impairment despite the rather prompt return of function to the stretched or shortened muscles. The impairment consists of an extra load on those muscles to maintain the erect posture.

Another common injury that involves predominantly cancellous bone is a fracture of the neck of the femur.[3,10] An *impacted fracture* of the femoral neck serves to depict the sequences of repair characteristic of such a fracture. The trabeculae follow a process of interdigitation similar to that observed for a compression fracture of the spine, but a mechanical factor, rotation, not usually at play in the spine, may serve to disimpact the fragments. Therefore internal stabilization may be indicated and can be accomplished simply by inserting any of several devices (e.g., threaded pins or cancellous bone screws).

Histology

Many specimens are available of femoral heads removed from patients whose medical situations contraindicated stabilization of a fracture of the femoral neck by internal fixation. When total arthroplasty was done in such cases, the removed specimens depicted the early and late stages of healing of that fracture, and they are used to illustrate the histological aspects of repair of cancellous bone, not available for compression fractures of the spine.

Case 3-2 The fracture first shows hemorrhage (in minimal amount) with disrupted trabeculae at the fracture surfaces (Fig. 3-2A), followed by formation of granulation tissue to replace the clot and invade the adjacent marrow spaces (Fig. 3-2B). The cortex of the femoral neck has little periosteum to participate in the formation of new bone, but the cells along the endosteal surfaces of the cancellous bone trabeculae form new bone within 2 weeks. This new bone unites with the new bone from the opposite cancellous bone surface (Fig. 3-2C). Assuming that the fragments remain stabilized, the process continues until a firm union has taken place, which occurs in a matter of 6 to 10 weeks (Fig. 3-2D). In an impacted (i.e., "undisplaced") fracture, the injury to major vessels sup-

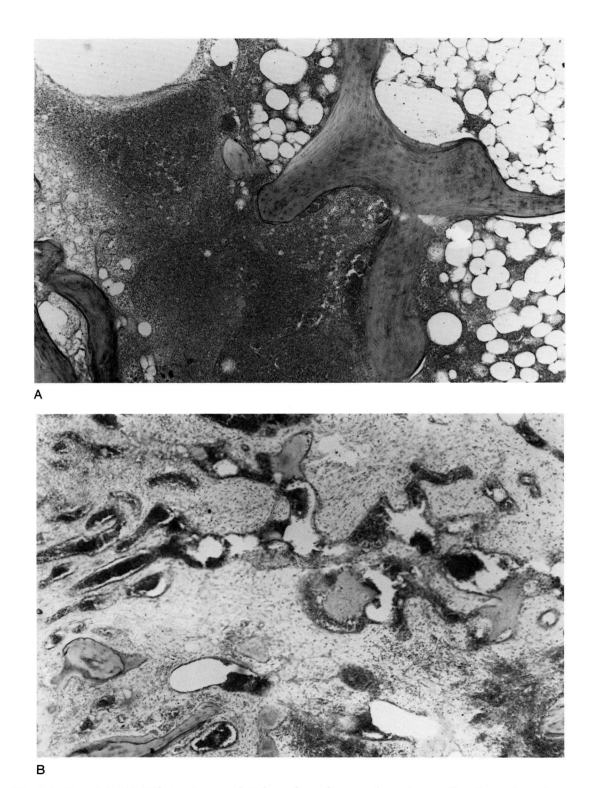

Fig. 3-2. Case 3-2. **(A)** A Photomicrograph 3 days after a fracture through cancellous bone shows hemorrhage within the marrow. (×59) **(B)** Granulation tissue with new bone that has formed along the trabecula at 1 week. (×59) *(Figure continues.)*

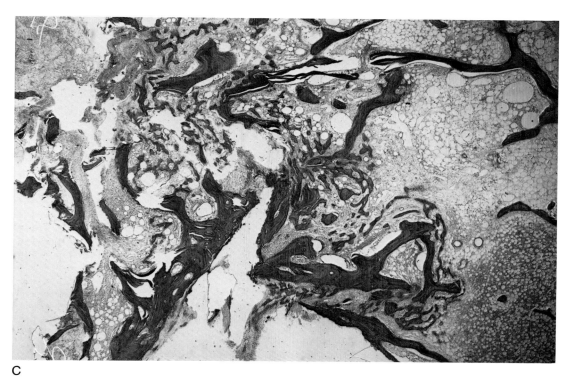

C

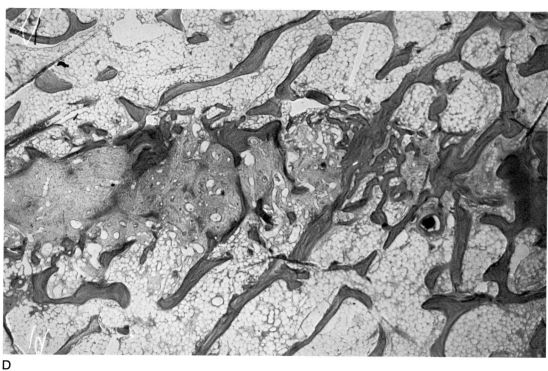

D

Fig. 3-2 *(Continued)*. (C) At the cortical margins of a 2-week-old fracture of the femoral neck and head, there are several fracture fragments, with callus surrounding and uniting some of them.(×15) (D) Cancellous bone healing with new bone connecting the trabeculae at 10 weeks. (×37)

plying the femoral head is minimal so that aseptic necrosis of the head of the femur ordinarily does not occur, and therefore that influence on fracture healing can be set aside (see Ch. 7). Of course there always is some injury to small vessels and therefore some necrosis, perhaps minimal, adjacent to the fractured surfaces. In the remodeling phase new trabeculae are reorganized to reconstitute the cancellous bone and the little cortical bone that is present at the junction of the head and neck. A similar anatomical situation prevails at other common sites of fractures involving predominantly cancellous bone, e.g., intertrochanteric area of the femur, distal part of the femur, proximal part of the tibia, and distal part of the radius.

The pathophysiological implications of these fractures through cancellous bone that have been emphasized relate mostly to the extent of derangement of vessels. Stability of the fracture fragments, when it is firm, really means that gross motion or even micro-motion does not occur and therefore does not repeatedly devascularize any viable trabeculae. The two examples discussed (spine and hip) were selected to illustrate (1) a situation where stability is ensured and (2) a situation where it might be at risk. The other sites just mentioned are influenced, in addition, by the important variable, the extent of displacement of the fracture fragments. The pathophysiological implications of displacement pertain not only to its intimate correlation with the extent of devascularization but also to dimensional considerations during therapy, repair, and residual impairment.

CORTICAL FRACTURES

Acute Events

A fracture in cortical bone is ordinarily accompanied by some degree of periosteal disruption. The important role of the periosteal new bone produced because of the disruption and involved in the repair of a cortical fracture is emphasized.[40]
Case 3-3 An 11-year-old boy, during sports, sustained a closed fracture of the proximal one-third of the femur with a moderate degree of displacement and overriding of the fragments (4 cm) (Figs.

3-3A–E). He was treated for 3 weeks in skeletal traction, the pin being inserted in the tibia. A plaster spica cast was then used for 5 weeks, after which repair of the fracture with periosteal and endosteal new bone was evident on the radiograph. The boy was then allowed to walk using crutches, but not bearing full weight on the affected limb. Full weight-bearing was first allowed at 12 weeks. At 5 months the fracture callus had remodeled to a moderate degree (Fig. 3-3D). Sixteen months after the injury the remodeling was extensive so that the medial and lateral parts of the cortex had been reconstituted and the medullary canal partially reestablished (Fig. 3-3E).

In this case, as in the previous ones, the mechanism of fracture involves a force applied to the skeleton at relatively low velocity and applied indirectly; that is, in all three cases the force is modified as it passes through a series of joints and is not directly applied to the involved vertebra or femur. As with most fractures, the direction and quantitation of the force at the fracture site must be deduced (approximated). The circumstances of the accident and the character and displacement of the fracture fragments constitute the evidence at hand. The deduction provides an interesting exercise in speculation, dear to the mechanical engineer but rarely of practical value. The plane of the fracture in this boy's case, as revealed in the radiograph, is spiral and oblique, as is often the geometry of the fracture plane in femoral fractures. That geometry has been attributed to a rotational rather than a bending, transverse, or axial force.

One should note, however, that the microstructure of the cortical bone has predominantly spiral components, and the geometry of the fracture plane may be attributed to them, rather than to the direction of the force of injury. How either possibility would affect any of the stages of response is difficult to imagine, so that discussion of these matters is academic. It also distracts one from the more important question of the extent to which the periosteum is torn. That dimension is best assessed initially by the extent of displacement of the fracture fragments. Their pointed shape assumes importance because the sharp points tend to extend periosteal tears. Other observations bearing on the periosteal injury are made during the next, second stage of injury. It should be pointed out that the

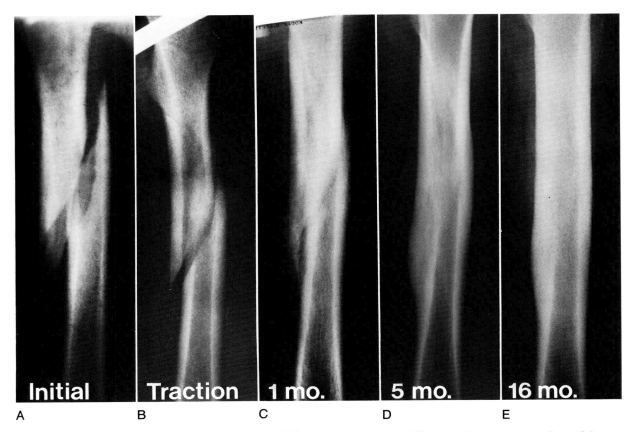

Fig. 3-3. Case 3-3. (**A**) Closed fracture of the left femur in an 11-year-old boy, with a 4-cm overriding of the cortical fragments. (**B**) After traction the gap is 1 cm. (**C**) At 1 month. (**D**) At 5 months the fracture is solidly healed. (**E**) At 16 months the radiographs show union and restoration of the medullary canal.

most important pathophysiological inference to be derived from the consideration of the periosteum is the likelihood that whatever the extent of the disruption of periosteum, given the closed nature of the fracture, the low velocity, and the thick musculature surrounding the femurs, important damage to soft tissues other than muscle at the fracture site is not likely. Whether important structures have been injured can and should be assessed immediately, the important structures at hazard being the superficial femoral and deep femoral arteries and the sciatic nerve.

If during the first-aid measures the limb has been inadvertently handled roughly, damage to the nerve and vessels may be the consequence; and if these structures had been slightly injured in the accident, the additional injury of rough handling

may change a slight injury to a severe one.[32] The large envelope of muscle may merely have been pierced by the sharp ends of the fracture fragments, and so only a small amount of muscle may have been significantly traumatized. Therefore it is not likely that there is massive necrosis of soft tissue. Nevertheless, there may have been severe extravasation of blood into the muscular envelope, and such a loss of blood, from a large artery or from smaller vessels, may easily be overlooked when the hematoma is deeply situated. Let us assume that there has been proper first-aid, i.e., effective splinting, immobilizing the fracture fragments.[33] During the physician's initial encounter with the patient, a detailed review of the first-aid should be recorded, including how the patient was moved from the site of injury to the emergency room of the hospital, how soon after the injury the splint was applied, if the leg was straightened and, if so, by traction or manipulation, and if a Thomas splint was used how hard a pull was exerted.

Answers to these questions might well affect the pathological situation that has to be assessed and might mandate prompt action even before radiographs are obtained. Suppose, for example, that the leg is observed to be in a Thomas splint with strong traction by means of a clove hitch around the ankle. If palpation of the dorsalis pedis and tibialis posterior pulses reveals no pulsation, even when the traction is released, the temperature of the calf and foot should be assessed to determine if the arterial circulation was compromised. If the foot *and* calf remain cold but the pulsations return within an hour or so, it leads one to suspect that the femoral artery may have been injured but not necessarily punctured or transected. When an artery is slightly traumatized by pressure or traction, the reflex vasospasm soon abates. Then there would be no further major concern about the integrity of the whole thickness of the arterial wall. The concern should be directed at the possibility of a lesion to the damaged intima of the artery or vein on which a plaque of platelets might form. This plaque might well be the site of formation of a thrombus, which might build up so gradually as to be silent for several days.

There are three possible courses for that lesion, in the following order of frequency: Most commonly by far, the plaque is covered by endothelium growing over it from the injured endothelium at its borders. Rarely, the plaque builds up to such a degree that it obstructs the vessel. Even more rarely, the plaque detaches from the vessel wall and becomes an embolus. If the affected vessel is an artery, the embolus lodges distally and obstructs the vessel. If the vessel affected is a vein, obviously the embolus passes into the lung. Clinically, this rare possibility conjures up the ominous threat of sudden death. Although that outcome has been reported, most often it does not happen, although it raises the question of what diagnostic measures are appropriate.

None of the presently available diagnostic modalities detect endothelial damage. Whether one should think of such tests as arteriography, venography, and computed tomography (CT) scans depend on the development of clinical signs or their evolution during the days after the injury. For example, arteriography is undoubtedly justified if the calf remains cold for several days, the pedal pulses after returning remain feeble, and Doppler tests show the arterial pressure to be consistently low.

These pathophysiological possibilities should remain under consideration and should ensure that continuing observations be directed at the circulation to the extremity. The foot, in particular, should be watched because of the possibility of arterial damage at the ankle by too tight a clove hitch on the splint.

Once the radiographs reveal the fracture (Fig. 3-3A), the displacement and overriding of the fracture fragments become the focus of attention. Those findings require pathophysiological interpretation, and some of the previously recorded facts must be kept in mind, i.e., the timing of the application of the Thomas splint, the conditions of the traction (force of pull, relaxation for assessment of circulation), and the period of time that elapsed between the injury and the time of the radiograph. If the traction was not strong, and if 2 to 3 hours had elapsed from the moment of injury, the extent of the overriding (4 cm in the present case) would be attributed to muscle spasm rather than to the force of the initial injury. If the traction seemed adequate but not excessive and only a few minutes had elapsed since the injury, it might well be deduced that one is dealing with a severe injury and might even entertain the possibility that some of the original displacement and angulation had been corrected.

When discussing the pros and cons of the treatment chosen, i.e., in case 3-3 skeletal traction through a pin drilled just distal to the tibial tubercle, the first advantage of that treatment is that it is safe.[5,39] Second, it permits strong (and adjustable) traction to be administered for the anticipated period that traction is needed, i.e., 2 to 3 weeks. Third, the surgeon, during the first day or two of fraction treatment, can observe the effects and deduce the extent of periosteal disruption, an important pathophysiological change. Because the periosteum in children is fairly thick—in fact, several times thicker than in the adult—it is less likely to be completely disrupted. Even when there is considerable initial displacement and overriding of the fracture fragments, strong traction does not permit distraction of the fragments within 1 day if even one-half of the circumference of periosteum is intact. If distraction of the fragments measuring a centimeter or more quickly becomes evident, one can deduce that the periosteum has been torn circumferentially around the femur. The potential influence of the tear in terms of maintaining axial alignment has been lost.

Another pathophysiological consequence may be predicted as well, i.e., the probable topography of the callus. If part of the periosteum is not torn, the callus that will be laid down internal to it will tend to establish a longitudinal bony continuity unless disturbed by excessive motion. In the event that the circumference is wholly disrupted, the callus that forms will tend to pile up maximally on the torn edge. It will resemble two ragged collars separated by a gap of a few millimeters, across which bony continuity will have to be established by elaboration of a considerably greater volume of callus then would have been required with lesser periosteal tears.

Intermediate Events

In case 3-3 the overriding was reduced to 1 cm by traction (Fig. 3-3); i.e., some of the periosteum at the site of the fracture must still have been intact. Two of the goals of the traction were prevention of gross motion of the fragments and proper axial alignment. In an 11-year-old child the slight residual overriding should be accepted, provided good axial alignment is attained. That some periosteum was intact is primarily important because it assures the surgeon that reestablishment of bony continuity will be rapid. Within 2 to 3 weeks the callus that will form under the intact stretch of periosteum will not only cross the fracture gap but also will bond proximally and distally to both fracture fragments. The considerable contribution of the periosteal fibers to stabilization of the fracture fragments has these therapeutic implications. It should be evident that skeletal traction at best restricts the motion of the fracture fragments relative to each other, but it does not immobilize them.

Parenthetically, it should be mentioned that the application of any cast, even one so extensive as to reach from the rib margins to the toes, with both extremities being encased, also does not immobilize the fracture fragments because muscle contractions can cause them to move somewhat. For the periosteum to contribute maximally to the stabilization, it should be stretched; and that maneuver should be done rapidly, before edema of the tissues or beginning organization of the hematoma become insurmountable obstacles to restoring the length of the bone. With these advantages, the treatment by skeletal traction leads to the expectation that only a short period of hospitalization will be needed, 2 to 3 weeks, for the traction phase of the treatment. In contrast to open treatment, the anesthetic and surgical risks have been reduced to the minimum. (The only important complication might be a pin tract infection, which is amenable to treatment.) The prospect for healing, then, is practically ensured, as shown by accumulated experience. From the socioeconomic viewpoint, the child will miss some weeks of school, which he or she usually can afford.

These arguments for traction treatment must be balanced against one important principle in the treatment of a fracture: Secure *immobilization* of the fracture fragments is essential. Why there is such an obvious exception to this principle—that it does not apply to fractures in children in whom stabilization of most fractures need not be nearly so firm as in adults—has given rise to much speculation, but the reason(s) still are obscure. In adults the principle has been responsible for the elaboration of many devices and several techniques for open reduction of femoral and other fractures.[22,23,26,27] These reasons do not constitute an argument that traction for fractures in adults, particularly for a fracture similar to the one under discussion, is not to be used in appropriate circumstances, however. The enormous armamentarium of devices for the fixation of fracture fragments should not so occupy the surgeon's thoughts that which device would be most appropriate is the first consideration. The first consideration should be the firm exception mentioned above, which incidentally applies not only to children but also to all the usual laboratory animals[2,6,11,15,18,34] and in fact to most other animals as well.[24,25] As a therapeutic principle, firm fixation for fractures, even in adults, has periodically been contested in a few specific fractures, e.g., those in the shaft of the tibia, for which there are advocates of closed treatment,[5,21,38] e.g., skin-tight walking casts, cast-braces, and external fixators.

Many interesting questions therefore arise, one of which is: What is meant by immobilization? To a physicist or an engineer, the surgeon's use of the word "immobilization" invites questions about measurements of the amplitude of motion, the direction(s) of the motion, its velocity, and its frequency. To a clinician, immobilization connotes a situation in which the amplitude of motion between the fragments never exceeds a low (perhaps very low) threshold; but in clinical practice and the laboratory, that threshold has not been demonstrated quantitatively. Whether it is millimeters or micrometers of axial, transverse, or rotatory motion, or whether tenths of a degree or only hundredths of a degree of bend or twist constitutes the threshold no one knows.

In the fracture under discussion, we could demonstrate radiographically several days after the injury that a displacement motion measuring centimeters could occur between the fragments, and that motion was possible even a week after the injury. The word "immobilization" (by traction), strictly speaking, is inappropriate, and perhaps *stabilization* is a better word. Any pathophysiological explanation of this exceptional situation in children, although entirely speculative, must include the probable participation of hormonal influences involved in the phenomena of growth. Callus, as is laid down in a child's fracture, is much more extensive and contains much more cartilage than does a similar fracture in an adult. The child's callus, and indeed his or her bones as well, are more flexible and at all stages of healing allow an amplitude of motion to occur that is greater by at least an order of magnitude without any of the usual events associated with gross motion of fracture fragments in adults: hemorrhage, edema, and necrosis. Empirical data, accumulated over centuries, have shown that fractures in children almost always heal even when only a minimal attempt or no attempt at all is made at stabilizing the fragments. Experience also has shown that, in a child, remodeling of a healed fracture of the femur in which there has been 1 to 2 cm of overriding and perhaps even severe angulation includes compensatory overgrowth and correction of the angulation. The younger the child, the more capable are the tissues to correct the discrepancy and angulation. Experience has shown that only rotational malalignment does not undergo substantial correction. The reason is unknown.

Most importantly, it is well known that even extensive residual displacement of the fracture fragments does not compromise completion of the healing of the type of fracture described, and the delay in the healing process is not excessive (i.e., as in adults, where delayed union may signify an interval of 3 to 6 months). However, if soft tissue has been interposed between the bony fragments, there may be not only a significant delay but even a lack of union. The time needed for repair of a fracture as in case 3-3 therefore is measured in weeks, whereas repair of the "same" fracture in an adult would require months. The appropriate treatment of that fracture in an adult therefore is different from that in a child.

In case 3-3 several considerations are important as they affect the magnitude and duration of the second stage of response, i.e., after the initial stage of hemorrhage, exudate, and necrosis. The first stage includes the few days from the moment of injury to the time during which hemorrhage and exudate would have peaked and then subsided; it also includes the time of splinting. It is obvious that bleeding, even if it ceases within a few minutes of the injury, will start again with each measure that disturbs the fracture fragments: the act of splinting, application of traction, and release of traction while positioning the patient or the extremity for radiography or for drilling the pin for skeletal traction. Each of these situations can be viewed as initiating a new stage of the response, and the hemorrhage that results evokes a proportional amount of exudate.

In addition to the amounts of hemorrhage and exudate, which are far greater in this case than in case 3-1, a vertebral fracture, the second phase of the response is more extensive in terms of the volume of tissue affected and the duration of the process. The most important difference, so far as therapy is concerned, principally concerns the extent of injury to and the reactions of the periosteum with respect to the volume of callus. It is this point that mainly distinguishes the two cases. In addition to the role of the periosteum during the second stage in regard to alignment of the fracture, as mentioned, it also governs the extent of necrosis to some extent because of the important contribution to the blood supply of the bone of periosteal vessels.[29-31] These vessels not only communicate with the haversian spaces but also are the principal supplier to the outer one-third of the cortex, which in children consists mainly of circumferential lamellae. The potential of cells in the periosteum to form callus rapidly and in large amounts close to or even within the fracture gap must also partly explain why fractures heal so much better in children than in adults.

There are four important differences between case 3-3 and case 3-1: the type of bone involved (the femoral fracture is cortical, the vertebral fracture is cancellous), the stability of the fragments (the femoral fracture lacks inherent stability), the displacement (extensive in the femoral case), and the ability of the child's bone, but not that of the adult, to be remodeled to the normal state during the growing years. Others that relate to the patient as a whole have been mentioned: The child requires little if any formal rehabilitation and tolerates better the discomforts of hospitalization, traction, or cast treatment. The surgeon rarely need tailor the treatment with socioeconomic considerations foremost in mind (employment, home care, compensation).

The "assured" favorable result notwithstanding, the possible complications in the treatment of any fracture must always be kept in mind. Those that are excessively rare (e.g., fat embolism or venous thrombosis in a child who has a single closed fracture) should not evoke so much concern that the surgeon orders multitudinous laboratory tests or, worse, prescribes ill-advised prophylaxis. Those measures that introduce risk should certainly be avoided unless there are strong clinical indications for their institution, as should most of the measures that introduce inordinate expense. The surgeon must have enough insight to realize that every needless test and every needless precaution raises the level of anxiety in the patient and the parents, a condition that may interfere with cooperation with the therapy.

In case 3-3 there was continuing good alignment and only slight residual displacement of the fragments relative to one another. The position was maintained after the first day of traction, as evidenced in the radiographs 1 month later. The films showed that the periosteum had not been completely torn; and where it was intact, callus had been produced by it on the side of the fracture. The amount produced in 1 month was sufficient to allow minimal load-bearing (with the protection of a cast or cast brace).

Cancellous Versus Cortical Fractures

In addition to the differences between cases that have already been discussed, a difference that causes stage 2 and particularly stage 3 of the healing period to be much longer in case 3-3 than in case 3-1 is that the bone affected is cortical. The femur has a thick cortex, perhaps the thickest of any bone in the body. The structure of cortical bone is designed for bearing heavy loads, and its formation or restitution takes many months, even in a child. In case 3-3 and in all fractures of cortical bone, all of the vessels in the endosteum and haversian canals would have been torn, and because of the overriding of the fracture fragments many of the blood vessels from the periosteum to the cortex would also have been torn. The result is ischemia of a considerable volume of cortical bone at the fracture site. The usual blood supply and even the collateral supply would have been destroyed, and so necrosis of some area of cortex in each fracture fragment therefore was inevitable. Although we cannot know how extensive those segments of necrosis were, it is likely that they extended at least several millimeters from the fracture line. The ischemia, however, presumably did not extend to the intact periosteum, and so its vessels could give rise to newly formed circulatory channels. A reconstructed vascular bed was needed in the fracture gap and marrow cavity, however, before healing could begin in that part of the fracture. It should not be assumed that as a prerequisite to healing all necrotic bone must be resorbed and replaced. Callus can be produced not only under the intact periosteum but also layered on the necrotic bone, which is in continuity with viable bone. Therefore the production of external and internal callus could proceed to the point where the injured segment was capable of bearing a load despite the presence of much necrotic bone. Any operative regimen of treatment probably would have increased the extent of injury to the circulation and the amount of necrosis. That risk was and should be avoided in view of the certainty that the fracture will heal in a relatively short period of time and functional use of the extremity will be possible long before healing is complete.

Histology

The microscopic aspects of cortical fracture healing are examined here. We consider what happens to the bone under a variety of conditions and how the various cells in bone, periosteum, endosteum, marrow, and blood vessels contribute to the process. There are many excellent descriptions of the histology of fracture healing available elsewhere,[6,8,9,11-18,22,28] and so the description that follows touches on only the essentials.

The reaction to bony injury soon after the immediate ones of hemorrhage and necrosis, like that for any tissue, is inflammation. All viable tissues adjacent to the injury participate in this process. To depict these patterns, a case of stress fracture is described.

Stress Fracture

Case 3-4 A 10-year-old boy complained that he had had pain in the calf for 3 weeks. He first noted the pain in the lateral aspect of his leg when he ran. The clinical diagnosis "shin splints" was offered without radiographs having been obtained. Because the pain persisted, especially after and during running and often when he was at rest, a radiograph was obtained about 1 month after the onset of symptoms. Because of some uncertainties at that time (several decades ago) about the exact diagnosis (one radiologist raised the question of Ewing's sarcoma) it was decided to remove a segment of the fibula en bloc. Although such a decision would today generally be condemned, it has afforded us an opportunity to examine histologically material that is today nearly impossible to come by.

The radiograph of the specimen reveals in better detail the features seen on the clinical radiograph (Fig. 3-4A). One of those features is an area of increased density on either side of a radiolucent line

traversing the fibula. Histologically, the radiolucent line is seen to consist of a barely visible gap in the cortex (Fig. 3-4B), and the gap consists of a narrow area of fibrochondroosseous callus. It also contains an area of residual (old) hemorrhage surrounded by a zone of organization (Fig. 3-4C). This pattern is entirely consistent with or even identical to the pattern that is found in an ordinary (i.e., not a stress) 4-week-old fracture of a thin long bone with minimal displacement.

What are the chronological implications of these findings? Obviously the hemorrhage occurred early, perhaps during the initial episode of overloading, although there might have been a series of small hemorrhages accompanying the cycles of stress. Histological evidence to support that possibility was not found in this case. Even though one sees many patients who have had several episodes of hemorrhage into one tissue site with clots that exhibit unequivocal evidence of different timing of the repair process, i.e., several bouts of repair, no such intermittence or repetition can be seen in the present case. Thus there is no positive answer to the question of whether each or several of the cyclic overloads caused separate hemorrhages. Nearby, however, the histological pattern represents a continuum of remodeling of the internal callus, from the most primitive stage (broad bands only faintly resembling trabeculae) to patterns that are more and more mature.

It is in the fracture gap that the continuum of maturation of fibroosseous callus is best recognized, and it is especially active in the center of the specimen. It would be expected that localization of the most advanced stage of maturation of the callus would correlate well with the site where the motion of the two fracture fragments relative to each other is least. The fibroosseous callus contains small foci of cartilage, as might be expected if one presumes that cartilage is prone to develop in a site where fracture fragments move on one another (Fig. 3-4E).

Another residual of stage 1 is evident, i.e., areas of necrosis of cortical bone with resorption cavities (Fig. 3-4D). Radiographically, these areas appeared somewhat radiolucent compared to unaffected cortex because of the foci of resorption. These areas somewhat resembled the motheaten areas of a Ewing's sarcoma and were responsible for the misdiagnosis by the radiologist. Radiographically, the areas of resorption at the site of the fracture are larger than the residual necrotic areas that remain.

In the subperiosteal area the attempt at repair is a constructive bridging from one fracture fragment to the other, and there are no signs of degeneration of the periosteal or muscular tissues. Necrosis was seen only in the small bony foci whose circulation was interrupted by the trauma. The new fibroosseous elements that cross from one fragment to the other have an orientation that is primarily longitudinal; they are influenced by the intact periosteum, their principal parental tissue, and are suitable for axial load bearing, their ultimate function.

The radiographic observation that there are longitudinal radiodensities on either side of the fracture fragments adjoining the radiolucent gap correlates well with the histological picture of layers of subperiosteal callus, more osseous than fibrocartilaginous, in those areas (Fig. 3-4F). The predominance of endosteal over periosteal callus (Fig. 3-4G) supports the idea that there has been little motion between fracture fragments. One cannot determine from the tissue patterns if healing has been impeded. Obviously, surgical removal or disturbance of the fibroosseous callus between the fragments would delay rather than promote healing. This subject is discussed further under nonunion and Phemister grafts (see Ch. 5).

The progressive pattern of remodeling of the cortex as examination proceeds from the fracture site proximally in the proximal fragment and distally in the distal fragment should also be noted. It represents a process of resorption, not only of necrotic foci but also of living bone. The cortex that has had its load-bearing pattern changed by the fracture responds to the alteration first by forming haversian spaces within the cortex and then, in those spaces, depositing new haversian systems. This remodeling of the haversian pattern in the cortical bone, rather than by creeping substitution, is the predominant feature of case 3-4 because so little of the cortical bone underwent necrosis. The resorption of bone and deposition of callus are most evident at the fracture gap, but callus in the gap has not yet restored continuity to the disrupted cortex. There is minimal bridging external callus, for reasons now to be considered.

The presence of a more and more mature but less and less voluminous callus in proportion to the distance from the fracture gap is an expression of the rate of elaboration of subperiosteal bone.The pathophysiological reason for the development of this pattern, which is common in fractures of any severity and is nearly always seen a few weeks after the injury, is the following: The most intense vascular dilatation occurs at the fracture site, in addition to the hemorrhage. The ensuing exudation tends to elevate the periosteum from the cortex. Under the stretched but intact periosteum, bone is laid down. The periosteum at a distance from the fracture site is also elevated by exudate but to a lesser extent and at a slower rate. Little remodeling then occurs in the essentially compact lamellae of periosteal bone compared to the remodeling of the immature callus produced adjacent to the fracture.

Radiography reveals deposition of subperiosteal bone that extends for nearly 4 cm on the cortex of bone fragments. The diameter of the bone is appreciably increased by the lamellae (Fig. 3-4B). This picture was also apparent radiographically in the fracture of the femoral shaft in case 3-3. The pattern of concentric layering of bone around the fibula in the present case is characteristic of periosteal callus in any location (because it is the response of periosteum whenever stimulated, not only by trauma but also by infection or tumor), and it was responsible for the misdiagnosis (tumor) in this case. The radiograph also revealed the resorptive process in the cortex, previously described in the histological phenomena.

The histological evidence presented was obtained from a stress fracture, but it corresponds in most respects to that found in any simple, relatively undisplaced, well immobilized fracture in which the periosteum has not been severely torn. The main differences might be greater degrees of resorption and necrosis at the fracture gap.

Obviously there was no possibility in the stress fracture of displacement of fracture fragments because there was no true fragmentation of the bone. The first injury probably was a microscopic rather than a gross hemorrhage and perhaps only a limited thrombosis of small vessels. One reaction to the vascular change would be zonal vasodilation perhaps accompanied by a more localized formation of granulation tissue at the site of hemorrhage or

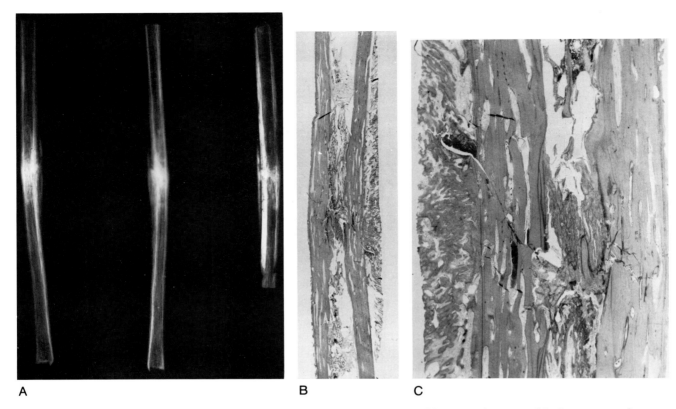

A   B   C

Fig. 3-4. Case 3-4. A 10-year-old boy complained of pain in the calf for 3 weeks. An en block segment of fibula was excised as a possible tumor. **(A)** Radiograph of a fracture of the fibula. Note the periosteal new bone and medullary density of a healing fracture. **(B)** Photomicrograph of the whole specimen shows the fracture resorption cavities within the cortices. (×2.2). **(C)** The fracture is seen more clearly in this higher power photomicrograph. Hemorrhage, cortical resorption cavities, periosteal new bone, and endosteal callus are present. (×10). **(D)** Fibrocartilaginous callus of stage 3. (×250). **(E)** Higher power view of the stage 1 hemorrhage. **(F)** Osteoclastic resorption of necrotic areas of cortex at the fracture site. Along with endosteal callus are fractures of several events occurring at the same time. **(G)** Periosteal new bone and the cutting resorption channel. (×40) *(Figure continues.)*

thrombosis. After one or at most a few weeks, the injured vessels would have been recanalized; they then could not be identified as injured vessels either histologically or physiologically. Perhaps there might be some slight necrosis and some resorption of cortex. Many assume that there is repeated micro-motion in the involved cortex when the leg was used. They conjecture that it is this motion, perhaps only a few degrees of bend or twist, that interferes with repair by callus between the fragments. Therapy then should allow callus the opportunity to form and remodel. It would be accomplished by minimizing motion, i.e., good im-

mobilization of the fragments even though weight-bearing might be permitted. One could expect external callus to be visible radiographically within 2 to 3 weeks if a cast or cast-brace were used,[33] and the cortex could be expected to be sufficiently reconstituted mechanically within a month so that the cast or brace would not be needed.[20]

The terms "stress fracture" and "fatigue fracture" are borrowed from engineers' description of the breakage of metal wires or rods subjected to repeated bending. These terms are somewhat inappropriate here in that the stressed metal shows a sequence of crystalline changes and none of the

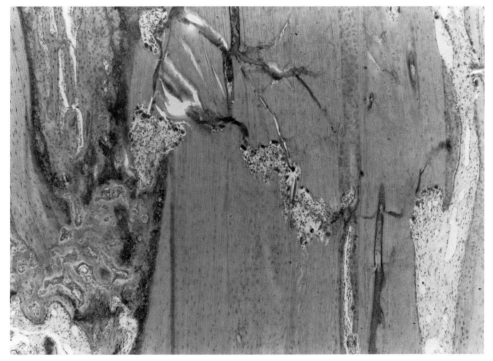

D

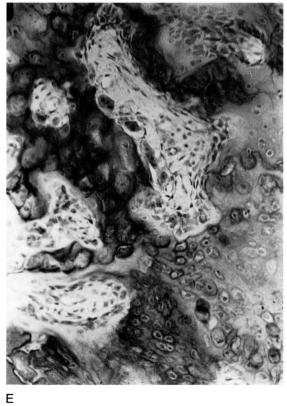

E

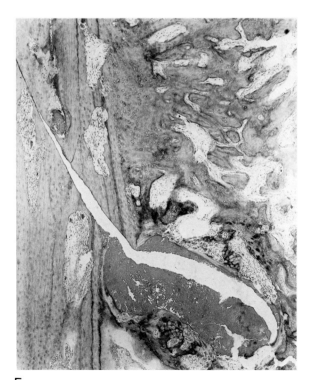

F

Fig. 3-4 *(Continued). (Figure continues.)*

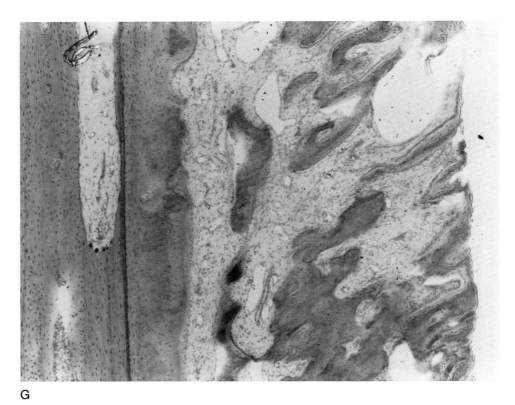

G

Fig. 3-4 *(Continued)*.

reactive processes (resorption and repair) that characterize the biological stress fracture. In particular, the radiolucent zone that characterizes the lesion radiographically represents a linear zone of resorbed cortex in which spaces that formerly were filled with compact bone are now occupied by radiolucent fibrovascular tissue. This zone has no counterpart in metallic fatigue fractures. In metal, any gap that may be demonstrated is due to beginning separation of the fragments long after the crystals that compose the metal have had induced in them marked stacking defects. Biological "stress" fractures should therefore not be viewed simply as the end result of a series of microfractures. Rather, they represent a continuum of injuries to an active repair process, including not only elaboration of callus but also resorption of necrotic bone and remodeling of the involved microstructures in the cortical bone and callus.

Perhaps an explanation is needed as to why a stress fracture was used here to portray the histological aspects of repair after injury. Ideally, a human specimen would have been used or many specimens of fractures of small bones (small, so as to show the complete specimen in one figure, e.g., Fig. 3-4). Those fractures should ideally show varying chronology, minimal displacement, good immobilization, and no complications. Such human specimens are practically unobtainable, however, for obvious reasons. There are important objections to the use of specimens from animals. The chronology of healing among species varies considerably, as do the variables of treatment. Compare, for instance, any one kind of immobilization that might be chosen for a fracture of the femur or fibula of a rat or fracture of a dog's radius.

The stress fracture has been used to represent the least cortical injury that can still be called a fracture; similarly, the vertebral fracture depicts the analogous (minimal) lesion in cancellous bone. If there is a lesser degree of injury, i.e., a direct blow to a bone, which laymen call a "bone bruise," it would be a small focus of hemorrhage subperiosteally, perhaps accompanied by a small focus of necrosis. Neither the resorption of those foci nor the evolution of the small volume of callus would allow a demonstrable solution of continuity of the bone, i.e., a fracture.

The case just discussed is unusual not only because of the availability of the specimen but also because the stress fracture occurred in a bone that rarely has a stress fracture. Note that in case 3-4, 4 weeks elapsed before the first radiographs were obtained. In most cases nowadays, a stress fracture is suspected and radiographic examination is done early. There has been much speculation, based on radiological data, on what the earliest histological changes might be. Most observers agree that there will be hemorrhage, thrombosis, and necrosis, as already mentioned. Because no specimens from such cases are likely to be available (and none has been described in the literature) there is no agreement as to the further changes that will occur. It has commonly been reported that in patients who ultimately developed the characteristic radiographic findings of stress fracture there are no radiographic changes whatsoever at the onset of symptoms or within a week or two thereafter. During that period, no gap exists in the involved cortex, but obviously the continuity of some haversian systems has been disrupted and some necrosis must have occurred. In contrast to other types of fracture, stress fractures show no displacement whatsoever, whereas all other (unimpacted or impacted) fractures have in common displacement on the order of millimeters or centimeters, with possible angular displacement of at least a few degrees.

If one considers that the thickness of the periosteum is about 1 mm, the diameter of the small nutrient arteries is at most 0.1 mm, and the diameters of the periosteal vessels are at most one-half that figure, i.e., 50 μm (the diameter of a strand of hair being 500 μm, or 0.5 mm), one can understand why a stress fracture is often called "hairline," although it differs from a hairline acute fracture (Fig. 3-5). With an acute fracture displacement approaching 1 mm surely would disrupt all of the vessels just mentioned, and the thrombosis that would follow would extend a few millimeters above and below the fracture gap. Even if part of the periosteum were torn and the rest stretched, the stretched fibers would be disrupted and some of the osteoblastic cells adjoining the cortex would be de-

stroyed. At first, the intact periosteum might not be displaced from the cortical bone, but what might displace it somewhat is the hemorrhage or some edema (Fig. 3-4C). There would be little inflammatory reaction and associated edema, although they would be much more extensive than in the developing stress fracture and would therefore cause much more pain.

Even though the tissue response after the acute inflammation in the two situations would be similar (beginning formation of vascular buds and fibroosseous callus), the acute fracture would be well protected from micro-motion (because such motion would aggravate pain that is already severe), whereas the incipient stress fracture would not be so protected. It is the effect of the micro-motion on the developing repair tissue, i.e., cyclic disruption of vessels and cyclic resumption of inflammation, that permits the sequence of events that yields the stress fracture.

It is evident that before there is radiological evidence of resorption enough callus must have been laid down to yield a positive bone scan, as even microscopic quantities of new bone pick up a bone-seeking radioisotope. One may infer therefore that an incipient stress fracture, diagnosed by clinical signs and symptoms but not by radiography, might be diagnosed by a bone scan (see Fig. 3-7B). Moreover, if it is treated promptly, i.e., if the cyclic trauma is terminated, it might heal without yielding radiographic evidence of an abnormality.

Any periosteal new bone response that would result from the fracture would be barely visible radiographically until a week or more after the first injury. If the periosteum were fully disrupted, there would be more disruption of periosteal vessels, which would contribute to the formation of a larger hematoma and more periosteal bone.

In the acute fracture with minimal displacement, the organization of hematoma and exudate ordinarily begins within 24 hours of the first injury, and new capillaries are provided by proliferation of the remaining periosteal capillaries, the process reaching a maximum 10 to 20 days after the injury. The cambium layers of the endosteum and periosteum provide the beginnings of new bone formation, callus, which therefore is intramembranous. It usually contains foci of fibrocartilage, after which endochondral sequences may be seen in those foci as

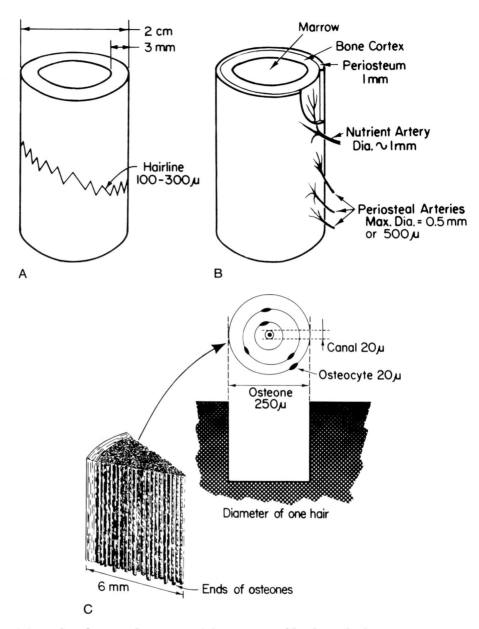

Fig. 3-5. (A) Hairline fracture dimensions. (B) Periosteum blood supply dimensions. (C) Osteone dimensions. *(Figure continues.)*

part of the callus, and new bone formation on each side of the fracture would bridge the fracture gap in a matter of 10 to 14 days. The callus would continue to remodel from that point onward, as noted earlier. As with the stress fracture, injury to the

callus within the first 2 weeks would be a major deterrent to the sequence of healing.

It must not be assumed that nearly all stress fractures demonstrate this so-called typical pattern of development of symptoms, radiological abnormali-

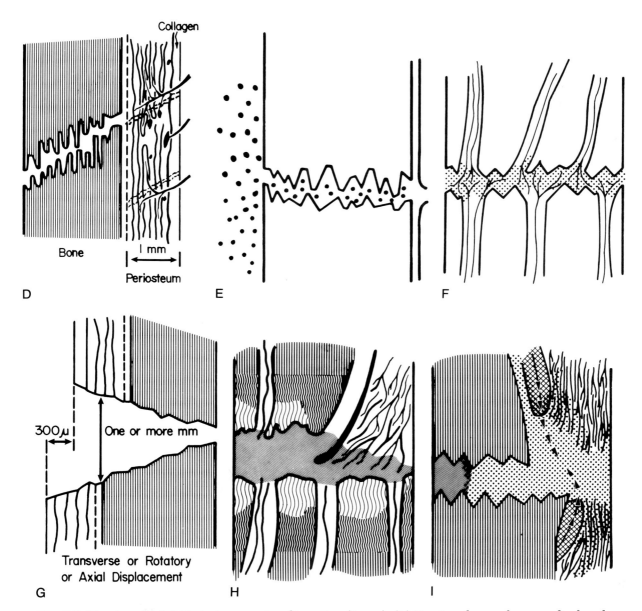

Fig. 3-5 *(Continued).* **(D)** Periosteum cortex disruption (1 mm). **(E)** Fracture hemorrhage, undisplaced. **(F)** Endosteal vessels, reanastomosed. **(G)** Displaced fracture. **(H)** Torn vessels, necrosis of bone ends. **(I)** Periosteal callus (crosshatched area).

ties, and repair process.[16,20] Another case makes this point.

Case 3-5 A 16-year-old girl complained of pain in the calf that had been present for 6 weeks and was worse whenever she was training for cross country races. Milder activity also produced some pain and a limp. Her tibia was tender at the junction of the

middle and proximal one-thirds, and she had pain at the same site when the heel was pounded. The radiograph showed some periosteal new bone posterolaterally at the entrance of the canal for the nutrient artery and one focus of cortical resorption; the intensity of the reactive new bone and the focus of resorption led the radiologist to consider osteoid osteoma in the differential diagnosis, but that diagnosis was considered unlikely in view of the symptoms: pain that worsened with activity, was not nocturnal, and was of relatively short duration.

A minimally displaced fracture was also considered but discarded as the probable diagnosis. With such a lesion, the periosteal new bone would be evident at 10 to 14 days, endosteal new bone would be detected within 3 to 4 weeks, and the fracture line would be radiodense at 14 to 21 days. By 4 weeks the periosteal callus would be fusiform and well defined, and the medullary callus would then be distinct. In this case none of these radiological features had progressed to the extent described over the 6 weeks of symptoms.

At the 6-week stage her radiographs showed a faint, irregular "hairline" radiolucency across all of the tibia (Fig. 3-6A). She was restricted from sports activity following the diagnosis of healing stress fracture, and its healing phase (Fig. 3-6B) because evident only after 2 months, at which time the patient was without pain or tenderness. Radiographically, at 5 months the callus had become more dense (Fig. 3-6C). In this case there might have been a need for further studies, e.g., radionuclide scans prior to the radiographic examination, which was done 6 weeks after the onset of symptoms.[10]

During the early stages the symptoms of stress fracture may be nearly identical with some traumatic lesions of soft tissue, e.g., partial tears of muscular attachments (see Ch. 6). With both lesions the radioisotopic scan may be positive, as it would

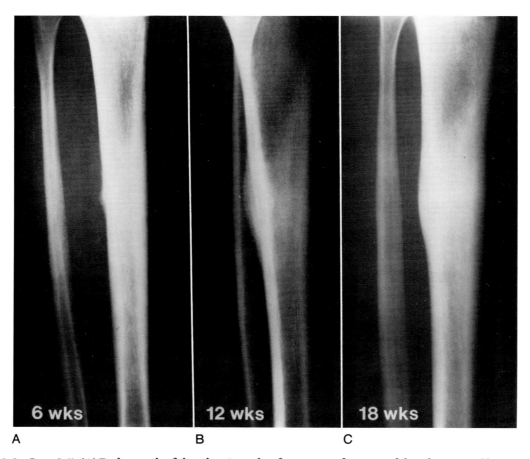

6 wks   12 wks   18 wks

A   B   C

Fig. 3-6. Case 3-5. (A) Radiograph of the tibia 6 weeks after a stress fracture of the tibia caused by running. (B) At 12 weeks the tibia is healing. (C) At 18 weeks it is healed.

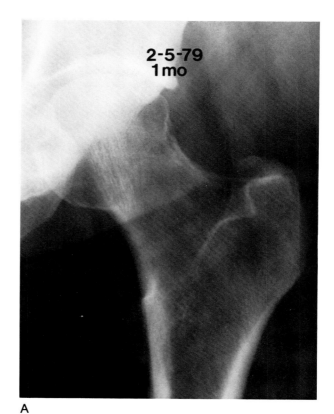

Fig. 3-7. Case 3-6. A 43-year-old woman was given steroids for 18 months for vasculitis. (A) Initial AP radiograph after the patient had reported having had pain for 1 month. Note the increased density medially and the suggestion of a step-off of a stress fracture. (B) Positive bone scan of the left femoral neck. (From El-Khoury et al.,[9] with permission.) *(Figure continues.)*

A

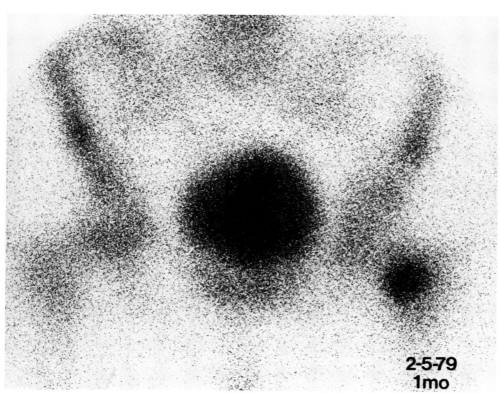

B

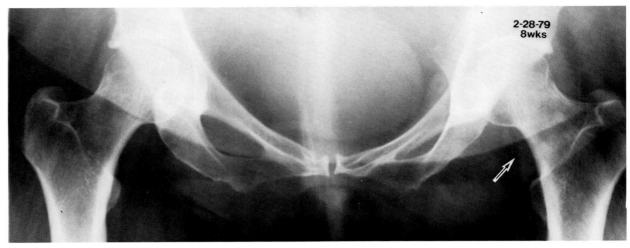

C

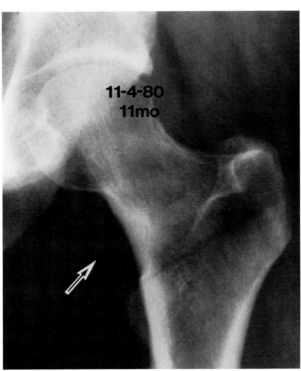

D

Fig. 3-7 *(Continued)*. **(C)** Increased density of the femoral neck site (arrow) at 2 months. **(D)** At 11 months the fracture has healed (arrow).

be with some periosteal tears or bruises without fracture. In many such cases positive patterns on the scan would differentiate the lesions, but the prognosis would be different (note, however, that identical therapy would be prescribed).

Delay in the diagnosis of a stress fracture, especially when it occurs in unusual sites (e.g., femoral neck) is not uncommon, and it is in such cases that a tomogram or a bone scan is of most value[10] (Fig. 3-7A,B). Either technique may reveal the repair process after conventional radiographs fail to do so because they allow callus of minimal extent to be identified.

Case 3-6 A 43-year-old woman who had been treated with steroids for 18 months for vasculitis developed pain in her left hip. The initial radiograph of the left hip was normal (Fig. 3-7A). A radionuclide bone scan performed on the same day demonstrated increased uptake localized to the femoral neck (Fig. 3-7B). Two months later the radiograph showed increased bone density in that same area (Fig. 3-7C). At 11 months the fracture is well healed (Fig. 3-7D).

We need not review the other sites of stress fracture, as they are well described in textbooks on fractures, and the features that are different in each are not especially important.

Treatment is rest for a sufficiently long time to permit union of the stress fracture. In military recruits with stress fracture of the calcaneus, a minimal period of 8 weeks was required for sufficient healing to allow the recruit to return to physical activities. Similar time periods are required for other sites.

GREENSTICK FRACTURES

Another type of fracture is the *greenstick fracture* (Fig. 3-8A,B). It resembles the stress fracture and vertebral compression fracture in that the fracture gap is small, and the fracture fragments have an inherent stability that requires no measures for im-

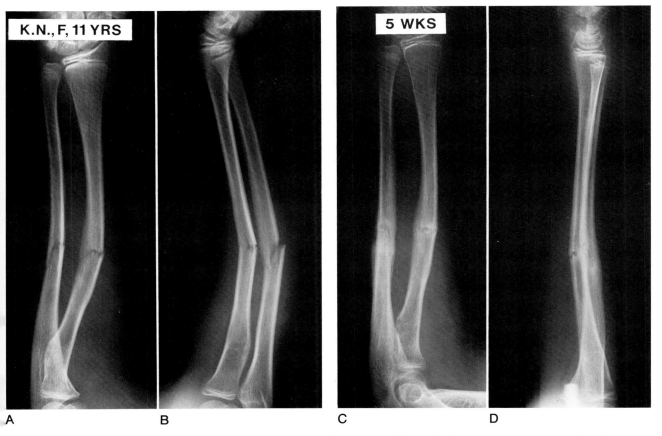

K.N., F, 11 YRS

5 WKS

A   B   C   D

Fig. 3-8. (A) AP and lateral radiographs of a greenstick fracture of the right forearm in an 11-year-old girl. (B) AP and lateral radiographs show the fracture healing at 5 weeks.

mobilization. It further resembles the stress fracture as well as the femoral fracture previously described in that the solution of continuity, i.e., the disruption is in cortical bone. Another feature it has in common with the stress fracture is that fracture "fragments" as such do not exist, the opposite part of the cortex at the fracture site being intact. All these similarities affect the repair sequences. The differences between those sequences in the stress fracture, as just described, and the greenstick fracture derive mainly from the fact that the latter is the result of one episode of acute trauma, whereas the former follows cyclic trauma applied over a period of weeks or longer.

The greenstick fracture essentially is an in situ bending, i.e., an indirect, low-energy injury; the main stage 1 processes, i.e., hemorrhage, edema, and necrosis, occur, but none is as extensive as with the femoral fracture. There is definite, but minimal, displacement of bone substance but no continuing motion at the site of injury.

This fracture commonly occurs in children, rarely in adults. The reasons are that a child's bones are flexible and the periosteum is thick and tough. Moreover, the child's joints are elastic and absorb much of the stress on the injured extremity, so that whereas one part of the cortex of the affected bone breaks the remainder retains its continuity despite the bending. In practice, it is impossible to reduce such a fracture perfectly without "completing the fracture." Simply straightening the bend in the remaining intact cortex as far as possible restores some of its alignment but not completely. On the side where there is a discontinuity in bone substance, attempts at reduction cause disimpaction and the formation of a small gap, filled by hemorrhage, and perhaps a few small necrotic fragments of bone substance. Even after the bone is straightened as far as possible with a firm manipulation, there is still some displacement of whatever torn ends of periosteum existed on the convex side of the diaphysis (Fig. 3-8A). The periosteum on the concave side is intact.

The repair of this fracture proceeds in some measure as described above for the stress fracture, but the increased hemorrhage and the periosteal tears lead to a much more rapid elaboration of callus. Its volume is easily revealed on radiographs but rarely is copious enough to be palpable.

Late Events

The callus that forms goes through the same stages of remodeling noted earlier, but fibro-cartilaginous components are prominent (Fig. 3-4E). As the hemorrhagic and necrotic tissues are replaced by the callus (Fig. 3-4C,D), the remodeling phase that ends in the restoration of structural continuity and elimination of all evidence of the fracture may be complete within a few months in a child (Fig. 3-3). There may be no evidence of the solution of continuity, but there may still be a slight residual bending deformity of the bone, rarely exceeding 20°. That deformity is the residual of the far greater bend that existed prior to the correction from manipulation of closed reduction. It may take up to a few years for the continuing remodeling of the cortex to correct all the bend and achieve true restoration of the bone to its normal contour.

An attractive but entirely speculative explanation of the uncommon complication of a permanent and increasing bending deformity after healing of such a fracture is axial growth of the cartilage foci in the fibrocartilaginous callus.

With the greenstick fracture and the femoral fracture previously described, there would be radiological or histological residual evidence of this fracture after healing and remodeling had been completed. With adult fractures (vertebral and fibular) some residual permanent evidence might well be recognized. With the vertebral fracture it would be a slight deformity in the form of wedging compression, whereas with the stress fracture it would not constitute a deformity but, rather, a change in the pattern of the haversian systems and perhaps a residue of remodeled callus. The latter might be recognizable radiologically as a line or narrow zone of radiodensity. Note, however, that there is no residual fibrous tissue in cases 3-1, 3-3, 3-5, or 3-8.

Any scar (i.e., fibrous) tissue that exists at the end of the healing process in tissues other than bone represents some inability of the injured tissue to return to its original state, but bone is unusual in that complete restitution is the rule, whereas most other tissue after an injury do not show total restitution of the normal structure. When restitution of the bone occurs, as happens rapidly in children, it proceeds to completion on both the gross and microscopic levels of the structure. In adults, even though the repaired bone may be grossly normal, some alteration in haversian structure of the bone substance may be evident after healing is complete. No gross scar is observable. The altered haversian systems at the fracture site may form a pattern reflecting the new load-bearing patterns of stress in the repaired bone. In cancellous bone the trabeculae may show a thickened, coarse pattern that, in essence, is the bony counterpart of a fibrous scar. The above histological residuals persist even though the bony matrix repair site is normal to chemical analysis and the cells are normal.

The formation of a loose fibrous tissue containing osteogenetic precursor cells, as well as fibroblasts, and capillary buds has been well described,[11,13,15,16] and this repair tissue occupies those areas from which hemorrhage and exudate have been or are being resorbed. Resorption of the necrotic marrow (and the hemorrhagic exudate) occurs rapidly — most rapidly when only a small area is affected and thrombosis of vessels has been minimal. The inflammatory and resorptive response with a fracture is identical to that with an injury to soft tissue, but differences become evident in the patterns of deposition of intercellular substance: fibrous, cartilaginous, and osteoid. It is the changes of those patterns over time that must be recognized if one is to understand how a fracture heals.[4,6,12–14,17–19]

Three of the cases that have been used to illustrate the basic principles of fractures caused by low-energy trauma also provide additional insights into the relation of the continuum of fracture repair to the therapy.

COMPRESSION FRACTURE

With compression fracture of an osteopenic vertebra, it has already been noted that a similar fracture, as judged radiologically, in a young adult may be much more serious for the following reasons. Because the cancellous bone in such an individual is not porotic, more energy would have been needed to cause the fracture, and one would therefore expect a larger volume of hematoma. Moreover, because in the young person the intact cancellous bone resists displacement better than bone

at the fracture site, a greater chance exists for some displacement of the fragments anteroposteriorly. This displacement plus the hematoma place the spinal cord and nerve roots at appreciable risk. Several implications can be drawn from this situation: The young individual must be monitored closely for neurological deficits (sensory loss, weakness or paralysis, reflexes, loss of sphincter control) and might well be examined by CT scan for evidence of encroachment of hematoma or fracture fragments on the neural canal or foramina (Fig. 3-1E–G). Although it was stated above that the impaction of the fragments promotes such stability to the fracture site that immobilization may be unnecessary, and mobilization of the patient would be advocated even before any callus is laid down, it may be advisable in the young patient to assure oneself of that stability and of the absence of additional fractures in the pedicles or laminae. These fractures often are difficult to see on routine radiographs, and CT scans therefore perform a double function of revealing occult fractures and demonstrating any stenosis of the spinal canal.

Compression fractures of a vertebral body rarely occur in children as the result of trauma, but they do occur, usually as the result of an eosinophilic granuloma of a vertebral body that is rendered porotic by the lesion. The long-term effects (known as Calve's disease or vertebra plana) (Fig. 3-9) are yet another example of the ease with which a fracture of cancellous bone heals in a young child, with few if any complications.

This ease of repair was also depicted in the femoral fracture already discussed, but that same type of fracture, viewed radiologically, in an infant aged 2 years or less, instead of age 12 as in the case described, would require a different treatment regimen: Skeletal insertion of a pin for traction not be required, thereby avoiding even the minor complications of that procedure. The fracture fragments need only be approximately aligned, and their motion must be minimally restricted because empirically it has been shown that healing is almost certain within a period of 3 to 4 weeks.

The two types of therapy meeting the above criteria are Bryant's traction and a plaster spica cast. The former — overhead traction on both lower extremities exerted through skin tapes — has the advantage of easy nursing care. It has the disadvan-

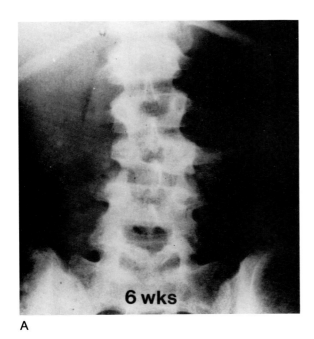
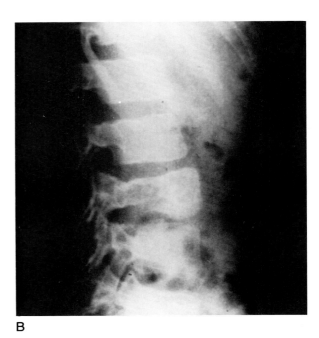

A   B

Fig. 5-9. AP (**A**) and lateral (**B**) radiographs obtained 6 weeks after the onset of sudden pain in a 10-year-old boy show a compression fracture and flattening of the posterior lateral and anterior aspects of the body of L3. The diagnosis of eosinophilic granuloma (Calve's disease) was established by biopsy and histological findings.

tage of requiring hospital care and is restricted to the infantile age group. The disadvantages of nursing an infant in a spica cast are obvious, and the possible complications (pressure sores) of cast treatment should be mentioned. In older children treated with Bryant's traction there is a considerable risk of Volkmann's ischemic contracture or other ischemic complications because of the stretch on the major blood vessels in the overhead traction position. Bryant's traction should not be used in children over age 2.

DIAPHYSEAL FRACTURE

Having considered the simple fracture of the femoral diaphysis briefly in infants and at some length in a child (applicable also to adolescents), the pathophysiological and other aspects of such a lesion in an adult are now discussed. Let us consider a situation comparable to that in case 3-3 (Fig. 3-3A) ex-

cept that the patient is not 12 years old but, rather, 25. One anatomical fact and one pathophysiological influence are of paramount importance for achieving repair of the fracture. Anatomically, the femoral cortex in the adult is so compact and so well differentiated that months if not years are needed for reconstitution of the microstructure. That reconstruction must be achieved, at least in large part, before load-bearing to the degree required can be effected. Pathophysiologically, the high levels of osteogenetic potential present in infants and children has markedly declined at skeletal maturity. However, one should not conclude that because children's fractures heal so easily there is progressive loss of healing potential with age. For reasons that are mostly socioeconomic and not pathophysiological, immediate and rigid immobilization becomes of prevailing importance in femoral fractures in adults, in whom any obstacle to healing must be minimized. The femoral fracture in a 70-year-old does not differ greatly from that in a 20-year-old in regard to the capability of elaborating callus. At either age, the better the immobilization, the better is the protection against repeated small injuries to the callus. This subject was discussed for the stress fracture but is equally applicable to all cortical fractures.

The implications of immobilization and osteogenesis are strongly influenced in adults by two aspects of the pathophysiology of repair of fractures that pertain to treatment of a fracture in an adult. One is the volume of callus needed to heal the fracture and the geometry of the callus vis-à-vis that of the fracture.[23,24] When the bony fragments are separated, the volume of callus needed is proportional to the extent of separation.[11,22,23,25] Hence the more accurate the reduction, the smaller is the volume of callus that is needed; moreover, the better the restitution of anatomical relations, the more effective is each cubic millimeter of callus. The second aspect is the amount of damage to soft tissue: the more extensive it is, the more thrombosis and resultant necrosis that result. The implications here are not so much directed to the trauma of the accident, which is discussed later, but rather to the trauma of any operative treatment.

The treatment regimens mentioned for the infant and child (skin traction, plaster cast, skeletal traction) are not usually appropriate for the adult, as illustrated in the present case (the 25-year-old man with a simple fracture in the mid-diaphysis of the femur). Any treatment regimen that might be considered applicable in the present case has its advocates, mostly for theoretical advantages than for demonstrated superiority. The pathophysiological implications of each is our major concern, but other considerations, often of overriding importance, should be mentioned. These considerations often take priority over the concept of the avoidance of risk; and arguments are usually advanced during the advocacy of each form of surgical device that take the form of offsetting one set of risks with another. The risks of anesthesia and one particular technique of surgery are allegedly offset by a lessening of the risks of delayed union, nonunion, and malunion.

An understanding of the pathophysiology of healing of simple closed fractures of long bones, treated by the various techniques that employ the devices most popular at present, should influence the choice of technique and device. However, it should be understood that the overriding considerations that usually prevail in the choice of any of the surgical treatments, i.e., the socioeconomic ones (hospitalization, employment, compensation) are compelling. Although such considerations readily pertain to comparisons of conservative versus surgical treatment, little effort has been expended to study them as they pertain to each of the advocated regimens of treatment and each device under advocacy. The neglect arises from the profusion of articles representing advocacy of one device or another. One is unable to address the difficulty, if not the impossibility, of conducting *controlled* trials of the advocated device. Even so common a fracture as in the illustrated case (a moderately oblique, two-fragment fracture) does not lend itself to randomized prospective scientific study because of the many unavoidable variables implicit in clinical situations. Not least in importance is the variable of technical expertise of even the small number of surgeons involved in such a study, so that technical imperfections, or even errors, often become important. It is especially true where small differences are under scrutiny (e.g., percent of union, time to resumption of function).[5]

The major pathophysiological advantage of treating the fracture with a plate (or more than one plate) and screws is that it allows more precise reduction than any other method.[22,23,26–28] It also offers the surgeon the capability of visualizing the security of the fixation, as well as supplementing the fixation, using whatever hardware is needed, to stabilize whatever additional fragments of bone exist in addition to the two principal ones. Finally, it reassures the surgeon that there is no interposed muscle or periosteum (or even nerves or arteries) between the fracture fragments, and that the repair to soft tissue requires surgical measures.

There are disadvantages of the above treatment regimen other than those discussed below with regard to pathophysiology: (1) Technical problems often arise because the hardware may not be ideal: The curvature of the bone may not conform to the available plate, the screws may not suit, and the surgeon's technical expertise in carpentry may not be ideal. (2) However well fabricated, all metal devices have real or potential engineering or metallurgical inadequacies that introduce a risk of failure. (3) Often the hardware, after it has served its purpose, must be removed, an additional operative risk.[28]

The ordinary (noncompression) plate has the advantages (and disadvantages) just mentioned. One pathophysiological aspect of applying such a device, in addition to those mentioned, is that only minor surgical trauma is applied to the *marrow* (insertion of the screws). This point is worth mentioning because, in contrast, the other (intramedullary) techniques are likely to devascularize the marrow entirely. An ordinary plate has certain mechanical advantages over the compression plates: It can more easily be made to conform to the contour of the bony fragments; and its application does not introduce some potential problems, e.g., distraction of fragments on the part of the cortex opposite to the plate. Because advocacy of compression plating in preference to use of ordinary plates often emphasizes supposedly superior pathophysiological sequences of repair, the subject merits scrutiny. The indications for choosing a compression plate ordinarily include clinical data that are favorable (e.g., the patient is young and healthy) and mechanical factors that are favorable (e.g., the fracture is transverse or only slightly oblique and is not fragmented).

The *mechanical* principles that make compression plating more effective than ordinary plating are (1) that properly applied, the fixation of the transected reduced fragments is firmer. The security of the fixation is in no small measure dependent on the topology of the fracture, and the slight irregularities on one fragment's surface interdigitating and congruent with the identical irregularities on the opposite fragment are essential to the process. Even minor fragmentation at the surface may nullify the effectiveness of the fixation. However, the compression per se has often been regarded as a pathophysiological advantageous process, whereas in all probability the opposite is true. Its disadvantages may be outweighed by the security of the fixation and by the fact that the gap between major fragments is reduced to the absolute minimum; nevertheless, the arguments to the contrary should be recognized.

The first disadvantage is that the technique necessarily increases the volume of necrotic bone that must be resorbed during the healing phase. The periosteum is further stripped from both fracture fragments, in addition to that part stripped by the injury. This disadvantage applies to ordinary (noncompression) plates as well.

The second disadvantage, however, does not apply to ordinary plates. Even if a "perfect" reduction of the fracture is evident by gross examination, it is well-nigh impossible for the fracture surfaces to fit in such a way that protruding haversian systems on the proximal (or distal) fragment will fit into the corresponding depression on the congruent surface (Fig. 4-5A,B). Unlike ordinary plates, compression plates exert sufficient pressure on some protruding haversian systems that have been juxtaposed to others, on the other fragment, to cause breakage of some of the asperities. The fit of one fracture surface on the other will be improved but at the price of additional microfragmentation of the surface. Although repair of the focal microscopic areas so involved may therefore be delayed because of the necrosis plus thrombosis, probably some other areas (perhaps adjoining them) may undergo minimum necrosis and thrombosis and may present minimal breadth of the fracture gap. Thus these areas present ideal conditions for callus formation. The key question is how extensive the areas are, and how long it takes for sufficient bone to form for weight-bearing. However, inasmuch as the plate takes on most of the function of bearing the load during the first 2 weeks postoperatively (only part of it is now dependent on the coapted fragments), the judgment of the surgeon as to when unprotected load-bearing can be prescribed depends on the highly variable geometry of the fracture. From the above discussion it is obvious that quantitation of any or all of the important elements in the situation in an experimental protocol in an animal, usually a quadruped and much smaller than humans, is precluded; and approximations can be arrived at only by extensive examination of clinical material.

The pathophysiological principles that relate to the other general approach to surgical treatment, intramedullary fixation, apply in some degree to each of the four techniques now used more or less widely, i.e., open nailing, closed nailing, nailing supplemented by one or more transfixion devices (Fig. 4-7), and Ender nailing. As might be expected, however, advocates of each method tend to ignore the similarities and emphasize the differences. The outstanding element the methods have in common is severe injury to the marrow. Even with a simple proximodistal nailing procedure, without reaming the endosteal bone, the trochanteric area is entered with a large instrument and the nail is hammered in. Whatever its design, it always has a cross-sectional configuration that displaces *all* of the marrow at the mid-diaphysis, the site of the fracture in the case under discussion. When the marrow cavity is wider, there is space for residual marrow; but it is doubtful if any substantial amount of marrow can remain viable, given the trauma of inserting the nail and the reduction of the fracture, which is being accomplished at the same time. It is also doubtful if there is any important difference between open reduction and closed reduction with regard to the severity of operative trauma in such a situation, disregarding the important element of the risk of introducing infection at the fracture site and focusing solely on the risk of additional devascularization of the bone.

The above considerations pertain mostly to simple insertion of an intramedullary nail, without reaming of the endosteal bone. They apply equally to situations where the nail is inserted from the trochanteric area or from below, i.e., just above the knee. The pathophysiological and empirical data that engendered the distal approach are (1) the larger risk of thromboembolism with an operation done at the hip region compared to one done at the knee, and (2) the increased surgical exposure with operations at the hip and the concomitant increased risk of infection. It was Ender who first developed the distal approach (usually involving lateral as well as medial incisions and nail insertions), but now there are devices of designs other than Ender's for the purpose. It is noteworthy that with the distal approach, whether one nail or several are inserted, the trauma to the marrow does not include that of reaming. In contrast to however minor a degree of reaming is needed or at least is used, it is applied during most nailing done from the proximal approach, with more trauma being the result. In recent years, recommendations about reaming have expanded the range so that the diameter of the nail to be inserted can be increased coordinately. Obviously, two mechanical considerations are responsible for this increase. One relates to the security of the fixation and the other to load-bearing. In essence, therefore, neither relates to the sequences of repair, considered below.

When an intramedullary nail is used to secure the fixation of the two principal femoral fragments, its intimate contact with an expanse of endosteal wall, on all the inner circumference, is needed. The longitudinal dimension of possible contact is most limited at the mid-diaphysis, where the medullary cavity is at its narrowest. Obviously, centrifugal enlargement of the cavity there expands the longitudinal dimension and so allows use of a thicker nail at the expense of loss of thickness of cortical bone. The practical limits of enlarging the cavity are not only the amount of cortex available to be reamed but also the need for the geometry of the final cavity to be close to cylindrical, i.e., straight-walled, whereas the anatomical characteristics of the marrow cavity (and the bone) include a slight anterior bow as well as a slight lateral bow. (The manner of introducing the nail requires that the cavity be nearly straight, so that the technical requirements of the procedure take precedence over the theoretical ones for anatomical restitution of the structure.)

With regard to the second consideration (load-bearing), thinner, more flexible nails have been shown empirically to fail (because of breakage) often enough for designers to include larger safety margins. The nail, as predicated for the therapeutic regimen outlined for it, takes nearly all the stresses of weight-bearing and ambulation not only on the short term (the first few weeks after insertion) but also for the many months during which the patient is reconstituting a femoral cortex. The stresses therefore can be anticipated to be mainly those of cyclic bending, with thousands of cycles to be anticipated.

Having summarized the more important of the mechanical considerations of intramedullary nailing procedures, let us turn to the consideration of pathophysiology, including repair.[29-31] Damage to the vessels of the marrow due to the trauma of the injury was assessed as minimal, but that due to the trauma of nail insertion was considerable if not total. Because damage to the periosteal vessels due to the injury and then to the reduction procedure was assessed as severe, devascularization of the cortex of both major fragments of the femur undoubtedly affected a segment of each fragment, extending at least a few centimeters from the fracture line. With extensive reaming, the longitudinal extent of the avascular necrosis measures many centimeters, and it even might involve *all* the diaphysis. Thus the patient will be walking on a femur that is well supported by metal but devoid of a blood supply, except for small segments at either end. This situation is not unlike that in patients with massive intercalated allografts, except for the fact that the latter patients may mount immunological reactions to the dead allografted bone, whereas the patients we are considering are not challenged by antigens from a graft. This patient's tissues, however, are challenged by the foreign bodies that are represented by the products of the reaming. They include the particles of reamed bone that could not be washed out, and, importantly, the devitalized bone that has been heated to such a degree by the reaming process, even if done slowly, as to consist largely of denatured proteins. It should be mentioned in this connection that denatured tissues evoke a more severe inflammatory reaction than do necrotic tissues rendered so by ischemia alone. (The same is true of necrotic tissues subjected to enzymatic denaturation, as by infection.)

A paradox therefore is immediately evident. Empirically, it has been shown that most patients with simple fractures of the femur treated by any of the intramedullary nailing methods described — provided the technical procedures are well done — do well and do not manifest the complications that might be expected from massive necrosis, i.e., prolonged delay in healing or even nonunion and increased risk of infection. It should be pointed out that the chronology of healing in such cases has not been documented well from the histological point of view, and the empirical evidence of successful "healing" relates mostly to resumption of function. Even radiological evidence of the chronology of reconstitution of the cortical bone of the diaphysis is not well documented. When an intramedullary nail is removed 1 to 2 years after it was inserted, radiological methods cannot distinguish between residual (and necrotic) cortex and new (and living) cortex, much less determine the extent of creeping substitution and haversian remodeling.

The histological details of the repair process beyond those already described above for less severe injuries are further considered in Chapter 4.

Also considered there, in cases to be described, are the features of fixation by special intramedullary nails and other forms of therapy.

REFERENCES

1. Allgower M: The healing of clinical fractures of the tibia with rigid internal fixation. p. 81. In Robinson RA (ed): The Healing Osseous Tissue. National Academy of Sciences, National Research Council, Washington, DC, 1967
2. Anderson LD: Healing of standard discontinuities of long bones in the adult dog. p. 41. In Robinson RA (ed): The Healing of Osseous Tissue. National Academy of Sciences, National Research Council, Washington, DC, 1967
3. Banks HH: Tissue response at the fracture site in femoral neck fractures. Clin Orthop 61:116, 1968
4. Brand RA: Scientific basis of orthopedic fracture healing. p. 289. In Albright JA, Brand RA (eds): Appleton-Century-Crofts, E Norwalk, CT, 1979
5. Cave EF: Fracture management injuries (Ch. 4). Healing of fractures (Ch. 5). In: Delayed Union, Non-union, Timetable for Healing by Bone and Age. Year Book Medical Publishers, Chicago, 1974
6. Cohen J: Cartilage production in human fracture callus. Lab Invest 5:53, 1956
7. Daffer RH: Stress fractures, current concepts. Skeletal Radiol 2:221, 1978
8. Eggers GWN, Shindler TO, Domerat CM: The influence of contact compression factor on osteogenesis in surgical fractures. J Bone Joint Surg [Am] 31:693, 1949
9. El-Khoury GY, Wehbe M, Bonfiglio M, Chow KC: Stress fractures of the femoral neck: a scintigraphic sign for early diagnosis. Skeletal Radiol 6:271, 1981
10. Enneking WF: Repair of complete fractures of rat tibias. Anat Rec 101:515, 1948
11. Ham AW: Early phases of bone repair. J Bone Joint Surg 12:827, 1930
12. Ham AW, Cormack CH: Histology. 8th Ed. JB Lippincott, Philadelphia, 1979
13. Ham AW, Harris WR: Repair and transplantation of bone. p. 337. In Bourne GH (ed): The Biochemistry and Physiology of Bone. Vol. 3. Academic Press, New York, 1971
14. Holden CEA: The role of blood supply in healing of diaphyseal fractures, an exploratory study. J Bone Joint Surg [Am] 54:993, 1972
15. Johnson LC, et al: Histogenesis of stress fracture. J Bone Joint Surg [Am] 45:1450, 1963

16. McKibbin B: The biology of fracture healing in long bones. J Bone Joint Surg [Br] 60:150, 1978

17. Mindell ER, Bobard S, Kwasman BG: Chondrogenesis in bone repair, a study of healing fracture callus in the rat. Clin Orthop 79:187, 1971

18. Misol S: Growth hormone in delayed fracture union. Clin Orthop 74:256, 1971

19. Morris GM, Blickenstaff LD: Fatigue Fractures, A Clinical Study. Charles C Thomas, Springfield, IL, 1967

20. Nicoll EA: Fractures of the tibial shaft. J Bone Joint Surg [Br] 46:373, 1964

21. Olerud S, Danckwardt-Lilliestrom: Fracture healing and compression osteosynthesis in the dog. J Bone Joint Surg [Br] 50:844, 1968

22. Perren SM, Rahn BA: Biomechanics of Fracture Healing. Vol I. Historical Review and Mechanical Aspects of Internal Fixation, Vol. II. Orthopedic Survey, p. 108, 1978

23. Pritchard JJ: Histology of fracture repair in modern trends. p. 69. In Orthopaedics. Vol. 4. 1964

24. Pritchard JJ, Ruzicka AJ: Comparison of fracture repair in the frog, lizard and rat. J Anat 84:236, 1950

25. Pulskamp JR, McFarland GB Jr: The effects of compression plate fixation on bone healing in dog femurs. Unpublished data, 1969

26. Rahn BA, Gallinaro P, Baltensperger A, Perren SM: Primary bone healing and experimental study in the rabbit. J Bone Joint Surg [Am] 53:783, 1971

27. Reynolds FC, Key JA: Fracture healing after fixation with standard plates, contact splints and medullary nails. J Bone Joint Surg [Am] 36:577, 1954

28. Rhinelander F: The normal microcirculation of diaphyseal cortex and its response to fracture. J Bone Joint Surg [Am] 50:784, 1968

29. Rhinelander F, Baragry R: Microangiography in bone healing. I. Undisplaced closed fractures. J Bone Joint Surg [Am] 50:643, 1968

30. Rhinelander F, et al: Microangiography in bone healing. II. Displaced closed fractures. J Bone Joint Surg [Am] 50:643, 1968

31. Rockwood C, et al: Emergency Care and Transportation of the Sick and Injured. Committee on Injuries, American Academy of Orthopedic Surgeons, 1971

32. Sarmiento A: Functional bracing of tibial and femoral shaft fractures. Clin Orthop 82:2, 1972

33. Sarmiento A, et al: Fracture healing in rat femur as affected by functional weight-bearing. J Bone Joint Surg [Am] 59:369, 1977

34. Teitz CC, Carter DR, Frankel VH: Problems associated with tibial fractures with intact fibulae. J Bone Joint Surg [Am] 62:770, 1980

35. Tonna EA: Source of osteoblasts in healing fractures in animals of different ages. p. 93. In Robinson RA (ed): The Healing of Osseous Tissue. National Academy of Sciences, National Research Council, Washington, DC, 1967

36. Urist MR, Johnson RW Jr: The healing fracture in man under clinical conditions. J Bone Joint Surg 25:375, 1943

37. Wilson JN (ed): Watson-Jones Fractures and Joint Injuries. 6th Ed. Vol. 1. Churchill Livingstone, Edinburgh, p. 23, 1982

38. Weiss C, et al: The application of structure-borne sound to the structural analysis of bone and fracture healing. J Bone Joint Surg [Am] 57:576, 1975

39. Young RW: The control of cell specialization in bone. Clin Orthop 45:153, 1966

40. Zuckerman J, Maurer P, Berbesson C: The effect of bone and periosteum in recent diaphyseal fractures. J Bone Joint Surg [Br] 50:409, 1968

4

Complex Fractures

In Chapter 3 only those fractures that can be regarded as injuries involving primarily osseous tissues were discussed; that is, coordinate injury to soft tissue was a minor component of the total damage. Among illustrative examples were a stress fracture, a greenstick fracture, and a simple two-fragment femoral diaphyseal fracture. Those fractures generally are produced by forces of low energy. In today's violent world, many injuries that involve the bones also involve the adjacent soft tissues, muscles and skin in particular; and it is these injuries, which we classify as complex, that are the subject of this chapter. As a class, they include injuries caused by high-energy forces (e.g., vehicular accidents, missile wounds), and they tend to cause damage to soft tissue that outweighs in importance the damage to the bone. Therefore the mechanical principles of treatment of the bony injury may have to be subordinated to, or at least coordinated with, principles of treatment for injury to soft tissues. Similarly, the pathophysiological aspects of the two classes of tissue injury, their natural chronology, and effects of treatment also must be regarded together. Treatment of the skeletal injury must not be pursued without regard for the injury to soft tissue and vice versa.

COMPLETE FRACTURE WITH CONSIDERABLE DISPLACEMENT

The variation in degree of injury to the two classes of tissue, separately and in combination, is so great that it is futile to discuss principles first and then their application to the panorama of cases. Instead, the effect of more severe injury to the skeleton than was considered in the previous chapter is introduced by considering several cases, the first being an extensively *comminuted closed segmented fracture* of the femur (Fig. 4-1).

Closed Fracture

Case 4-1 A 19-year-old man was riding a motorscooter when he was struck by a car and was thrown for a distance of 15 feet. He sustained injuries to both lower limbs, but we consider here only the more severe injury—that to his right leg and thigh. In the proximal part of the thigh, at the site of impact, there was an extensive contusion and a large subcutaneous hematoma. A defect was palpable in the fascia, and through it a palpable fragment of the right femur was penetrating, although it had not broached the skin (Fig. 4-1A,B). There was a laceration of the right knee. Skeletal traction to both lower extremities was applied and maintained for 3 weeks with adjustments. The alignment of the bony fragments of the right femur that was obtained then was satisfactory.

When conceptualizing the pathophysiological elements of the damage to the tissues of the thigh in this case, it is convenient to consider first the radiological determinations of the extent of displacement. They must be assessed with attention to chronology and to all attendant relevant circumstances. The initial radiographs, obtained about an hour after the injury, reveal a displacement that had been considerably reduced from that which existed at the time of injury, reduced by manual

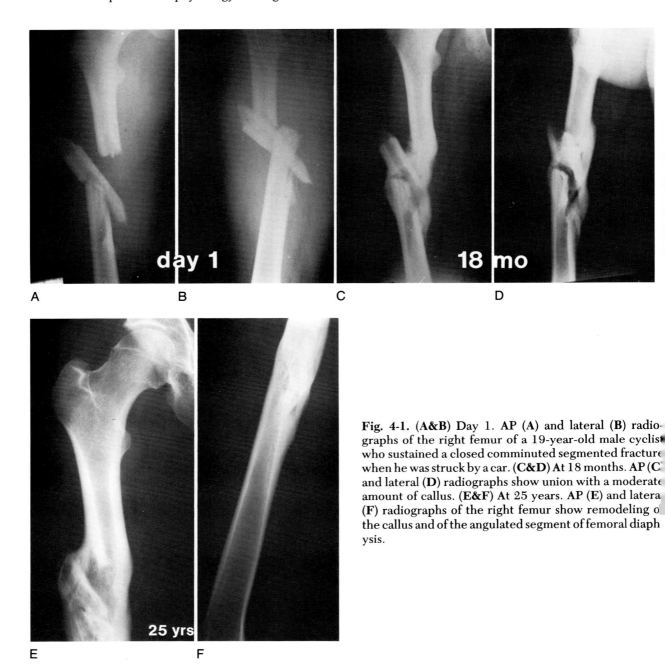

Fig. 4-1. (A&B) Day 1. AP (A) and lateral (B) radio-graphs of the right femur of a 19-year-old male cyclist who sustained a closed comminuted segmented fracture when he was struck by a car. (C&D) At 18 months. AP (C) and lateral (D) radiographs show union with a moderate amount of callus. (E&F) At 25 years. AP (E) and lateral (F) radiographs of the right femur show remodeling of the callus and of the angulated segment of femoral diaphysis.

traction administered by the paramedical person-nel and maintained by a splint during the patient's transport to the hospital. To some extent, of course, spasm of the muscles of the thigh, which is always severe shortly after such an injury, might have in-creased the displacement. The traction therefore may well have lessened the effect of the spasm and decreased the actual displacement. Subsequent ra-diographs during the period of skeletal traction in the hospital, which revealed only minor improve-ments in the extent of the displacement (overrid-ing) but major correction of alignment, might lead to an assessment, as in case 3-4, that some part of the periosteum remained intact, were it not for two important findings on physical examination. One was that the proximal fragment of the femur was palpable subcutaneously. The other was that there was a defect in the fascia. These findings led to the following conceptualization of the injury: As the femur fractured, the proximal fragment was driven distally through the anterior musculature, engaging its fascial elements and tearing them as the fragment progressed distally, resulting in an extensive defect in the fascia. The progress of the pointed fragment subcutaneously halted when the energy of the injury had been absorbed. It was to be expected therefore that the manual traction and later the skeletal traction probably would not restore the injured soft tissues to their normal anatomical relations. With regard to the bony fragments in particular, the hematoma would have interfered with their alignment and coaptation. The amount of hemorrhage, as indicated by the degree of swelling, probably was severe at first and may have intermittently increased until definitive (skeletal) traction was applied. The probability therefore is that (1) there would be some muscle tissue as well as clot between the fragments at the moment when definitive treatment was begun; (2) the periosteum was stripped to a major degree, and none of it presented longitudinal continuity; and (3) major injury to soft tissues as well as bone had occurred. Whether that injury included an injury to the major vessels, despite the absence of signs of such an injury (no abnormalities of pulse, coloration, or temperature in the foot) could only be inferred by sequential observation.

The choice of skeletal traction for definitive treatment had the following major pathophysiological objectives: (1) It permitted sequential observation; (2) it permitted treatment of the concomitant ipsilateral injury (laceration of the knee) as well as of contralateral and systemic injury; and (3) it added no important further trauma (surgical) to the extremity. An advantage that accrued was that no surgical option for treatment was foreclosed.

During traction the soft tissues of the thigh continued to be markedly enlarged, and some swelling of the calf and leg developed as well, indicating that there indeed had been an injury to one or more large veins. The conceptualized lesion therefore is thrombosis, which limited the venous drainage from the distal part of the limb. The range of motion (ROM) of the knee remained severely restricted, and the conceptualized reason for that limitation influences the choice of treatment. Consider first the laceration at the knee. If the wound entered the joint and elicited a mild infection, not evidently suppurative, the limitation might be attributed to synovial inflammation. If the laceration involved one or more of the many bursas around the knee or extended into the planes between tendons, the incipient scars in those structures might well be responsible for limiting the motion. Lastly, if the perforation of the muscle and fascia by the femoral fragment caused enough necrosis of muscle to have an extensive axial scar, that too might be the cause of the restricted motion. It was common knowledge that when femoral fractures, whatever the severity, were not treated surgically, as a rule the outstanding impairment in end-result studies was restricted motion of the knee. The early finding of restricted motion in this case should constitute a warning if any of the above lesions was diagnosed; barring a conceptualization that infection was the cause, efforts to increase ROM to the knee should be instituted as soon and as vigorously as possible by active flexion and extension of the knee in traction. In today's mechanized world, the physical therapist might supplement the manipulations and exercises with a flexion-extension machine after the traction is removed.

However, in this case one physical finding tilted the probable diagnosis away from those lesions and toward another. It was the continued swelling of the thigh and especially the calf. The other lesion was massive edema of the musculature caused by thrombosis of a considerable part of the venous network. With any fracture and soft tissue injury, some thrombosis occurs, if only as a mechanism to stop the hemorrhage. With most such injuries the thrombosis is not extensive enough to obstruct the venous return in this extremity. Here it was. The implications as they concern therapy first is that it serves to emphasize the wise surgical choice of skeletal traction. No other therapeutic choice, early on, would have provided so well for detecting the swelling. Second, the edema and thrombosis would argue for *gentle* mobilization of the knee, avoiding any possible force that might lead to embolism. It should be understood that some of the other (conceptualized) lesions might also have contributed to the restricted ROM.

The skeletal traction pins were removed 6 weeks after the injury, and skin traction was used for another 6 weeks. At that time the fracture site, on palpation and manipulation, did not seem firm, and a bridging callus was not unequivocally evident on the radiograph. There was only 90° of flexion at the knee, although full extension could be achieved actively. There was considerable discomfort in the musculature of the thigh where swelling was still evident. Swelling of the calf also remained, but it was on the decline. A hip spica was applied to permit the patient to walk with crutches, with the hip spica protecting the thigh. Partial weight-bearing was permitted. The radiograph 4 months after the injury had shown tenuous bridging of the comminuted fracture fragments; although the callus did not present a broad zone of repair bone, it was considered sufficiently solid to allow load-bearing of limited degree. In the soft tissues the adjacent region was thought to contain a mixture of the residual necrotic muscle that had not yet been resorbed and perhaps some residual hematoma, in addition to the fibrous repair tissue that had been elaborated. Although one might have expected the repair to show some evidence of differentiation toward callus at this long interval after the injury, such an expectation would be conditional on a fairly rapid reconstitution of the vasculature. In this case, there must have been considerable necrosis of tissues, muscle as well as bone, because of the severity of the injury; and much more time (months) would be needed before the vascular bed could support the production of internal callus. Therefore union of the femoral fracture was considered precarious. Only at 18 months after the injury was there a moderate amount of callus accompanied by minimal remodeling of the segmented fragment (Figs. 4-1C,D). There was residual swelling in the right calf but none in the thigh. The ROM of the knee had not improved. Some induration was palpable in both thigh and calf, and all the musculature, although functional, had less than normal strength and endurance. All of these abnormalities, pathophysiologically, were attributed to diffuse scar formation in all the tissues distal to the site of injury. The scarring is an inevitable

consequence of long-standing, continuous (i.e., not intermittent) edema, the result of the venous obstruction in the thigh. This patient continued to have swelling of the leg because of chronic deep vein obstruction from soft tissue scarring of the thigh 4 years after his injury.

The patient was followed for 25 years after the injury, at the end of which time he had an improved but limited range of knee motion, from 0° to 95°, and atrophy of the thigh musculature. The radiographs showed incomplete remodeling of the fragments without restoration of a medullary canal (Figs. 4-1E,F).

One should refrain from overemphasizing the importance of extensive necrosis in segmental fracture fragments during assessment of the repair process. More importantly, in case 4-1 the extent of soft tissue injury was a major factor in causing the protracted (18 month) period needed until there was adequate healing; even after 24 years the repair was incomplete.

Reviewing this case with the purpose of determining if there were better options of treatment than the one pursued, we immediately faced the problem of how important was each of the components of the injury (e.g., hemorrhage, necrosis of bone, periosteal disruption, interposition of muscle between bony fragments). The vascular injury has been emphasized. Would specific attention to it have been worthwhile? Consider what that would entail. Even if diagnostic tests demonstrated obstruction of major vessels in the thigh, which might be repaired or made patent, the odds would be overwhelmingly against a successful endeavor. The major veins in the thigh are not large, and the injury would have caused thrombosis in the network of small veins that could not be cleared. If the next component of the injury, hemorrhage, is considered, and removal of the extensive clot is judged to be a favorable maneuver in conjunction of course with surgical stabilization of the fracture fragments, the major contraindication is that the surgical procedure would convert a closed wound into an open one in an area of such extensive necrosis (muscle as well as bone) as to constitute a major risk of infection. Even recognizing the desirability of removing the interposed muscle, minimizing the distances between bony fragments, restoring the relative positions of periosteum, and imposing rigid stabilization of the fracture fragments by whatever device and technique might accomplish that formidable task, they do not cumulatively outweigh the major risk. Arguments that introduce considerations of the patient's general condition, treatment of other injuries, and possibilities for delayed surgical treatment simply cannot prevail because the necrotic tissue and tissue with a precarious circulation can so easily form a culture medium for bacteria introduced by the surgical procedure. These tissues can even become infected hematogenously via the transient bacteremias that are the rule even in a healthy, uninjured individual. If a surgical procedure has been done, moreover, it could well be blamed for a hematogenous infection.

It will be instructive also to compare the case just discussed (case 4-1) with that presented at the end of the last chapter. Both cases involved young male subjects who had been in vehicular accidents that caused a fracture of the femur. The ages of the patients, 19 and 12, respectively, strongly affected not only the prognosis for healing but also the therapy. Were the ages to have been reversed, a two-fragment femoral fracture with relatively unimportant injury to soft tissue in a 19-year-old would undoubtedly have been strongly considered for surgical treatment with an excellent prognosis. In contrast, although the 12-year-old with the more severe injury would have had the identical conservative (i.e., nonoperative) treatment that was given to the 19-year-old, the prognosis for healing would have included a much shorter time and the knee joint would have been much less severely limited. The improved prognosis would be strongly dependent on the ability of younger tissues (both skeletal and fibrous) to remodel. The outstanding difference between the two cases, however, is attributable to the energy difference, which in turn can be held responsible for the major damage — that to the soft tissues. Although the energy involved must be inferred from the details of each accident and from the physical and radiographic findings in each case, the contrast between the two cases becomes instructive concerning the multifactorial influences on the character of the lesions, the therapy, and the prognosis.

It is an important diagnostic principle that even before initial radiographs are taken one should check carefully if the arteries and nerves of the limb are intact. The proximity of the superficial and profundus branches of the femoral artery and veins and the sciatic nerve to the fracture place those structures at risk. From the radiographs it is obvious that there has been major disruption of periosteum and small vessels to the injured parts of the bone. The radiographs also reveal that one should expect more extensive necrosis of bone, which delays remodeling of the callus. The elaboration of repair therefore takes longer (5 months for the 12-year-old and 18 months for the 19-year-old). Lastly, repair bone, laid down alongside the dead bone that is slowly being resorbed but that therefore persists in large amounts, inhibits reconstruction of the continuity of the bone and does not provide sufficient structural strength to allow early weight-bearing without protection. This situation may prevail over a period of years and must be recognized from the beginning. Appropriate protection and rehabilitative measures may be necessary for years. The appropriate time for unprotected weight-bearing varies with each fracture, but in general the continuity of callus uniting all fracture fragments should be the first prerequisite for beginning weight-bearing. It should begin on a partial weight-bearing basis in a cast or a cast-brace, graduating to full weight-bearing only when all evidence of local tenderness of the bone has disappeared and the radiographic appearance indicates a continuous dense callus without evidence of radiolucent lines traversing the callus. The correlation of the clinical features of bony union (i.e., lack of pain or tenderness, or motion at the fracture site) plus the radiographic evidence of bridging callus provide the basis for cessation of protective weight-bearing. If one is uncertain about the solidity of the union, it may be checked by testing the site with tomograms to show if radiolucent gaps are present in the callus.

A fracture through dense cortical bone that shows marked displacement and comminution presents several reasons for the surgeon to worry. There is a large volume of tissue damage: vascular, muscular, and osseous. The amount of hemorrhage tends also to be large, and therefore the subsequent exudate and inflammatory reaction are also extensive.

The volume of bone and soft tissue that is necrotized affects the cleanup time and the progressive mechanical adequacy of the callus. The repair of a fracture when there is a large necrotic bone fragment introduces interdependent circumstances that have important influences on the repair process: (1) the space occupied by the dead bone interferes with the production of live bone that can be remodeled; (2) the resorptive process that must go on therefore causes weakened microscopic foci in the dead bone; and (3) there are interfaces between dead bone and live bone that have less strength than either the long bone or the necrotized foci. Each of these features poses a risk of refracture of the bone at the site of remodeling where the dead bone is undergoing replacement.

If there is a concomitant extensive soft tissue injury, particularly necrosis of muscle from vascular interruption, as well as associated extensive periosteal disruption and bone necrosis, callus formation is delayed or prevented.[18] Periosteal integrity with viable and vascular attached muscle and fascia are important to the repair of fractures. Therefore the muscle with its blood supply should not be damaged during any surgical procedure, and any stripping of periosteum that must be done to carry out a fixation procedure should be kept to a minimum.

The quantitative importance of displacement becomes apparent when one considers the degree of disruption of both the periosteal and endosteal blood supply that accompanies even small displacements. The amount of necrosis of bone is variable depending on the location and the severity of the fracture. Although in case 4-1 the fracture healed to the extent that the limb could be used to bear weight 18 months after the repair, the segmental fragment had undergone necrosis; and 25 years later (Figs. 4-1E,F) it still shows evidence of incomplete replacement. The radiolucent gap between the distal fragment and the distal end of the previously separated segment of diaphysis is evidence of a deficiency in the repair of the fracture. In fact, the present radiograph still shows evidence of continued resorption and remodeling of the segment with reorganization of the bridging callus.

Repair of the displaced fracture in case 4-1 follows the classic model of osseous and fibrocartilaginous bridging callus described in experimental animals, but the extent of soft tissue and bone injury alters quantitatively the repair process. The differ-

ent topographical pattern of the granulation tissue in the two cases also makes for fundamental changes in the repair process and therefore what would be appropriate therapy. In the 12-year-old boy the granulation tissue, which contains fibroblasts and their precursors as well as the rudiments of the collagen framework of the natural repair mechanism, within a week or two bridges the gap between fracture fragments. That action quickly (within 2 to 3 weeks) stabilizes the previously unstable fragments. The gaps in question, measuring several millimeters or perhaps 1 to 2 cm, i.e., the distance from viable bone in one major fragment to viable bone in the other, become progressively more stable as more fibrous tissue forms and as the fibers become thicker and better oriented. In contrast, in the 19-year-old, the repair tissue that is being elaborated may well be so situated as to fail to bridge the gap or, at best, require several weeks to do so. The gap to be bridged here is much larger — several centimeters. That gap is filled with hematoma undergoing degradation and with necrotic tissue, and these elements decrease the rate of progress of the granulation tissue. A third factor that further impedes healing is as follows: Fibrous tissue always obeys a natural chronology of formation and maturation. A crucial element in that maturation is contraction of the fibers, the well known shrinkage of a scar. On the microscopic level that shrinkage, which reaches a peak 2 to 3 weeks after the granulation tissue has begun to form, is accompanied by a decrease in its blood supply. Many of its capillaries are so squeezed as to lose their patency. The result is that the center of the gap, where granulation tissue has not yet formed, has a poorer prospect for being bridged.

The consequences of these negative influences on natural stabilizing of the fracture fragments in the 19-year-old are obvious. A longer, much more vigorous therapeutic program of stabilization of the fracture is needed. A long period (months) must elapse before the fracture is united. In regard to the timing and adequacy of the several components of that process (resorption of hematoma and necrotic tissue, formation of granulation tissue, elaboration of callus, remodeling), all of the components are still represented. The hematoma, much larger in volume than in the case of the 12-year-old also permeates soft tissue more extensively so that resorption is slower. Similarly, the necrosis is more extensive and not only requires more time (weeks) for resorption but concomitantly further delays the essential process by limiting the blood supply necessary for resorption, even of the hematoma. Therefore the topographical anatomy of the granulation tissue at the fracture site differs in important ways in the two cases. In case 4-1, the 19-year-old, healthy granulation tissue forms a shell around the damaged tissues, and as days and weeks go by the shell becomes thicker and more fibrotic. Within it, depending on what soft tissue and bone retains a blood supply, granulation tissue also forms on the surfaces of that viable tissue while resorption of the nonviable elements — hematoma, necrotic fascia, and bone — occurs at the interface. However, owing to the limited potential for elaboration of granulation tissue, parts of the hematoma endure for weeks within the shell of the repair, and that hematoma undergoes deteriorative sequences. The clot changes from a gel to a liquid, as enzymatic breakdown proceeds, and denaturation of proteins also occurs in extensive foci. Thus the process of resorption is changed in a fundamental way. In the 12-year-old most of the hematoma (serum proteins, hemoglobin, and even intact erythrocytes) easily finds its way back into the active circulation, the cells doing so by diapedesis. In the 19-year-old more cells are required to permeate, resorb, and replace the larger volume of hematoma and necrotic soft tissue and bone before the repair tissue becomes a stabilizing callus. The end result, although satisfactory in the sense that the fracture healed and acceptable function was achieved, involved a long period of recumbency and included considerable impairment. These adverse considerations have assumed greater importance today, as contrasted with those in effect when the patient was initially treated, about 30 years ago; in particular, the escalating cost of hospitalization assumes so important a role in treatment that it alters risk – benefit calculations in favor of surgical treatment. One option for such treatment has been strengthened by the development of new techniques and devices. Thus a brief consideration of the case of this 19-year-old patient as to the alteration in pathophysiological processes involved in more modern treatment is necessary.

Recall that the man had fractures of *both* femurs, one being a less severe, simple, uncomminuted break. That fracture was dismissed from consideration for the purpose of this presentation except to imply that its treatment would also have included a considerable period of recumbency (as did the contralateral fracture). In recent years manual or motorized reamers have been developed that shape the endosteal surface of the femoral cortex into a cylinder that can be engaged along much of its length by any of several designs of nails. Therefore when the fracture has been reduced, immediate and secure fixation of the fragments would be obtained; and the extremity would be able to bear weight within a week or two. Similarly, devices have been developed to secure, by internal fixation, the other femur's fractures.

This subject is considered further below, but it introduces a new pathophysiological implication as to treatment: the possibility of surgically removing much of the hematoma and necrotic soft tissues. Such a surgical cleanup would reduce the volume of material that required phagocytic cleanup; and because the patient's potential for producing histiocytes is limited, the period needed for resorption would be reduced from the several weeks or months described above to a few days or, at most, a week or two. What it means is that, coordinately, the amount of fibrosis also would be reduced. Most important, however, is the fact that the natural devascularization of the fibrous tissue (scar) by contraction occurs during a different phase of the healing process, i.e., at a time when that fibrous tissue is not integral to the secure fixation of the fracture fragments and when the granulation tissue no longer is essential to cleanup of the hematoma. Although secure fixation at the time of operation can be reliably mediated in this case by an intramedullary nail to stabilize the most distal fragments and attach them to the proximal fragment, that secure fixation requires more than a month or two for development of the healing biological repair tissue (callus) to make up for some loss of fixation attributable to resorption of devascularized bony fragments and fracture surfaces. Nevertheless, the adverse effects of excessive and prolonged scarring are avoided, and the positive effects of early function are implemented early in the repair process.

Case 4-1 illustrates the interdependence of several influences on the healing of any fracture, in

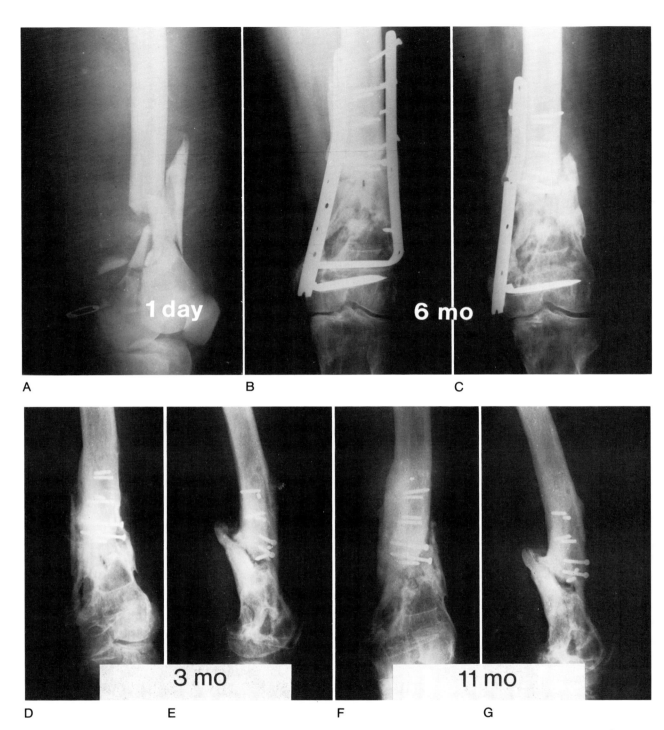

Fig. 4-2. Case 4-2. **(A)** Oblique radiograph of the distal right femur shows extensive comminution of a closed fracture incurred by a 43-year-old farmer when a tree fell on his limb. The soft tissue was severely contused and swollen. Neurovascular structures were intact. Open reduction was done and a blade plate inserted. **(B)** AP radiograph at 6 months shows that the blade plate inserted on the lateral side has broken. **(C)** A second fixation device was placed on the medial side. Iliac bone grafts were added across the supra-condylar component of the fracture. **(D&E)** After 5.5 years AP and lateral view of the fracture shows the removal of both plates and the radiolucent gap of a nonunion at the mid-fracture area. **(F&G)** AP **(F)** and lateral **(G)** radiographs 11 months after a tibial onlay bone graft shows union of the fracture. *(Figure continues.)*

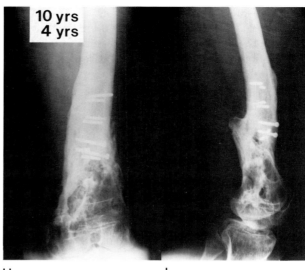

Fig. 4-2 *(Continued)*. (**H&I**) At 10 years after the fracture and now 4 years after the tibial bone graft, the union is solid. Knee motion is 70° of flexion.

particular the pathophysiological factors (hemorrhage, necrosis, resorption, callus formation) and the mechanical factors (security and efficacy of fixation, the latter being strongly affected by variables in the elements of treatment).

Case 4-2 As a more compelling illustration of that interdependence and as an illustration of other therapeutic principles, case 4-2 (Fig. 4-2) merits discussion. The nature of the fracture includes certain important features: First, it is a high-energy injury, i.e., one may expect much necrosis and much displacement of bony fragments. Second, it involves not only cortical bone but a considerable volume of cancellous bone as well. Third, the lines of fracture enter the knee.

Considering the last feature first, as it relates to treatment, we note that the intraarticular fractures are considered in detail in Chapter 5. Therefore we dismiss this patient's interarticular injury with a brief comment. The optimal ultimate function of the limb, as ideally projected, requires good motion of the knee joint, which in turn requires reconstruction of the femoral articular surface, now disrupted, and, in turn, coaptation of the broken fragments of cartilage. Because this objective can only be met operatively under direct vision, an early operation with that objective as the focus must be (and was) done. The second feature concerns the anatomy of the fracture. As the radiographs show and as was evident grossly at operation, the cortical bone has been splintered extensively to a point several inches above the joint. Concomitantly, some of the cancellous bone has been fragmented into crumbs, and there are only two large fragments, each of which (fortunately) includes the articular cartilage of a femoral condyle. It is this feature of the fracture that must be clearly understood in regard to therapy; in the present case, the lack of appreciation of the details just mentioned was responsible for the failure of therapy. One may regard all of the small fragments of bone, splinters and crumbs alike, as devitalized. Probably the two large condylar fragments retained their circulation and were sufficiently large and sturdy to support the screws that are needed to maintain the congruity of the articular surface after the principal segments were reduced. So far, so good. The error in judgment of the surgeon, then, was the estimation that the condylar fragments would also be sturdy enough to support a right-angle blade plate, inserted to stabilize the proximal fragment of diaphysis, vis-à-vis the condyle, the intervening several inches, and the crumbs of devitalized bone.

Although one may easily condemn the surgeon on this point and propose other, possibly more appropriate devices, what is basic to the problem is not how one might secure adequate fixation but, rather, what would be the alternative in this case (and similar ones) if the bony fragments just cannot be secured. Surgeons should avoid the all-too-common posture that their expertise is so all-embracing they can fix anything. In this case there was a significant degree of risk that the fixation would become insecure during the immediate postoperative weeks, when some resorption of bone had to occur at the periphery of the blade of the blade plate. The surgeon desired to mobilize the knee quickly but ignored the fact that the motion would impose too large a moment of force on the device because the fracture site inherently was unstable. The error therefore resulted in cyclic micro-motion at the fracture site just at the time when such motion should be minimized.

Before considering what would be more effective treatment (in retrospect, admittedly, but supported by valid principles), the first feature of the fracture, its high energy mechanism, should be mentioned. The expectation of much necrosis always conjures up the probability that healing will be slow, which in turn leads to planning a therapeutic regimen that may take several or many months.

When planning such a regimen, as in this case, the most common mistake is to attempt to do too much at once. Staging the therapy should always be considered as a way of avoiding risky maneuvers. Therefore considering, first, the need to retain the function of the knee, the surgeon should recognize the option of deferring the mobilization routine for a few weeks, although immobilization of the knee for 2 months or more (in an adult) is likely to lead to iatrogenic loss of motion. Thus the surgeon might consider an option of limiting the operation to reconstruction of the articular surface and then using, for several weeks, a technique to immobilize the components of the fracture proximal to the joint (e.g., traction or cast). After those several weeks, during which time the condyles should unite and some repair tissue should develop proximally, the options for treating the other elements of the fracture depend on how healing was progressing.

Given the likelihood that the above restricted intraarticular operation and limited period of immobilization are best for the knee, what would be best for the other elements of the fracture? Three basic variables may be entered into the equation

devised to answer that question: maintaining good alignment, avoiding shortening, avoiding micromotion of fragments. Each of these elements varies in degree and, at present, cannot be measured objectively. All physicians would agree, however, that the priority is immobilization, and that the most secure method to immobilize the fracture site today is probably use of an external fixator device that couples the proximal femoral fragment with the tibia. This method would reliably avoid shortening and maintain femoral length and alignment. The splinters and crumbs of bones would act as autogenous bone grafts for the 6 weeks (or so) during which the device is in use, and the patient could well be ambulatory (and not hospitalized) for most of that period.

It is not our purpose here to follow the patient through the possible regimens of treatment. We recognize that even if the regimen described above for the stages of treatment up to the 6-week milestone were used, it might fall short of reaching the goal of incipient union of the fracture and might require choices of an additional operative intervention or a nonoperative (e.g., cast-brace) treatment for many months. The emphasis that is paramount is that the pathophysiological sequences must be understood, both in regard to the nature of the injury and the therapeutic maneuvers, and the planned regimen must not be devised with only one set of principles in mind.

Open Fractures

When there is an open wound, as when a markedly displaced fracture fragment penetrates the soft tissue envelope and the skin, an *open fracture* is the result. In such cases a significant risk of infection is introduced, the risk being increased as the degree of contamination rises.[2,4,6,10-15] Once infection occurs, there may be sequestration of fracture fragments. The complex interaction of the many factors involved is depicted in case 4-3.

Case 4-3   A 20-year-old man fell from a second story window, sustaining a severely comminuted open fracture of the shaft of the femur with marked displacement of the fragments. The proximal fragment protruded 2 cm through a small wound in the skin, perforated his clothing, and had gone into the ground for 10 cm or more. Extensive soft tissue damage, especially of the quadriceps muscle, was noted during the débridement, but no bone was débrided. The proximal fragment was stripped for a distance of about 10 cm. There was mud in the medullary canal of the bone. No bleeding from that canal was seen until the dirt was curetted from it; there also was no evidence of bleeding from the cortex of the stripped bone. The distal fragment bled freely, but the free fragment did not. There was dirt on the quadriceps musculature on all sides of the wound, and it was excised. Traction was applied to the femur through a pin inserted in the proximal tibia, and the fracture fragments were aligned in good position (Figs. 4-3A,B). The wound was then packed open, and routine intravenous antibiotics were administered, not specifically targeted at all the various organisms cultured from the wound. The drainage continued. Further débridement was needed after 2 weeks, at which time 350 ml of purulent material was surgically removed and the femur was noted to have purulent material in the medullary canal. One week after that, further débridement of bone and soft tissue was performed, and a catheter was inserted for continuous local administration of antibiotics. A spica cast was applied, but the wound continued to drain, and it became evident that there was osteomyelitis of all three major bony fragments. After 1 year it was clear that the denuded fragments were going to sequestrate (Figs. 4-3C,D). Two years after the injury, sequestrectomy of all the necrotic segments was performed, which led to cessation of the drainage (Fig. 4-3E,F).

This case raises many points as to what the treatment achieved and in what way it failed. As regards the fractures, the traction that was applied initially was successful in that all bony fragments were aligned adequately. However, treatment of the open wound, from the moment of transport of the patient from the site of injury to the hospital, bears close scrutiny. Because the patient's proximal femoral fragment was withdrawn from the hole it made in the earth, as the patient's history revealed, all would agree that not only was the fracture a high-energy injury but also the contamination of the wound must have been maximal. Then, when the contaminated, pointed end of proximal diaphysis was pulled back into the wound by ambulance personnel, there was contamination of a considerable tract of soft tissue, although the appearance of the soft tissue and skin might well be misleading in that they looked healthy, except for traces of dirt. The detailed history, then, plus the extensive impaction of dirt into the medullary canal of the proximal fragment should have alerted the surgeon to the fact that there was a maximal potential for infection. Routine débridement, as for surface contamination, would therefore be insufficient to remove most of the contaminating organisms. Furthermore, the extensive stripping of periosteum and the presence of a large butterfly fragment would auger for extensive necrosis of bone on the basis of ischemia. The question then arises as to what would be the proper degree of débridement.

Here the surgeon may have little in the way of gross recognition of tissue changes other than active hemorrhage, clot, and dirt particles for guidance and so should be diligent in the application of principles to supplement the tissue changes observed.[10] Having been alerted to the probability of extensive damage (by the history), the surgeon's first operative move would be excision of a small rim of skin around the wound, the objective being removal of the tissue into which particles of earth had been driven. This maneuver routinely would be preceded by copious lavage of the area before routine preparation by antiseptics, as is done for all surgical procedures. One surgical principle should be kept in mind, however: the probability that lavage (or indeed any invasive maneuver) disseminates some bacteria, even if it is designed to remove a local highly contaminated focus. The lavage therefore should not be directed into the wound. Following excision of a limited amount of skin, the surgeon would realize that a small portal would not provide the requisite exposure for proper handling of the bony injury. Extensile prolongation of the wound distally and proximally would be the next maneuver, and that is what was done.

In the description of the case, the degree of débridement of soft tissue was termed "extensive." Such description called for excision not only of a rim of quadriceps muscle around the buttonhole made by the femoral fragment but also of all of the clotted material, any purplish discolored muscle around the bony cortex, and any shred of tissue that had dirt adhering to it. That having been done and

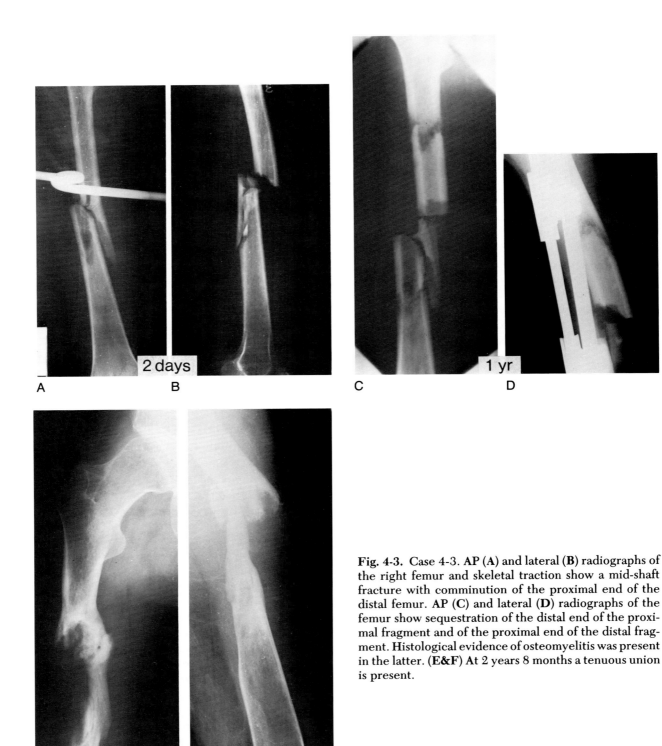

Fig. 4-3. Case 4-3. AP (**A**) and lateral (**B**) radiographs of the right femur and skeletal traction show a mid-shaft fracture with comminution of the proximal end of the distal femur. AP (**C**) and lateral (**D**) radiographs of the femur show sequestration of the distal end of the proximal fragment and of the proximal end of the distal fragment. Histological evidence of osteomyelitis was present in the latter. (**E&F**) At 2 years 8 months a tenuous union is present.

additional lavage having been directed at removal of any dirt not grossly apparent, the surgeon then directed attention to the bony fragments. One principle that was violated in this case (and that may have led to the catastrophe to be described) is that any measure that would avoid spread of contamination must be adopted. In this case the surgeon should have realized that attention to the proximal femoral fragment, obviously crammed full of dirt, should consist in isolating that dirt from the remainder of the exposed tissues. Instead, an attempt was made to remove the dirt, not realizing that any subsequent handling of other fragments would contaminate them. Although there may be no quarrel with vigorous curettement of the medullary cavity, preceded and followed by copious lavage, that maneuver should have been preceded by isolation of the end of the bone perhaps by a rubber glove over a sponge tied by a ligature around the bone. It also should have been preceded by an extensile incision of the quadriceps muscle to allow access to the distal fragments of femur; instead, the surgeon "took care of" what was an obvious and necessary débridement. The incision was then extended into the muscle, mostly in a distal and lateral direction, with the following ideas in mind: First, the fracture fragments, now cleaned of all dirt, could be aligned. Second, possible damage to the innervation of the quadriceps muscle could be avoided or minimized. Third, a good avenue for the drains, whose insertion was anticipated as a final surgical maneuver prior to a loose suture of the wound, would be provided. It should be emphasized here that it was this surgical plan, which did not envision a final open packing of the wound, that precipitated a series of maneuvers that created the anatomical bases for the catastrophic infection — the deadspace.

When the distal fragments were exposed, the surgeon took care that the butterfly fragment was not further stripped of periosteum and was properly aligned, as was the other distal fragment. The entire cavity was then profusely lavaged, and the proximal fragment was replaced in aligned position. Several drains were inserted, and the skin incision was loosely sutured.

Three points may be discussed with reference to the above "definitive" initial handling of the wound. One is that the surgeon did obey the princi-

ple that the less foreign material that is introduced (no metal device in this case), the less the risk of infection.[5] Were an attempt made to fix the three bony fragments by any device whatsoever, not only does the device constitute an element of risk, but so does the maneuver of its insertion, because contamination attends every incision and every drill hole. In particular, any thought about using an intramedullary nail in this case should be accompanied by a vision of microscopic particles of dirt spread up and down the medullary cavity and, if it were reamed, driven into the endosteal surface of the cavity from end to end. Pursuing that train of thought, if any device is used, the surgeon must anticipate how the wound will be handled once the device is in place. If, as we suggested, open packing of the wound was a preferable alternative to closure over drains, the latter alternative would usually be inappropriate, especially if the period of open packing was planned for weeks and not for only a short interval (as with delayed closure of the wound).

The second point has to do with the deadspace, an inevitable anatomical consequence of the injury and the débridement procedure. The surgeon's decision to use drains to allow evacuation of exudate and hematoma was predicated on the anticipated elimination of the deadspace by the pressure of the muscular envelope during the several days following the débridement. The drains were removed after a week, not after the usual 2 days as is customary following elective surgical procedures, because in those procedures the viable tissues elaborate enough fibrin and fibrous tissue around the drain to render the drains ineffective. During that week, the muscular envelope did lessen the volume of the deadspace, but inevitably some deadspace remained, and an egress of exudate from that space was impeded more and more by the healing of the incision. The result was an accumulation of exudate (pus in this instance); and in view of its volume at 2 weeks (350 ml), the pus must have been under pressure and undoubtedly constituted one more step in the catastrophic course of the lesion.

The third point that should be discussed briefly is whether removal of all visible dirt from the proximal fragment by curettement of its medullary canal was sufficient in regard to débridement. Although ideally all dead tissue is excised, cortical bone constitutes an exception to that principle for several reasons. One is that grossly visible indications are absent as to what area is dead and what area is alive, so that the decision to remove some bone in this case is either arbitrary or based on inference: The periosteum on the fragment was stripped for 10 cm or more, and the dirt was impacted for a similar distance. The cortex therefore had to be ischemic for several centimeters at least, even allowing for some intact intracortical circulation through the axially oriented haversian systems. A second reason for conservatism when excising cortex is that it constitutes a poor medium for growth of pathogenic bacteria, having a minimum of soft tissue components and little free aqueous solution. A third reason is that bone excision is more traumatic than excision of soft tissues (nibbling bone with a chisel or osteotome versus clean cuts with a scalpel) and less easily guided by provocation of bleeding or color changes in the tissue. With these reasons in mind, radical removal of bone would be foolhardy. In the present case, it came to mind only in retrospect. Bone excision here permitted proper immobilization to be maintained, while the wound could be observed daily and dressed appropriately. After the first week elapsed, drainage from the wound ceased, and further dressings were not needed. The drains were then removed, but over the next 2 months it became apparent radiologically that a large part of the proximal fragment of bone was undergoing necrosis because of disruption of the medullary and periosteal blood supply; clinically, it was apparent that there was local osteomyelitis. It took a year for radiographic evidence to delineate the resorptive demarcation zone between the living and dead bone in the proximal fragment. It also became evident that the butterfly fragment was necrotic but surrounded by callus. Necrosis was apparent in the distal fragment, with some evidence of a motheaten endosteal surface, indicative of osteomyelitis.

The extent of the necrosis of all three fragments and the slow evolution of the demarcation explains the marked delay (more than 2 years) before it was decided to excise the sequestered fragments. The fracture then proceeded to heal albeit in tenuous continuity. Additional periosteal new bone formation that had been evident around the sequestered segments that were left in situ established the con-

tinuity (Fig. 4-3E,F). Once that union had been achieved, it was recommended that bone grafting be performed to augment the cortex, but the patient failed to return for that procedure.

It should have been apparent at the time of the injury that the extensive soft tissue and bony injury to this patient's thigh would delay his achieving any functional result, and the advent of infection, which did not help matters any, contributed to the delay in uniting the fracture; primarily, however, the delay was attributable to the extensive damage to the blood supply to the soft tissues and the bony fragments at the fracture site. The infection and the ischemic loss of bone magnified the problem of reconstruction of the tenuous union. The case demonstrates that fractures do unite in the presence of infection provided there is no major vascular damage to the healing components. However, in view of the likelihood of major impairment (flexion of the patient's knee now is about 70°) and an additional year or two of morbidity for reconstruction of the femur, the case can well be termed a catastrophe.

Three of the essential principles of débridement have been emphasized: All dead soft tissue and debris must be removed, leaving minimal deadspace and insertion of fixation devices must be avoided, and drainage must be encouraged. There are principles pertaining to the initial weeks of treatment of open severe fractures[2,3,5,7,8,13-16] in addition to those already discussed in case 4-3 and for less severe cases discussed previously that are brought out in case 4-4, which illustrates a common injury often requiring prolonged treatment and often causing severe impairment. (For the purposes of the presentation, the case is only summarized, selecting certain details of the patient's course of treatment that are needed for exposition of principles not yet discussed. Too elaborate an account would merely distract the reader.)

Case 4-4 A 21-year-old motorcyclist sustained an injury to his leg that consisted in the loss of skin and underlying soft tissues over perhaps one-third of the anteromedial aspect of his leg, with associated markedly comminuted fractures of the tibia and a closed uncomminuted fracture of the fibula (Fig. 4-4). Once his systemic condition had stabilized, during which period his leg was splinted and protected in sterile dressings, an external fixator was

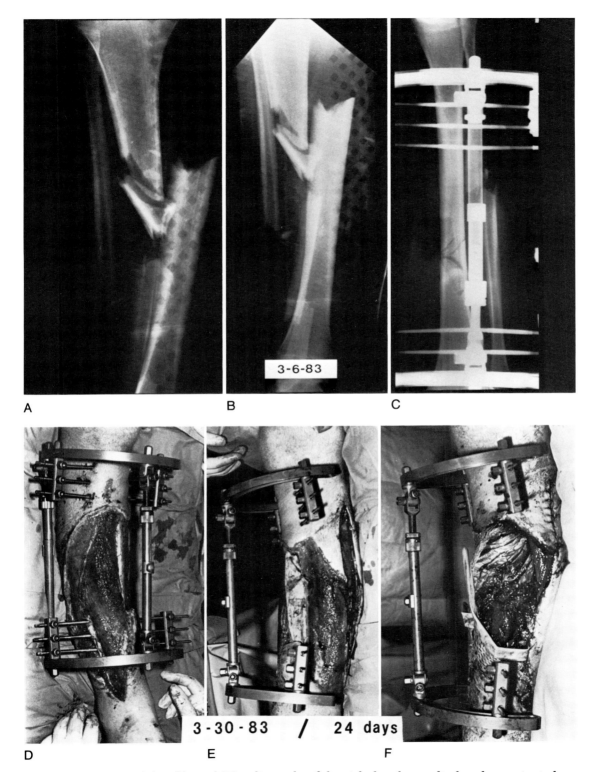

3-6-83

3-30-83 / 24 days

A   B   C

D   E   F

Fig. 4-4. Case 4-4. AP (**A**) and lateral (**B**) radiographs of the right leg show a displaced comminuted open fracture of the tibia and a minimally displaced fracture of the fibula. (**C**) AP radiograph of the fracture in an external fixation frame after débridement and reduction. (**D–F**) A 15 × 10 cm soft tissue defect remained on the anteromedial aspect of the leg with an exposed tibia. A low grade *Pseudomonas aeruginosa* infection complicated a soleus muscle flap. *(Figure continues.)*

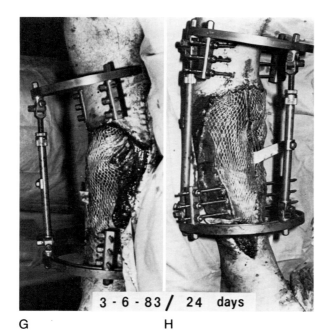

G

H

Fig. 4-4 *(Continued).* **(G&H)** Skin graft closure of the muscle flap wound. **(I&J)** AP radiographs of the tibia at 14 weeks before **(I)** and after **(J)** excision of dead fragments because of a persistent low grade infection. **(K&L)** AP radiographs of healing at 6 and 7 months. *(Figure continues.)*

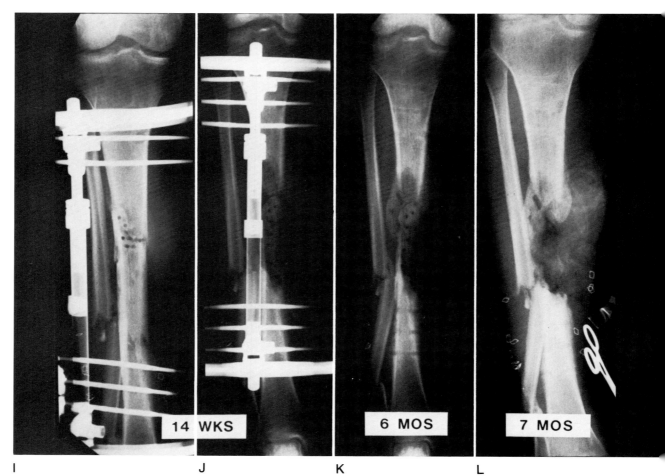

I

J

K

L

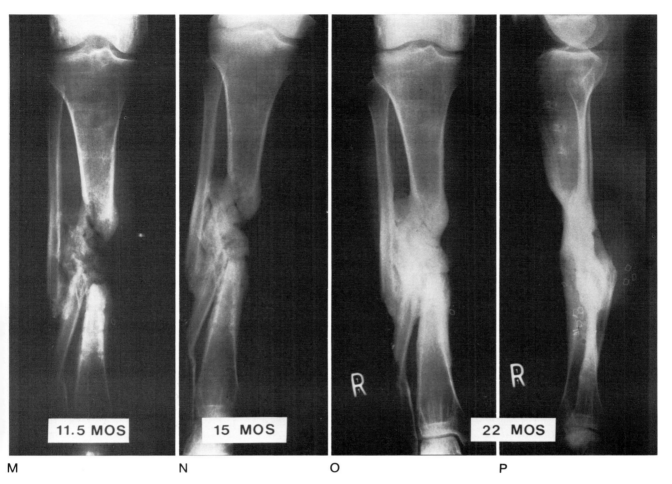

M N O P

Fig. 4-4 *(Continued).* **(M&N)** AP radiographs at 11.5 and 15 months and O&P at 2.2 months show healing. **(O&P)** AP and lateral radiographs at 22 months show solid union of the tibia and of the tibia with the fibula after two more sequestrectomies, a period of 2 months of no drainage, and insertion of iliac bone grafts in the defect between the fibula and the tibia.

applied, and the wound was cleaned, lavaged, and débrided. The débridement procedure differed somewhat from that in case 4-3 in that the dirt was more superficial and therefore more easily (and completely) removed, and there was no need for extending the wound. However, as emphasized in case 4-3, the plan of treatment had to be premeditated, so that every step would not only fit the plan but also carry it forward.[7]

The errors in the plan for case 4-3 have been discussed. In the present case there were no errors. The initial débridement was conservative, not so much because so much soft tissue had been lost but,

rather, because the remaining tissues (and bone) were available for examination and further sequential débridement procedures should gross evidence of necrosis become apparent. No bone was removed during the débridement. There was no question here of how the wound should be treated during the first week or so; but there was one question that was not raised in the previous case: What would have to be done to close the wound, and when could the procedure that was chosen be scheduled? In passing, it should be mentioned that had there been evidence of vascular injury (to the tibial or popliteal artery) or evidence of injury to the tibial nerve (see Ch. 5), or a compartment syndrome of serious degree associated with the fractures and loss of soft tissue, the best decision might have been to do a below-knee amputation. Such a decision would be based on the high probability of failure of one or more of the reconstructive procedures that would be needed, the prolonged morbidity, and the ultimate result, which would at best include not only impairment but also a continuing risk of more complications.

The patient of case 4-4, under standard conservative treatment to the wound, rapidly developed granulation tissue over most of the exposed tibial bone. Some diaphyseal areas, however, particularly on the ends of the major tibial fragments, assumed the dead-white color characteristic of ischemic bone. The plan of treatment did not include removal of this ischemic bone but was flexible with respect to two possible contingencies. Should there have been signs of infection the infected tissues would be excised, and should the granulation tissue be unhealthy (i.e., edematous, pale, and succulent) it too would be excised. Under sterile dressings and firm, even pressure, healthy granulation tissues spread over all but two small foci; then, for a week or more, the wound remained in status quo, and no systemic or local evidence of infection developed. It seemed obvious then that delaying the decision about how the wound should be epithelialized would merely make things worse. There would be more scarring in the interval and a greater risk of infection given the obviously necrotic ischemic bone that was still in evidence. (See case 4-3 for a discussion of removal of cortical bone.) However, mere epithelialization of so extensive an expanse of denuded bone and muscle would not only pose risks, in view of the exposed and necrotic foci, but also would be unsatisfactory as an end result because the thin covering of the bone would be so vulnerable to trauma. Split-thickness skin grafts in such a situation could be considered only interim therapy, preliminary to covering the bone with a more substantial layer of soft tissue.

Discussion of the several options for coverage of the wound, all with advocates who emphasize the advantages of the method they prefer, is beyond the purview of this book, and the reader is referred to the references[4,5,8,9,23–25] for such discussions.

Suffice it to say that the method used ultimately was successful but not without a prolonged regimen of treatment and many operations (Fig. 4-3).

The additional principles illustrated in this case are as follows: Severe injuries that include myocutaneous damage and severe open fractures should be treated under a plan that envisages from the start the several stages of therapy and that allows for all contingent events.[2,3,5,8,10,14,16] Repeated débridements always play an important role in such a plan, as does daily observation of the wound under sterile conditions. Selecting a device for immobilizing the fracture fragments must allow for the débridements and observation. Selection of the device and the considerations attending its application and maintenance must also envisage its use for at least several weeks or perhaps months. It must also envisage mobilization of an adjacent joint, which could surely lose motion if kept immobile. Extending this principle, which is the interdependence of the various technical maneuvers that constitute therapy, the device must be such as to allow any of the possible grafting methods, referred to by citation, to be implemented when events permit. In this case, the patient's fractures did not begin to show signs of repair until the dead cortex was excised and the *Pseudomonas* infection was cured. Meanwhile, mobilization of the muscle and joints, which were free to move in the external fixator, minimized permanent impairment. Recovery of function took more than a year. Despite the loss of much soft tissue and bone, a low grade infection that was unavoidable because of the necrosis and prolonged exposure of the injured tissues, and the need for several operations to restore the viable tissues to a healthy, functional state (including reconstructive procedures), the functions of the foot, ankle, and knee were maintained, and the limb achieved a function close to normal.

The 21-year-old man of case 4-4 highlights the delay in bone healing for almost 2 years because of extensive soft tissue injury to the leg after he sustained an open tibial fibular fracture in a motorcycle accident. The loss of soft tissue and disruption of the muscle attachments and blood supply to bone not only affect the function of the soft tissue structures but have deleterious effects on bone repair. The frequent procedures required to achieve healing of the soft tissues and bone and limited function of the foot and ankle as an end result over a 2-year period makes consideration of early amputation, i.e., within 3 months, a reasonable alternative, particularly if there is a neurological deficit as well.

PATHOPHYSIOLOGY OF OPEN REDUCTION

One must recognize that any operation on bone causes some hemorrhage or, if there was a preceding injury increases the amount of hematoma already present. It therefore thromboses some vessels in addition to transecting others, and it at least temporarily displaces some soft tissue by the accumulated hematoma. If a fracture is reduced as an open procedure, ordinarily the clot that has been present is removed and a lesser amount accumu-

lates; but because of the improved topography (reduction of the fragments, improved alignment, restoration of soft tissue anatomy, and of course immobilization) the amount of clot at the fracture site should be minimal. When an internal fixation device is used, complete contact of the fracture surfaces of the fragment is rarely obtained even when there is no comminution and a so-called hairline reduction is achieved, as determined by gross observation.[19] The fracture surfaces are in contact at small points, where the asperities of the roughened fracture surface abut against asperities on the other surface (Figs. 4-5A,B). The areas not in contact permit vascular tissue to fill the spaces that exist at the ends of the broken cortex, and the medullary canal in both fragments is gradually invaded by the vascular tissue. When a bone plate is used to join the fragments (in the simplest case, only two fragments), in most instances the points of contact, or asperities, are most numerous near the plate.

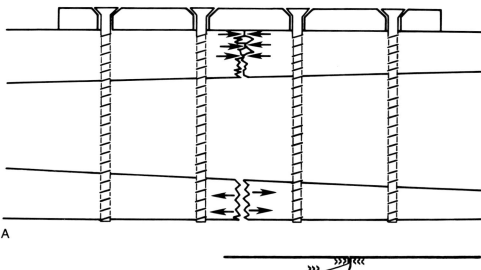

A

Fig. 4-5. (A) Internal fixation with a compression plate. (B) Contact points of the cortex with a compression plate.

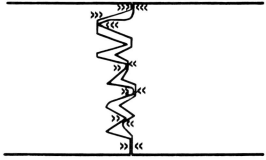

B

That part of the bone cortex on the opposite side tends to present a gap that may not be large enough to be apparent either to the naked eye or on radiographs. The gap offers easy access to the initial repair tissue, as during the initial stages of fracture healing already described (i.e., hemorrhage, resorption of hematoma and necrotic tissue, and beginning callus formation).

The new bone that forms in the gap may be layered on the surface of ischemic bone, or it may be produced in the "cutting cones" (Fig. 4-6). As newly formed blood vessels invade the necrotic bone as vascular buds, they are preceded by a loose mucoid tissue containing histiocytes and osteoclasts that are brought in and resorb the necrotic bone. New bone also is formed in the foci on the walls of the resorption front. Initially, the mass of new bone is oriented mostly in line with the fracture gap, but gradually the callus changes from its immature coarse structure and helter-skelter orientation to a more ordered trabecular pattern, with individual elements more longitudinally oriented.[19,20]

Immobilization by plating has the effect of minimizing the amount of external callus compared to the amount of callus elicited during conservative treatment (i.e., traction, plaster cast, or brace immobilization). Most of the experimental studies on the use of internal fixation with plates seems to indicate that the "rigidity" of fixation is not absolute but, rather, connotes the situation in which there is but little motion between the bony fragments. However, no one has been able to quantitatively define that motion, e.g., as to longitudinal excursion (in micrometers?), lateral angulation or rotatory displacement (in degrees), or cycles per unit of time.

Because plates of varying design and materials

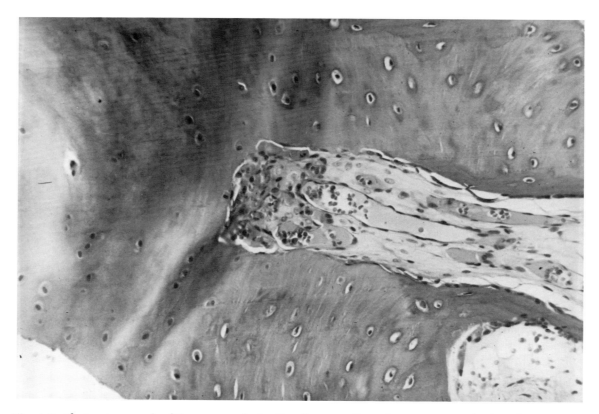

Fig. 4-6. Photomicrograph of the cortex of a healing fracture. Note the "cutting" cylinder of osteoclasts, capillaries, and osteoblasts removing live bone of the callus as part of remodeling. (×250)

are in use and under investigation, their relative "rigidity" (more appropriately their elasticity) strongly influences the efficacy of the restriction of motion of the fracture fragments. Nevertheless, this relative inelasticity is a critical influence on stabilizing the fragments and may be potentiated by compression to provide a load-bearing capability in the limb.

The sequence of repair can then proceed, but one should not conclude that "rigid" fixation is the overriding influence that allows quick repair. It probably is true that there is an inherent chronology of repair as it pertains to microscopic elements, e.g., how long it takes for precursor cells to become osteoblasts, how long it takes for an osteoblast to secrete bony matrix, how long it takes for a blob of matrix to be remodeled into a trabecula. That inherent chronology probably cannot be appreciably accelerated by mechanical means, but it certainly can be slowed and even brought to a halt. What plate "immobilization" does is to provide a situation where, first, the volume of the space between bony fragments is drastically reduced compared to the space present with some other forms of treatment, including open reduction without internal fixation. Second, the excursions of one fragment relative to the other (micro-motion) are not sufficiently large to elicit repeated small hemorrhages, as would be the case with greater excursions. Third, it provides a means of allowing early physiological muscular action as well as load-bearing long before the callus that forms would permit the same. Although this influence is difficult to study in animal experiments and probably impossible in the human, it is a general observation that in all subjects with fractures who use the injured extremity, animal or human, hematoma is more rapidly resorbed and less edema occurs, i.e., the early phases of the reaction to trauma are shortened. Thus repair can be more rapid.

When the internal fixation device is an *intramedullary rod*, the amount of callus elaborated depends on the stability provided by the rod as it abuts against the endosteal surface. A greater amount of fibrocartilaginous callus is produced with a loose-fitting rod than with a well-fitted rod, which engages a wide area of cortex distal and proximal to the fracture site(s). With a loose-fitting rod there is extensive intramedullary callus in the areas where

there is no contact, but elaboration of that callus requires several weeks at least until motion of the rod is sufficiently limited to allow the interfragmental callus to be adequate for load-bearing. With a tight-fitting rod even a small amount of peripheral callus of periosteal origin helps stabilize the fragments early. Although more necrosis is inevitably produced by extensive reaming of the endosteal bone in order to get a tight fit, that disadvantage is more than offset by the immobility achieved by the better instrumentation (see case 4-5).

Case 4-5 A 22-year-old man sustained a comminuted closed fracture of the mid-shaft of the femur (Fig. 4-7A,B). After a few days in skeletal traction, during which time other minor injuries were attended to, he underwent a "closed" procedure of intramedullary fixation; because of the comminution we planned to use a rod with cross-fixation screws drilled through the rod proximally and distally. We also planned to ream the femur to the size of the rod. The rod itself would stabilize the fracture anteroposteriorly and laterally, and the interlocking screws would prevent collapse and shortening and would control rotational displacement (Fig. 4-7C–E). A small amount of periosteal callus was evident on radiographs 3 weeks postoperatively, and there was no change in the position of the fragments compared with the immediate postoperative position. Therefore limited weight-bearing was prescribed, which was followed by uncomplicated healing of the fracture. The patient, a highly reliable individual, was encouraged to move his knee in its full range and to walk with crutches as soon as comfort permitted. It was intended that the distally placed screws be removed after 2 months, when it became evident that sufficient callus was present to prevent the fragments from telescoping on the nail.

It is convenient to discuss, at this point, the pathophysiological considerations that were important with regard to the surgeon's conduct of those 2 months of therapy. First, with reference to mechanical questions regarding the device to be used and its insertion, the choice of device has already been mentioned. The device has the disadvantage of requiring a good deal of surgical expertise, especially in terms of the precision required when inserting the interlocking screws; even with ideal image intensifier technique, much experience is

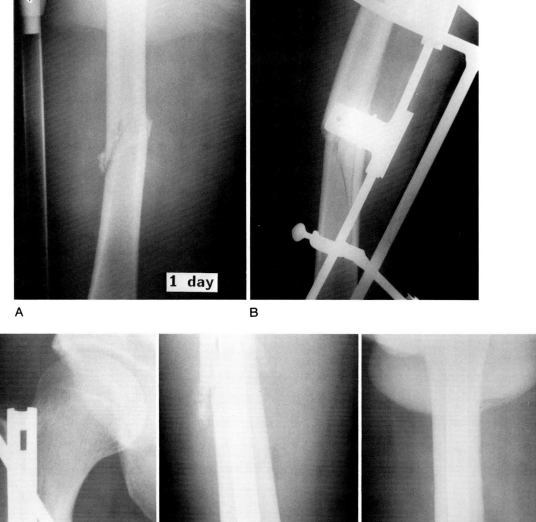

Fig. 4-7. Case 4-5. AP and lateral radiographs of a femur fracture treated with an intramedullary locking nail with cross screws (Brooker-Wells). (A&B) Initial radiographs. (C–E) Postoperative radiographs. *(Figure continues.)*

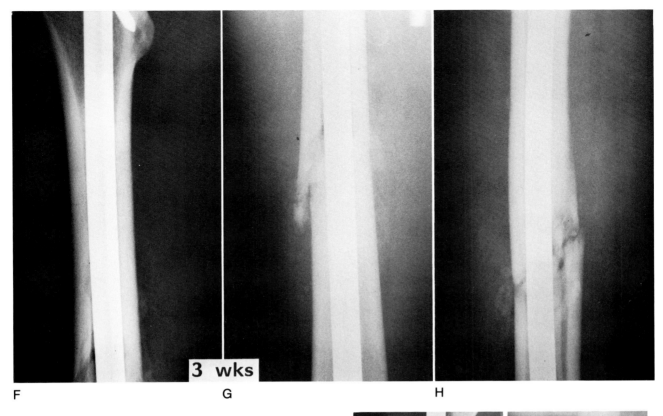

F   G   H

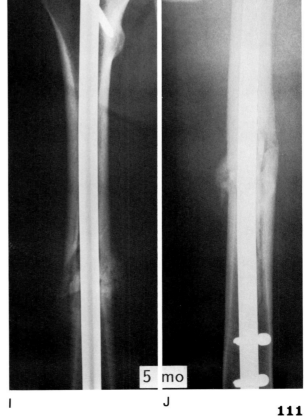

Fig. 4-7 *(Continued)*. (**F–H**) At 3 weeks. (**I&J**) At 5 months.

I   J

111

needed to aim the screws so they hit the target of the holes in the rod. The advantage of the security of the assembly, once achieved, outweighs this disadvantage, however. The closed intramedullary reaming also requires expertise, particularly in a case such as this one, where there was a large butterfly fragment, not easily amenable to adjustment of its position. Because its cortex on one side was missing, the surgeon thought the fragment would not be markedly displaced during the reaming process, so it would not introduce the risk of intraoperative difficulties. Of course, one great advantage is that the site of the fracture is not directly exposed, so surgical trauma to the soft parts and added damage to the vessels in the fracture site are avoided. In addition, the risk of bacterial contamination is not greatly magnified; but even though the procedure is popularly called "closed rodding," the incisions proximally and distally (for the rod and the screws), strictly interpreted, render the procedure an open one, and from the proximal incision the reamer might easily introduce contaminating organisms.

If those mechanical problems did not become manifest, the pathophysiological potential for healing, according to the principles discussed in the plating situation above, would be maximal, and the prospect would be for a short period of morbidity and a superlative result. One should factor into the equation the minor disadvantage of requiring the operative removal of the nail and interlocking screws. However, should there be mechanical problems, the surgeon must be prepared for them, as with a premeditated fall-back position and with the availability of the appropriate instruments. The most usual fall-back position in this case would be to convert the closed to an open "rodding." With that maneuver, the butterfly fragment could easily be repositioned and fixed with cerclage wiring if necessary.

At 2 months after the fracture the patient did not have the two distal interlocking screws removed as had been originally planned predicated on the idea that there would be enough callus at the fracture site to prevent deformity but there was not enough to take up the entire load of weight-bearing without crutches. Removal of the screws would have allowed some telescoping despite physiological patterns of loading on the callus and therefore accelerated remodeling. The result at 5 months was

entirely satisfactory (Fig. 4-7I,J), and it was decided that the components of the device were to be removed after a year or so.

Mention must be made of the reliability of the patient, because this elective therapeutic plan requires that the patient comply with the surgeon's advice concerning protection of the extremity even though after 2 to 3 weeks the patient might well believe that unlimited use is in order because he would have no symptoms to indicate otherwise. Therefore important considerations other than purely mechanical ones enter into planning the therapy, and it may be a more important precept for orthopedic surgeons than for physicians in other specialties.

PATHOPHYSIOLOGY OF CLOSED REDUCTION

Just as open reduction of fractures affects the repair process, we can expect that closed methods of treatment (e.g., cast-brace, pins and plaster, and external immobilizer) influence fracture healing.

The cast-brace method, popularized by Sarmiento, and other traditional splinting methods have essentially the same immobilization properties as does a standard plaster dressing with the exception that the adjacent joints are permitted a ROM as the patient tolerates the movement without pain. The evidence seems to suggest that the fracture healing is not delayed and may in fact be accelerated slightly, as experimental evidence has suggested.[22] The principle involved is that of weight-bearing in the cast-brace, with lateral and longitudinal compressive effects of the soft tissue mass on the bone during weight-bearing to provide stabilization that, although not rigid, is more nearly physiological. The same principle applies to upper limb fractures, where muscle forces act on the fracture site. The reader is referred to publications on the subject before undertaking this method, which requires meticulous attention to detail.

Pins used to reduce a fracture are sometimes incorporated in plaster to maintain the length and alignment of the fracture, a method mostly replaced in large medical centers by skeletal fixation devices (frames). This technique prevents the com-

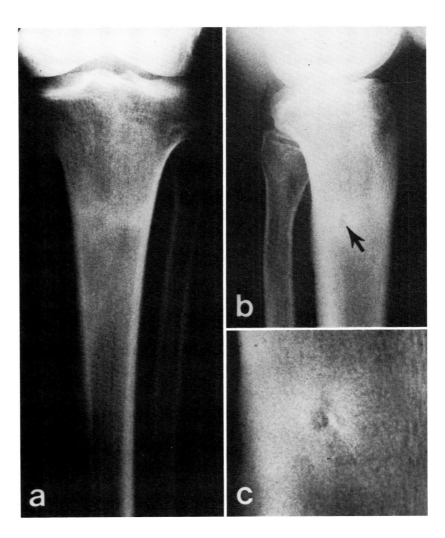

Fig. 4-8. AP (**A**), lateral (**B**), and spot (**C**) radiographs of a tibial "ring sequestrum" pin tract infection (arrow) secondary to infection, necrosis, and sequestration in the proximal tibia.

pression effect of muscle action within the plaster dressing so that as resorption at the fracture site occurs there may be interference with the callus formation at the fracture surfaces. The peripheral callus is not particularly troubled beyond the interference caused by the nature of the injury and the damage to the periosteum and soft tissues. It is therefore imperative that the pins are removed as soon as is practical to prevent the distraction effect of their presence, as there is a high incidence of delayed union or nonunion in long bone fractures treated by this method. For example, with a fracture of the shaft of the tibia, such pins should not be in place longer than 6 weeks.

Several types of external immobilizers that re-

quire pins have come into use since the 1940s. They have the advantages of achieving reduction and providing free access to soft tissue wounds for dressing changes and limited surgical procedures during the course of treatment of open fractures, as depicted in case 4-4 (Fig. 4-4). The method has the same disadvantage as pins and plaster in that a high incidence of delayed union or nonunion is associated with their prolonged use. The opportunity for distraction of the fracture site is great and should be recognized and countered. Similarly, the opportunity to apply compression in a noncomminuted fracture is present so that fracture callus could be enhanced in that circumstance.

It goes without saying that with any method in

which pins project from bone through skin the potential for bacterial organisms to produce infection at the site is increased (Fig. 4-8). Any surgeon who uses pins to traverse soft tissues to fix bones should be aware of the risk of additional damage to vessels and nerves in those soft tissues.

SOFT TISSUE INJURY

Except with stress fractures and minimally displaced fractures, soft tissue injury is a component of most fractures. It is therefore appropriate that we briefly consider the injury to soft tissue associated with fractures. Whenever there is a disruption of any tissue, the same things occur in soft tissue as in bone. Mainly there is hemorrhage and exudate as well as damage to one or all the components of soft tissue: muscle, fascia, tendon, blood vessels, and intermuscular connective tissue. With open fractures the skin and subcutaneous fat are damaged as well.

The initial aspects of any tissue injury are similar, depending on the nature of the wound. How it is incurred is obviously important in both soft tissue and bone. It is obvious that an open injury takes on a different dimension than a closed one; but even a closed fracture has wide variability, as has been seen for fractures produced by motor vehicle accidents. In the latter case, mechanical injury is imparted to the bone and soft tissues, in contrast to that seen with a stress fracture, with which there is essentially no soft tissue component.

The open wound varies again with the kinetic energy of the injury. A minimal, low-energy, localized blow that produces a contusion and a local hemorrhage and may break the bone is different from a high-energy injury such as a high-velocity gunshot wound. Extensive soft tissue damage may result from the 1,800 to 2,500 feet/second velocity bullet compared to damage seen in a low-velocity gunshot wound, where little or less soft tissue damage is produced.[1,10,17]

The classification[12-15] of the soft tissue wounds associated with open fractures divides them into three types: (1) clean wounds less than one centimeter in length; (2) lacerations longer than one centimeter without extensive flaps, avulsions, or damage to the subcutaneous tissues; and (3) lacerations with the above-mentioned lesions. Special categories of type 3 are gunshot wounds, wounds requiring microvascular repairs, etc. The sequences of the response to all three types of soft tissue injury, in any of the structures damaged, are the same as those described for bony injury (Ch. 3). For convenience of description, they are divided into the same four stages, hemorrhage and necrosis; organization of the hematoma; elaboration of fibrous tissue; and remodeling of the fibrous tissue. These stages, as in bone, represent a continuum, characterized as the repair process, but, in soft tissues that process differs from repair in bone in two respects. One is that the only new tissue produced is fibrous (scar), whereas in bone it may be fibrous, cartilaginous, or osseous. The other is that the end result never is the restitution of the affected structures to their previous state—the scar, however remodeled, is permanent. This repair process, for the various structures in the soft tissue, skin, fat, muscle, tendon, etc., is further described in Chapter 6.

For the repair to proceed well, the vascular network must be regenerated from the viable parts of blood vessels that have been transected or thrombosed. Blood flow must be established promptly, to nourish any of the viable structures and to support the high metabolic processes involved in the repair—the multiplication of cells, and elaboration of collagen.

The disrupted arteries, veins, and capillaries regenerate by forming solid columns of cells at their ends and sides and then these columns grow into and across the wound. The buds join adjacent proliferating buds and mature vessels and become canalized so that blood flow is reestablished. The lymphatics follow a similar path to canalization.

At the same time fibroblasts appear in the wound, originating in part from fixed cells that have survived and, for the most part from precursor cells brought to the wound through the blood. They produce the collagen fibers that ultimately will be the scar of repair. Muscle that is injured also must be repaired and collagen is needed for its endomysium and perimysium as well as for the fascial septa. Likewise, the fat will contain collagen fibers when the repair is complete.

Only a small portion of the muscle that is injured

will be restored to normal. Those fibers in which the sarcolemmal tubes remain intact will have the actual sarcoplasm regenerated. Perhaps a few muscle fibers will recover from a brief period of hypoxia, but most do not. The residual scar in muscle and fat develops over a period of weeks, and undergoes reorganization for several months.

One of the important aspects of the repair of the soft tissues is the restoration of the gliding planes between muscles, tendons and the other tissues (skin, fat, bone). The feature that distinguishes scar from normal connective tissues (e.g., tendon, fascia) is that the collagen fibers have a random orientation, whereas the normal structures have collagen bundles disposed in directions appropriate for their mechanical function. As the scar is forming, and especially in the first week or two after the wounding, movements of the injured tissues will influence the ways in which the collagen is laid down, whereas complete immobility of the tissues allows the fibers to be oriented in random fashion. Therefore, if gliding movements of the muscles and tendons are to be restored, one should not completely immobilize the part, except for the first few days after the injury. That immobilization serves the purpose of protecting the thrombosed vessels from reinjury, and it also protects the fragile newly formed vessels. Early motion, after the short period of complete protection minimizes the task of reorganization of the scar. The repair of the individual connective tissue structures will be further discussed later (Ch. 6).

When there is a severe injury to the soft tissues, with concomitant impairment of the blood supply to the part, there is an effect not only on the repair mechanisms in the soft tissues, but also on the healing of the injured (fractured? necrotic?) bone. Thus there frequently is a need for procedures to accelerate the restoration of the blood supply to the part. For this purpose, transposition of muscle, or a skin flap, with blood supply intact may be indicated, or a pedicle graft, or a microvascular anastomosis. None of these procedures can be pursued without concomitant attention to the other important components of the injury besides the wound in the soft tissues. One prerequisite for success of any of the procedures mentioned will be stability of the fracture fragments and therefore the means chosen to stabilize them must be one that does not inter-

fere with (or perhaps doom) the soft tissues. Other injuries, e.g., to the contralateral limb, or to viscera, may dictate the course of therapy and may, indeed make it impossible to pursue what would be considered the ideal regimen for the part, if it were the only injured area. Then the surgeon's choice may be the deferring of definitive procedures until the ideal regimen is possible, or the choice of a suitable, but not ideal alternative.

When a fracture fails to heal the accepted convention is to designate the circumstance as "delayed union" if not more than six months have elapsed from the time of injury. After nine months failure to heal is called a nonunion. More often than not a delayed union or nonunion cannot be confidentially attributed to a single pathophysiological deficit, and often one assigns to the complication a multifactorial etiology. The usual factors adduced by the surgeon are: inadequate immobilization of the fracture fragment; inadequate reduction; excessive soft tissue injury, possibly causing vascular insufficiency; necrosis of a large area of bone as caused by either the injury, or the early treatment rendered; infection; and systemic disease. Since nonunion tends to occur most frequently in a few locations and hardly ever in others, some have speculated that local deficiencies in the potential of tissues to repair occur at those sites (e.g., lower part of the tibia, carpal navicular). That speculation has resulted in therapy designed to stimulate local tissues to increase their elaboration of cells and matrix. Two of the therapies designed on that rationale are the application of an electric current or potential across the area of nonunion, and the injection of so-called inductor substances into it. The substances, which are derived from chemical or enzymatic processing of bone, theoretically stimulate the osteoblasts in repair. Neither of these therapies as yet have been subjected to rigorous controlled testing.

A histological description of a nonunion helps to put in perspective the five factors just mentioned (excepting infection). Since the site of the nonunion, even in so small a bone as the carpal navicular, is much too large for photomicrographic illustrations of adequate magnification, only a few details need be provided to portray the essentials of the pathophysiology. The predominating tissue always is fibrous, and, because months of fibrosis have elapsed, the scar always is firm, and it forms a continuous layer covering the two fracture surfaces. The scar however reveals some inflammatory activity in focal areas, and that undoubtedly is caused by the preternatural motion of the ununited fragments. The adjacent bone will manifest some measure of formation of new bone-callus and if that measure is large, the non-union is termed hypertrophic while, if small, it is termed atrophic. If motion has been considerable, a synovial-lined sac may be found between the fracture fragments — a pseudoarthrosis. Finally, in addition one may encounter residuals of the original injury — old hematoma or necrotic areas in the bones, or in small fragments. Delayed union and nonunion are considered in more detail in Chapter 5.

In adults, as we have indicated, even though normal bone substance and no scar may be the endpoint of repair, there may still be some microscopic abnormality of haversian systems in the fracture site in either the cortical or trabecular bone or gross evidence of a healed fracture. Such repair may continue for many years, as noted by an active radioisotope scan in a fracture healed for 26 years (Fig. 4-9).

As we have noted in the examples above, the quantitative aspects of fracture repair account for (1) variations in the rate and quality of fracture healing; (2) a rational basis for the recognition, prevention, and treatment of complications of fractures; (3) recognition of repair processes simulating tumors; and (4) treatment decisions.

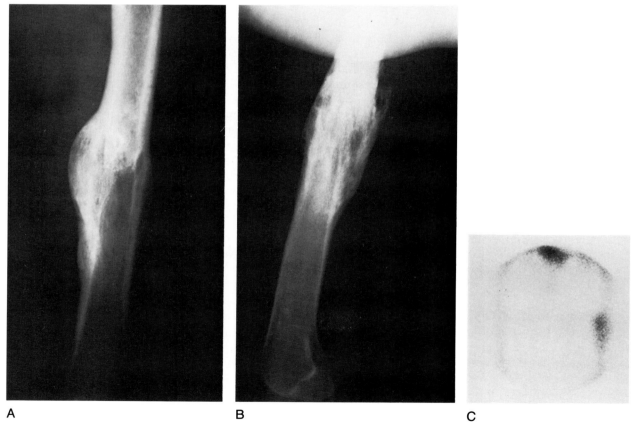

A   B   C

Fig. 4-9. AP (**A**) and lateral (**B**) radiographs and a ^{99m}Tc DP bone scan (**C**) of a fracture of the femur after 26 years.

DECISION-MAKING IN THE THERAPY OF FRACTURES

From the material covered in Chapter 3 and the foregoing parts of this chapter, it should be apparent that there are numerous considerations that influence the choice of therapy, whether the fracture is simple or complex. Which one should have priority is the key question. Should function be regained in a short period of time even if the long-term result is somewhat compromised? If so, does the phrase "a short period of time" mean a week or a month when other considerations, e.g., economics, govern the choice? Is the risk/benefit ratio the overriding consideration?

Because so many variables exist in the characteristics and approach to any one fracture, general principles in therapy are difficult to enunciate, but one paramount principle should be emphasized: The surgeon must plan the therapy step by step, not all at once. In many relatively straightforward cases, the step-by-step process may be accomplished quickly, perhaps within an hour or two. For complicated cases, however, the step-by-step process may take weeks or months, each step being governed by what has transpired before, what the present options are, and what the options will be in the future. When choosing any one present option, the surgeon must take into account whether future options are being preserved or one or more important ones are being eliminated.

Even step 1, evaluation of the patient at presentation, requires the exercise of options. Obviously, any potentially fatal condition (bleeding, shock) are immediately attended to. Then, with a straightforward uncomplicated case, e.g., one that presents with no other injury but a closed uncomminuted fracture in an extremity, step 1 would be immobilizing the fracture in some sort of splint for the patient's comfort while a physical examination and radiographic examination are done. Even then, *rigid* adherence to a formulated step progression (an algorithm) is to be condemned because that program requires that *every* contingency be included in the formulation and that each contingency be accessible in quantitative terms. There is no provision for the possibility that an unforeseen event might either alter or invalidate the progression. There is no possibility of expressing quantitatively all the aspects of each contingency.

Consider a situation where step 1 as described above, is not yet completed; i.e., the initial finding in the case just mentioned on physical examination is a pulseless extremity, but the remainder of the physical examination has not been done and the radiographs have not been obtained. Obviously, pulselessness has absolute priority over any fracture in that its cause must be found and the appropriate measures taken to restore the pulse. Yet, even if pulselessness were included in the algorithm, its duration, the reliability of its assessment, and so on cannot be stipulated. Nevertheless, pursuit of a stepwise plan, not so detailed as to be called an algorithm, in most cases has great advantages. It allows determinations that often are difficult to obtain in the urgency of the immediate post-injury climate — determinations, for example, of the probability that the patient might not be cooperative with a program that required his or her active participation, or that an important medical condition existed that was not evident on physical examination and not revealed in the history. Either of these determinations might exercise an important influence on the choice of the definitive therapy.

Equally important in the step-by-step elaboration of the therapy is the recognition of probable stages in the pathophysiology of the lesion. In the straightforward case now under consideration, for instance, step 1 includes immobilization of the extremity in a splint. That measure mostly is designed to avert a more copious hematoma at the fracture site. Rarely is a patient seen so soon after injury that clotting of the extravasated blood has not had time to occur; and if the interval is an hour or more, enough time will have elapsed that most of the ends of the large vessels have retracted and are occluded by a thrombus. The immobilization is designed to prevent dislodgement of the thrombus and additional injury to vessels. Moreover, it is easy to picture the sharp fracture fragments as destructive agents if they are allowed to move through reflex contraction of musculature or are forced here and there during manipulation of the extremity.

If the injury is more complex, as was described in

the case of the compound fracture of the tibia (case 4-4), the act of immobilization would also be part of the therapeutic regimen, but it probably would not constitute step 1. If there was still active bleeding when the patient was first treated, step 1 would be application of a tourniquet; and in view of the extensive open injury to soft tissues, step 2 would be protection of the area from further contamination. Only then would immobilization be the step indicated. The further sequence of steps, in that case, has already been summarized under the considerations that govern débridement. However, the pathophysiological interpretation of the severity and progress of the lesion must include an assessment, for severe injuries, of probabilities as to whether the treatment, appropriately designated in such severe cases as salvage, will be worthwhile. Hansen[16] aptly considered the options:

> With the advent of highly sophisticated internal and external fixation devices and the enormous attention paid to severely injured patients in recent years, it is often thought that almost any extremity can be salvaged if the technique is good. Further medical advances such as free tissue transfers and the refined skills developed by some microsurgeons tempt us even further to seek triumphs of technique over reason.
>
> The decision to amputate or not to amputate has significant repercussions medically, economically, socially, and medicolegally . . . there is no question that prolonged hospitalization and recumbency have a negative effect on the total individual both physically and mentally. The patient suffers economically as he or she is unable to continue earning a living, but prolonged hospitalizations are also extremely costly to society since these patients frequently remained disabled and do not become productive citizens after the injury . . . after two years there is almost 100% probability that the patient will never return to work. Reconstruction of the limb in order to salvage it after this type of injury can easily take two or more years . . . if the individual is the head of a household, which is often the case, this role is taken away, at least temporarily. If this continues for a long period of time, the individuals self-image, ego and position in the family may be forever destroyed.
>
>   . . . in the event that salvage attempts are continued over a long period of time and the final

result leads to a late amputation, the patient may realize that he or she is much better off after the amputation is finally done, but that everything has been lost during the duration of the treatment. The surgeon may then be criticized for prolonging the treatment program and adversely affecting the patient's family and lifestyle as a result.

Two of the cases (4-3 and 4-4) described above are excellent illustrations of just that problem of assessment. After several years — the fracture of the femur having healed but the extremity being of little use because of the scarring — the patient (case 4-3) desired and obtained an amputation. The patient in case 4-4 has union of the tibia but with extensive scarring of the soft tissues of the leg and limited function of the foot and ankle, and he may yet come to amputation.

The insertion of screws to fix fracture fragments or a plate creates an additional problem that may have clinical consequences. The use of a drill and insertion of a screw generates heat and local necrosis of bone estimated at 0.5 mm. Resorption of the dead bone may loosen the screw(s) and plate. If the surgical field is infected, the areas of dead bone may sequester to form "ring sequestra." The removal of plates, screws, and sequestra is necessary, as the incidence of delayed or nonunion is higher in the infected fractures.[14] The insertion of smooth or threaded pins for traction or for external fixation methods produces the same potential for heat, necrosis, infection, and "ring sequestrum" (Fig. 4-7). After removal of an internal fixation device, particularly a plate and screws, sufficient time with protection of the bone from stress must be allowed to avoid refracture through a screw hole that acts as a stress raiser until the hole in response to Wolff's law is repaired with bone, usually 4 to 6 weeks. This protection is in the form of plaster immobilization or splinting of the bone with graduated activity permitted or by increasing weight-bearing with crutches or cane for lower limb bones.

Complications associated with surgery (open reduction) of fractures are more serious than those seen with fractures treated by nonsurgical methods (e.g., closed reduction and plaster immobilization or cast-bracing, closed reduction and fixation with an external pin fixation device). Fractures do heal with each of these methods, but each has particular requirements for optimal effectiveness. The physician must be familiar with the principles of fracture repair before selecting any method of treatment for a specific fracture.

REFERENCES

1. Barach E, Tomlanovich et al: A pathophysiologic examination of wounding of firearms. I & II. J Trauma 1986
2. Byrd HS, Spicer TE, Cierney G III: Management of open tibial fractures. Plast Reconstr Surg 76:719, 1985
3. Caudle RJ, Stern PJ: Severe open fractures of the tibia. J Bone Joint Surg [Am] 69:801, 1987
4. Chapman MW, Hansen ST Jr: Part III. p. 199. In Rockwood CA, Green DP (eds): Current Concepts in the Management of Open Fractures. JB Lippincott, Philadelphia, 1984
5. Cierny G, Byrd HS, Jones PE: Primary vs. delayed soft tissue coverage for severe open tibial fractures: a comparison of results. Clin Orthop 178:54, 1983
6. Cooney WP III, Fitzgerald RH Jr, et al: Quantitative wound cultures in upper extremity trauma. J Trauma 22:112, 1982
7. Edwards CC: Staged reconstruction of complex open tibial fractures using Hoffman external fixation: decisions and dilemmas. Clin Orthop 178:130, 1983
8. Ger R: The management of open fractures of the tibia with skin loss. J Trauma 10:112, 1970
9. Ger R: Muscle transposition for treatment and prevention of chronic post traumatic osteomyelitis of the tibia. J Bone Joint Surg [Am] 59:784, 1977
10. Gregory CF: Open fractures. p. 169. In Rockwood CA, Green DP (eds): Fractures in Adults. 2nd Ed. JB Lippincott, Philadelphia, 1984
11. Gustilo RB: Management of infected fractures. p. 105. In Evarts CMcC (ed): Surgery of the Musculoskeletal System. 2nd Ed. Vol. 4. Churchill Livingstone, New York, 1989
12. Gustilo RB: Management of infected nonunion. p. 135. In Evarts CMcC (ed): Surgery of the Musculoskeletal System. 2nd Ed. Vol. 4. Churchill Livingstone, New York, 1989
13. Gustilo RB, Anderson JT: Prevention of infection in the treatment of 1025 open fractures of long bones. J Bone Joint Surg [Am] 58:453, 1976
14. Gustilo RB, et al: Problems in the management of type III (severe) open fractures: a new classification of type III open fractures. J Trauma 24:742, 1984
15. Gustilo RB, Simpson L, Nixon R, Ruiza: Analysis of 511 open fractures. Clin Orthop 66:148, 1969
16. Hansen ST Jr: Type IIIC tibial fracture. J Bone Joint Surg [Am] 69:799, 1987 (editorial)
17. Hennessy MJ, Banks HH, et al: Extremity gunshot wound and gunshot fracture in civilian practice. Clin Orthop 114:296, 1976
18. Holden CEA: The role of blood supply in healing of diaphyseal fractures, an exploratory study. J Bone Joint Surg [Am] 54:993, 1972
19. Olerud S, Danckwerdt-Lilliestrom: Fracture healing and compression osteosynthesis in the dog. J Bone Joint Surg [Br] 50:844, 1968
20. Pulskamp JR, McFarland GB Jr: The effects of compression plate fixation on bone healing in dog femurs. Unpublished data, 1969
21. Rhinelander F: The normal microcirculation of diaphyseal cortex and its response to fracture. J Bone Joint Surg [Am] 50:784, 1968
22. Rockwood C, et al: Emergency Care and Transportation of the Sick and Injured. Committee on Injuries, American Academy of Orthopedic Surgeons, 1971
23. Stern PJ, Neal HW, Gregory RO, et al: Function reconstruction of an extremity by free soft tissue transfer of the latissimus dorsi. J Bone Joint Surg [Am] 65:729, 1983
24. Weiland AJ, Moore JR, Hotchkiss RM: Soft tissue procedures for reconstruction of tibial shaft fractures. Clin Orthop 178:42, 1983
25. Wood MB, Cooney WA, Irons GB: Lower extremity salvage and reconstruction by free tissue transfer. Clin Orthop 201:151, 1985

5

Special Fractures and Injuries

There are certain variations inherent in several special but common clinical situations. They have been chosen for discussion here to emphasize the modifications of the repair process. While that process is still capable of permitting some part of the healing of the fractures, even when conditions are suboptimal, attention to the pathophysiological influences is needed for the repair to be successful.

FRACTURES INTO JOINTS

Whenever a bone is fractured near a joint, the surgeon must envisage the possibility that a plane of the fracture enters the joint. In fact, even when the bone seems to have been the structure that bore the brunt of the injury, it should be suspected that there might have been a break in the articular surface. That suspicion is intensified if, within minutes of the moment of injury, a large effusion develops. That effusion—blood in all likelihood—is more likely to come from the vascular subchondral bone than from any of the other intra-articular structures. After all, the cartilage itself has no vessels; and ligaments, either intra-articular or extra-articular, have only a few small vessels. The suspicion leads the surgeon to appropriate radiographic studies, e.g., special views, arthrography, and CT scan.

Transarticular fractures are those in which one or more fracture fragments include not only a substantial amount of the cancellous subchondral bone and the covering articular cartilage but perhaps some adjoining cortical bone as well. A special type of transarticular fracture is the so-called osteo-

chondral fracture, where there is only a flake of cancellous bone in continuity with the detached fragment of hyaline articular cartilage.

Transarticular fractures present special problems for the patient and the physician. Because cartilage repair in animals and humans occurs by formation of fibrocartilage, not hyaline cartilage, the goal is to minimize the size of the gap in the articular cartilage that must be bridged, so as to provide the best functional articular surface. A study in rabbits[4] suggested that accurate coaptation of the cartilage with compression fixation after an intra-articular fracture was induced produced repair by a tissue that closely resembled hyaline cartilage. Otherwise there was repair by fibrocartilage. The surgeon is rarely faced with such an ideal situation for treatment because of complicating factors, illustrated in case 5-1.

Case 5-1 A patient suffered a closed fracture of the radial head during a fall. At presentation, less than an hour after the injury, the elbow was markedly swollen. Although the patient tolerated minor passive flexion and extension of the elbow, any pronation or supination of the forearm elicited severe pain. These findings are pathognomonic of a fracture of the radial head. The details of the radiographs contribute two main items of information that have pathophysiological implications: (1) The head of the radius has been broken in two parts, so that one part is displaced a few millimeters from the other and has been pushed distally a few millimeters; and (2) the fragment described above constitutes about one-half of the radial surface of the radiohumeral joint.

The pathophysiological implications of this displacement, beyond those that pertain to repair of the gap between fracture fragments of bone (cancellous and cortical), already discussed in Chapter 4, concern the articular surfaces of the radius, one of which bears on the articular surface of the lateral condyle of the humerus and the other on the lateral articular surface of the ulna and on the annular ligament. In the unreduced state, the first articular surface, instead of being saucer-like, able to glide back and forth over the rounded lateral condyle, and able to rotate on that structure for 180° when the forearm supinates or pronates, now is not congruent with the condyle. One-half of it is in position, but the other half is displaced, presenting the fracture edge as a sharp ridge that cuts into the condyle on all of the motions just mentioned. With respect to the second (radioulnar) joint that has been disrupted, the ring-shaped articulation of the radius lacks a firm abutment against the annular ligament and ulna for nearly one-half its circumference. If allowed to heal in the unreduced state, the fibrocartilaginous expanse that will bridge the gaps will make incongruous the articular surfaces of both of the joints.

Case 5-1, dating back many years, was chosen because a specimen was available for histological study. The surgeon's decision, because of other injuries in the patient caused by high voltage electricity, was to accept the position of the fragments (Fig. 5-1A&B) when attempts at closed reduction were unsuccessful. Parenthetically, it is agreed that with such a large free fragment the surgeon's decision should be to attempt an open reduction, so that the cartilaginous articular surfaces would be restored, with only hairline fracture gaps and fixation of the fragments, thereby stabilizing the fragments firmly enough to allow early motion of the elbow and forearm. In case 5-1, the fracture united by fibrocartilage (Fig. 5-1C–G), but after 5 months secondary post-traumatic degenerative arthritis (Fig. 5-1H) and synovitis (Fig. 5-1I) impaired the function of the radiohumeral and radioulnar joints to such an extent that the pain and restricted motion required treatment, i.e., excision of the radial head.

The subchondral bone of an intra-articular fracture undergoes repair as described in Chapter 3 under Cancellous Bone Repair. Granulation tissue, including its fibrous tissue component, first fills the gap between the two fragments, including their bony and cartilaginous components. The fibrous tissue formed in the gap in cartilage may develop into fibrocartilage; and if the size of the defect or gap is small, the fibrocartilaginous area of repair may function well.[1,5] This prognosis holds true for the well reduced fracture, with minimal post-traumatic degenerative arthritis in most patients being the expected result. It is particularly important to reduce accurately the major articular fragments in the load-bearing area of all diarthrodial joints. This measure is as true for the femoral condyle and tibial plateau as for the radius, as illustrated. Accurate reduction is desirable but not as critical at the margins of joints or for certain articular structures (e.g., radial styloid process, medial malleolus, or olecranon process), where apparently lesser loads permit some irregularity of the articular surface to persist without major impairment of the joint.

Certain intra-articular fractures occur for which compromises must be made because perfect restoration of the articular surface is impossible. Examples are comminuted fractures of the tibial plateau, the talar surface, or the acetabulum. With such fractures there are many fragments of cortical bone as well as cancellous bone, and some of the fragments are covered by articular cartilage. The fragments of bone unite readily by intramembranous and enchondral ossification, whereas the articular fragments with cartilage unite by fibro-cartilage.[1-3] When the comminution is especially severe, it may be impossible to approximate all the fragments in their anatomical positions.

The individual cases vary greatly, not only with regard to the extent of comminution of articular fragments and their displacement, but also with respect to two other important aspects of the injury, i.e., the extent of the bony injury and the extent of the injury and also of the surgery on soft tissues. To achieve the goal of minimal impairment of the extremity, a treatment regimen must be chosen that orders and coordinates the priorities properly. As noted later in Chapter 6, the dangers of infection in open fractures take some priority over all other considerations, but that priority is not absolute or overriding. If during the first week after the injury those dangers can be eliminated, the need for early motion of the joint to allow the irregularities of the joint surface to be molded can be met. If a regimen of several weeks of treatment to

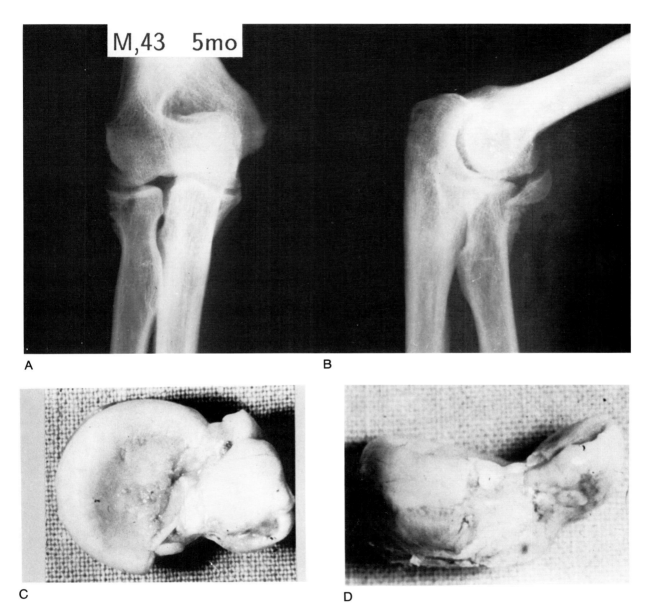

A

B

C

D

Fig. 5-1. **(A & B)** Comminuted articular fracture of the radial head in a 43-year-old male secondary to electrical injury. **(C & D)** Surface and side views of the gross specimen. *(Figure continues.)*

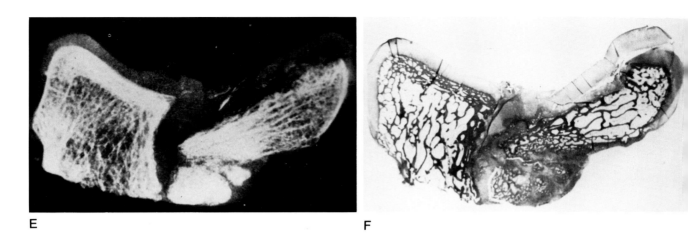

E

F

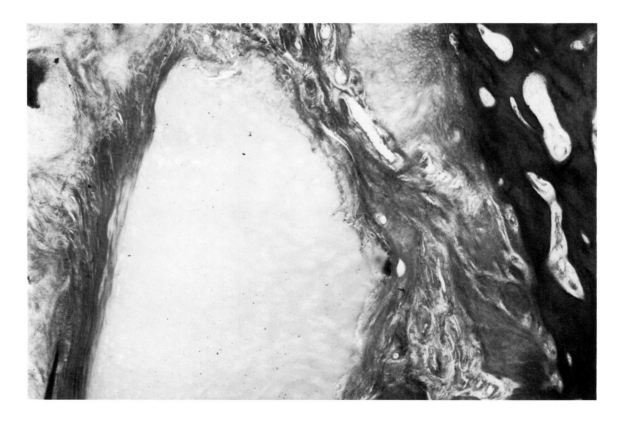

Fig. 5-1 *(Continued).* **(E)** Lateral radiograph and **(F)** photomicrograph of a coronal section of the specimen showing the malunion. (×1). **(G)** Fibrocartilaginous and osseous repair of the articular surface (×100). *(Figure continues.)*

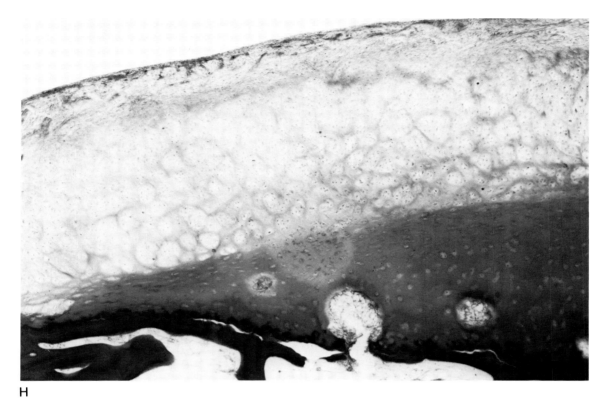

H

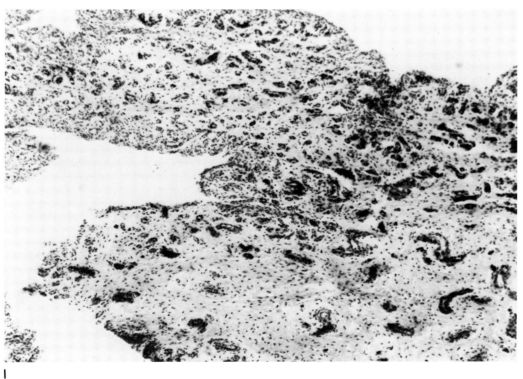

I

Fig. 5-1 *(Continued).* (H) Post-traumatic degenerative changes: proliferation of hyaline cartilage cells and subchondral cortex vascular invasion (×100). (I) Post-traumatic synovitis (×40).

avoid infection is planned, it must be done with the calculated loss of the benefit that early motion can provide for molding the repair fibrocartilage. If the extent of the bony injury adjacent to the joint is so great that the required level of load-bearing potential is not attained when healing is complete, that requirement may have to be met by extensive bone grafting or internal fixation devices. Here too the temporal consideration is important if not paramount. Unless motion of the injured joint can be started about a week after the injury, the benefits of molding of the fibrous and cartilaginous repair at the articular surface are sacrificed.[2,3,5]

It should be evident that the many trade-offs in the priorities of treatment are matters of clinical judgment. The surgeon's opinion, not only of the anatomical and pathological details inherent in the particular case but also of his or her own role vis-à-vis those details, plays a crucial role in the choice of treatment. In case 5-1, the surgeon could have opted for operative reduction, as mentioned, but with the anticipation of having to use a device for fixation of the fragments. With so small a bony fragment, screw fixation might well be impossible and might lead to further fragmentation of the subchondral bone. In addition, the likelihood that the orbicular ligament would have been torn and would need extensive repair should be seriously entertained. Such considerations might weigh so heavily in the surgeon's judgment that it might well be decided to see what conservative therapy can do because the other alternative, immediate removal of the radial head, is not an attractive one. Furthermore, that option would still be available whatever regimen of early treatment was chosen.

Osteochondral fractures, a special category of intra-articular fractures, are characterized by the fact that the fragment either has a small flake of bone with articular cartilage lining one face (at the time of injury) or it consists entirely of cartilage. The special pathophysiological features of this kind of fracture, in addition to what has already been said about healing of articular surfaces, can be categorized into two groups for the purpose of reviewing clinical implications. The grouping depends on whether the osteochondral fracture is discovered (diagnosed) soon after injury or much later.

In the first instance the clinical signs of injury implicate the joint (immediate massive hemoarthrosis), but the osteochondral fragment, even if recognized, plays a secondary role to the ligamentous injury. The pathophysiological consequence of ligamentous injury in the ankle or knee, where most osteochondral fractures occur, is an unstable joint unless measures are taken to ensure healing of the ligaments without elongating them. On the other hand, the pathophysiological consequence of loss of a small sector of the articular surface, particularly if it is not in a site essential to the most important part of the arc of motion of the joint, may be of small impact.

In instances where the osteochondral fragment is not discovered until long after the injury (months or years perhaps) two pathophysiological facts assume clinical significance. One is that small fragments of cartilage introduced freely into the joint do not undergo necrosis or resorption. They survive, nourished by the synovial fluid, and tend to grow. Regardless of whether this fragment contains a bony flake (which undergoes necrosis and slow resorption), the loose body, then, over many months, grows and even manifests the sequences of endochondral ossification so that in the center there may be a new nubbin of cancellous bone. The sequela of having a loose body in the joint is either locking of the joint when this loose body is caught between the articulating surfaces or damage to those surfaces by abrasion. However, on many occasions the loose body stays in contact with the synovial membrane and may even become attached to it, so the situation simulates synovial chondromatosis. That condition, in which the synovial membrane elaborates *multiple* nodules of cartilage by metaplasia, is only rarely confused with a traumatic osteochondral fracture because the fracture rarely contributes many cartilaginous free fragments in the joint. However, when synovial chondromatosis nodules free themselves from the membrane and become loose bodies, there is an obvious problem in the differential diagnosis and a parallel problem in treatment. In traumatic cases, all that is needed is removal of the fragment(s). When there is metaplasia, the involved membrane itself should also be removed insofar as that is feasible.

With certain osteochondral fractures a flake of subchondral bone separates from the mass of cancellous bone adjoining the articular cartilage, which itself is not broken through entirely. The small disc of bone that separates is not displaced, and, at its periphery at least, an arc of the overlying cartilage remains in continuity even though its basal layer is cracked. The crack usually is angled away from the bony disc so the cartilage of the fragment is larger than the bony disc. The best explanation for this situation is that the involved area of cartilage has been forcibly compressed to the point where the less compressible bone underneath it is compacted. As the trabeculae fracture, further compression permits a crack to develop at the periphery of the compacted bone, and that crack progresses into the cartilage for a variable distance in the various sections of the circle of involved bone. If the crack becomes complete, a free fragment is formed that can be extruded into the joint. If it remains incomplete throughout, the osteocartilaginous fragment remains in situ and is recognizable grossly by the fact that it is overly compressible against the bone. With time the cartilage changes color, from blue-gray to yellowish. Sections of the periphery may show extension of the crack into the joint, and in that event an arthrogram reveals penetration of the medium under the fragment.

The pathophysiological consequences of this train of events, in terms of the bony part of the fragment, are that (1) it undergoes necrosis; (2) callus forms in the viable area of the bony bed; (3) as the necrotic area is invaded by vessels and resorption can occur, the fragment unites with its bed, provided the fragment remains in place and motion is interdicted. In this situation motion means not so much the angular motion of the joint but, rather, compression and decompression, i.e., weight-bearing. The clinical implications for therapy are obvious. If the fragment is not free, all that is needed is the prevention of weight-bearing on the involved spot (e.g., plaster cast immobilization with the joint at the appropriate angle). If the fragment is free and can be restored to its position, it can be fixed there (by a nail or two). It should be remembered that here too most of the cartilage remains alive, nourished by synovial fluid.

Fracture dislocations present particular problems for treatment related not so much to fracture repair as to the complications of the injury that stem either from the vascular anatomy adjacent to the joint or, when the injury is an open one, the strong propensity of the tissues of the joint to become infected when foreign bodies are introduced. Aseptic necrosis of a fracture fragment is a common feature with fractures of the carpal scaphoid, lunate, humeral head, femoral head, and body of the talus. The repair of aseptic necrosis with or without an associated fracture is dealt with in Chapter 7.

EPIPHYSEAL INJURIES

Epiphyseal fractures belong in this chapter in special situations for a pathophysiological reason that does not pertain to any other of the injuries considered so far — the effect of the injury and the repair process on the growth of the bone(s) (Fig. 5-2A) and therefore on the function of the extremity once repair is complete.[6,12,18–21] For this reason the injuries in question are divided according to their risk in regard to disturbance of growth (Figs. 5-2B–D).

Low Risk Epiphyseal Injuries (Class I)

When the location of the fracture is anywhere through the metaphysis, including the zone of calcified cartilage, it occurs at a level that is mechanically weak so far as the bone and cartilage are concerned. A thick layer of periosteum–perichondrium supplements the hard structures. Figure 5-3 shows a block of bone removed at the time of an epiphyseodesis procedure. It reveals the site at which the calcified cartilage and bone form a junction.

Pathophysiologically, this zone of weakness is witness to two normal, active processes. One of these processes is resorption of the residual cartilaginous struts and the primordial layers of bone deposited along those struts; the other is deposition of new trabeculae of bone, replacing the primordial structures. In other words, remodeling of bone in the metaphysis is ongoing — the metaphysis being the location where primary spongiosa is replaced by secondary spongiosa; i.e., the trabeculae become coarser, thicker, and stronger. Whenever a generalized disease (e.g., leukemia, renal rickets) causes wholesale resorption of bone, the

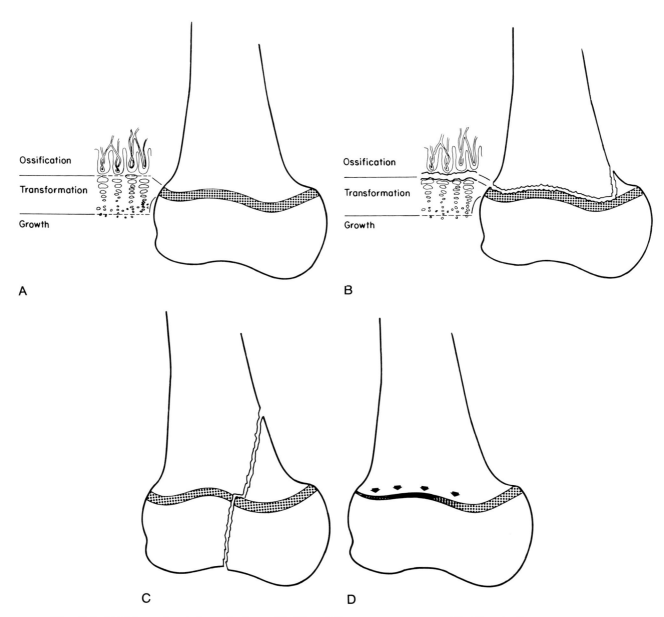

Fig. 5-2. (**A**) Normal epiphyseal plate. (**B**) Class I fracture-separation. (**C**) Class II fracture-separation: transepiphyseal fracture. (**D**) Class II crush injury: epiphyseal fracture.

metaphyses display the maximal effects, and the weakness of those areas is then exaggerated.

The natural hyperactivity of children leads to many skeletal injuries, a good many of which are epiphyseal fracture separations; only minor displacement of the fragments occurs owing to the strength of the periosteum-perichondrium (which is stretched but not torn). Repair of the fracture in this situation is that of cancellous bone, with no anticipated disturbance of the epiphyseal growth (Figs. 5-4 and 5-5).

Minor displacements are generally caused by

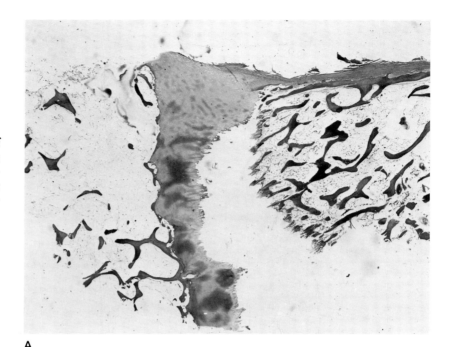

Fig. 5-3. (A) Site of separation of normal epiphyseal plate specimen removed at an epiphysiodesis procedure (×4). **(B)** Separation occurs at the calcified cartilage–bone junction (×100).

A

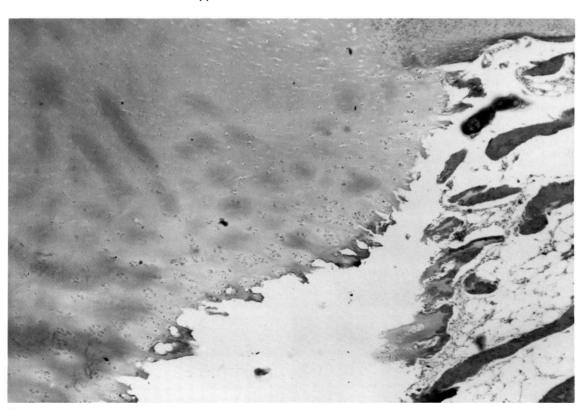

B

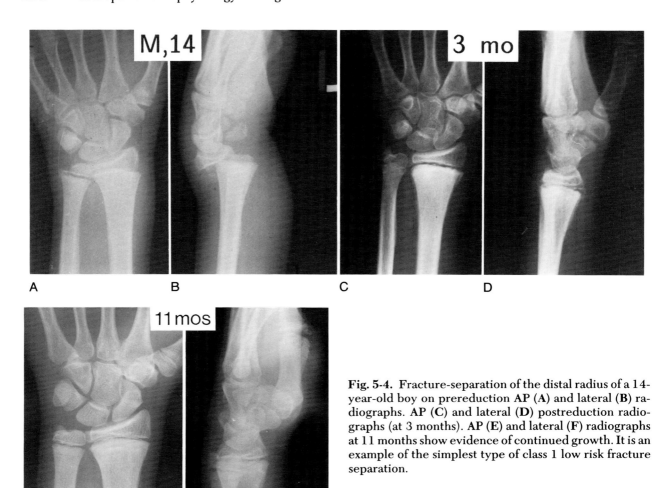

Fig. 5-4. Fracture-separation of the distal radius of a 14-year-old boy on prereduction AP (**A**) and lateral (**B**) radiographs. AP (**C**) and lateral (**D**) postreduction radiographs (at 3 months). AP (**E**) and lateral (**F**) radiographs at 11 months show evidence of continued growth. It is an example of the simplest type of class 1 low risk fracture separation.

trauma that is not severe, and such displacements generally are spontaneously corrected as a function of growth and remodeling.[6,9,14–16,21] Into that function must be factored the number of years of growth to be anticipated; even severe displacements, e.g., birth injuries (Fig. 5-6) or infantile abuse trauma (as with fracture trauma), are followed by complete restitution of normal alignment with no discrepancy in the length of the bone when compared to that on the contralateral, uninjured side.

High Risk Epiphyseal Injuries (Class II)

Certain types of injury are at high risk for disturbed growth: (1) those that result from severe trauma; (2) those that affect only a small sector of the epiphysis-metaphysis (mainly a segment of the periphery); (3) those that cause a fracture plane to traverse the epiphyseal plate, displacing one part of it to an important extent (more than 1 to 2 mm); (4) those in which the fracture plane — traverses not only the epiphyseal cartilage but also the epiphysis

Fig. 5-5. AP (**A**) and axillary (**B**) views of a fracture-separation of the proximal humerus. (**C–E**) Progression of healing, including remodeling of the proximal humerus without growth disturbance.

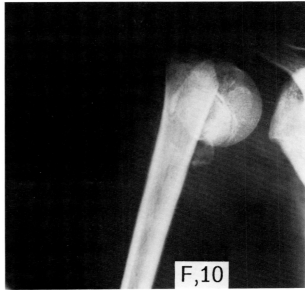

A

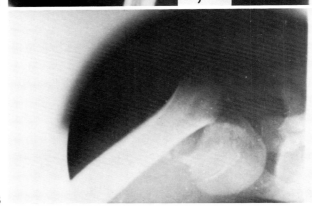

B

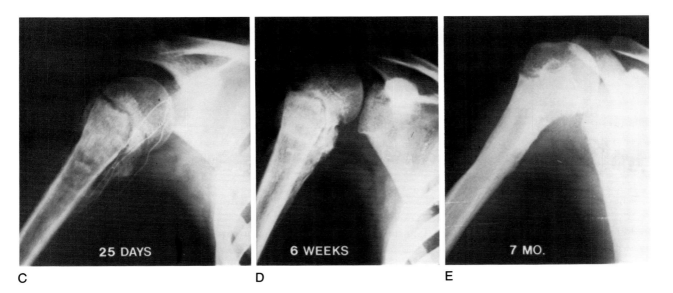

C   D   E

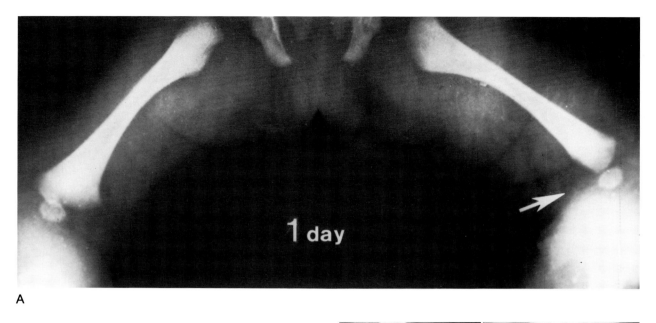

A

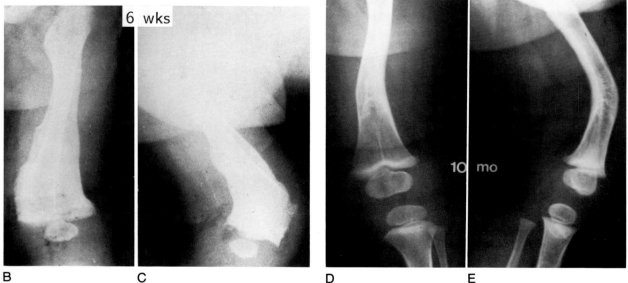

B   C   D   E

Fig. 5-6. (A–H) Sequence of radiographs of a fracture-separation of the distal left femoral epiphysis at a breech delivery to show remodeling of the unreduced fracture separation over 13 years. *(Figure continues.)*

and articular cartilage; (5) those in which the epiphyseal cartilage is severely crushed, regardless of whether there is displacement of fracture fragments (Fig. 5-2C); and (6) those peripheral injuries that occur close to the age of skeletal maturation and tend to cause closure of one section of the epiphyseal plate whereas the remainder of the plate continues to grow.

The Harris-Salter classification[14-16,19] of epiphyseal injuries into four categories serves as a convenient way to regard these injuries, particularly in terms of radiographic appearances. As far as its util-

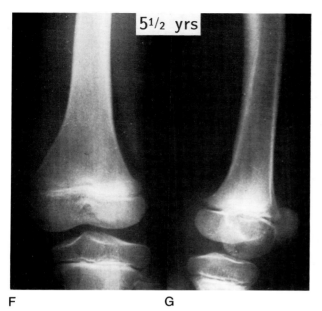

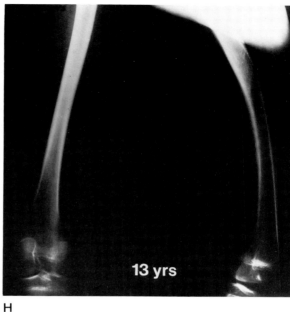

F   G   H

Fig. 5-6 *(Continued)*.

ity for prognosis of disturbances of growth, it does not take into account several of the pathophysiological phenomena just mentioned (e.g., age of the patient and severity of the injury). Moreover, the relative risks of any one of their four classes of injury are not sufficiently discriminative to indicate differences in terms of treatment of the acute injury. In our opinion, few of the epiphyseal injuries require any treatment other than gentle manipulation (closed) reduction. Open reduction or forceful manipulation may well increase the severity of the injury to the growing area of cartilage and further devascularize the already ischemic metaphysis. It should be recalled that there are several small vessels that course into and out of the epiphysis and metaphysis via the metaphyseal cortical segment, and the smaller vessels in that site are terminal vessels with a slow rate of flow. This area therefore is particularly susceptible to vascular injury (see Ch. 2).

When the high risk injury producing an epiphyseal fracture separation is in the distal femoral or proximal tibial location, it results in premature closure of the medial[20] or lateral side of the plate, which in time causes a varus (Fig. 5-7) or valgus

deformity. There is crushing of a portion of the plate along with the vertical fracture. Therefore growth continues from the uninjured remainder of the plate, and the progressive angular deformity begins to develop. The entire plate closes prematurely, so linear growth is decreased. The severity of the angular deformity and inhibition of linear growth depends on the age of the patient, the location of the injury within the plate, the particular epiphysis involved, and the severity of the injury. An injury to the epiphyseal plate of the distal femur (Fig. 5-8) or proximal humerus can result in greater deformity and loss of length if it occurs in a young child rather than in an adolescent who is near the time of skeletal maturity. If the injury involves the distal epiphyseal plate of the tibia, which has less growth potential than the proximal plate, it causes less of an angular deformity and inhibition of growth. An open injury to the epiphyseal plate by violent trauma, e.g., a power lawnmower injury, is certain to cause closure of the plate because in such a case fragments of the plate are lost along with skin and soft tissues, and some of the plate probably is devitalized (Fig. 5-9). Such an eventuality should not deter the surgeon from achieving as accurate a

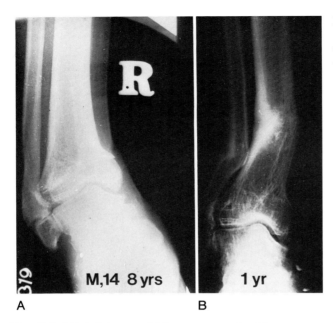

Fig. 5-7. (A) A 14-year-old boy presented with a varus deformity of the right ankle from a crush injury to the distal tibial epiphysis 8 years earlier. He had a class 2 high risk epiphyseal injury. **(B)** One year after tibial osteotomy to correct the deformity.

reduction as possible; the surgeon must try to ensure that the optimal position of the joint will persist with the remaining growth. The bony bridge that tends to develop in the fracture gap through the epiphysis may be kept small, and complete arrest of the growth plate may be delayed until near the end of the growth period (Fig. 5-9).

It should thus be apparent that knowledge of how bones grow and when and how epiphyseal plates close is important before one contemplates a surgical procedure where there is a length inequality or an angular deformity following an injury to an epiphyseal plate.[12,19] Two examples illustrate the pathophysiological principles that underlie the treatment of the sequelae of epiphyseal injuries.

Case 5-2 A 4-year-old girl suffered a closed fracture at the distal tibial epiphysis 9 months prior to the date of presentation. The fracture had been well reduced and the ankle immobilized in a cast for 6 weeks. The presenting complaint was developing varus at the ankle, so that excessive wear was evident on the lateral aspect of the sole of her shoe.

From the radiographs it is evident that there is narrowing of the epiphyseal plate of the tibia medially. The process at work here is development of a bony bridge, not yet apparent on the radiograph. The inhibition of growth medially has caused varus of the ankle; and because the patient is so young, one may expect further, considerable varus to develop, until all growth from the involved epiphysis ceases.

The first measure is to compare the tibias with two radiographic techniques: The first ascertains if the lateral half of the distal tibial epiphysis is somewhat narrow (perhaps less so than the medial half), and the second ascertains the tibial lengths precisely. If either or both of these examinations reveal that there is substantial growth inhibition of the entire epiphysis, the surgical plan will differ somewhat from that to be followed if no such findings exist. Given those findings, the following facts pertain: (1) The growth in tibial length, attributable to the distal epiphysis, is 0.7 cm per year of growth; in a 4-year-old child it amounts to 5 to 6 cm of total inhibition. If at the 9 months postinjury examination there already has been 0.5 cm of inhibition, two conclusions may be drawn. One is that the increase in varus at the ankle would progress little during growth. If this increase is tolerable, a surgical approach to prevention of more varus would be unnecessary, and correction of the varus might also be deferred — to a time when some measure might be substituted to correct the leg length discrepancy, which would surely be formidable. The second conclusion concerns the discrepancy, which if it exceeds a few centimeters should be corrected by epiphyseodesis on the contralateral side (see below) or possibly by tibial lengthening (indicated especially if the child promises to be of short stature. It should be noted that the conclusions depend on an evaluation of a discrepancy of approximately 0.5 cm. So small a distance, as measured on radiographs, brings to the fore the problem of the accuracy of the technique used to expose the radiographic films. Least accurate are ordinary films taken of each leg. Most accurate is an orthoroentgenogram. This technique involves a single film with a tube-to-film distance of 6 feet; a metal rule is strapped to each leg, and separate exposures are targeted at the knees and ankles. Other techniques (ordinary 6-foot films, scanograms) yield results of intermediate accuracy. It

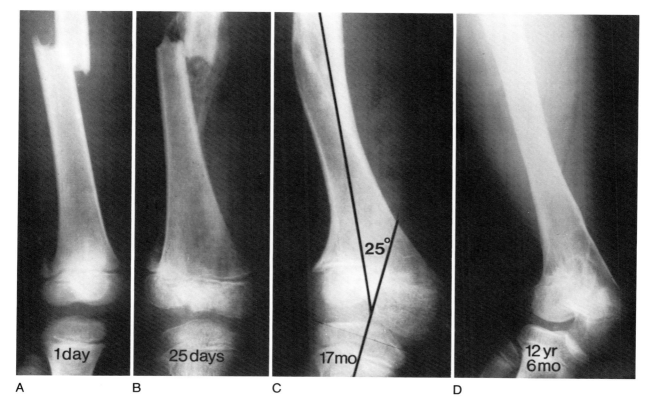

A   B   C   D

Fig. 5-8. A 7-year-old boy sustained a fracture of the shaft of the femur and an epiphyseal fracture-separation of the distal femoral epiphysis in a motor vehicle accident. AP radiographs of the femur including the knee show the initial injury, the union of the fracture of the femur, and closure of the lateral epiphyseal plate as a result of the injury. A varus deformity developed, which was treated by an osteotomy at 17 months followed by a fat graft at the epiphyseal plate laterally with no effect on the correction at 12.5 years.

should also be noted that the accuracy of the orthoroentgenogram is ±1.0 mm.

It has been stipulated that the length discrepancy was 0.5 cm. Suppose now that the discrepancy was a good deal less, possibly zero. What are the pathophysiological implications? The first is that the ankle varus would be progressive, and the second is that the projected leg length discrepancy might not be such as to require equalization of leg lengths. The promise of increasing angulation at the ankle or an already symptomatic varus justifies a rationale of surgical interference with the varization mechanism, namely, the incipient bony (and fibrous) bridge that is forming on the medial aspect of the tibial. Mere excision of that bridge would be followed by scarring and formation of a new bony bridge. Some means is needed to inhibit the growth of those repair tissues elaborated after the bridge is excised; such a technique (first invented by Langenskiold[11]) is interposition of a substance that occupies the position of the repair tissue replacing the bridge. Langenskiold used fat, although other substances (e.g., silicone) have been tried.[8] The existing varus could, at the same time, be corrected by an osteotomy through the metaphysis.

The question can be raised as to whether 9 months was too long an interval, in case 5-2, to wait before conducting the evaluation. Could decisions have been made shortly after the injury, or even at the time of acute treatment? Probably not, because it would be difficult if not impossible to gauge the severity of the injury to the epiphyseal cartilage, as

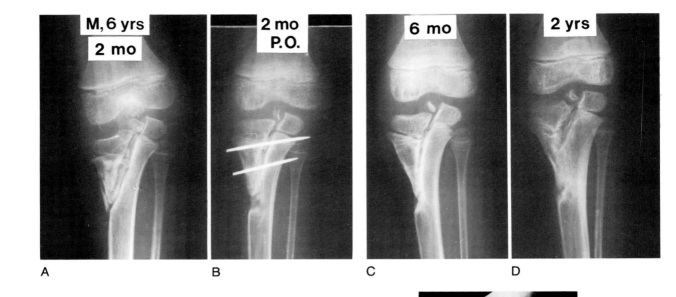

A   B   C   D

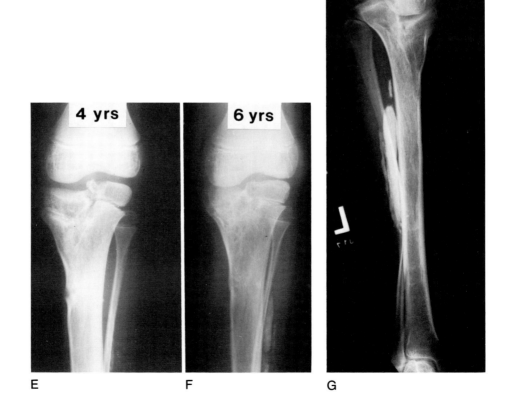

E   F   G

predictive of the degree of disturbance of growth. Moreover, measures such as the interposition operation are much too serious to use for routine prophylaxis. It is far better to allow an interval of time to pass to enable the surgeon to make a more accurate prediction and act accordingly.

Case 5-3 A 12-year-old boy with a closed fracture separation of the lower femoral epiphysis was treated acutely by closed reduction and plaster cast immobilization for 6 weeks. He presented 1 year after the injury for a routine check-up. Many of the pathophysiological considerations just discussed pertain somewhat but with differences. A major difference is that the epiphysis under scrutiny is one that grows at about double the rate of the distal tibial epiphysis (1.2 cm versus 0.7 cm per year of growth). Another is gender. A boy's maturation would be expected at a later age (2 years later), so that the total growth to be expected from the injured epiphysis would be about 5 cm. The important problems in the previous case — varus and leg length discrepancy — might also pertain here, as the fracture development indicated greater injury to the medial side of the epiphysis than to the lateral side. The same two radiographic examinations as for case 5-2 would therefore be done, but the (asymptomatic) varus (or valgus) could be evaluated on the orthoradiograph (or perhaps on films taken with the patient standing). Although a minor degree of varus, or decreased valgus, could well pass unnoticed, it should be evident on physical examination and it should be measurable on radiographs. In the present case, the differences between the extremities were 3° of varus at the knee and 0.8 cm in the length of the femurs. The varus,

asymptomatic and not nearly as important functionally as almost the same degree of varus at the ankle, would predictably increase somewhat, coordinate with the degree of increase in discrepancy in femoral length. However, that increase would be calculated as 67 percent (0.8/1.2) and therefore is less than the rate in the previous case (0.5 in 9 months, i.e., 0.5/0.6). Some allowance should be made for temporary overall growth inhibition attributable to systemic effects after a major injury or illness that would be present in both cases. The cosmetic aspect of the varus (less important in a boy) would also support observation of the varus over the next few years with no planned treatment. It is not so, however, in regard to the discrepancy of femoral length. The actual shortening must be projected over the period of growth (perhaps $0.8 \times 5 = 4$ cm), and the calculation must be based on a determination of skeletal age. Repeated measurements are mandatory every 3 to 6 months at first and then every 3 months during the year prior to the projected time of femoral epiphyseodesis. That operation is considered standard treatment because it is effective and safe, and because a discrepancy of more than 4 cm is considered too large for conservative treatment (adjustment of height by a heel lift). The skeletal age adjustment allows the surgeon to choose the ideal time for the epiphyseodesis so that the lengths of the femurs are equal at maturity.

Each epiphyseal plate normally closes gradually at skeletal maturity. Vascular ingrowth occurs on both the metaphyseal and epiphyseal sides of the cartilaginous plate (Fig. 5-10), and new bone is formed along the vascular channels. A bony bridge

Fig. 5-9. A 6-year-old boy sustained an injury to his proximal tibial epiphysis when a lawn-mower blade lacerated the lateral aspect of his leg into the knee joint. He had vascular and neural injury at the time. The vascular injury was repaired; the neural injury was not. No attempt was made to reduce the depressed lateral tibial plateau and epiphyseal plate until 2 months later. **(A)** The depression of the lateral tibial plateau with partial healing is evident; Surgery was attempted to correct the depression. **(B)** Radiograph shows partial elevation of the tibial epiphysis fixed with two Kirschner wires. **(C)** At 6 months there is union of the tibia, with continued growth from both fragments of the proximal tibial epiphysis. **(D)** At 2 years that growth continues. The femoral condyle is now overgrowing to accommodate the depressed medial aspect of the proximal tibia. **(E & F)** AP views at 4 years and 6 years. Note the calcification of the lateral compartment muscles. **(G)** AP radiograph at 23 years after the injury shows calcification of the anterolateral compartment but, more importantly, the modification of the tibial femoral joint over that period with preservation of the articular cartilage space. An equinovarus deformity secondary to the neuromuscular injury required a triple arthrodesis at age 12 with a lateral wedge resection. Shortening of the leg was accommodated with a shoe lift and epiphyseal arrest of the right proximal tibial epiphysis.

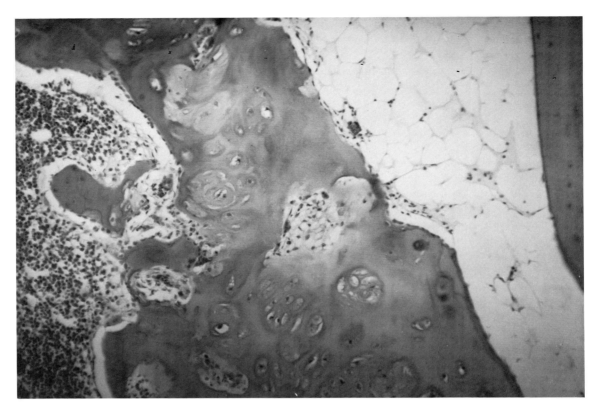

Fig. 5-10. Case 5-3. Photomicrograph showing the residuals of an epiphyseal plate with vascular end growth into the epiphyseal cartilage and bony bridging at one corner of the segment (×100).

then unites the two sides, and its lack of elasticity slows the growth of the part of the plate that is still growing. This bridge occurs in the central portion of the plate first. The process of bridging by bone is the basis for the operation of surgical closure of the plate, or *epiphyseodesis,* by the Blount[7] or Phemister[13] method.

With the *Blount procedure,* staples are inserted across the plate either on the convex side of the deformity to correct varus or valgus, or on both sides to slow down overall growth. In the former instance the staples slow down the growth of the cartilage cells for a long enough time to allow the cells on the unstapled side of the epiphyseal plate to grow and correct the angular deformity. When staples are used on both sides, all cartilage growth gradually ceases. However, the staples must be inserted somewhat earlier than with the Phemister procedure to yield equal correction of the discrep-

ancy. Premature arrest may result if during insertion of the staple there is direct injury to the growth plate; such injury must be guarded against if stapling is done to correct a deformity. In case 5-3, the deformity being mild, stapling would not be used unless during the period of observation the deformity increased. In that event the projected epiphyseodesis might be done after the affected side had had the varus corrected. The plan would then be to remove the staples and allow resumption of growth of the epiphyseal plate on the affected side.

The *Phemister procedure* works by producing a bony bridge on both sides of the epiphysis. Premature closure of the entire epiphyseal plate is the result. With this procedure, two blocks, one on each side, are removed from the epiphyseometaphyseal area. For the contralateral femur, each block includes a rectangular segment of epiphyseal cartilage and bone that measures approximately 2 to 3 cm, with the metaphyseal side slightly longer. Removal of the block allows the surgeon to visualize residual epiphyseal cartilage, which is curetted (subtotally to ensure prompt and symmetrical closure of the plate). The blocks are then replaced after they have been rotated 180°. For some unknown reason, epiphyseal cartilage whose directional orientation is reversed does not grow or at least has not been known to grow (thicken). The blocks rapidly reattach to their beds and form bony bridges across their periphery, and the curetted areas fill in with callus so that within a matter of weeks a large bony bridge is formed and growth ceases in the remainder of the plate because of the compression from the bony bridges vis-à-vis expansion. When a discrepancy in leg lengths *(anisomelia)* is to be corrected, a limb lengthening procedure occasionally is appropriate, perhaps supplemented by arrest of the corresponding epiphyseal plate of the opposite limb, a contralateral bone-shortening procedure, or both. These therapeutic combinations are rarely appropriate in cases of traumatic epiphyseal injuries and pertain most often when the affected limb is grossly abnormal and the surgeon does not want to operate on the normal extremity.

The bone bridges do not unite firmly until more time has elapsed. As experience has shown, inhibition of growth is more gradual when the Blount method is used than with the Phemister method. It is known that in experiments with animals central defects cause less disturbance of growth than do more peripheral injuries. Moreover, a smooth pin inserted in the center of an epiphysis and into the diaphysis after correction of a displacement is less likely to result in premature closure of the epiphyseal plate because it affords less purchase for the bony bridges.[9]

SLIPPED CAPITAL FEMORAL EPIPHYSIS

There are important differences between the pathophysiology of slipped capital femoral epiphysis and that of post-traumatic epiphyseal fracture separation, although in several respects the phenomena are similar.

Slipped capital femoral epiphysis is one of the most common causes of disability of the hip in adolescents, and its sequelae in adults not infrequently lead to a need for total hip replacement.[22,23,25,27]

Case 5-4 A 12-year-old boy began to limp spontaneously. There was no history of a fall or other trauma. After a year of the painless limp a radiograph was obtained (Fig. 5-11A) and the diagnosis suspected. Two months later he had an episode of acute pain localized mainly in the knee (Fig. 5-11B). Previously he had had no pain in either the hip or the knee. Physical examination revealed that motion of his right hip was restricted (about 50 percent) in all directions except external rotation, which was the position of comfort. The diagnosis (made on the basis of the above findings, which are typical) was of acute slipping of the right femoral capital epiphysis superimposed on chronic slipping. It was confirmed on radiographs (Fig. 5-11).

This condition, as portrayed anatomically, is usually characterized as small, repeated displacements of the capital femoral epiphysis posteromedially on the femoral neck through the epiphyseal plate (Fig. 5-12). When there is a complete, acute separation of the epiphysis, it is usually attributed to an episode of acute but not severe trauma. The pathogenesis of the condition is not completely understood. Observations of core biopsies and the whole-mount sections of the upper end of the femur[26,28] (Fig. 5-13) portray the displacement as occurring through the proliferating zone and the hypertrophic cartilage cells of the growth plate, i.e., one or two epiphyseal plate zones away from the site of epiphyseal fracture separations and of the usual site that occurs with traumatic displacement of a subcapital fracture of the neck of the femur (see Fig. 7-25A&B).

Some of the difficulties of the diagnosis are those responsible for the 1-year delay in diagnosis of case 5-4.[22,27] A limp in a child aged 8 to 16 should always alert the physician to the condition; but often when the limp is painless, the child and the parents tolerate or ignore it. Moreover, when the symptoms have an insidious onset, they do not invite much attention until, perhaps again as in case 5-4, a more sizable displacement of the epiphyseal plate, compared to previous displacements, occurs evoking acute symptoms. In case 5-4 the acute episode was the initial appearance of pain as a symptom. Patho-

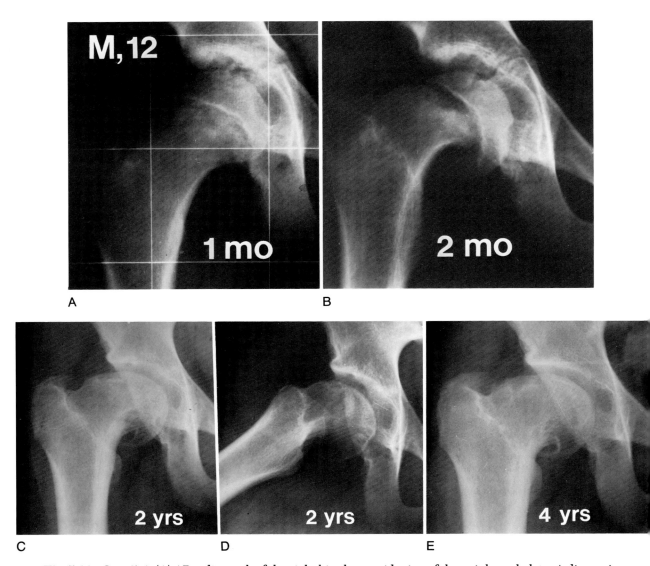

Fig. 5-11. Case 5-4. (A) AP radiograph of the right hip shows widening of the epiphyseal plate. A diagnosis of slipped capital femoral epiphysis was suspected and was confirmed after an episode of acute pain 1 month later. (B) At 2 months there is obvious displacement of the femoral neck on the capital femoral epiphysis. (C–E) Progression of the spontaneously healed slipped epiphysis and secondary deformity including an osteophyte along the anterior aspect of the femoral neck.

physiologically, this pain is attributable to stretching of the perichondral-periosteal membrane that surrounds the epiphyseal cartilage and marks the attachment of the synovial membrane and capsule of the hip joint. Presumably, the previous displacements were so small that the membrane that is well innervated was not stretched to the degree that

would excite the sensory innervation. Case 5-4 also illustrates the fact that the innervation may be provided by the obturator nerve; and because that nerve also innervates the medial aspect of the knee, referred pain to that part is not uncommon with slipped femoral capital epiphysis. It is understandable that the patient and parents might focus their

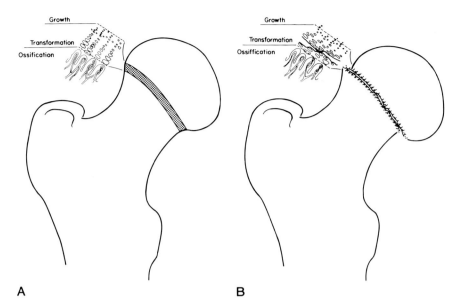

Fig. 5-12. (A) Proximal femur with a normal epiphyseal plate configuration and zones of the physis. (B) Slipped epiphyseal plate, with the slip depicted through the proliferating and hypertrophic cartilage cell zone.

attention on the painful knee and ignore the real culprit; but the physician, having found no positive physical signs in the knee, should pay particular attention to a physical examination of the hip. Only too often the knee is the focus of concern even to the point of radiographic examination, and the hip is ignored.

The physical findings in this study case have

pathophysiological implications that bear on diagnosis and are important to treatment. Had this boy had a physical examination prior to his acute episode, the findings would have been a disturbance in the range of motion of the hip far less severe than the limitation that was elicited (50 percent). The actual findings are attributable to spasm of the pericoxal muscles and, in particular, those closest

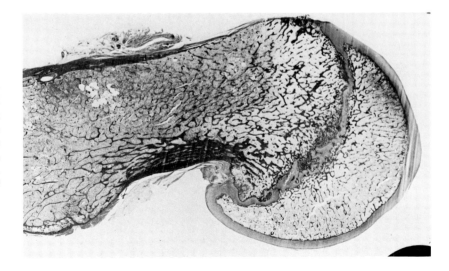

Fig. 5-13. Whole-mount photomicrograph of a slipped capital femoral epiphysis shows the alteration within the substance of the physis. The femoral neck is displaced anteriorly to correlate well with the classical lateral radiograph of hip to show displacement. (From Mickelson et al,[26] with permission.)

to the capsule of the hip joint, the small external rotators. Prior to the acute slippage, there would have been little or no component of muscle spasm —such reflex spasm being usually associated with pain. The restriction of motion then would pertain mainly to internal rotation and would be attributable to the malposition of the femoral head.

The difficulties that may be encountered in radiographic diagnosis (as when the clinical findings are not conclusive) stem from situations not evident in case 5-4 (where both clinical and radiographic findings were definitive). The patient whose hip is in spasm may have had "routine radiographs" that do not represent views in two projections at 90° to each other; and in many cases the so-called lateral view is the one that is most likely to be diagnostic. Often the technician finds that the patient can not assume the "frog-leg" position, or there is trouble with the exposure factors. A true cross-table lateral view is preferable, safer, and more comfortable for the patient. Whatever the reason, the inadequacy of the lateral view, which provides the crucial evidence of the degree of displacement, is the most frequent reason for radiographic misdiagnosis.

The biomechanics of the condition have been studied in detail possibly because the facts involved are so similar to those that pertain to subcapital fractures of the femoral neck and to total replacement arthroplasty (see Ch. 5 and 10). It is well known that the femoral neck is a structure that has a high predilection for fracture, but that the predilection does not extend to the adolescent age group. In fact, subcapital fractures in that age group, ascribable to known (and often severe) trauma, are uncommon. Furthermore, such fractures usually do not traverse the entire epiphyseal plate in one plane, and their displacements differ considerably from those of slipped epiphysis. Nevertheless, most early studies on fracture of the femoral neck (until about 1920) included some cases of slipped epiphysis.

The pathogenesis of the slip therefore cannot focus on trauma as the essential mechanism, even though any displacement, whatever its essential nature, involves action of forces: With slipped femoral capital epiphysis, the forces may well be those considered physiological rather than traumatic. This speculation is supported by the fact that in perhaps 20 percent of patients the contralateral hip is observed to have, or to develop, what is known as a "pre-slip."[27] That condition, symptomless and presenting *no* abnormal physical findings, is diagnosed on radiographs, which show a widened radiolucency just distal to the epiphysis as if the cartilage were thickened or the metaphyseal struts of calcified cartilage and trabecular bone were, at least in part, resorbed. In a few instances there is slight anterior displacement of the femoral neck on the head on the lateral view. To our knowledge, however, no specimen of such a "pre-slip" has been studied histologically.

The existence of the pre-slip must be kept in mind when theories of pathogenesis are considered. Several theories have been promulgated. One evokes an anatomic peculiarity—the oblique orientation of the epiphyseal cartilage during adolescence compared to a more horizontal orientation in younger children. That theory also emphasizes the high prevalence of obesity in patients with this lesion. Another group of theories state that the condition is based on an endocrine abnormality. However, studies of endocrine gland functions in these patients have not succeeded in producing reliable evidence of malfunction despite several provocative bits of clinical evidence. There is a 3:1 prevalence of the condition in boys, and lesions are often found in patients who have hypopituitarism or hypothyroidism (Fig. 5-14) and delayed closure of the epiphysis; the predilection of the lesion is for girls of average age 12 and boys of average age 14 (the time of the growth spurt). However, all these bits of evidence do not consider one essential aspect of the condition, i.e., the fact that a *single site* is most often affected in otherwise healthy children in whom an endocrine abnormality would be expected to produce generalized effects.

Certain pathophysiological implications regarding treatment follow from the postulated pathogenetic mechanisms: (1) no endocrine or metabolic treatment is based on firm ground; and (2) the biochemical mechanisms have little relation to rational treatment regimens. More important logical consequences follow from the fact that the slip, which is an area of discontinuity (resembling a fracture gap) but situated in a zone of epiphyseal cartilage (Fig. 5-15), heals either by reconstitution of the metaphyseal structure as the cartilage grows

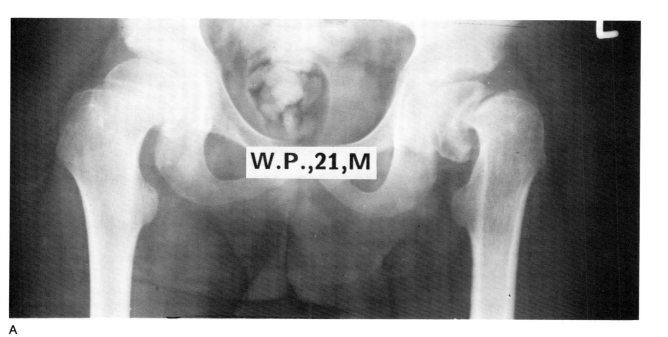

A

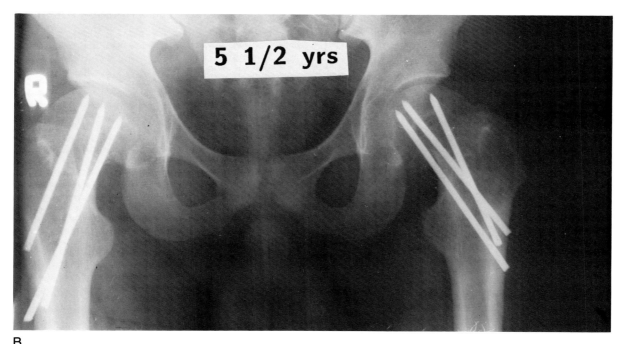

B

Fig. 5-14. (A) A 21-year-old man with hypopituitarism, hypothyroidism, and delayed closure of the epiphysis developed slipped capital epiphysis bilaterally; it was acute on the left side. These defects were treated by gentle reduction and internal fixation using threaded pins on the left and in situ threaded pin fixation on the right. (B) At 5.5 years both epiphyseal plates are closed.

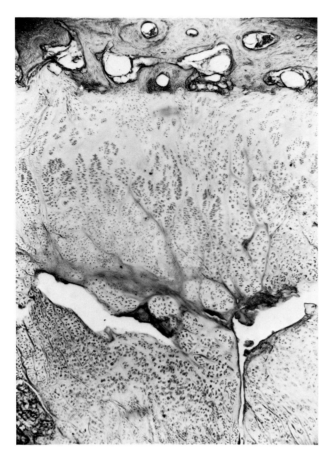

Fig. 5-15. Photomicrograph of the epiphyseal plate. The cartilage cells are disorderly and separated by fibrillated septa. A large cleft is seen filled with small amounts of amorphous debris (×50). (From Ponseti and McClintock,[28] with permission.)

or by closure of the epiphyseal plate. The result is as much as 2 cm of residual shortening of the affected limb if the patient is young, i.e., 12 years of age, but usually much younger. However, these processes require several weeks or months for the gap to heal and the fragments to stabilize. Prior to arranging for that long-term objective, the acute spasm of the hip must be dealt with for reasons that will soon become apparent. Spasm is best relieved by immobilization, as in case 5-4, using traction for a few days. That hiatus allows the surgeon time to determine just how much internal rotation and flexion are possible with the displacement at hand. If the distal fragment has pushed anteriorly to form

a sharp ridge that, on flexion, abuts against the anterior lip of the acetabulum, flexion is limited; and if that fragment has rotated externally to a great extent, internal rotation to neutral is impossible. These clinical observations bear strongly on the therapeutic alternatives because if the child has 15° of internal rotation and more than 90° of flexion, the safest, most satisfactory regimen of treatment includes the decision not to attempt altering the position of the fragments. All too often that decision is predicated on the radiographic measurements that indicate that the slip is minimal (i.e., 2 cm or less) (Fig. 5-16). Case 5-4 reveals why the radiographic measurement may be a poor criterion on which to base treatment. The chronic series of displacements and the repair bone that was deposited in response to those displacements interferes with the measurement between the medialmost edges of the epiphysis and metaphysis.

Mention has already been made of the factor of safety during treatment. The problem primarily is the lack of safety during a procedure that aims to replace the epiphysis in its proper orientation on the metaphysis, whether that procedure is a "gentle" manipulation or an operative reduction.[25,27] Experience has shown that there is an unacceptable percentage of patients who develop aseptic necrosis of the femoral head after even a gentle manipulation. That maneuver, which is attractive but seductive and often fatal to the femoral head, carries the risk of further stretching or tearing the epiphyseal vessels that enter the epiphysis precisely at the perichondral-periosteal ring at the epiphyseal line. Those vessels may well have been compromised by the acute slip as well as by scarring that followed the previous small slips. The manner by which manipulation may further compromise the vessels is the distraction of the femoral neck from the proximal fragment: Its projecting ridge acts as a lever and the acetabular margin as the fulcrum. The thigh is so long and heavy a lever arm that palpation cannot reveal the tearing of the delicate tissue.

Some authors judge a slip minimal when the radiographic projection (either lateral or anteroposterior) shows 2 cm or less of slippage. Others use a criterion of one-third the width of the epiphyseal plate.[22]

With minimal slips there remain two objectives

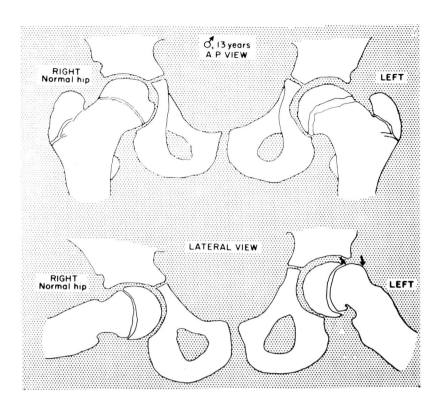

Fig. 5-16. Drawing of AP and lateral radiograph to depict a minimally slipped epiphysis, bordering on a moderate degree of slip. (From Bonfiglio,[22] with permission.)

of treatment: acceleration of closure of the discontinuity and prevention of further slippage. Both of these goals can be attained with fixation of the fragments in situ preferably by a screw or several screws (or threaded pins).[22,23] Screws are preferable to nails[25] inasmuch as they can (and should) impose a measure of compression to help nature's closure of the epiphyseal plate. Another reason for using screws is that use of a nail, particularly a fixation nail, has on occasion led to distraction of the fragments. The robust cancellous bone of a healthy teenager offers a good deal of resistance to the nail, and pounding on it, even under image-intensifier control, may be as risky to the vascular supply of the epiphysis as manipulation.

Aseptic necrosis is so devastating a complication in the age group under consideration, as illustrated in the radiographs of a 14-year-old boy (Fig. 5-17), that even a small rate of incidence is to be avoided. The pathophysiological reason for this conclusion is that after the age of 8 the acetabulum can no longer remodel its shape to articulate acceptably with a deformed femoral head. Moreover, the en-

suing two decades of maximal physical activity lead to a severe traumatic arthritis in a hip affected by aseptic necrosis, so that almost certainly a reconstruction procedure will be needed for such a hip. Total hip replacement arthroplasty is least successful in patients under the age of 30. It is far better therefore to emphasize the indications for fixation in situ so that the operative regimens to be mentioned below are only used under exceptional circumstances.[23] Should one find the range of motion of the hip treated by fixation in situ too restricted because of the ridge of femoral neck that is protruding, that ridge can be removed.

When the slippage is more than minimal (Fig. 5-16), i.e., one-half or more of the width of the epiphyseal plate, it is technically difficult to insert screws into the epiphysis without having them enter the hip joint en route; that consideration, as well as the more severe disturbances of the articular relation, compared with those caused by minimal slips argue for a treatment designed to correct to some extent the anatomical abnormality. Some have advocated osteotomy of the femoral neck, and

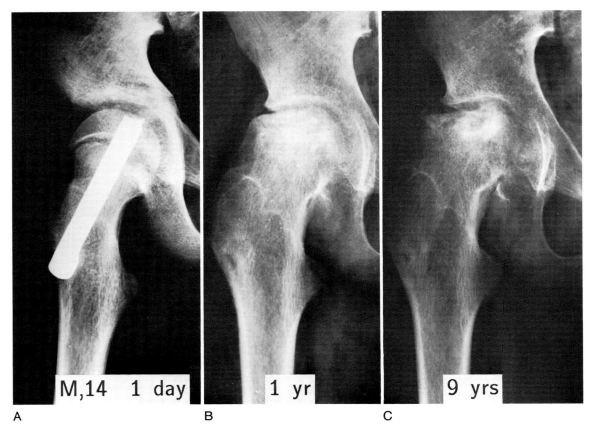

Fig. 5-17. A 14-year-old boy with an acute slipped capital femoral epiphysis had a "gentle" reduction of the slip and internal fixation with a Smith-Peterson (SP) nail. **(A)** AP view with the SP nail in place one day after insertion shows slight distraction of the epiphyseal plate. **(B)** AP radiograph at 1 year shows collapse of the weight-bearing aspect of the hip secondary to aseptic necrosis of the epiphysis. **(C)** Epiphyseal plate has closed. Secondary degenerative joint disease is present at 9 years. At age 34 the patient had had enough pain and functional impairment to undergo a cup arthroplasty.

one study has shown that if a wedge of bone is removed the osteotomy performed in the subcapital area can restore the normal position of the epiphysis on the neck. However, the pathophysiological precaution that should be taken if this regimen of treatment is chosen is to allow the vessels, stretched by the acute episode of slippage, to adapt to the stretch by keeping the patient in traction for a week or two instead of operating immediately. If the osteotomy is done in the proper spot, Phemister-type epiphyseal arrest can be added to accelerate closure of the epiphyseal cartilage.

Sites of osteotomy distal to that just mentioned have also been advocated, the most common being at the level of the trochanter. Various techniques have been used—hexagonal cuts, dome-shaped cuts, removal of a wedge—but all of them emphasize the avoidance of aseptic necrosis and minimize the fact that one deformity is being treated by creating another.

Two other points deserve mention before leaving this subject. One is the complication of chondrolysis, a puzzling and happily uncommon sequel to the slippage that seemingly is not brought on by the treatment.[24] Yet, because it appears shortly after treatment, patients (and the surgeon as well) may associate the two, considering chondrolysis as resorption of the articular cartilage of the femoral head, epiphyseal plate, or both; the problem is seen in perhaps 5 percent of the patients. With the resorption (detected on radiograph) there is profound, long-lasting irritation of the joint, resulting in severe restriction of motion, despite any form of treatment. A major impairment of the joint ensues possibly due to the long-lasting disuse of the periarticular muscles. The pathophysiology of the condition is unknown, and to our knowledge its histology has not been studied. Chondrolysis has a predilection for black individuals with slipped femoral capital epiphysis.

The final point is that, in general, when a series of cases is reported in which many of the patients are black, the results of treatment tend to be worse, and this predilection does not seem to be associated with genetic hematological abnormalities. It should be recalled that those abnormalities may themselves predispose a patient to aseptic necrosis of the femoral head. Conservatism of treatment in black patients therefore is especially indicated.

AVULSION FRACTURES

With the burgeoning of sports activities by youths and physically active adults, avulsion fractures have become increasingly common, often recognized by early complaints of "weak ankles," "groin pulls," "hamstring pulls," "hip pointers," and so on.[32,34,36] Even before sports commanded so much attention, however, avulsion fractures were some of the most common injuries treated by orthopedic surgeons; and such injuries have assumed increasing importance as occupational and medicolegal problems. An avulsion fracture may be defined as a break in the continuity of the bone at the attachment of a ligament, tendon, or muscle caused by a forceful pull in the attaching fibers.

From one pathophysiological point of view in regard to bony repair, these fractures are merely instances of cancellous bone surfaces facing each other across a small gap filled with hemorrhage at first and then fibrochondroosseous callus. The width of the gap varies, of course; and if it can be reduced and the fragment immobilized, whether by manipulation and an externally applied device (bandage, cast, or percutaneous wire) or by opera-

tive internal fixation, rapid union of the fragment can be expected.[36] Conversely, if the fragment is separate and not immobilized, nonunion can be expected frequently (see below).

From another pathophysiological point of view, some avulsion fractures often contain a considerable expanse of articular or apophyseal cartilage,[33] and in those cases the repair follows the principles already summarized for osteochondral fractures (above). In particular, malleolar fractures at the ankle, fractures of the tibial spine in the knee,[36] and fractures of the olecranon illustrate the importance of the repair of the cartilage. It is thus evident that with some avulsion fractures precedence as to the objectives of treatment may be accorded either the chondral or osseous pathophysiological processes of repair. However, the importance of the structure that avulsed the fragment is the focus of this section, and restoration of its function may take precedence in treatment. It is obvious that if the avulsing force has been applied by a ligament, as by forceful subluxation of a joint, the subluxation may be minimal (and transient). The ligament, having been stretched maximally, has an ultimate tensile strength that is greater than the tensile strength of the substance of the bone, so it is the bone that "gives way." It may not be assumed that the ligament has not been lengthened in the process; therefore the total lesion may be a composite of the fracture plus some fibrous tearing within the ligamentous substance.

The most important objective of treatment of such a lesion (not merely the fracture) is to restore stability to the joint. For guidance as to what is needed, the amount of instability present must be assessed. It can be done by physical examination for the most part; in some instances, an intra-articular injection of local anesthetic allows assessment of a joint that would normally be impossible immediately after an acute injury. Stress radiographs, using the contralateral extremity as a standard, are also useful at times. Given an unacceptable instability, an operation to strengthen and shorten the affected osseoligamentous element would then address the pathophysiological defect.

Similarly, an avulsion fracture caused by the pull of a tendon poses the same pathophysiological situation and implications. The lesion on a distal phalanx where the extensor digitorum tendon attaches

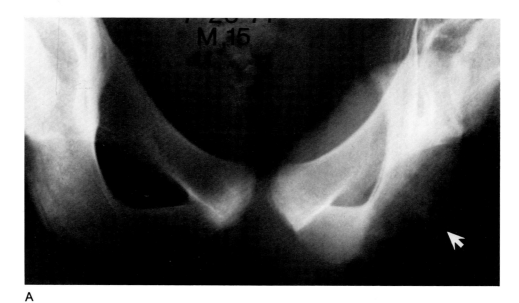

A

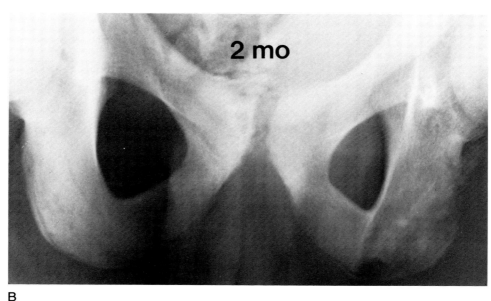

B

Fig. 5-18. Case 5-5. (A) Radiolucent area of the left ischium, the site of avulsion of hamstring muscle origin. (B) At 2 months, mottled ossification and radiolucency are present at that site. *(Figure continues.)*

is a case in point. The physical finding there is not instability of a joint but, rather, inability of the distal digit to extend fully. The required goal of treatment for manual function may be of the essence for individuals who require dexterity (e.g., musicians), whereas in others the cosmetic goal may be the most important factor. Healing of the fracture, if

the gap between the fragment exceeds 1 mm or so, may yield an unacceptable impairment, which in an adult is permanent. (Children often, over a few years, regain the lost arc of motion.) Therefore, if by appropriate positioning of the finger (hyperextension of the distal metaphalangeal joint and flexion of the proximal and metacarpophalangeal

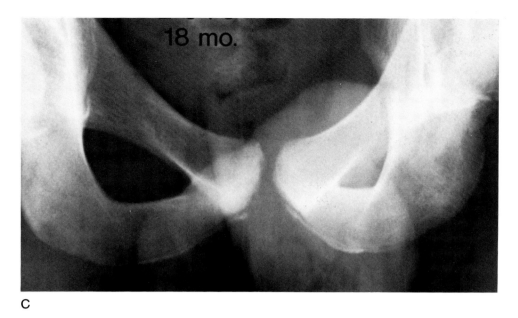

C

Fig. 5-18 *(Continued).* (C) At 18 months, reossification has occurred.

joints) the fragment cannot be restored to an acceptable position, operative restoration is indicated.

In both types of ligamentous or tendinous avulsion cases just discussed, one may ask if, with time (years), the injured soft tissues (e.g., the stretched ligament and tendon) will develop contractures, so that slow improvement can be anticipated. It may well be the situation for stretched ligaments that have not compromised the stability of the joint. If those ligaments are not further traumatized (and in their weakened state secure protection is needed) over a long period, healing may be complete. Such protection is not practical for tendinous lesions, however, inasmuch as all function would then be interdicted for a long time. It also is probable that the tendon has not been stretched beyond its physiological limit, given the limitations of the muscular force, in contrast to the greater forces possible with ligamentous avulsion.

Some avulsion fractures present difficulties in diagnosis. Sometimes the diagnosis depends on identification of a fragment of bone so small or so situated as to be inapparent on radiographs. Such a problem is illustrated in case 5-5.

Case 5-5 A 15-year-old boy noted the onset of pain in his left buttock and upper thigh posteriorly

while in the middle of a sprint. He was unable to finish the race. His pain subsided with rest or walking. About 2 months later he still had pain but only while running.

On deep palpation tenderness was elicited at the ischial tuberosity, where the suggestion of a mass was noted. A radiograph of the pelvis showed a mottled radiolucency in the left ischium (Fig. 5-18A), and a profile radiograph of the ischial rami showed, in addition, irregular areas of increased density medial to the ischium, that were interpreted by the radiologist as possibly a chondromatous tumor. This possibility was discounted because the patient was gradually improving with restriction of activity (Fig. 5-18B). The clinical diagnosis was avulsion injury of the origin of the left medial hamstring muscle. After 18 months the radiograph showed remodeling of the ischium (Fig. 5-18C), and the patient returned to long distance running.

The radiographic sequences of the repair process suggested that there was cartilage formation in the callus that had undergone partial ossification. In an avulsion of the ischial apophysis one would expect fracture callus composed of fibrous tissue, fibrocartilage, and new bone, all of which are components of a fracture repair. The original avulsion

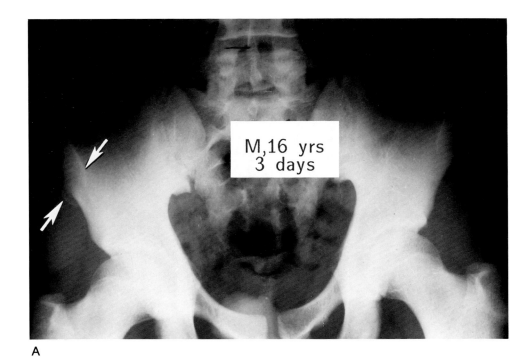

A

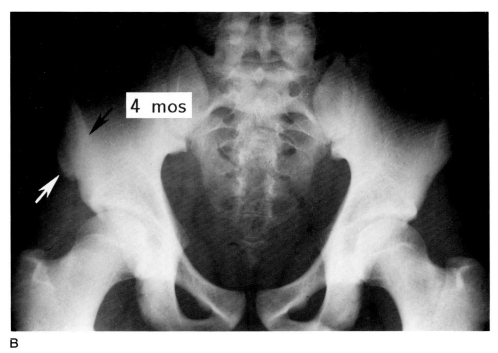

B

Fig. 5-19. (A) Three days after sudden onset of pain during a sprint, a radiograph of the pelvis shows avulsion of the anterosuperior spine of the right ilium. (B) At 4 months, the fragment has united to the ilium (arrows).

may well have included a flake of ischial bone that could not be demonstrated on the early radiographs.

Such an apophyseal avulsion usually reunites, and the callus remodels to the nearly normal state. Specimens of musculotendinous attachments have been removed by biopsy when a malignancy was suspected. In such cases, particularly in adolescents, the fracture callus resembles myositis ossificans because some adjacent muscle fibers are included in the biopsy; in the absence of clinical information, the picture may seem ominous. The clinical data and radiographs should dispel any doubt as to the proper diagnosis.

Similar avulsions occur in children at the medial epicondyle of the humerus ("little leaguer's elbow") and at the tibial tubercle (Osgood-Schlatter's disease).[33-35] Other sites of avulsion fractures are associated with apophyses of the ilium: the anterior superior spine[32] (the hip pointer), the crest,

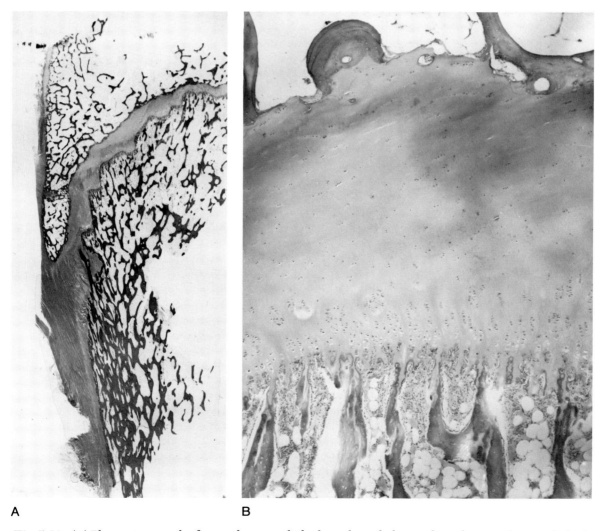

A   B

Fig. 5-20. (A) Photomicrograph of normal proximal tibial epiphyseal plate and epiphysis with normal tibial tubercle insertion of the patellar ligament ($\times 2$). (B) Normal physis and metaphysis with normal growth. Specimen was obtained from the limb of a 14-year-old boy who underwent amputation for sarcoma of the femur ($\times 30$).

and the anterior inferior spine (Fig. 5-19). Other sites are the lesser trochanter of the femur, the bicipital tubercle of the radius, and the base of the fifth metatarsal. After healing, these lesions usually are not symptomatic; and even if bony union does not occur there is no impairment, as the strong fibrous repair functions adequately and the muscle adapts to a shorter distance from its origin to its insertion.

The mechanism of injury is a tensile force — a sudden uncoordinated contraction of the muscle attached to the particular apophysis. One presumes that other muscles whose function it is to diffuse the area of application of the force fail to do so. It is difficult to explain otherwise how a muscle could exert a force in excess of the physiological maximum. Confusion with an osseous or cartilaginous tumor occurs when the radiographic appearance of the callus suggests to the radiologist that the irregular foci of increased density are associated with a cartilaginous tumor. No misdiagnoses should occur when a series of radiographs are obtained at intervals of one to several weeks. Meanwhile symptoms are relieved by restricting activity.

Osgood-Schlatter's Disease

The radiographic characteristics of Osgood-Schlatter's disease were well described separately by Osgood and Schlatter in 1903, and the lesion was then considered an "osteochondritis," i.e., an inflammatory condition. Prior to the availability of radiographs, it was considered a traumatic disorder — either an acute avulsion fracture that was difficult to heal or a series of fractures. An understanding of the development of the tibial tubercle provides a clue as to why this disorder occurs during late childhood. The secondary ossification center of the proximal end of the tibia has a tongue-like anterior projection that projects inferiorly. The patellar ligament attaches broadly at its inferiormost point, and that attachment extends past the epiphyseal cartilage to the metaphysis. Closure usually takes place by age 15 in girls and age 17 in boys, and therefore the mainly cartilaginous tibial tubercle is essentially a focal point for the forceful action of the quadriceps femoris, which acts via the patella and the patellar ligament[34,35] (Fig. 5-20).

Kicking a ball, forcefully jumping, or rising from a squatting position places maximal tension on the attachment of the patellar ligament so that the causative mechanism in this disorder begins as a partial avulsion of the attachment of the tendon to the tibial tubercle. In some patients there is no clear-cut history of a single important injury at the onset of the pain, yet the clinical and the radiographic features are indistinguishable from those in patients who clearly recall an injury. Some patients who present with the characteristic physical finding — a tender projecting tibial tubercle — have no complaints of pain on extension of the knee; and on occasion patients with that clinical pattern show no avulsed fragment radiographically. However, the radiograph then shows inflammatory changes in the infrapatellar fat pads, a finding that is almost uniformly present so long as the lesion is painful. Some patients have pain only when they kneel, and that is true not only of patients with the acute process but also those whose lesions have healed. The projecting callus is responsible for the pain in those cases. Avulsion fracture of the proximal tibial epiphysis occurs acutely and involves more than the anterior tongue of epiphysis, which is considered by some to be a distinctive and uncommon injury[35] (Fig. 5-21). However, more than one-half of the patients studied with that lesion had a history of Osgood-Schlatter's disease.

Radiographically, most cases show only one small fragment of bone separated from the remainder of the tibial epiphysis, but a few cases have several fragments. During the healing process, which may occupy a period of 2 years or even more, there is gradual coalescence of the fragments(s) with the rest of the tibial epiphysis and with the metaphysis as closure of the epiphyseal plate proceeds. This radiographic pattern is somewhat different from the pattern of callus seen when an ankle fracture unites, and it differs as well from the pattern of healing of a stress fracture.

Case 5-6   A 14-year-old boy had had pain in both knees intermittently for 1 year. He was active in sports and noted more discomfort in the right knee with running and jumping. He developed marked

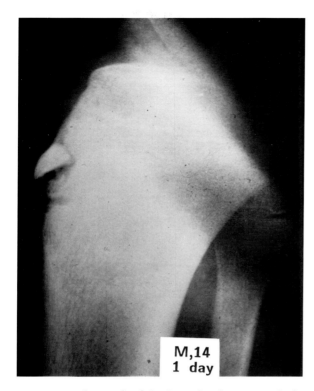

M,14
1 day

Fig. 5-21. Radiograph of the lateral right proximal tibia with an acute avulsion fracture of the tibial tubercle.

prominence and more tenderness of the right knee. The radiographs (Figs. 5-22A & B) show bilateral Osgood-Schlatter's disease but with a more prominent right tibial tubercle. Because of this prominence the right tibial tubercle was excised. The specimen radiograph (Fig. 5-22C) shows a double radiolucent gap of the avulsion fracture and at the tip of the secondary center of ossification. The photomicrographs (Figs. 5-22D–H) show the avulsion fracture (Fig. 5-22E), the repair bone (Fig. 5-22F), and necrosis of the tip of the tubercle (Figs. 5-22G&H).

The avulsion usually consists of the tendon along with small areas of cartilage, or it may include the cartilage and some of the bone. The amount of tendon, tissue, cartilage, and bone, the degree of fragmentation, and the depth of the injury vary from case to case. Following the injury or multiple injuries there is a wide spectrum of reparative responses involving all the tissue involved. Such response can result in excess tissue and protuberance, and on occasion it has caused a pseudoarthrosis between one or several cartilaginous or bony ossicles and the remaining cartilage and/or base of the tubercle, including necrosis of fragments that have lost their blood supply. It is not surprising that the literature reflects confusion about these reparative processes: It often refers to Osgood-Schlatter's disease as heterotopic ossification, tendinitis, tenosynovitis, osteochondritis, and intratendinous dysplasia.

As one would expect, relative to the development of the tibial tubercle, the onset of the disturbance usually occurs in children 10 to 15 years old and there is occasional bilateral involvement. The radiographs reflect the pathological changes, showing irregular areas of increased and decreased density depending on the position of the fracture of the avulsed fragments and manifestations of reparative bone and soft tissue.

The treatment of Osgood-Schlatter's disease is essentially the same as that for a sprain or an avulsion fracture. Protection from strain for a reasonable period of time to allow repair is usually all that is needed. The operative treatments with bone pegging, excision of fragments, and injection with steroids attest to the temperament and judgment of the surgeons who apply them. Until the epiphyseal plate and apophysis have closed, surgery is not indicated. Genu recurvatum has been reported after bone pegging that crossed and fused the epiphyseal plate anteriorly.

Because of continued muscular pull on the fracture site, repair may be incomplete and leave an ununited bone fragment. Excision of residual ununited ossicles after maturity provide relief of persistent pain and tenderness in the area of the tubercle[33] (Fig. 5-23).

Post-traumatic Avulsive Cortical Irregularity in the Distal Part of the Femur

An unusual variation of this process results when an avulsion injury at the insertion of the adductor magnus muscle into the supracondylar ridge of the

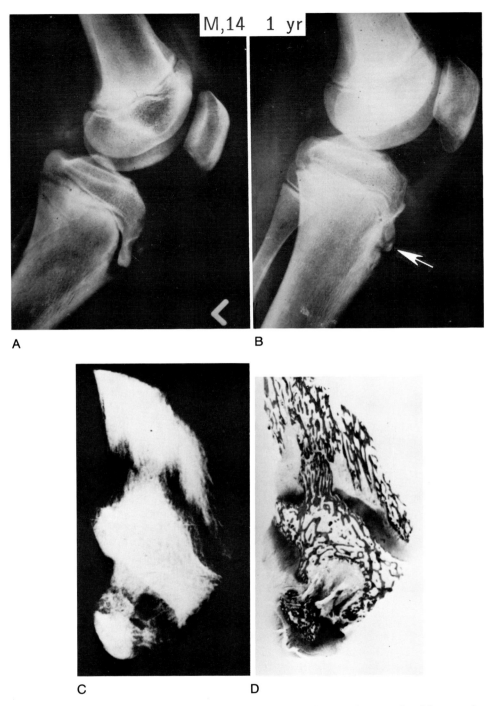

M,14　1 yr

A

B

C

D

Fig. 5-22. Case 5-6. **(A)** Lateral radiographs of both knees show bilateral Osgood-Schlatter's disease with fragmentation of each tibial tubercle and partial avulsion of the left proximal apophysis with widening of the physis. **(B)** Because of pain of the left tibial tubercle that persisted for 1 year, the tubercle was excised. Radiographs of the specimen showed a radiolucent separation between the proximal and the distal fragment at the tip of the tubercle (arrow). **(C & D)** Specimen shows the apophysis, the epiphyseal plate with a tongue of repair bone crossing it distally at the insertion of the patella ligament fibrous tissue replacement of the secondary center of ossification (×2). *(Figure continues.)*

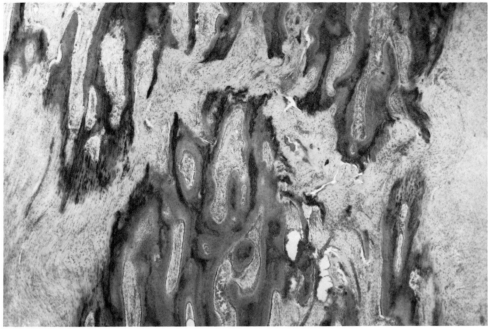

E

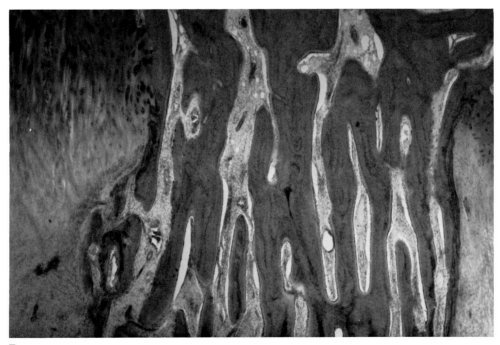

F

Fig. 5-22 *(Continued).* **(E)** Photomicrograph of the fracture at the proximal epiphysis and tibial tubercle fracture site shows fibrovascular connective tissue and new bone formation corresponding to the radiolucent zone (×40). **(F)** Tongue of bone repair across the physis (×40). *(Figure continues.)*

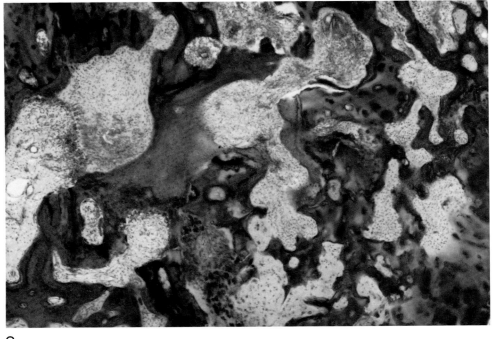

G

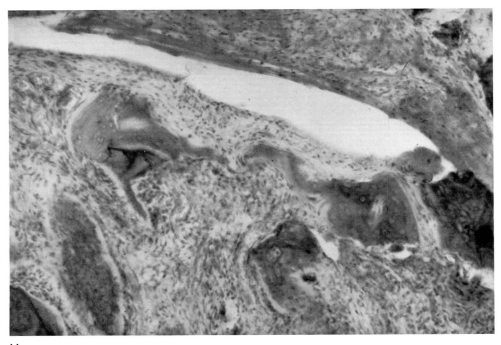

H

Fig. 5-22 *(Continued).* **(G)** Photomicrograph of the tip of the tubercle shows the necrosis undergoing repair. A mixture of bone and epiphyseal cartilage is present (×100). **(H)** High power view of the apophysis shows a cleft within fibrovascular repair tissue and osteoclastic resorption of the residual necrotic bone (×250).

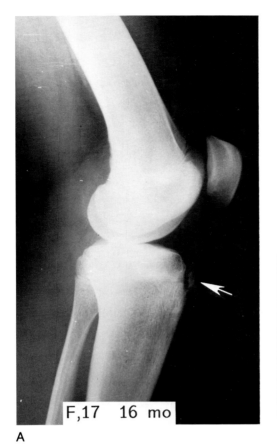

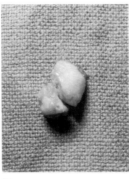

A   B

Fig. 5-23. (A) Lateral radiograph of an ununited fragment of the tibial tubercle (arrow) in a 17-year-old girl with persistent pain in the area. (B) Fibrocartilaginous fragment was excised as an ununited ossicle. The pain was relieved.

distal femur produces a cortical irregularity that can be confused with tumor radiographically and histologically.[29-31] The reaction has been termed a cortical, periosteal, or juxtacortical desmoid. None of these terms is appropriate.

The lesion, composed of mature fibrous tissue and periosteal new bone (Figs. 5-24E&F), is seen as a radiolucent irregular defect accompanied by periosteal bone at the distal insertion of the adductor magnus on the supracondylar ridge of the medial aspect of the distal femur. It occurs in athletic boys in their mid and late teens after strenuous physical sports activity. The patient may complain of pain with use but does not recall an acute episode. Radiographs show the radiolucent irregular cortical defect (Fig. 5-24A–D), and often the contralateral femur has a similar lesion.

Once it is recognized, the patient should restrict those activities that aggravate the symptoms. Biopsy is not required for confirmation. The lesion is not a true neoplasm but the result of an avulsive injury of the insertion of the adductor magnus along the supracondylar ridge of the medial femoral condyle. One may therefore expect a spectrum of alterations from acute to chronic injury in what is a common abnormality.

In the mature skeleton one should be aware of avulsion fractures at insertions of tendons and ligaments that occur with sprains or dislocation. These fractures do not present problems of interpretation

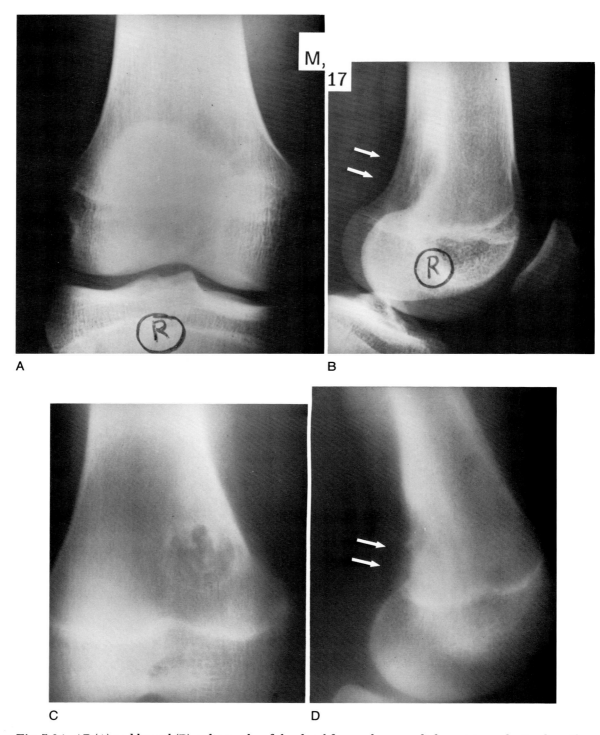

Fig. 5-24. AP (**A**) and lateral (**B**) radiographs of the distal femur show a radiolucent irregularity along the posteromedial aspect of the femur, best seen on the lateral view. (**C & D**) Tomograms of the same area as in **A** and **B** show the defect more clearly. *(Figure continues.)*

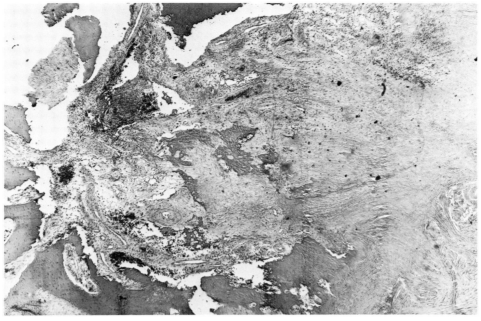

E

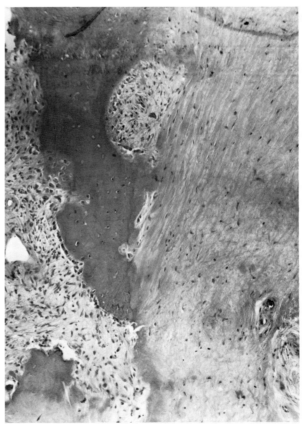

Fig. 5-24 *(Continued)*. **(E)** The lesion is composed of mature fibrous tissue and periosteal new bone. The central portion of the lesion shows reparative granulation tissue with bits of necrotic bone (×40). **(F)** Periosteal fibrous tissue at the insertion of the adductor magnus at the supracondylar ridge (×100).

F

but may give difficulty when decisions are needed about the best treatment. Such lesions include avulsion fractures (1) of the extensor tendon, (2) at the insertion into the dorsal aspect of the proximal phalanx of the finger at the interphalangeal joint of the thumb, (3) at the femoral attachment of the medial collateral ligament (Pelligrini-Stieda's disease), (4) of the tibial spine with the anterior cruciate ligament, the medial malleolus, and the base of the fifth metatarsal, and others too numerous to mention. Orthopedic textbooks describe the various methods of treatment, and so the subject need not be discussed here. In many instances stress on these sites interferes with completion of the bony repair, so if a nonunion results without serious functional impairment, treatment may be unnecessary.

UNUNITED FRACTURE (DELAYED UNION, NONUNION, PSEUDOARTHROSIS)

Some fractures unite slowly, and some do not unite at all (Table 5-1). In this section we examine some of the reasons for this biological aberration of the repair process and how they relate to various aspects of fracture healing discussed to this point. We define the problem, the frequency and particular sites of occurrence, and the clinical, radiographic, and pathological features of nonunion. In particular, we focus on the treatment of ununited fractures.

The incidence of ununited fractures varies from none in Watson-Jones series[62] of 800 consecutive femoral and tibial shaft fractures to as high as 4 to 5 percent.[49] The overall estimated incidence for the entire skeleton is less than 3 percent,[42] being higher for selected sites such as the tibia.[40,60,64] It is our purpose to discuss why fractures do not unite and what to do about it. Because healing of a frac-

Table 5-1. Ununited Fractures

Definitions
    Delayed union
    Pseudarthrosis
    Atrophic nonunion
    Hypertrophic nonunion
Diagnosis
    Clinical: symptoms and signs
    Radiographic
    Pathological
Etiological factors
    Injury-related
        Anatomical dimensional components
        Segmental bone loss
        Extensive soft tissue damage
        Blood supply to one or more fragments
    Treatment-related
        Reduction
        Distraction
        Immobilization
        Infection
Treatment
    Prevention
    Benign neglect
    Orthosis—brace
    Bone grafts
    Combinations with internal fixation
    Plate fixation
    Electrical stimulation

ture is a continuous process until repair of bone is complete, any disturbance of that repair prior to the time of expected union can be interpreted as an ununited fracture—the accepted terminology is "delayed union" during the early phase or "nonunion" or "pseudarthrosis" during the late phase.[44] Clinical examples are useful for illustrating this range of manifestations.

Case 5-7 An AP radiograph of the femur of a 31-year-old adult illustrates *delayed union* 9 months after plate fixation of a fracture of the left femur. The patient presented with minimal motion and pain at the fracture site at the junction of the mid-

Fig. 5-25. Case 5-7. (A) AP radiograph obtained 9 months after internal fixation with a plate and screws for a fracture of the femur in a 31-year-old man. Gaps persist at the fracture site, which is at the junction of the middle and distal thirds of the femur. (B) Photomicrograph of the nonunion site shows fibrous tissue with small amounts of immature new bone within it (×100). AP (C) and lateral (D) radiographs at 7 months after an onlay bone graft on the posterolateral aspect of the nonunion site shows union along the posterior and lateral cortex.

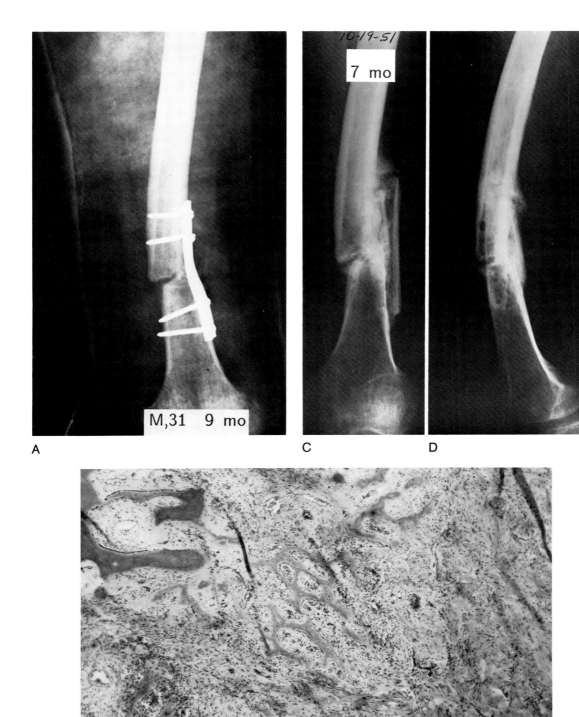

A

M,31   9 mo

C

10-19-51

7 mo

D

B

dle and distal thirds of the femur. The radiographs showed a broken screw and a radiolucent gap at the anteromedial aspect of the fracture site (Figs. 5-25A&B). This gap is either secondary to a failure to maintain contact of the bone ends in the application of the plate or to resorption of the bone ends over time. In this instance, it appears as though the plate has served to prevent the physiological compression of the fracture fragments. The plate and screws, including the broken screw, were removed, and tibial bone grafts were applied to the posterolateral aspect of the femur.

Delayed union was confirmed by the histological section prepared from tissue from the fracture site, which revealed fibrous tissue and intramembranous bone deposition. There was no evidence of a fluid-filled gap (Figs. 5-25B). Seven months later the femur is clinically united. A radiograph now shows union along the graft and on the posterolateral cortex of the femur (Figs. 5-25C&D). Bridging callus is present anteromedially where the widest gap had been preoperatively.

Case 5-8 *Delayed union* occurred in a 23-year-old woman with a fracture of the junction at the proximal and middle thirds of the ulna. The fracture was treated by simple plaster immobilization applied intermittently. The patient had pain localized to the fracture site with springy motion at that site. The radiograph shows a zone of radiolucency at the junction of the proximal and middle thirds. Within that radiolucency are small areas of soft, fluffy, increased densities. There is marginal periosteal new bone on the ulnar and radial aspects of the ulna. In addition, increased density within the medullary canal has narrowed the canal at the fracture site (Fig. 5-26A).

The fracture was treated with an onlay iliac crest bone graft. The fracture site histologically shows evidence of new bone formation on either side of a zone of fibrocartilaginous tissue, within which are small areas of new bone with marrow corresponding to the rounded densities in the radiolucent zone (Fig. 5-26B). The persistent attempt at repair by fibrocartilagenous endochondral bone formation without evidence of a cleft at the nonunion site would still classify it as a delayed union (Fig. 5-26C). Within 5 months after the bone grafting, the fracture united by ossification of the intermediary callus.

Case 5-9 There was little doubt that a *nonunion* existed when marked motion (80°) was demonstrated in the AP and lateral radiographs of the right femur 1 year after a supracondylar fracture incurred in a 60-year-old arthritic man (Figs. 5-27A–C). The patient had osteoporosis secondary to his arthritis for which he had undergone proximal tibial osteotomy to correct a varus deformity. The supracondylar fracture was treated by traction for a few days followed by a cast-brace for 1 year. This nonunion was considered *atrophic*. Because of the patient's general condition, he was treated with a lightweight long leg brace (Figs. 5-27D&E). The nonunion site was minimally symptomatic. Two years later he was still walking with a brace and a walker.

Case 5-10 A 43-year-old woman had an ununited fracture of the proximal end of the tibia of 2 years' duration. The AP and lateral radiographs demonstrated the radiolucent zone between the major fragments of the proximal end of the tibia and bony union of comminuted fragments within the proximal fragment (Figs. 5-28A&B). The tissue removed from the medial aspect of the fracture site at the time of the combined inlay—onlay tibial bone grafting showed the characteristic fibrous nonunion of such an atrophic type of *nonunion* (Fig. 5-28C). Union resulted gradually within a year.

Hypertrophic pseudoarthrosis lies somewhere between the two extremes of delayed union and true nonunion. It has features of both types with a synovium-lined gap between the persistent attempts at fibrocartilaginous and osseous repair at the margins. The gap gives the lesion its name.

Case 5-11 A 28-year-old man had had a fracture of the left femur treated with an intramedullary nail 18 months earlier. Clinically, the patient complained of pain on walking, and the site was tender to palpation. The bony reaction on either side of the fracture site indicates a periosteal attempt at repair but failure to bridge centrally along the endosteal areas of the cortex (Figs. 5-29A&B). Motion of the distal fragment is evident by the radiolucent area in the metaphysis between the nail and a reactive zone of new bone density; this picture has been called the "windshield wiper" sign radiographically.

At the time of onlay tibial bone grafting, the hypertrophic callus was evident. Histologically, it was

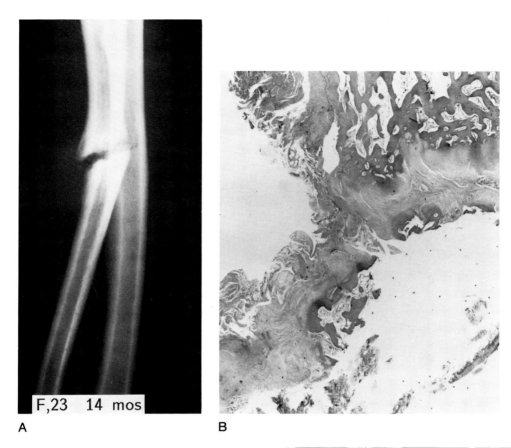

A

B

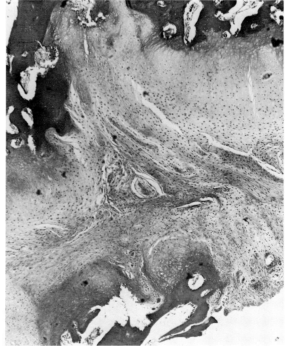

C

Fig. 5-26. Case 5-8. (A) AP radiograph of the forearm shows a 4-mm radiolucent gap in the ulna at the junction of the proximal and middle thirds with small densities within it. There is periosteal new bone on either side of the gap and endosteal new bone. (B) Photomicrograph of the margin of the nonunion site shows fibrocartilaginous tissue with evidence of new bone at the edges and within the cartilaginous tissue corresponding to one of the densities in the radiolucent zone (×25). (C) Fibrocartilaginous endochondral bone formation without evidence of a cleft is seen at the delayed union site (×100).

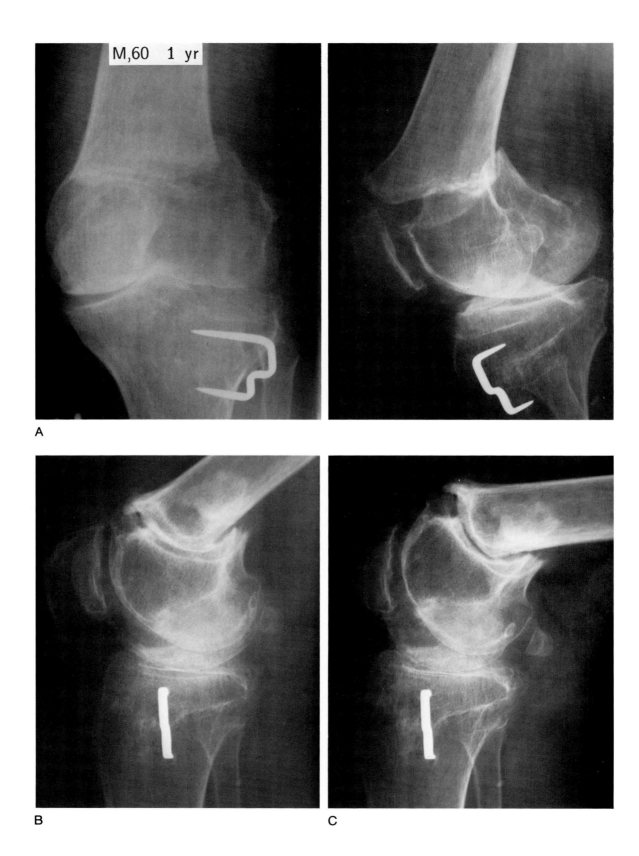

A

B

C

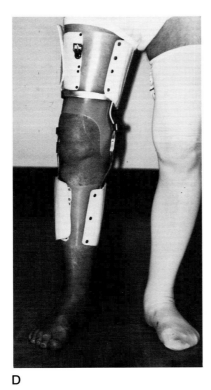
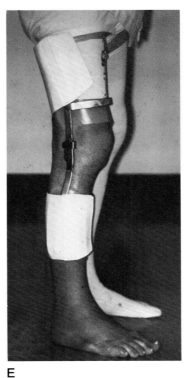

D   E

Fig. 5-27. (Case 5-9. (A) AP radiograph shows nonunion of a supracondylar fracture of the femur. Flexion (B) and extension (C) lateral radiographs demonstrate the range of motion at the atrophic nonunion site. (D & E) The patient had minimal symptoms with the use of a long leg orthosis.

composed of bone peripherally and fibrocartilage centrally with a cleft of synovium-like tissue to characterize this hypertrophic pseudoarthrosis (Figs. 5-29C&D). The *nonunion* began to heal uneventfully within 4 months, with new bone formation. Definitive union was evident 2 years later (Figs. 5-29E&F).

All definitions of nonunion must perforce be arbitrary but are important if one is to assess the results of different forms of treatment in terms of an end result. As noted from the examples cited, one must assess the clinical, radiographic, and pathological aspects in each case.

Definitions

It is much easier to define union of a fracture than nonunion. Clinically, a *healed fracture* is nontender to pressure and rigid on attempts to manually stress

the bone; and the bone transmits sound with a tuning fork or other sound source.[57,65] Radiographically, osseous continuity is present in at least two planes.

A delayed union is said to be present when a fracture has not healed within the time expected for that fracture.[44,60] This statement obviously presupposes a timetable for the proper sequence of repair for a given fracture and for a given fracture treatment method. Such a timetable must be imprecise because of the difficulties posed by the multifactorial nature of the problem. Such a timetable would need to consider the types of bone (cancellous, cortical, corticocancellous) and the location of the fracture (e.g., neck of the femur,[37,41] neck of the talus, carpal navicular[52,56]). In addition, the dimensional aspects would affect the healing time, particularly if displacement of fracture fragments such as bone penetration through the fascia or out of the compartment, bone loss, or increased

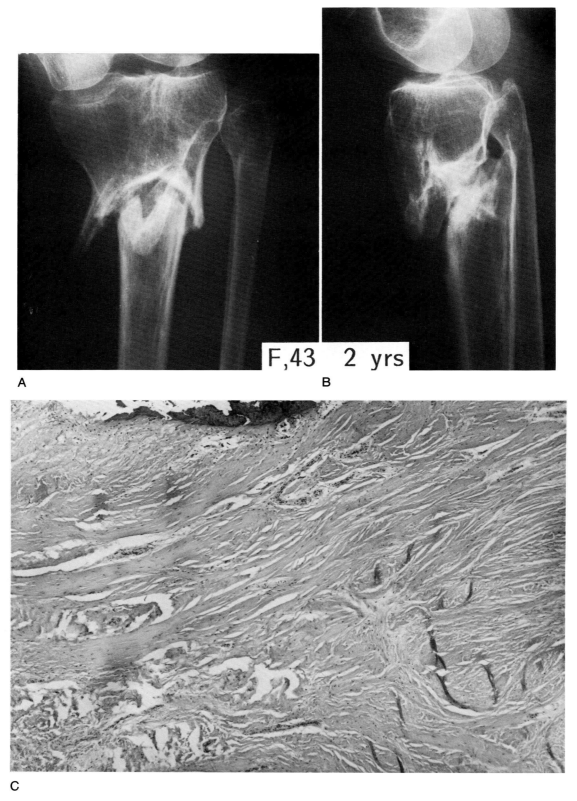

A

B

F,43 2 yrs

C

Fig. 5-28. Case 5-10. AP (**A**) and lateral (**B**) radiographs of the proximal tibia with atrophic nonunion. (**C**) Fibrous nonunion, atrophic type (×40).

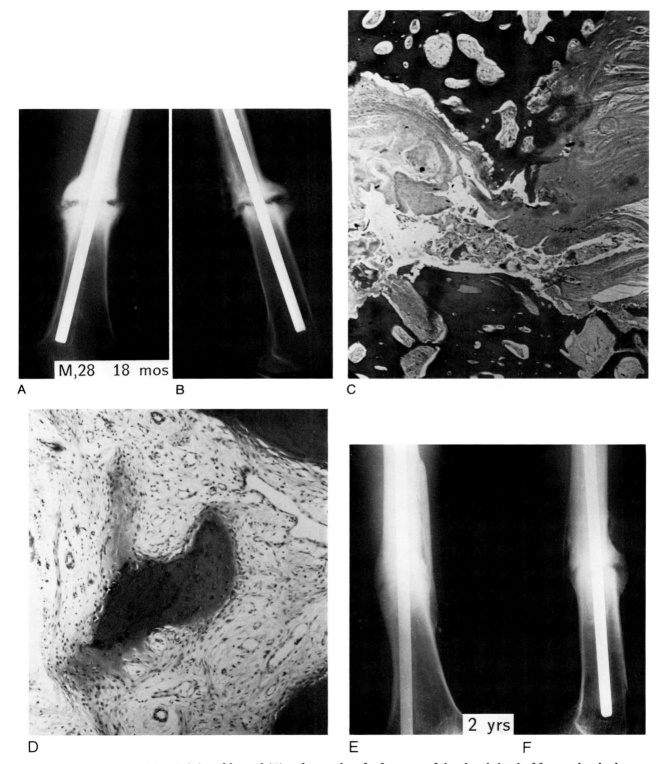

Fig. 5-29. Case 5-11. AP **(A)** and lateral **(B)** radiographs of a fracture of the distal third of femur that had been treated 18 months earlier with an intramedullary rod. Note the "windshield wiper" sign at the end of the nail in the AP view. **(C)** Photomicrograph of the nonunion site shows a cleft filled with synovial-like fibrous tissue at the margins of the bone ends (×30). **(D)** A margin of the pseudarthrosis in which new bone is being formed (×100). AP **(E)** and lateral **(F)** radiographs 2 years after an onlay bone graft from the tibia with healing of the site.

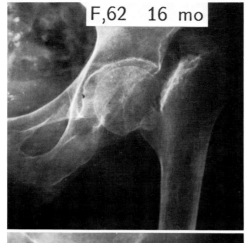

A

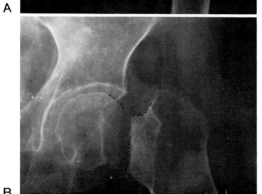

B

Fig. 5-30. Case 5-12. AP (**A**) and AP in traction (**B**) radiographs of the left hip of a 62-year-old woman 16 months after fracture of the femoral neck, atrophic type. (**C**) Photomicrograph of the fibrous nonunion site with little evidence of new bone formation at its attachment to the femoral head (×100). *(Figure continues.)*

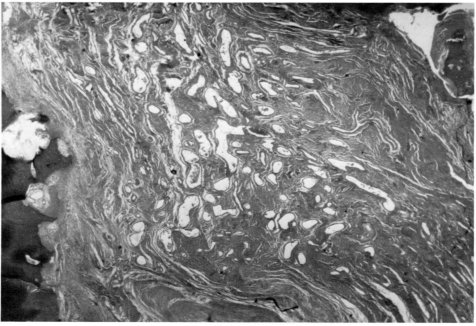

C

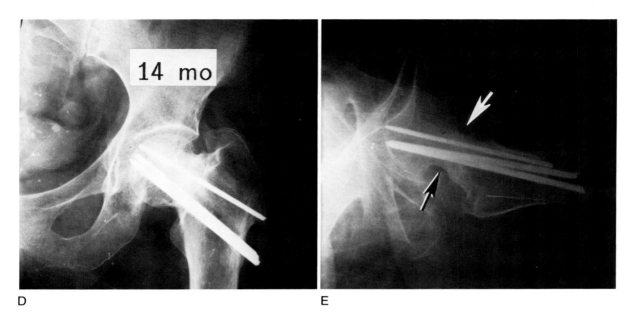

D   E

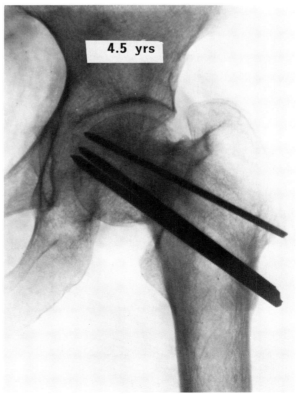

Fig. 5-30 *(Continued).* **(D & E)** Lateral radiograph obtained at 14 months shows reconstitution of the neck of the femur with restoration of continuity. **(F)** AP radiograph of the hip shows union of the neck of the femur with maintenance of the articular cartilage space 4.5 years after surgery. (A, B, E, & F from Bonfiglio and Bardenstein,[41] with permission.)

F

motion or distraction when handling the fracture is part of the situation. It is apparent that such a wide disparity of situations makes a timetable for fracture healing almost impossible for it to be practical.

Clinically, *delayed union* is characterized by tenderness and some motion (springy or a few degrees) at the fracture site. Sound transmitted across the fracture site is decreased (dampened by this fibrocartilagenous tissue) compared to that between two points in normal bone.[57,64] Radiographically, bony callus is present in variable amounts with a radiolucent gap of a few millimeters. The callus is both periosteal or medullary in location, usually of a softer primary bone density (Figs. 5-25B and 5-26B&C). Most of these fractures are united 4 to 18 months after injury.

A *nonunion* or *pseudoarthrosis* is readily identified by the presence of pain and tenderness at the site; there is also palpable motion of the fracture fragments well past any reasonable estimate of healing time (e.g., 18 months or longer). Some untreated fractures, particularly intra-articular fractures are considered ununited after shorter time periods. Sound is poorly transmitted across the fracture site. A gradual change occurs in the fibrocartilaginous callus of a delayed union. There is degeneration of the fibrocartilage to form a cleft, with fluid being elaborated in the site of the pseudoarthrosis. The continued attempt at repair at the margins leads to the club-like ends of a pseudoarthrosis noted radiographically. A translucent gap is surrounded by dense periosteal intramedullary bone callus, which seals the medullary canal, rounds off the ends, and extends well beyond the cortex (Figs. 5-29A&B). A bone scan remains positive wherever a blood supply and new bone is forming in the medullary canal or subperiosteally, but the scan may be "cold" at the gap.

Radiographically, two types of pseudoarthrosis are identified. An *atrophic pseudoarthrosis* is really a fibrous union such as occurs in the diaphysis of the humerus or in femoral neck fractures (Figs. 5-30A&B). The other, more classic type, *hypertrophic pseudoarthrosis*, and consists of fibrocartilaginous callus and a synovial fluid-containing cavity between the bone ends (Fig. 5-29C).

There are many factors that predispose to nonunion. Some of them are injury-related, e.g., anatomical dimensional components including segmental bone loss, extensive soft tissue damage, and loss of blood supply to one or more of the fragments. Other factors are treatment-related and include reduction, distraction, and the period of immobilization.

It is obvious that fracture and treatment factors combine to interfere with repair by competent cells, which have to be stimulated by physiological compression and biomechanical and bioelectrical forces. When these biological factors are interfered with, as for example, by infection, the result may be an ununited fracture.

Those factors that are related to the injury are important to keep in mind during treatment of the fracture, as they may well alter the method, as well as the length, of treatment. Allowances must be made for the anatomical alterations from the injury and loss of repair potential. When the injury is severe enough, it can cause extensive stripping of the periosteum and *extensive damage to the soft tissue* and its blood supply, which in turn can lead to extreme scarring about the fracture site and thus impairment of the repair process. If a large amount of soft tissue interposed between the fracture ends is displaced from the periosteal envelope, the delay in fracture healing is slight if reduction and alignment are achieved. Small amounts of tissue are readily resorbed and replaced by callus.

If there is *loss of bone*, however, which leaves a gap, there is increased potential for delayed repair. Key,[50] Robinson,[54] and others have demonstrated that only gaps in diaphyseal bone at least 1.5 times the diameter of the diaphysis can produce a pseudoarthrosis in animals. When possible, filling the gap with a bone graft aids in the restoration of continuity and union of the bone if the soft tissues covering the bone are adequate for the situation. The other alternative is to accept shortening by permitting the bone ends to come closer together; this method is sometimes used for an open fracture when infection may be a problem.

Probably the most significant injury-related factor leading to nonunion is *impairment of the blood supply*. Specific examples of sites where impaired blood supply are associated with a high incidence of nonunion are fractures of the neck of the femur with loss of circulation to the femoral head, fractures of the carpal scaphoid, and fractures of the neck of the talus. These fractures do unite, but the fracture should be protected longer according to the size of the area of necrosis, thereby allowing appropriate treatment to promote restoration of the blood supply and prevent late sequelae of this complication (see Ch. 7). In addition, fractures at the junction of the middle and distal thirds of the tibia may have a high incidence of nonunion due to interference with the medullary blood supply of the diaphysis at that level.[62] Similarly, the diaphysis of the humerus and femur may be affected because of interference of the medullary blood supply, although in those long bones the periosteal blood supply is so rich that it is not as critical a factor as distraction and poor apposition of bone fragments.

Although the factors related to the extent and location of the injury may not be under the control of the treating physician, recognizing the problems before undertaking appropriate treatment should minimize the occurrence of nonunion.

The most important treatment-related factors in terms of healing or nonhealing of the fracture are *reduction* and *immobilization*.[62] Watson-Jones[61] adamantly stated that "the cause of nonunion is inadequate immobilization." Nearly all the problems can be overcome, provided stringent immobilization is maintained in one axis, i.e., the weight- or load-bearing axis. Rigid immobilization in all planes is an extreme measure that may be desirable but not necessary. The immobilization must be appropriate for the particular fracture — in regard to both type of fracture and, importantly to Watson-Jones, the duration of the immobilization. The period of time must be long enough to permit maturation of the callus from a primary type of bone to a secondary type of bone, i.e., lamellar and osteonal.

That *reduction* is critical to healing of fractures goes without saying, as fractures with wide displacement (e.g., penetration of a bony fragment through fascia or into a muscle compartment) have a higher incidence of delayed union or nonunion. As another example, poor reduction of femoral neck fractures lead to a high incidence of nonunion. *Distraction* of fracture fragments is detrimental to union, as noted for bone loss, fracture gaps, and the use of external fixation devices during healing. During the treatment of fractures of the shaft of the femur by skeletal traction, distraction for days to weeks reduces the blood supply to the healing fracture by occluding capillary flow, which interferes with callus formation.

Compression is said to stimulate bone repair.

Physiological compression (i.e., the action of muscles about the fracture site compressing the reduced fracture fragments) is considered the most important factor. The mechanical effect of reducing the fracture gap to a minimum improves the immobilization, which may be the principal factor in healing when the compression principle is put into effect by various methods, e.g., weight-bearing with casts, or braces, or the use of compression plates.[61]

Observations on the electrical properties of bone, reported in 1954 by Yasuda et al.,[65] revealed that when bone is compressed in vivo new bone formation is stimulated. When bone is distracted, the reverse is true. Excessive pressure, however, has been shown to cause bone necrosis, and it may produce trabecular or osteonal microfractures and areas of focal necrosis.

[The *piezoelectric effect* was referred to earlier regarding the effect of compression on bone.] Whether electrical factors play a role in good fracture treatment is yet to be determined. There is some suggestive evidence that the use of electrical stimulation promotes the healing of delayed union and in some instances of nonunion, as is discussed later.[38,39,43,46,63]

Each of these factors must be taken into consideration along with the location and type of bone fractured.[40] It is recognized that an isolated fracture of the tibia in an adult predisposes the tibia to a high rate (26 percent) of nonunion or varus malunion because of the biomechanical distracting effect of the intact fibula.[59] The effect is less severe in patients under 20 years of age, where because of the flexibility of the fibula in this age group, varus malunion ensues, and a bent fibula may also be associated with the tibial deformity in some cases.[59]

Biological factors (i.e., systemic) are said to be important, but only extreme starvation or debility from concomitant disease has interfered with fracture healing. The minimum subsistence levels with regard to nutritional factors essential for life are apparently all that is required to heal a fracture. Callus appears to hold a high priority for use of all tissue building materials that are in transport. The body metabolizes other tissues in order to meet the requirements necessary for repair of a fracture. In the presence of rickets or osteomalacia, the material of repair may be primarily osteoid tissue rather than mineralized tissue. Corticosteroids in large doses presumably delay fracture healing, as they do for all tissues.

Infections can delay or even prevent healing. When extensive areas of bone necrosis exist, they may require sequestrectomy, which in turn may leave a gap in the bone. Adjacent soft tissue infection also interferes with repair. Infected fractures heal if they are immobilized for prolonged periods. Fracture healing can be benefited by controlling the infection, but it is not the infection per se that prevents healing. Infection interferes with fracture repair by imposing loss of blood supply to the fracture sites in addition to the loss caused by the injury. After operative treatment of the fracture periosteal stripping involved in the application of internal fixation causes an additional loss of blood supply. Although delayed healing of the fracture may result, the application of good principles in the care of the infection and the fracture usually permit healing of both the infection and the fracture.[40,47-49,51,53]

Treatment

The age and specific needs of a patient can determine the most favorable method of treatment for nonunion. Identification of the most frequent sites of nonunion in the large studies mentioned earlier, have led to development of several treatment methods that applied to fresh fractures minimize the frequency of nonunion.

Prevention
For example, few would treat a fracture of the femoral neck by plaster immobilization, as internal fixation with threaded pins or compression devices has markedly reduced the incidence of nonunion.[37] It is now accepted that fracture of the lateral condyle of the humerus is best treated by internal fixation. Thus prevention becomes a significant strategy for reducing the incidence of delayed or nonunion of fractures at those sites. Prolonged distraction of long bone fractures treated by traction is avoided whenever possible, as it is known that fractures that heal with a small amount (2 cm or less) of shortening cause minimal impairment of function. Shortening of an upper limb bone more than 2 cm causes little trouble. For the lower limb, shoe lifts

can compensate for more severe shortening. Physicians and patients should be willing to accept a less than perfect anatomical result to prevent nonunion or other complication (infection, bone loss, or loss of limb) in lieu of surgical intervention pursued to achieve an anatomically perfect result.

Continued immobilization by external means for long bone fractures in well molded plaster dressings applied to minimize the shearing effect on the fracture site and to maximize the axial loading by muscle ("physiological compression") or weight-bearing compression permits most fractures to heal. The principle involved is to avoid interruption of the repair process until union is achieved.

Advocates of cast-brace treatment of fractures and internal fixation or external fixation of fractures must be skilled in the application of each of those methods to prevent delayed union or nonunion. Watson-Jones stated that "nonunion is due to failure of surgeons much more than failure of osteoblasts."[61] Blumenfield, after a review of the Iowa experience with 346 cases of pseudoarthrosis, reported in 1947 that, "nonunion is an avoidable complication in the treatment of fractures."[40]

Numerous methods are employed to treat nonunion. The treatment may range from benign neglect to rigid internal fixation with or without bone grafts, to bone grafting, to electrical stimulation with implanted electrodes or external coils.

As noted earlier, the end result, or prognosis, with a given method depends on the biological state of the nonunion at the time of treatment. The closer to a delayed union the situation is, the better are the chances of achieving bone union.

Benign Neglect
Painless nonunion of a medial malleolus with no associated ankle instability may be neglected and left untreated. Other ununited avulsion fractures such as fracture of the ulnar styloid process, the base of the distal phalanx of a finger, or the base of the fifth metatarsal, or a stable medial collateral ligament avulsion fracture from the femur may be ignored unless symptomatic.

Braces, Orthoses
An elderly person with a fibrous nonunion of the humerus can perform the functions of daily living

with a long arm brace. A long, lightweight leg or-thosis was used in the patient with nonunion of the supracondylar femur fracture (Case 5-9; Figs. 5-27D&E). Patellar tendon bearing or cast-braces may permit a patient with a tibial nonunion reason-able weight-bearing function.

Bone Grafts

The most widely employed treatment for nonunion is some form of bone grafting. Principles involved are based on knowledge of the biological aspects of the healing of fractures and the pathological fea-tures of delayed union or pseudoarthroses.

Phemister firmly established the principle of onlay bone grafting without removing the interme-diary callus.[53] A strong graft, usually of cortical-cancellous bone from the proximal part of the tibia or occasionally, for use in fractures of smaller bones from the ilium, is placed across the prepared flat-tened surface to bridge the fracture site.

The key to proper bone grafting of a long bone is preparation of the recipient surface so that the graft has good contact on either side of the un-united fracture site. The periosteum is stripped for 4 to 5 cm on either side of the nonunion site to expose the nonunion site. The protruding mass is chiseled off in line with the cortex on either side so that a flattened surface at least 4 to 6 cm long and 1.5 to 2.0 cm wide is available on each side of the fracture. The remaining intermediary callus (fi-brous, cartilaginous, or osseous) need not be re-moved. If the nonunion is near the curve of the metaphyseal area, a trough made through the cor-tex into the medullary canal to receive the graft allows better contact across the fracture site (Fig. 5-29). The cancellous bone trimmed from the end-osteal surface of the graft is packed about the non-union site and along the graft before closing the soft tissue envelope of periosteum and muscle. It may be necessary to make a longitudinal relaxing inci-sion of the periosteum and soft tissue envelope to allow closure over the bone graft without tension.

Ununited fractures of the femoral neck require two tibial grafts 1 to 2 cm wide by 8 to 10 cm long inserted as intramedullary supports with or with-out internal fixation.[41] A few clinical examples are illustrated to highlight the principles involved and the variations encountered because of anatomical differences.

Case 5-12 Tibial bone grafts were used for fibrous nonunion (Fig. 5-30E) of a fracture of the neck of the femur in this case. A 62-year-old woman had had an ununited fracture of the left femoral neck of 16 months' duration (Figs. 5-30A – F). It is appar-ent that the two tibial grafts hypertrophied by 14 months to reconstitute the femoral neck (Figs. 5-30D). In such an unstable situation, the addition of threaded pins or some other form of internal fixation is useful. Some surgeons prefer a fibular graft for the neck and head of the femur for treat-ment of nonunion. In any case, the success of any method of bone grafting depends on the early union of the bone graft to the bone surface, in this case the channel with which it is in contact (Fig. 5-31).

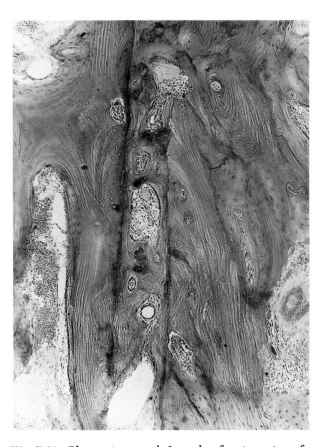

Fig. 5-31. Photomicrograph 3 weeks after insertion of a tibial bone graft into a channel of the neck of a femur of a dog shows union of the head and graft to the margin of the channel ($\times 100$).

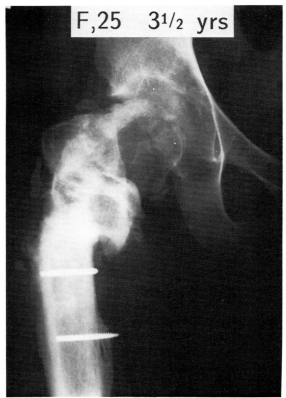

A

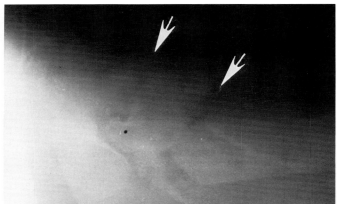

B

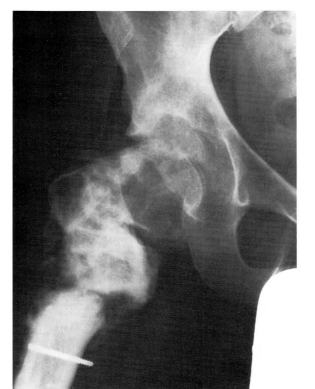

C

Fig. 5-32. Case 5-13. **AP (A)** and lateral **(B)** radiographs of the proximal femur show a double nonunion (arrows) —the base of the neck and subtrochanteric area— 3.5 years after fractures incurred in a motor vehicle accident. **(C) AP** radiograph with abduction of the thigh shows pseudarthrosis at the subtrochanteric region. *(Figure continues.)*

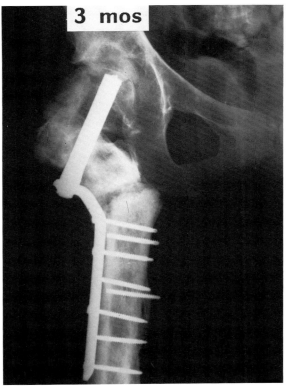

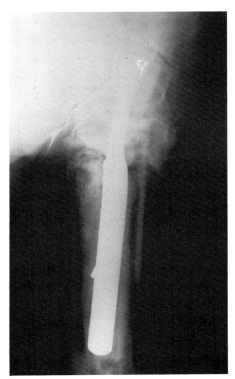

D

E

Fig. 5-32 *(Continued)*. AP **(D)** and lateral **(E)** radiographs of the proximal femur at 3 months show the inlay graft in the neck and head and an onlay bone graft along the anterior aspect of the femur and trochanter. **(F)** AP radiograph at 2 years 3 months shows union of all the sites treated. However, secondary post-traumatic degenerative arthritis is present in the hip joint.

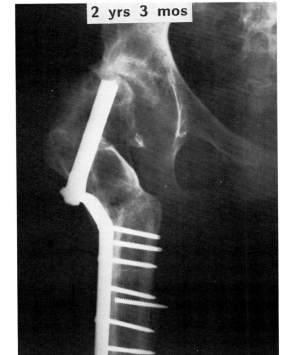

F

Case 5-13 A 25-year-old obese woman with a double nonunion site of the proximal femur in the region of the femoral neck and the subtrochanteric region was treated with onlay and intramedullary bone grafts 3.5 years after her initial injury (Figs. 5-32A&B). She had a true pseudarthrosis in the subtrochanteric region (Fig. 5-32C). The tibial graft was onlayed anteriorly along the proximal part of the femur and inlayed across the nonunion site into the intratrochanteric region in a channel prepared for it. A second tibial graft was inserted into a channel cored from the trochanteric region across the femoral neck nonunion into the femoral head, and a nail plate was applied for stability of both sites. Because of a failure of earlier internal fixation in the treatment of her initial injury, the patient was treated in a single hip spica for 1 month to add external protection of her nonunion sites.

A photomicrograph of tissue from the subtrochanteric nonunion site shows the typical synovium-like pseudarthrosis. At 3 months the radiographs of the hip and proximal femur showed early union of both fracture sites and union of the tibial graft anteriorly (Figs. 5-32D&E). At 2 years 3 months after the bone grafting procedure, the patient had minimal difficulty with the hip related to secondary degenerative arthritis. Both of her fracture sites were solidly united (Fig. 5-32F). It is obvious that bone grafting procedures require adaptation to the clinical situation in each instance in order to obtain the optimal result.

The onlay bone graft without fixation may need to be altered when the ununited segment of a fracture is malpositioned. The next patient illustrates this point vividly.

Case 5-14 A 20-year-old man suffered a severely comminuted fracture of the humerus in a motor vehicle accident. Some of the fracture fragments united, but there was failure of union of the flexed distal fragment with the central and proximal diaphyseal fragment (Figs. 5-33A&B) 9 months after injury. Clinically, there was motion at the nonunion site and restricted motion of the elbow joint.

Using an anteromedial approach, the nonunion site was exposed subperiosteally, lifting the brachialis muscle and retracting it laterally, dissecting the neurovascular bundle, and retracting those structures medially and posteriorly. The angulation was correctable without osteotomy. A tibial graft was applied as a rigid splint anteriorly and held in place with screws. The arm was immobilized in a long arm plaster dressing, which was attached to a plaster band about the patient's body in order to prevent external and internal rotation of the arm. At 8 weeks all immobilization apparatus was removed, and the patient was permitted to begin gentle motion of the shoulder and elbow. The radiographs showed that the position of the fragments and the graft maintained proper alignment, and there was early union of the bone graft to the fragments (Figs. 5-33C&D). The patient gradually recovered full range of motion of the shoulder and elbow and at 8 months showed evidence of solid union of the fracture fragments.

An example of the use of only iliac grafts in an ulnar fracture was cited earlier (Fig. 5-26). Iliac bone grafts served well because stress on the nonunion site was minimal. The intact radius served to splint the ulna. Iliac grafts provided the osteogenic stimulus required for union.

The reflected periosteum and muscles are firmly sutured over the graft, and then the fascia, subcutaneous tissue, and skin are sutured over that layer. When needed, a relaxing incision of the deep portion of the periosteum permits closure over the increased mass of graft tissue. The graft is thereby firmly held as a rigid splint against the bone so it does not become displaced. External plaster immobilization of the limb for 2 to 3 months permits bony union in a high percentage (94 percent) of cases with few complications.[53] Some surgeons prefer strips of cancellous bone from the ilium packed about the fracture site.[51]

The biological principles underlying the rationale of the operation are as follows: (1) the osteogenic cells of the graft and the reactivation of the repair process stimulate the intermediary fibrous or fibrocartilagenous tissue to ossify by endochondral and intramembranous bone formation. (2) The graft is long enough and thick enough to splint the fracture mechanically, and the tight periosteal envelope and close fit of the graft along a flattened bed are prepared to bridge the fracture site. (3) Elimination of motion as a result of periosteal bony union between the graft and fracture fragments occurs within a few weeks. The splinting effect of iliac grafts is less than that afforded by cortical bone, although the osteogenic potential is theoreti-

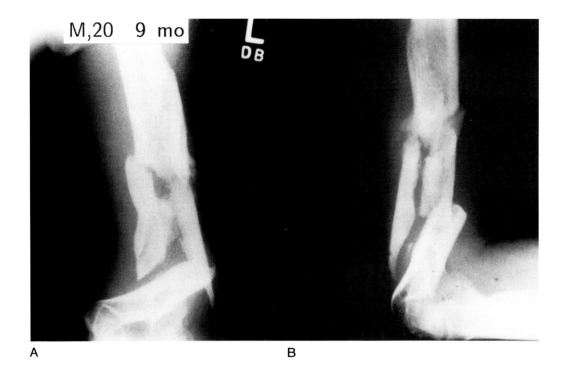

A   B

Fig. 5-33. Case 5-14. AP (**A**) and lateral (**B**) radiographs of the distal humerus show a severely comminuted fracture with nonunion and malposition of the distal fragments 9 months after injury. AP (**C**) and lateral (**D**) radiographs of the distal humerus and elbow 1 year after open reduction and internal fixation with an onlay tibial bone graft. There is solid bony union.

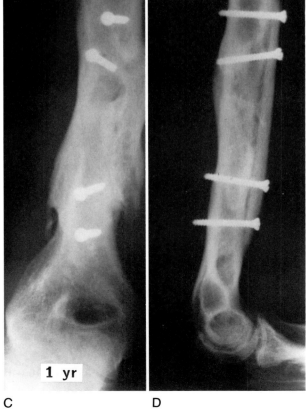

C   D

cally greater (Figs. 5-25, 5-26, 5-28, 5-29, 5-30, 5-32).

Union of the graft to the host bed occurs along all contact points between graft and bone. The callus is first seen subperiosteally at the ends of the graft at 10 to 21 days. Thus physiological immobilization, afforded by union of the graft across the fracture site, allows uninterrupted growth of vascular buds into the fibrocartilaginous callus to replace the old callus with new bone. It requires at least as long as for initial fracture union and additional time for reorganization of the fracture site (several months to a year or more). Gradually increased stress on the involved but protected limb permits the necessary remodeling without a breakdown of the repair.

Union occurs in a high proportion of ununited fractures treated by bone grafting: 88 to 94 percent in a series reported by Boyd et al.,[42] 94 percent in a study by Phemister,[53] and 96 percent in a series of nonunions of the scaphoid reported by Murray.[52]

The failures usually resulted from infections, improper grafting, or inadequate immobilization. A number of surgeons advocate the use of internal or external fixation along with onlay bone grafts as a means of achieving immobilization. In some situations, screws have been used to fix the cortical grafts, either single or dual, in lieu of plate fixation. This method is particularly useful for fractures of the radius or ulna and in instances of a malunion and nonunion of the distal humerus where correction of the alignment is required (Fig. 5-33).

Combinations with Internal Fixation

The addition of interfragmentary screws or a plate or intramedullary rod does not alter the principle on which bone grafting is based but does add to the risks of the additional surgical trauma, i.e., tissue necrosis or infection. This approach is particularly useful, however, when bony defects complicate the treatment of acute fractures or when treatment is delayed, as shown earlier (see Fig. 4-4).[64]

Compression Plate

In recent years advocates of compression plate treatment of fractures have used that system for treating nonunion of fractures without bone grafts. The relatively rigid immobilization permits the fibrocartilaginous callus to convert to bone by endochondral ossification.[64]

Electrical Stimulation

A number of reports since 1953 have noted the effect of electrical energy to stimulate bone healing.[38,39,43,63] In 1977 Spadaro[58] reviewed the literature on the subject. Variable success in the treatment of delayed union or nonunion has been reported using electrical energy applied by implanted electrodes (invasive) or by externally induced current (noninvasive). Most investigators have employed direct current, but alternating currents seem to be equally effective.[46] The reports indicate that a favorable effect on repair is predictable in cases of delayed union but not so in bones where a pseudoarthrosis with a fluid-filled cavity is present.[7] The exact percentage of union varies in different reports because of the lack of a clear definition of nonunion; success in treatment ranges from 50 percent for pseudoarthroses to 90 percent for delayed unions, but no control studies are available to compare prolonged immobilization as the treatment with immobilization plus electrical stimulation. There was considerable variation in the properties of the electric current or potential applied and the time schedules used. For the invasive techniques, the composition, size, and shape of the electrodes are still under study.

DeHass and Watson[46] reported that a relatively simple noninvasive method of electrical stimulation by pulsed magnetic fields (induced alternating current) to treat ununited fractures of the tibia led to union in 15 of 17 patients whose fractures had not healed for 9 to 60 months. Most of these patients had had failed bone graft surgery. The time to union was shorter, less than 6 months, when compared to a group of conventionally treated ununited fractures. The suggested mechanism of action is increased revascularization at the fracture site followed by gradual intermediary callus ossification based on radiographic observations. The pulsed magnetic field across the fracture induces a portion of the current across the fracture sufficient to stimulate bone formation. Once appropriate clinical trials have been completed, this method may be included in the treatment of some ununited fractures. The accumulating evidence is strongly suggestive, on empirical grounds, that there is a stimulating effect of electrical energy on repair, but the pathophysiological mechanism is speculative at best.

PATHOLOGICAL FRACTURES

A wide variety of conditions including prenatal and developmental abnormalities, infections, metabolic processes, radiation effect, lesions simulating tumors, benign and malignant tumors, and tumors metastatic to bone are responsible for the occurrence of pathological fractures. Any condition affecting the skeleton that weakens the trabecular or cortical structure of bone may predispose to a pathological fracture.

Those most frequently encountered by the physician and the orthopedic surgeon occur in patients with osteoporosis or tumors metastatic to bone. The evaluation and treatment of these areas are given greatest emphasis here. In addition, however, the orthopedist is occasionally called on to consider fractures in patients who have undergone radiation therapy for tumors and in whom the skeleton has been affected by the radiation, as well as patients with Paget's disease. Examples from each of these groups form the basis of this section.

Osteoporosis

Compression fracture of the spine in an older person is probably the most common fracture in humans. It often occurs repeatedly and is responsible in part for the loss of height many people show after age 45 in women and after age 60 in men. It differs from the acute compression fracture that occurs after more severe injury (see Ch. 3).

Case 5-15 The thin trabeculae that produce the typical radiographic appearance, depicted in the 76-year-old woman with senile osteoporosis shown in Figure 5-34, undergo microfractures with collapse of the vertebral body end-plates to give the characteristic biconcave appearance to the vertebral body, which resembles a "codfish vertebra" (Fig. 5-34A). Some vertebrae also have a wedge-shaped compression fracture similar to that of the post-traumatic compression fracture. In some patients with osteoporosis it probably results from no more trauma than muscular contraction, such as might occur with a sneeze or when bending to pick up a small object.

The vertebrae, which have been greatly altered

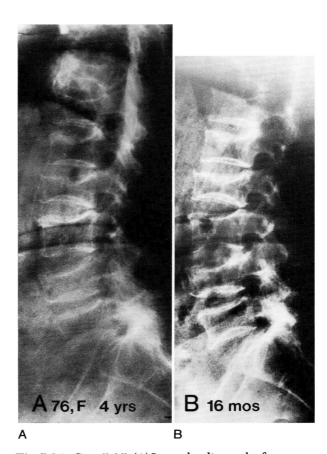

Fig. 5-34. Case 5-15. (**A**) Lateral radiograph of compression fractures in an osteoporotic 76-year-old woman. (**B**) Lateral radiograph 16 months after treatment with exercise and fluorides. The patient has no symptoms.

by osteoporosis, either undergo a single gross compression fracture or serial microfractures that cumulatively lead to deformity of individual vertebrae or, in most cases, several vertebrae successively as noted in this patient.[70,83]

With medical treatment, such patients can obtain symptomatic improvement and in some instances a slight increase in bone density; usually there is no further decrease in bone density if drug treatment is successful.[73] This patient was treated with sodium fluoride 25 mg twice daily and vitamin D calcium lactate capsules along with a program of increased activity, including walking and mild daily exercise. The radiograph obtained 16 months after the earlier ones showed an increase in the bony

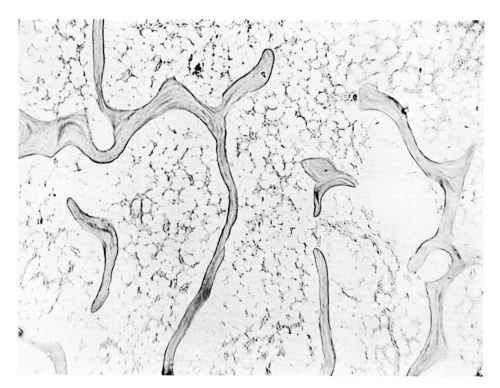

Fig. 5-35. Photomicrograph shows thin trabeculae of osteoporosis (×100).

density of the vertebral end-plates of the thoracic and lumbar spine (Fig. 5-34B).

Case 5-15 represents an example of senile or involutional osteoporosis. The condition is indistinguishable from postmenopausal osteoporosis, except for its later onset. Both forms should be distinguished from the many specific treatable other forms of osteopenia or loss of bone density secondary to hormonal deficiencies such as hyperparathyroidism, hypercortisolism (Cushing's syndrome), or osteomalacia of either chronic nutritional or renal origin.[73]

A discussion of calcium and phosphorus metabolism is beyond the scope of this section other than in general terms as it applies to the pathophysiology of the examples cited (references on the subject are appended).

Suffice it to say that, should clinical findings suggest a metabolic disturbance, appropriate hormonal assays may be indicated in addition to the usual serum calcium, phosphorus, and alkaline and acid phosphatase values needed to determine the

nature of the problem. The orthopedic surgeon is frequently asked by medical colleagues to perform a bone biopsy to assess the change in trabecular structure caused by the condition in question. Most studies have used iliac crest full-thickness trephine 10- to 20-mm samples for routine histological and histomorphometry evaluation. The histological features of simple osteoporosis (Fig. 5-35), osteomalacia (Fig. 5-36), and hyperparathyroidism (Fig. 5-37) are easily differentiated and often are more readily diagnostic than some of the more complicated biochemical studies.

The histological features seen in these figures do *not* indicate the cause of the trabecular thinning but do differentiate the normal but thin trabeculae of osteoporosis from the bone-resorption disease of primary or secondary hyperparathyroidism and from the osteoid seams of nutritional or other forms of osteomalacia. Once that determination is made, the evaluation can be directed toward elucidating the cause and appropriate treatment.

The prevention of postmenopausal osteoporosis

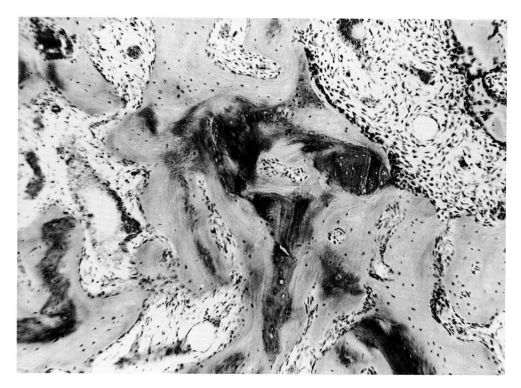

Fig. 5-36. Photomicrograph of osteomalacia with wide osteoid in the seams (×200).

is as difficult as its treatment. Evidence has accumulated that replacement estrogen therapy reduces the rate and amount of bone loss. Thus bone density in treated women is greater and the incidence of vertebral and femoral neck fractures is lower than in women so treated.[74] The use of estrogens in women with osteoporosis after age 60 has not been shown to increase bone formation once the loss in bone mass has occurred; suggests that the bone loss due to aging is not only hormonally dependent but also is attributable to reduced physical activity, inadequate calcium intake, and perhaps a decrease in osteoblast function.

For these reasons most treatment regimens include increased physical activity, increased calcium intake, and vitamin D, perhaps supplemented by fluoride, Estrogens, when used in low doses, seem to improve the patient's well-being and acceptance of the combined regimen. Thus maintenance and improvement of bone density minimize the number and frequency of fractures.[73,74]

It is apparent that should the diagnosis be pri-

mary or secondary hyperparathyroidism, the search for parathyroid hyperplasia or tumor in the former and renal disease in the latter would be in order.

Nutritional osteomalacia is an uncommon problem except in Third World countries where nutritional deficiencies are pervasive. Some women with low calcium intake and little exposure to sunshine exhibit osteopenia secondary to mild degrees of osteomalacia combined with senile or postmenopausal osteoporosis.

Whatever the cause of the pathological fracture, in this group of conditions repair occurs within the usual time for the site, whether it is the vertebral body, the distal radius, or the neck of the femur.

However, the associated osteopenia strongly influences the surgical aspects of treatment in two ways. One is mechanical, the other systemic. The mechanical properties of an osteopenic bone may be so compromised that any ordinary means of fixation of fracture fragments will be precarious or ineffective, so that implanted hardware or external

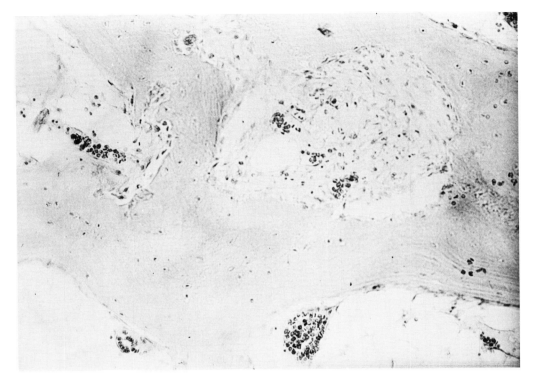

Fig. 5-37. Secondary hyperparathyroidism shows fibrovascular marrow, marginal osteoclasts, osteoblasts, and osteoid along poorly mineralized trabeculae (×250).

devices (including plaster casts) will fail. Unusual methods of fracture fixation, e.g., supplementation of hardware with polymethyl methacrylate may have to be resorted to, if the surgeon considers fixation to be mandatory. If any surgical fixation is deemed too risky on mechanical grounds, other options can be pursued.

Two of the commonest fracture situations in osteoporotic bones other than in the vertebrae illustrate these options. One is fracture through the neck of the femur, the other Colles' fracture of the radius. With the former, one option, now considered standard practice, is removal of the proximal fracture fragment, followed by hemiarthroplasty or total hip replacement arthroplasty. In some contrast, with a Colles' fracture of the radius associated with severe osteoporosis, the surgeon may accept a mild or moderate deformity, or reduce a severe one, but refrain from efforts at fixation in order to pursue a regimen that provided a good chance of retaining the mobility of the wrist, namely, early

motion. If that objective is achieved, the deformity would be acceptable as a small price to pay.

The systemic influences on the surgical options for treatment of a fracture can be summed up as assessment of the patient's general condition. That includes judgements of the degrees of risk of anesthesia, operation, protracted bed rest, etc., factored in with the probable life expectancy and the predicted quality of life with each regimen of treatment. The osteoporosis is one factor in the assessment but it is so closely related to depressed levels of physical activity, and often is associated with medical abnormalities that are concomitant but not related, that it cannot be viewed in isolation as a systemic influence.

Radiation Effect

Osteoporosis secondary to the effects of radiation therapy for tumors such as carcinoma of the cervix, in particular, leads to spontaneous fracture of the

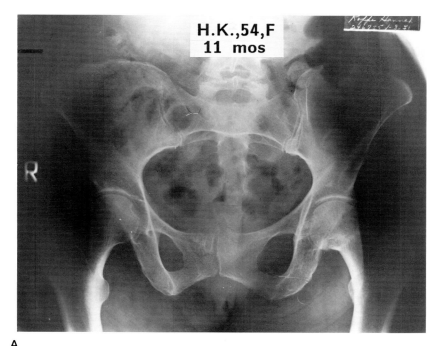

Fig. 5-38. **(A)** AP radiograph of the pelvis shows a stress fracture of the left femoral neck in a 54-year-old woman treated for carcinoma of the cervix with external irradiation. **(B)** Photomicrograph of a trabecula from the femoral head shows capillary resorption along this viable trabecula within the femoral head (×400). (From Bonfiglio,[69] with permission.)

A

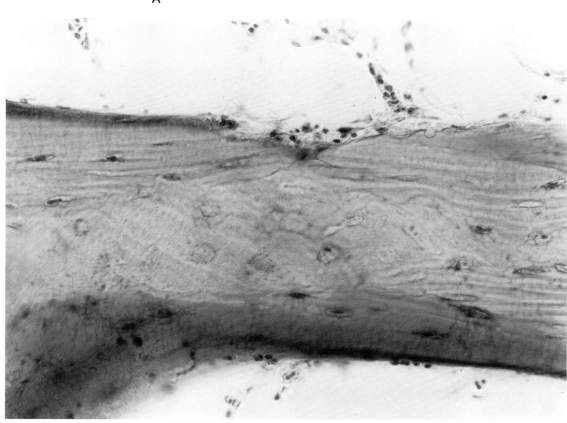

B

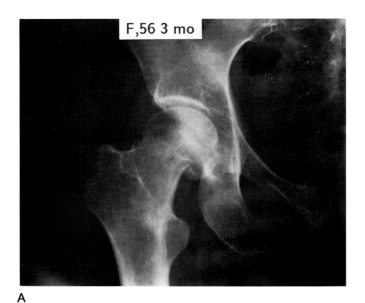

A

Fig. 5-39. **(A)** AP radiograph of the right hip with a fracture of the femoral neck secondary to irradiation for carcinoma of the cervix in a 56-year-old woman who had had pain for 3 months. **(B)** Photomicrograph of the fracture site from a core biopsy shows fracture callus around the thin trabecular fragments. (From Bonfiglio,[69] with permission.)

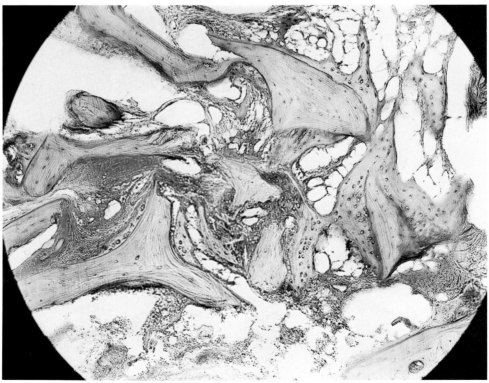

B

neck of the femur in about 1 to 2 percent of patients[69,79] (Fig. 5-38). The ribs, clavicle, and scapula are at risk in patients who receive radiation for treatment of breast cancer.[94]

The pathological findings after megavoltage irradiation depend on the dosage. When there is bone atrophy it predisposes the bone to fractures[69] (Fig. 5-39). The reparative aspects then include bone resorption, bone formation, and in some instances bone necrosis with the usual changes of fragmentation during the resorption of the necrotic bone.

Because, with low or moderate doses of radiation adequate callus occurs at the fracture site, indicat-

ing a good repair response, the fracture should be treated without special regard to the cause. Many of the fractures are of the "stress type," through the osteoporotic trabeculae. When the dose is below 4,500 rad, the potential for repair of the fracture is good. When the dose exceeds 4,500 rad, the secondary radiation osteitis and necrosis may delay or prevent healing. If segmental collapse occurs in the femoral head or the acetabulum, as in the 48-year-old woman in Figure 5-40, a reconstructive procedure may be needed.

Other complications of therapeutic x-irradiation that may be encountered include skin changes in the form of chronic dermatitis, scarring, or epider-

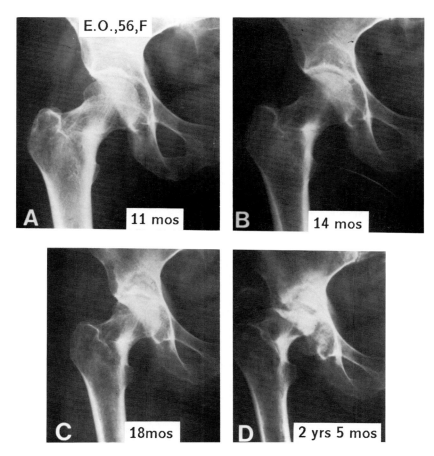

Fig. 5-40. AP radiographs of a 48-year-old woman who was treated with radiation for carcinoma of the cervix. **(A)** Eleven months. **(B)** Fourteen months. **(C)** Eighteen months. **(D)** Two years, five months. These radiographs demonstrate the progression of radiation changes in the acetabulum and the femoral head, indicating segmental collapse along with necrosis of the bone for a radiation dose that exceeded 4,500 rad. *(Figure continues.)*

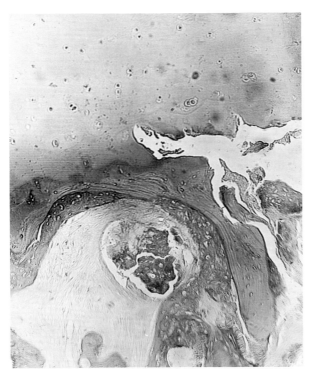

E

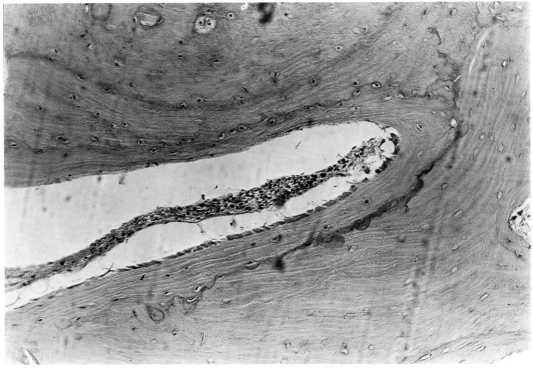

F

Fig. 5-40 *(Continued)*. (E) Articular cartilage in underlying subchondral cortex shows necrotic changes with partial repair with new bone (×90). (F) Necrotic bone is undergoing replacement by vascular invasions, bringing osteogenic cells (×170). (Figs. A–F from Bonfiglio,[69] with permission.)

moid carcinoma. [The outdated practice of reducing fractures under fluoroscopy predisposed the physician to such a risk. Fortunately, physicians rarely do so nowadays.]

A rarer complication is radiation-induced sarcoma.[95] The average latent period is about 8 years, with a range of 2 to 30 years. The threshold dose of 3,000 rad seems to be the dose for the induction of a malignant tumor; however, that dose has been exceeded in most reported cases. A pathological fracture may herald the presence of the sarcoma. Once encountered, the prognosis after treatment, usually surgery, is poor, and the surgery is thus generally palliative.

The physician should be aware that irradiation of growing bone results in growth disturbances that bear a direct relation to the radiation dose and the age of the patient, ranging from minimal or no growth retardation to complete growth arrest.[70,83]

Paget's Disease

A pathological fracture of the tibia or femur may be the first problem that brings a patient with Paget's disease to seek medical attention. Commonly, however, other manifestations of the disease, e.g., pain or progressive anterolateral bowing of the tibia or femur, may bring the patient to the physician. Repeated episodes of pain usually accompany the deformity. Such pain results from pathological stress (infractions or fissure) fractures, which heal spontaneously but add to the length and deformity on the tension side of the bone as it fills in with new bone (Fig. 5-41).

The radiographic descriptions of fractures in patients with Paget's disease, e.g., "banana" fracture or "chalk" fracture, reflect an extension of these fissure fractures after minor trauma to a long bone.[83,96]

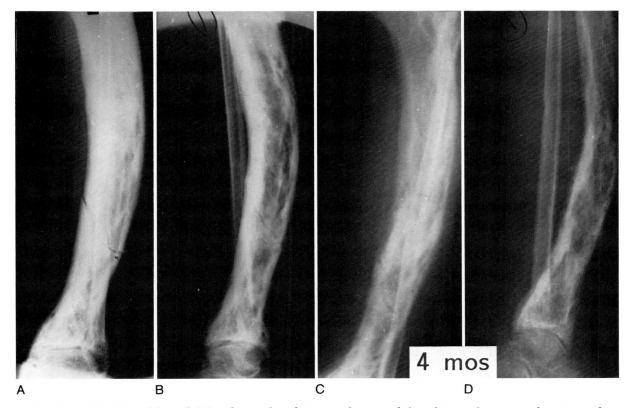

A   B   C   D

Fig. 5-41. AP (**A**) and lateral (**B**) radiographs of Paget's disease of the tibia, with anterior bowing and fracture of the junction of the middle and distal thirds. (**C & D**) At 4 months the fracture is healed.

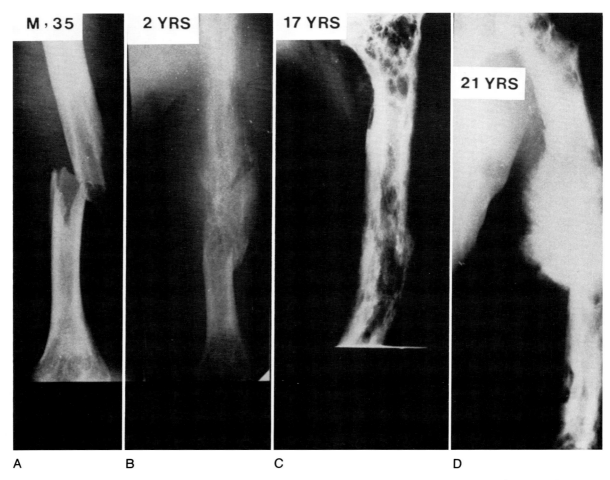

Fig. 5-42. Case 5-16. **(A)** Pathological fracture through an advancing radiolucent zone and Paget's disease. **(B)** At 2 years the fracture is healed. **(C)** At 17 years, note the changes of long-standing Paget's disease. **(D)** At 21 years a sarcoma in mid-humerus arises at the site of the original fracture.

Case 5-16 A 56-year-old man characterizes the problems encountered in patients with Paget's disease. At age 35 the patient sustained a fracture of the humerus after minimal trauma (Fig. 5-42A). The fracture healed without difficulty, but at 2 years (Fig. 5-42D) changes suggestive of the mottled appearance of Paget's disease were apparent. At 17 years the humerus clearly depicted the pagetoid pattern of resorption cavities within the cortices and coarse trabecular remodeling of the cancellous bone (Fig. 5-42C). This patient, at 21 years after the onset, developed an osteosarcoma of the humerus and at three other sites: the skull, femur, and second lumbar vertebra. He died within 6 months after he presented with pain and swelling of the humerus secondary to the osteosarcoma (Fig. 5-42D).

Case 5-17 A 45-year-old woman presented with a transverse fracture of the proximal third of the femoral shaft with minimal displacement (Fig. 5-43A). At 11 months the fracture healed with remodeling into pagetoid bone. This fracture would probably be treated today by internal fixation rather than the method chosen 40 years ago. This case is used to illustrate the repair of fractures in Paget's disease and the continued progressive involvement of the femur by the advancing radiolucent wedge, as shown in Figure 5-43B.

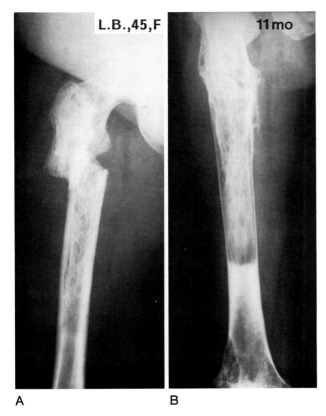

A   B

Fig. 5-43. Case 5-17. **(A)** Fracture of the proximal third of the femur in a patient with Paget's disease. Note the lucent advancing edge in the mid-shaft. **(B)** Eleven months later the fracture is healed, and the radiolucent changes are more pronounced in the diaphysis.

Paget's disease manifests by repeated episodes of osteolysis of unknown cause followed by excessive attempts at repair with a particular type of inferior bone that does not orient along lines of stress.[70,83,84] The result is a weakened, deformed skeleton susceptible to pathological fractures.

The disorder begins as small foci in bone, spreading gradually over months and years in long and flat bones. The disease may remain asymptomatic and monostotic, discovered only incidentally, or it may disseminate extensively throughout the skeleton. Schmorl[93] found a 3 percent incidence of pagetic changes in cadavers over age 40, most commonly involving the skull, lumbar spine, sacrum and proximal femurs. The incidence based on a hospital admission diagnosis is estimated at about 1 per 1,000.

The osteolytic phase is most apparent in the skull, with patchy disseminated areas of radiolucency in the outer table that slowly enlarge until the outer table is indistinct and hazy (this condition is called osteoporosis circumscripta cranii).[77,83] Opacities then appear within the lucent areas to give a cotton-wool appearance as the osteoblastic repair ensues; the outer table enlarges as the periosteum forms a thick, porous cortex with coarse spicules of condensed bone. The inner table remains fairly normal, and the dural surface is smooth. Eventually, the tables and diploë cannot be distinguished.

The base of the skull is also affected, with the skull flattening under its own weight causing dorsal inclination of the foramen magnum. With basilar invagination, the odontoid projects up into the posterior cranial fossa to create nerve root tension. Periosteal new bone formation about the cranial nerve foramina results in visual loss, deafness, and other cranial nerve defects.

Softening and thickening of the sacrum and ilii with settling and development of protrusio acetabuli produce a waddling gait. Eventually there is coxa vara of the femurs. The trabeculae in the innominate bones are apt to be prominent and coarse.

In the thoracic spine there is wedging of vertebral bodies with decreased height of the bodies, increased height of the discs, exostoses, and kyphoscoliosis resulting in stenosis of the spinal canal with possible spinal cord pressure. There is lateral flattening of the ribs with an increased anteroposterior diameter and dyspnea.

In long bones the disorder tends to develop as a small radiolucent focus at the proximal end and work its way gradually as a wedge-shaped arc to the other end. Affected long bones are dense and compact with coarse trabeculae; the cortex is thickened and lamellated with bowing and pseudofractures. The femurs develop coxa vara and anterolateral bowing; the knees show genu varum; the tibias bow anteriorly with thickening of the anterior cortex to form saber-shaped shins. Throughout the process, the medullary canal remains intact unless there is excessive repair. Anemia is therefore uncommon. However, the bones are susceptible to transverse fractures with slight trauma; they most commonly occur in the femur and tibia. The fractures heal slowly with pagetic bone. Infractions are more common than complete transverse breaks, and histologically they resemble fatigue fractures. This pattern accounts for the anterior bow of the femur and tibia as each tension fracture heals and fills the break with new bone.

Histologically, during the osteolytic phase the trabeculae exhibit Howship's lacunae with prominent osteoclasts (Fig. 5-44A). In the cortex, Howship's lacunae and osteoclasts also are seen on the walls of haversian canals. The scalloped resorption cavities are filled with vascular fibrous connective tissue (Fig. 5-44A).

With portions of osteones irregularly resorbed, osteoblasts lay down bone on these surfaces with-out regard to haversian pattern. Spicules of bone may have osteoclasts on one side and osteoblasts on the other. The osteoid is composed of a coarsely fibered matrix lining large, thin-walled vascular spaces (arterial and venous sinuses). Because of the arterial hyperplasia (and not arteriovenous shunting) the blood flow may be 20 times normal. The increased cardiac output leads eventually to ventricular hypertrophy with resulting congestive heart failure, hypertension, and arteriosclerotic cardiovascular disease.

At the margins of the resorption areas, there are cement lines where new bone is laid down. In "cooled off" areas of bone, there is less osteoclastic activity and less fibrous vascular matrix. The mo-

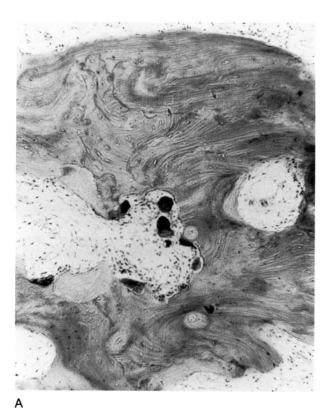

A

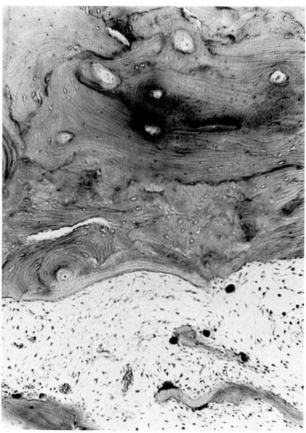

B

Fig. 5-44. (A) Osteoclasts in Howship's lacune are absorbing pagetic bone × 400). (B) Cortex with classical mosaic pattern in fibrovascular marrow with a thin trabecula (× 200).

saic pattern is the histological hallmark of Paget's disease (Fig. 5-44B).

The cambium layer of the periosteum forms spicules of coarse, primitive bone. The periosteal new bone widens the bone as a whole but does not encroach on the medullary space, which is invaded instead by fibrous tissue. As surface infractions appear, the periosteum forms pagetic callus; and with bowing, cancellous bone is replaced by compact pagetic bone.

With regard to laboratory values, the serum calcium is within normal limits. It is elevated only if the patient is immobilized for treatment of fractures or if there is concomitant myeloma or hyperparathyroidism. The serum phosphate level is normal, and the alkaline phosphatase level is elevated (if very high, it is an indication of either extensive involvement or a supervening sarcoma). The acid phosphatase level is normal, allowing differentiation from the blastic lesions of prostatic carcinoma, particularly when a solitary metastatic focus in the spine or pelvis resembles Paget's disease radiographically.

About 5 percent of patients with extensive involvement develop sarcomas,[66,70,83] which may be multicentric and are heralded by pain and swelling; radiographs show irregular lucent areas against a pagetic background. The sarcomas range from hypocellular fibrosarcomas to highly cellular anaplastic sarcomas with tumor giant cells. Two-year survival is rare, as most patients succumb to lung metastases.

There is no specific curative treatment for the disease, but the use of analgesics, e.g., high-dose aspirin, does control symptoms. Calcitonin, diphosphonates, and mithromycin for hypercalcemia may improve the symptoms but do not reverse the pathological process.[78]

Treatment of the fractures should be the simplest that is required to maintain the position of fracture fragments and to immobilize the patient for as short a time as possible, thereby minimizing the increase in serum calcium from prolonged immobilization in bed or in plaster. Internal fixation with intramedullary rods or plates is fraught with complications such as excessive bleeding because of the high vascularity of pagetoid bone. The use of cast-braces as soon as the fractures permit is a reasonable alternative to internal fixation. The fractures have no predilection to nonunion.

Tumor in Bone: Primary or Metastatic

A discussion of pathological fractures would hardly be complete without discussion of those occurring as a consequence of primary tumors in bone or, in particular, tumors metastasic to bone from other organs and tissues.

Pathological fracture may be the first event indicating that a tumor — primary or secondary, benign or malignant has involved a bone. That event occurs with sufficient frequency to alert the physician to that possibility.[68,71,75,88–90] The benign tumors that are prone to such an event include enchondroma, giant cell tumor of bone, chondromyxoid fibroma, and rarely the stalk of an osteocartilaginous exostosis. The malignant tumors likely to metastasize are fibrosarcoma, chondrosarcoma, reticulum cell sarcoma, and plasma cell myeloma. However, in terms of frequency, metastasis to bone from carcinomas heads the list.

The incidence of cancer metastatic to the skeleton is probably much higher than initial reports indicate. Early reports of 10 to 28 percent incidence are in contrast to that of 70 percent, reported by Jaffe based on extensive autopsy studies.[84] As medical and surgical care of cancer patients improved the survival time, the disease has run a more extended course and has thus resulted in a higher incidence of bone metastases and pathological fractures. The effort to treat patients so affected are targeted at relief of pain and maintenace of function. The mean survival time following a pathological fracture of a long bone has gradually increased to nearly 19 months. It is longer for patients with metastases from prostate or breast cancer and shorter for those with metastases from carcinomas of the kidney or lung.

The incidence varies for each type of primary tumor. Cancer of the prostate, breast,[68,75] thyroid, kidney, and lung are those that most frequently metastasize to bone, although any cancer may do so. Some bones are more frequently involved by metastatic tumor than others. Bones having red-marrow, such as bones of the axial skeleton (the thoracic and lumbar spine), as well as the proximal ends of the long bones, are those most commonly invaded. The problems presented to the orthopedic surgeon vary considerably from simple undisplaced fractures to those from multiple metastases in the same bone causing extensive loss of bone substance. Examples of these problem sites at risk, e.g., the proximal femur, humerus, and vertebral body, are illustrated to characterize the range of problems encountered.

In general, it is unusual to find metastases distal to the elbow or knee. When they do occur at those sites, those cancers from junctional areas such as transitional cell carcinoma of the genitourinary tract or epidermoid carcinoma of the lung, must be considered. Some primary cancers have predilections for spread to specific bones, such as cancer of the prostate to the ilium and the lumbar vertebrae, and breast cancer to the ribs, thoracic spine, and skull.

Four routes of metastases exist for cancer to affect bone. They are direct extension, embolism through arteries, spread through the vertebral vein complex, and spread by lymphatics. Spread through the vertebral vein complex known as Batson's plexus deserves special comment. Batson[67] showed that the vertebral vein complex has rich, valveless ramifications that allow forward as well as retrograde flow of blood. These ramifications can trap tumor emboli within the veins of the vertebral body.

Whatever the method of spread, it is essential to recognize that appropriate treatment depends on (1) accurate diagnosis of the primary tumor, and demonstration whether the metastasis is solitary or multiple, and (2) assessment of the condition of the patient. The prognosis is based on probable response to adjunctive therapy and that depends on the specific tumor involved. [The purpose of treatment is to relieve pain, prolong life, and improve function.]

Case 5-18 This case illustrates a relatively straightforward approach to treatment of a pathological fracture due to metastases. A 65-year-old woman who had had a carcinoma of the breast removed previously, had metastases to the proximal left humerus and proximal right femur and had acute pain in the left humerus and aching in the proximal right thigh of several weeks' duration. The radiograph shows an oblique fracture without displacement in the mid-shaft of the humerus (Fig. 5-45A). It was treated simply by coaptation splint of the humerus and a sling on the arm. She was comfortable within a few days, and the fracture healed within 39 days (Fig. 5-45B). The large lytic metastases of the proximal diaphysis of the femur were treated by closed intramedullary rod fixation. Both sites received palliative radiation therapy with excellent relief of pain and reossification of the cortex at 18 months (Fig. 5-45C&D). She remained functional for 2 years after her metastases began.

An alternate method for treating this fracture might be internal fixation with an intramedullary rod and methylmethacrylate, and this method would be appropriate if conservative treatment failed. In this instance, the diagnosis of metastatic breast cancer was confirmed by tissue histology, and the presence of several sites of involvement was a compelling indication for conservative treatment.

We pursue the question of evaluation of lesions responsible for pathological fractures in Chapter 9.

If a pathological fracture is present, tissue from the fracture site is preferably obtained away from any existing hematoma. It should be carefully handled to avoid the crushing effect of curets and so on. When a closed nailing is performed, as in case 5-18, use of a long curet is a practical, acceptable alternative for biopsy in preference to a second incision.

A tissue specimen adequate for histological examination may be obtained by needle biopsy, or open biopsy. Needle biopsy under fluoroscopic control is an appropriate method to differentiate tumor from other conditions that produce lesions suspicious of metastases. There are advantages and disadvantages to each method that should be clearly understood. Needle biopsy is less traumatic but open biopsy allows a frozen section inspection, one can thereby determine the adequacy of the sample of tissue; it also provides the opportunity to obtain specimens to determine the hormonal or chemotherapeutic sensitivity of a tumor, which in turn may direct the adjunctive treatment.

Case 5-19 A 58-year-old woman who had had radical mastectomy for carcinoma of the left breast 2 years prior to the onset of pain in the right hip region illustrates another approach to treatment.

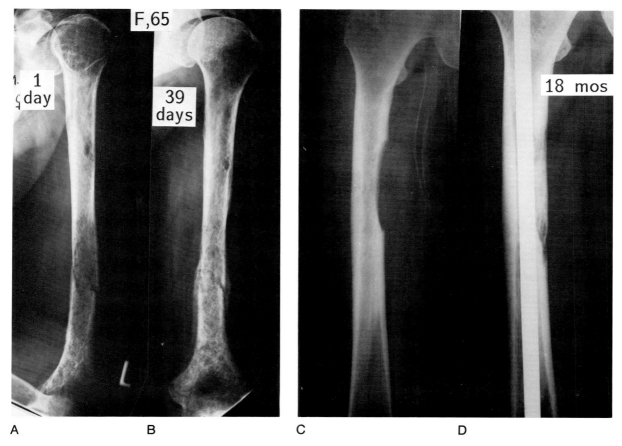

Fig. 5-45. Case 5-18. (A) AP radiograph of the left humerus shows motheaten areas of reduced density, with a fracture at the junction of the middle and distal thirds. (B) At 39 days after simple splinting of the humerus the fracture is united. (C) Preoperative AP radiograph of the right femur shows a lytic cortical defect in the proximal diaphysis. (D) At 18 months after intramedullary rod fixation and radiation therapy the lesion has ossified.

Radiographs of the hip had revealed a fracture of the femoral neck that had been treated by Hagie pinning 4 months earlier (Fig. 5-46A). Because of persistent pain the Hagie pins were removed and a Zickel nail was inserted. Then 2,000 rad were administered to the hip region. Tissue removed at the time of the Zickel procedure indicated that the tumor was hormonally dependent, and so she received hormone therapy in addition to the radiation. Insertion of the Zickel nail in the area of extensive metastatic disease immobilized the fracture fragments, and permitted the patient's fracture to heal within a year and allowed her to walk soon after the nailing without aids. Despite generalized

bone pain, she was still able to walk with a walker 4 years 9 months after her surgery (Fig. 5-46B).

Case 5-20 Another approach to fracture of the femoral neck is excision of the head and insertion of a prosthesis, as was performed in a 76-year-old man with metastasis secondary to cancer of the prostate (Figs. 5-47A&B). He was able to go from bed to chair within 24 hours of the hemiarthroplasty and to walk with a walker thereafter while his metastatic disease was being treated by hormonal and chemotherapy.

The prophylactic use of internal fixation to prevent a pathological fracture is appropriate in selected cases of metastatic cancer of bone.[90] The

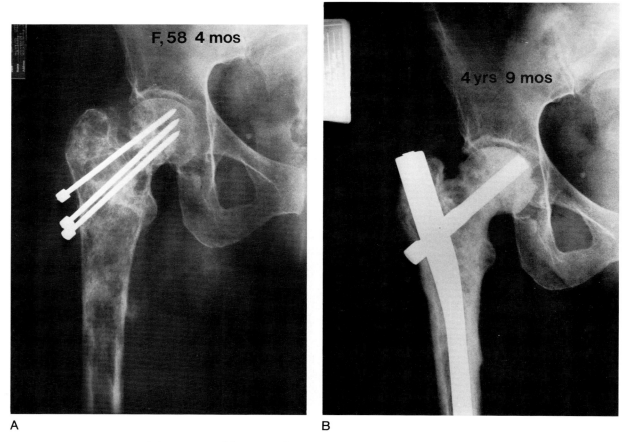

A   B

Fig. 5-46. Case 5-19. **(A)** Fracture of the neck of the right femur secondary to carcinoma of the breast. Four months after insertion of a free Hagie pin the fracture is not united. **(B)** At 4 years 9 months after insertion of a Zickle nail and radiation therapy (2,000 rad) there is healing of the femoral neck fracture and an increase in the density of the metastasis to the proximal femur.

patient in case 5-18, with a fracture of the humerus from metastic cancer of the breast, also had a lytic lesion in the proximal third of the femur that destroyed more than 50 percent of the cortex[89] (Fig. 5-45C). This lesion was treated with an intramedullary Küntschner rod followed by radiation therapy. The lesion healed sufficiently after radiation therapy to permit weight-bearing for 2 years (Fig. 5-45D).

The diagnosis of metastatic cancer, however, may present many problems. It is important to differentiate metastatic tumors from primary tumors of bone, inflammatory processes, or various metabolic diseases. The history of a previous malignant

disease is often helpful. In one of six patients the initial manifestation of a cancer is a metastasis, which is evident even before the first symptoms or clinical signs of the primary tumor appear. A suspected lesion metastatic to bone should follow the American Joint Cancer Commission protocol for evaluation discussed in Chapter 9 for tumors in general.[1] In addition to the usual history and physical examination, proper radiographic evaluation includes films of the sites identified by the history and physical examination. In fact, a biopsy should be done early in the course of the evaluation once routine radiographs identify a lesion; the biopsy results give direction to studies that might identify

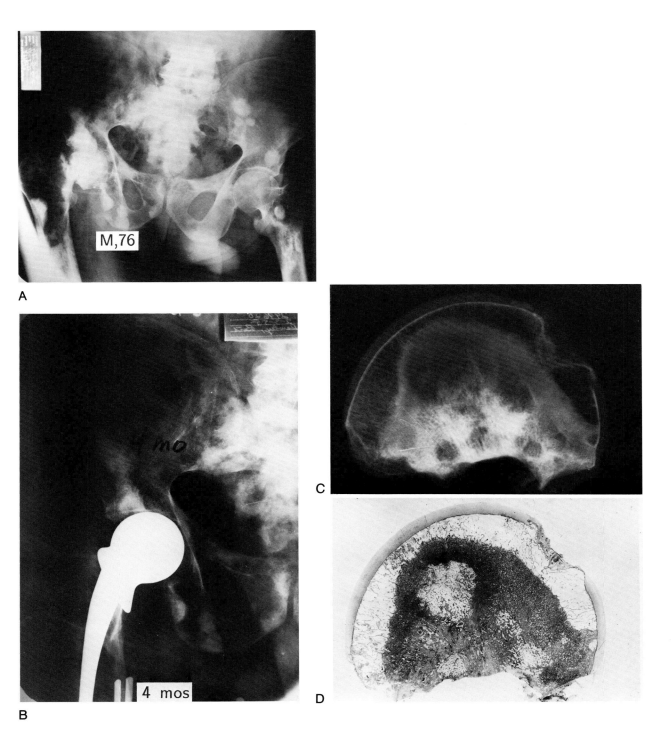

Fig. 5-47. Case 5-20. (**A**) Pathological fracture neck of right femur secondary to osteoblastic metastasis from carcinoma of the prostate. (**B**) Prosthesis after resection of the femoral head. (**C**) Radiograph of the specimen shows the lytic and blastic components of the metastasis within the femoral head. (**D**) Histologic section shows the extent of the metastasis and the site of the fracture through the osteoblastic component of the metastasis (×2).

the primary lesion and may obviate the necessity of extensive and expensive diagnostic tests, e.g., intravenous pyelogram or barium enema.

When the site identified is not easily accessible for biopsy, a radioisotope scan may identify a more readily accessible site of less risk to the patient. However, if the involved bone is weight-bearing bone and requires surgery for internal stabilization, the scan need not be obtained prior to performing the biopsy. Only when resection of a solitary metastasis is contemplated should computed tomography or magnetic resonance imaging be performed to outline the anatomical parameters of the metastasis.

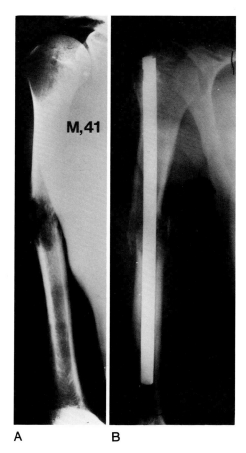

A   **B**

Fig. 5-48. (A) AP radiograph of the right humerus with a pathological fracture through a lytic lesion of the midshaft. (B) Postoperative radiograph shows of a 41-year-old man an intramedullary nail anchored proximally and along the channel with **PMMA.**

For each site of metastatic disease that results or threatens to result in a pathological fracture, the surgeon must use a method appropriate to the situation.[68,71,75,76,80–82,85–89,91,92,97] Problem areas include fractures of vertebrae, which threaten neurological integrity. In such cases, excision of tumor-bearing bone by resection[86] or curettage is appropriate, followed by reconstruction with bone grafts or polymethylmethacrylate (PMMA) and posterior fusion in the cervical spine.[72] Anterior interbody fusion with fixation rods contoured posteriorly for lesions in the thoracic or lumbar spine has been employed.

In the upper limb, maintenance of function in an affected arm may allow the patient to perform the activities of daily living that require the use of both arms. To that end a fracture of the humerus can be stabilized by internal fixation with an intramedullary rod or plates supplemented, perhaps, by polymethyl methocrylate inserted in the medullary canal or in the head of the humerus only to anchor the nail (Fig. 5-48).

Similarly, a patient at high risk for pathological fracture of the proximal end of the femur can be helped prophylactically as regards relief of pain, ease of nursing care, and bed-to-chair activity — by a combination of devices for internal fixation, e.g., wire mesh, threaded pins, and polymethyl methocrylate. Acetabular insufficiency secondary to metastatic disease has been treated using variations of these same surgical principles.[97]

REFERENCES

Joint Fractures

1. Bennett GA, Bauer W: Further studies concerning repair of articular cartilage in dog joints. J Bone Joint Surg [Br] 17:141, 1935
2. Landelle JW: The reaction of impaired human articular cartilage. J Bone Joint Surg [Br] 39:548, 1957
3. Mankin HJ: The reaction of articular cartilage to injury and osteoarthritis. N Engl J Med 291:1285, 1974
4. Mitchell N, Shepherd N: Healing of articular cartilage in intra-articular fractures in rabbits. J Bone Joint Surg [Am] 62:628, 1980
5. Salter RB, Simmons DD, Malcolm BW, et al: The

biological effect of continuous passive motion on healing of full-thickness defects in articular cartilage. J Bone Joint Surg [Am] 62:1232, 1980

Epiphyseal Injuries

6. Baxter MP, Wiley JJ: Fractures of the proximal humeral epiphysis. J Bone Joint Surg [Br] 68:570, 1986
7. Blount WP, Clarke GR: Control of bone growth by epiphyseal stapling. J Bone Joint Surg [Am] 31:464, 1949
8. Bright RW: Surgical correction of partial epiphyseal plate closure in dogs by bone bridge resection and use of silicone rubber implants. J Bone Joint Surg [Am] 54:1133, 1972
9. Campbell CJ, Grisolia A, Zancomato G: The effects produced in cartilaginous epiphyseal plate of immature dogs by experimental surgical traumata. J Bone Jont Surg [Am] 41:1221, 1959
10. Cooperman DR, Spiegel PG, Laros GS: Tibial fractures involving the ankle in children (the so-called triplane epiphyseal fracture). J Bone Joint Surg [Am] 60:1040, 1978
11. Langenskiold A: Operative treatment for growth disturbance after epiphyseal injury. Acta Orthop Scand 38:520, 1967
12. Ogden JA: Injuries to the growth mechanisms of the immature skeleton. Skeletal Radiol 6:237, 1981
13. Phemister DB: Operative arrestment of longitudinal growth of bones in the treatment of deformities. J Bone Joint Surg 15:1, 1933
14. Poland J: Traumatic Separation of the Epiphyses. Smith Elden, London, 1898
15. Salter RB, Harris WR: Injuries involving the epiphyseal plate. J Bone Joint Surg [Am] 45:587, 1963
16. Shapiro F: Epiphyseal growth plate fracture-separations: a pathophysiologic approach. Orthopedics 5:720, 1982
17. Siffert RS: Current concepts review — lower limb lengths discrepancy. J Bone Joint Surg [Am] 69:1100, 1987
18. Siffert RS: The effect of trauma to the epiphysis and growth plate. Skeletal Radiol 2:21, 1977
19. Siffert RS, Gilbert MD: Anatomy and physiology of the growth plate. In Rang M (ed): The Growth Plate and Its Disorders. Churchill Livingstone, Edinburgh, 1969
20. Tong JS, Pavlov J, Morris VB: Salter-Harris type III fracture of the medial femoral condyle occurring in the adolescent athlete. J Bone Joint Surg [Am] 63:586, 1981
21. Williams DJ: The mechanism producing fracture separation of the proximal humeral epiphysis. J Bone Joint Surg [Br] 63:102, 1981

Slipped Capital Femoral Epiphysis

22. Bonfiglio M: Slipped capital femoral epiphysis. J Iowa State Med Soc April:189, 1955
23. Boyer DW, Mickelson MR, Ponseti IV: Slipped capital femoral epiphysis. J Bone Joint Surg [Am] 63:85, 1981
24. El-Khoury GY, Mickelson MR: Chondrolysis following slipped capital femoral epiphysis. Radiology 123:327, 1977
25. Klein A, Reidy JA, Hanelin J: Roentgenographic changes in nailed slipped capital femoral epiphysis. J Bone Joint Surg [Am] 31:1, 1949
26. Mickelson MR, Ponseti IV, Cooper RR, Maynard JA: The ultrastructure of the growth plate in slipped capital femoral epiphysis. J Bone Joint Surg [Am] 59:1076, 1977
27. Ponseti IV, Barta CK: Evaluation of treatment of slipping of the capital femoral epiphysis. Surg Gynecol Obstet 86:87, 1948
28. Ponseti IV, McClintock R: The pathology of slipping of the upper femoral epiphysis. J Bone Joint Surg [Am] 38:71, 1956

Avulsion Injuries

29. Barnes GR, Gwinn JL: Distal irregularities of the femur simulating malignancy. Am J Roentgol Radium Ther Nucl Med 122:180, 1974
30. Bufkin WJ: The avulsive cortical irregularity. Am J Roentgenol Radium Ther Nucl Med 122:487, 1971
31. Denham WK, Marcus NW, Enneking WF, Haren C: Developmental defects of the distal femoral metaphysis. J Bone Joint Surg [Am] 62:801, 1980
32. Khoury MB, Kirks DR, Martinez S, Apple J: Bilateral avulsion fractures of the anterior superior iliac spines in sprinters. Skeletal Radiol 13:65, 1985
33. Mital MA, Matza RA, Cohen J: The so called unresolved Osgood-Schlatter lesion. J Bone Joint Surg [Am] 62:732, 1980
34. Ogden JA: Injuries to the growth mechanisms of the immature skeleton. Skeletal Radiol 6:237, 1981
35. Ogden JA, Southwick WO: Osgood-Schlatter's disease and tibial tuberosity development. Clin Orthop 116:180, 1976
36. Zaricznyj B: Avulsion fracture of the tibial emi-

nence: treatment by open reduction and pinning. J Bone Joint Surg [Am] 59:1111, 1977

Ununited Fractures

37. Banks HH: Nonunion in fractures of the femoral neck. Orthop Clin North Am 5:865, 1974
38. Bassett CAL, Mitchell SN, Gaston SR: Treatment of ununited tibial diaphyseal fractures with pulsing electromagnetic fields. J Bone Joint Surg [Am] 63:511, 1981
39. Bassett CAL, Mitchell SN, Schink MM: Treatment of therapeutically resistant nonunions with bone grafts and pulsing electromagnetic fields. J Bone J Surg [Am] 64:1214, 1982
40. Blumenfeld I: Pseudoarthrosis of the long bone. J Bone Joint Surg [Am] 29:97, 1947
41. Bonfiglio M, Bardenstein M: Treatment by bone grafting of aseptic necrosis of the femoral head and non-union of the femoral neck. J Bone Joint Surg 40:1329, 1958
42. Boyd HB, Lipinski SW, Wiley JH: Observations on nonunions of the shafts of long bones, with a statistical analysis of 842 patients. J Bone Joint Surg [Am] 43:159, 1961
43. Brighton CT: The treatment of nonunions with electricity; current concepts review. J Bone Joint Surg [Am] 63:847, 1981
44. Cave EF: Healing of fractures (Ch. 4). Delayed union, non-union, timetable for healing by bone and age (Ch. 5). In: Fracture Management Injuries. Year Book Medical Publishers, Chicago, 1974
45. Cooney WP III, Dobyns JH, Linscheid RL: Non-union of the scaphoid. J Hand Surg 5:343, 1980
46. DeHaas WG, Watson J: Non-invasive treatment of ununited fractures of the tibia using electrical stimulation. J Bone Joint Surg [Br] 62:465, 1980
47. Freeland AE, Mutz SB: Posterior bone grafting for infected ununited fractures of the tibia. J Bone Joint Surg [Am] 58:653, 1976
48. Hanson LW, Eppright RH: Posterior bone grafting of the tibia for nonunion. J Bone Joint Surg [Am] 48:27, 1966
49. Hey-Groves EWH: Ununited fractures with special reference to gunshot injuries and the use of bone grafts. Br J Surg 6:203, 1918
50. Key JA: The effect of local calcium depot on osteogenesis and healing of fractures. J Bone Joint Surg 16:176, 1934
51. Luckey CA, Adams CO: The use of iliac bone in bone grafting and arthrodesis. J Bone Joint Surg 28:521, 1946

52. Murray G: End results of bone grafting for non-union of the carpal navicular. J Bone Joint Surg 28:749, 1946
53. Phemister DB: Treatment of ununited fractures by onlay bone grafts without screw fixation and without breaking down of the fibrous union. J Bone Joint Surg 29:946, 1947
54. Robinson RA: Healing of bone discontinuities in puppies and dogs. J Bone Joint Surg [Am] 53:1017, 1971
55. Ruby LK, Stinson J, Belsky MR: The natural history of scaphoid non-union. J Bone Joint Surg [Am] 67:428, 1985
56. Russe O: Fractures of the carpal navicular, diagnosis, non-operative and operative treatment. J Bone Joint Surg [Am] 42:759, 1960
57. Sekiguchi T, Hirayama T: Assessment of fracture healing by vibration. Acta Orthop Scand 50:391, 1979
58. Spadaro JA: Electrically stimulated bone growth in animals and man. Clin Orthop 122:325, 1977
59. Tietz CC, Carter DR, Frankel VH: Problems associated with tibial fractures with intact fibulae. J Bone Joint Surg [Am] 62:770, 1980
60. Urist MR, McLean FC: The pathogenesis and treatment of delayed union and non-union. J Bone Joint Surg [Am] 36:391, 1954
61. Watson-Jones R: Repair of fractures, p. 23. In Wilson JN (ed): Fractures and Joint Injuries. 6th Ed. Churchill Livingstone, New York, 1983
62. Watson-Jones R, Coltart WD: Slow union of fractures with a study of 804 fractures of the shaft of the tibia and femur. Br J Surg 39:260, 1943
63. Weber BG, Brunner C: The treatment of nonunions without electrical stimulation. Clin Orthop 161:24, 1981
64. Weiss C, Gruber Swett R: The application of structure-borne sound to the structural analysis of bone and fracture healing. J Bone Joint Surg [Am] 57:576, 1975
65. Yasuda I, Noguchi K, Sata T: Dynamic callus and electric callus. J Bone Joint Surg [Am] 37:1292, 1955

Pathological Fractures

66. Barry HC: Sarcoma in Paget's disease of bone in Australia. J Bone Joint Surg [Am] 43:1122, 1961
67. Batson OV: The vertebral vein system as a mechanism for the spread of metastases. AJR 48:715, 1942
68. Beals J, Smell WE: Breast cancer metastatic to the femur. J Bone Joint Surg [Am] 45:660, 1963

6

Soft Tissue Injury and Repair

Acute injury accompanying skeletal injury was lightly covered in Chapters 3, 4, and 5, and cases were illustrated in which there were three grades of mechanical injury to the skin, muscles and sometimes tendons, and vessels and nerves. We now focus on these soft tissue injuries. Obviously, the soft tissues that are injured undergo repair concurrently with the skeletal wounds, but the chronology of repair for each tissue differs, as does the end result of the repair process in each of these tissues, as well as the totality.

WOUND HEALING AND SURGICAL TREATMENT

Injury to any of the soft tissues evokes one response common to all the tissues in question, i.e., activation of local cells capable of reparative changes. In the regional sense, there is hemorrhage and necrosis followed by mobilization of circulatory cells that remove hematoma or dead tissue. Other cells that are competent to elaborate the fibrous tissue components essential for repair are similarly concentrated in the injured focus. The objective of treatment is to guide the repair process so that return of the focus to as nearly normal an anatomical and functional state as possible is accomplished as rapidly as possible.

The early, common tissue responses relate to inflammation and the later ones mainly to fibrosis. We previously used the example of a nonspecific synovitis in the knee with its clinical response of pain and effusion to illustrate the early process (see

Ch. 1). In this chapter we consider certain aspects of the early reactions of other tissue elements. The brief descriptions of the acute soft tissue injuries that accompanied the fractures in cases 4-1 and 4-3 are therefore amplified here to include the surgical implications with regard to the acute injuries to nonskeletal structures and their treatment.

In case 4-1 the patient sustained a closed fracture of both femurs when he was struck by a car and thrown from his bicycle. The skin and subcutaneous tissue of the right thigh were severely contused, particularly at the areas of impact. They were then progressively deprived of blood supply by the force of compression by extravasated blood and by the disruption of the vessels between the muscle, fascia, and deeper layers of subcutaneous tissue. The extent of the eventual necrosis of each of these layers would depend on the progression of the hemorrhage, the nature of (and injury to) the collateral circulation, the size and time for resolution of the underlying hematoma within the envelopes of skin and subcutaneous tissue and fascia, and the amount of contused, crushed, and torn muscle. In addition to the initial ischemic contusion and necrosis of tissue from direct impact, further necrosis may be cyclically produced by hemorrhage into the extremities as the fracture fragments are moved during the care of the patient at the site of the accident or during transport. It is impossible for the surgeon, observing the patient during the first few hours after the accident, to delineate the area of skin that may ultimately undergo necrosis. The same may apply to the other soft tissues in the region. However, it can be estimated roughly by measuring the circumference of the thigh and observing the buttocks to see if active

201

hemorrhage is occurring, as has already been mentioned (see Ch. 3 and Ch. 4). Active life-threatening hemorrhage would be the only indication for any emergency surgical procedure in this case. Retention of an intact envelope of skin, albeit some of it may later prove to be necrotic, is highly desirable inasmuch as it is the best prophylaxis against secondary infection. Therefore in the absence of definitive evidence of massive internal hemorrhage (rapid enlargement of the thigh or buttock, with progressive shock unresponsive to transfusion, or disappearance of pulses at the foot), a suspicion of continuing hemorrhage requires that an arteriogram be done followed, if necessary, by selective embolization of the injured vessels, balloon control of the hemorrhage, or an arterial repair. Skeletal traction was used in case 4-1 to stabilize the fragments of femur and the thigh, and the bleeding into the soft tissue promptly ceased. The mechanism for that fortunate event was spontaneous retraction and thrombosis of the severed vessels, aided perhaps by tamponade by the intact soft tissue envelope. The contusion and ecchymosis gradually resolved within a week or two, and the basal layer of skin did not undergo necrosis to any extent. The necrotic collagen of the ischemic parts of the dermis and fascia were replaced by fibrous tissue, as were the necrotic foci of subcutaneous fat. In this case, no signs of injury to major nerves or vessels were apparent at any time.

Recall that during the 6-week period after the accident the patient's fractured right femur was in skeletal traction, but the knee was being actively and passively moved through a pain-free (subtotal) range of motion. This treatment was predicated on the rationale that the scar tissue that replaces the necrotic foci should not be permitted to permeate the region as it would if the leg were kept immobile. It would then render immobile those tissues (e.g., muscle, fascia, fat) whose proper function includes (indeed requires) a gliding motion coordinate with the diarthrodial motion of the adjacent joints. Any loss of gliding of tissues along their planes (subcutaneous fat and fascia, fascia and muscle) may be analogous to losses observed during repair of a laceration of the flexor tendons of the hand (described below). The need is for passive motion as early as a range-of-motion manipulation regimen can be tolerated to keep the scar (fibrosis)

from tethering the soft tissues and to ensure that a functional range of motion be retained. The formation of scar tissue is not diminished, and in fact it may be slightly augmented by the motion; but instead of the disorderly configuration of collagen fibers that ordinarily occurs in scars, there is a tendency for the scar to form with fibers parallel to the tissue planes, not across them.[21,29,64]

In this patient, a fragment of the diaphysis of the femur tore through the muscle and into and through the external fascia of the thigh. With traction, that fragment returned to a position of alignment with the other fragments of the femur, and within a few weeks a bony union of the fragments was in process. The tear in the fascia was invaded by fibroblasts, as was the hematoma in muscle during the cleanup phase. Initially and up to 3 weeks, when motion of the knee was markedly limited by pain, the fibroblasts and collagen fibers in the tear and the muscle were arranged randomly; but during the maturation and remodeling phases, beginning about 3 weeks after the injury, as in the tissue planes mentioned above, the fibers become realigned in a more nearly anatomical configuration. During the subsequent weeks, because of the stresses of muscle tension and the motions of the hip and knee, the scarring allowed nearly normal alignment of all the tissues in the thigh, but there remained strands of scar connecting all the tissues undergoing fibrosis, including the callus of the fracture, subcutaneous fat, dermis, and muscle.[20,66] These strands may persist indefinitely but may be stretched by motion of adjacent tissues.

The next case, case 4-3 (see Fig. 4-4), is that of an open injury of the leg with loss of skin, subcutaneous tissue, muscle, blood vessels, and nerve as well as fractures of the bones. (For the assessment and treatment of a nerve lesion the reader is referred to appropriate texts.)

Although there was an obvious neural deficit indicating an injury to the peroneal nerve, the blood supply to the foot — as indicated by pulses and the color and temperature of the skin — was not critically diminished. An area of skin and subcutaneous tissue measuring 15 × 20 cm was completely avulsed from the anteromedial aspect of the leg. The remaining skin was severely crushed over the lateral and anterior tibial compartments, and the fractured tibia was exposed throughout the middle third of the leg. The exposure was more extensive after the initial major débridement. Over the next 3 days two further minor débridements were done to remove obviously necrotic tissue (see Fig. 4-4D).

As described previously (see Ch. 4), an external fixation apparatus was used to immobilize the fracture fragments. This device was chosen specifically to enable the surgeon to care for the soft tissue lesions, which required daily dressings and observation.

At 24 days, a soleus muscle flap was prepared and transposed to cover the bone, and a split-thickness meshed skin graft was applied over the cutaneous deficit. The rationale of that treatment was to epithelialize the wound once there was minimal danger of infection as observed directly by formation of healthy granulation. Further reconstructive procedures, including those targeted at the bones and the injured nerve, were deferred. The bare areas of muscle and granulation tissue were expected to be epithelialized by coalescence of the outgrowth of epidermal cells from the margins of the wound and from the grafts.[61] It was not expected that the subcutaneous layer would return to a normal state, and it and the muscle substance were expected to undergo considerable fibrosis.[5,7]

The status of the injured leg following application of skin grafts and a soleus flap represents a holding pattern designed to allow the surgeon the option of a variety of procedures, contingent on the sequence of events that transpire. As noted in Chapter 4, despite all precautions there was minor necrosis of grafted skin (ischemia), and despite antibiotic prophylaxis an infection (osteomyelitis) supervened, first with staphylococci and later with *Pseudomonas* organisms. The fixation apparatus allowed easy débridement of soft tissues and surgical removal of sequestra once necrosis of these fragments became apparent. As mentioned, there was drainage of pus from the osteomyelitis and continuing, but slow, spread of the infection in the soft tissues and bone, with evident scarring of the overlying soft tissues, until a chronic status quo (steady state) was reached. The residual open areas of the wound, except for the drainage tract, had healed by epithelialization from their margins. All obvious sequestra had been sloughed or removed, and drainage was minimal and inconstant.

The steady state in this case and in case 4-1 in regard to this permanent (chronic) condition in the injured soft tissues was as follows: In case 4-1, a mild non progressing fibrosis involved the area of the right thigh extending from the bone at the site of union of the fracture to the overlying skin, but that fibrosis consisted merely of strands of scar, which caused only slight restriction of excursion of the quadriceps muscles so that the hip could not be fully extended and the knee could not be fully flexed.[5,7]

In contrast, case 4-2 represents a common pathophysiological set of circumstances in regard to soft tissues that require treatment. This situation may occur with a variety of nontraumatic lesions as well as after fractures. Burns, frostbite, radiation injuries (particularly iatrogenic radiation injury), venous stasis from varicose veins or arterial insufficiency affecting the smaller vessels, even a Volkmann's ischemic manifestation are examples of common similar lesions with different etiological mechanisms.[2,8,31,36] What is common to them all is the fact that there is progressive fibrosis, attributable mainly to a low grade infection, and sequential episodes of necrotic foci that are being rendered ischemic by the normal contraction of the scar constricting the small blood vessels.[45] That constriction may even be sufficient to cause patches of skin to become necrotic; and in all of the conditions mentioned, the likelihood that a patient will develop chronic ulcers can be explained in this way. Naturally, with a precarious blood supply healing of such ulcers may be a prolonged process, and it may have to be preceded by physiological resorption of the necrotic soft tissue, as well as resolution of the accompanying infection. Even with heroic measures (bed rest for prolonged periods, repeated skin grafts, prolonged administration of antibiotics), the basic deficiency (pervading and progressive scarring) is not addressed and often cannot be. For a relatively small area so affected when no nerve vessels or tendons are involved, it may be possible to excise the scar, even down to bone, and replace it with healthy (unscarred) tissue, as with a cross-leg pedicle graft or a microvascularized soft tissue composite from another site.

In addition to the lesions mentioned, pressure or ischemic skin necrosis commonly occurs at many sites for a variety of reasons that are just mentioned here, without discussion. A common occurrence in a diabetic patient is the development of an ulcer anywhere on the foot or ankle.[45] A favorite spot is on the dorsum of the great toe at the metacarpal phalangeal joint or on the plantar aspect of the distal phalanx. Pressure sores under a plaster cast or sacral, ischial, and trochanteric decubitus sores in the bedridden patient, especially if emaciated, or in a patient who has lost sensation in the part, e.g., paraplegics, are other instances. Other sources of ischemic necrosis are venous thrombosis at sites of injection and electrical injury.

Inasmuch as the discussion here pertains mainly to the pathological changes in the soft tissues after a severe mechanical injury, and not to the other etiological categories that have been mentioned, "good judgment" in regard to the extent of fibrosis is based on one's appreciation of how dense is the scarring under the epithelialized traumatized area and how far it extends in three dimensions. That appreciation, in turn, must take into consideration the length of time the fibroblasts have been at work, how extensive and severe was the inflammation, and how long it was allowed to proceed. Similar considerations concerning the necrosis obtain. All of these considerations tend to widen the spectrum of findings, especially when the time frame, post injury, is lengthened by weeks or months. Despite that variable spectrum, at least one general principle applies in regard to therapy: There must be a good blood supply to the affected tissues.[19–21,61,62,66]

Whatever the fundamental cause for the lesion—be it direct vascular injury, neuropathy, or chemical, thermal, or radiation damage—the treatment depends on the extent of the inflammation, and of the necrosis (which includes loss of skin ulceration) and fibrosis. For success, the therapeutic plan must be based on good judgment of these three processes, whatever therapeutic approach is chosen. One approach may be simply to apply conservative means that foster spontaneous healing. If the ulcer is small and there is minimal necrosis of subcutaneous tissue and muscle, and if minimally active inflammation is evident, one would tolerate the fibrosis and would promote epithelialization by conservative means including frequent dressing changes and local pressure dressings. The rationale for each of those elements for this

course of action rests on the decision that the vascular status at the time of therapy is adequate for healing and later will not be precarious so as to risk breakdown of the repair, i.e., recurrence of the ulcer.

If the vascular status of the injured extremity is precarious or demonstrably inadequate, amputation may be necessary, as discussed below. Thus the spectrum of treatment may range from conservative measures to ablative surgery; and the pathophysiological basis for the surgeon's choice of treatment must depend on the assessment of the three aforementioned processes occurring in the lesion. In addition, such aspects as the lesion's size, location, and vulnerability along with important aspects of the patient as a whole must be considered (e.g., age and occupation as it refers to use of the affected part). Between the two ends of the spectrum, many types of surgical treatment, e.g., the grafts described for case 4-2, may be appropriate.

Even though it may seem obvious to the reader that the conservative therapeutic measures just mentioned constitute elementary precepts in the care of wounds, their pathophysiological rationale should be stressed. All too commonly, wound healing is delayed or even prevented when these measures are not carried out precisely and diligently. Frequent changes of a dressing may mean a change every day or two, or even a few times a day, depending on the amount of exudate. The exudate of an ulcer or open wound is an optimal medium for bacterial growth. If a dressing accumulates the plasma proteins and the bacteria, even if they are not virulent, the toxins cause enough irritation and inflammation to defer epithelial growth. When a lesion becomes crusted over, the ingrowth of epithelium at its edges may not proceed, and a heaped-up epithelial edge is the result. The obvious ideal is a wound as clean of exudate as possible. It should be remembered, however, that blood is also an excellent culture medium; and if when removing crust capillaries are torn and the wound is covered with blood, even in small amounts, not much has been accomplished by the dressing change.[19,61]

The pathophysiological rationale for a pressure dressing has received little attention, aside from warnings about arterial occlusion by the pressure.

It has long been observed that mild, even pressure on an ulcer causes the granulation to become firm and reddish, where without pressure it tends to be jelly-like and purplish gray, and to exude serum. One other effect of firm pressure on the edges of an ulcer is to minimize heaping up of the epithelium, the edge of which, under pressure, then tends to spread on the ulcer's surface, as do fibroblasts or other cells in tissue culture.[61,66] Removal of the obstacles to spread (e.g., a crust or excessive granulation tissue) further facilitates healing.

It has been shown that an arteriosclerotic patient, with a necrotic lesion of the lower extremity, is better served in terms of blood supply to the lesion if the involved extremity is not elevated but, rather, is maintained on a level with the torso.[45] This observation does not apply in general to a patient with a wound of an extremity who does not have arteriosclerosis. There the elevation serves the important purpose of minimizing edema. Although edema plays an important role in the body's defenses against infection during the acute post-traumatic interval, after several days it becomes an adverse influence on healing and thus should be held to a minimum by elevating the injured extremity.

Because so many of the patients who have had soft tissue damage are those who have been involved in accidents, we emphasize the principles of treatment for the composite wounds they incur, although the treatment of soft tissue lesions arising from other causes should follow similar principles. The pathophysiological sequences in the two groups of wounds are similar, but the open wound from an accident is nearly always a more acute therapeutic problem for the surgeon. How it is solved deserves elaboration. The principles are as follows: (1) Prevent contamination, or if the wound already is contaminated prevent further contamination. (2) Ensure that the setting for anticipated débridement and toilet of the wound is ideal (e.g., anesthesia, operating room). (3) See to it that the débridement process is just adequate: do not remove healthy tissue, do not allow active bleeding to persist, and do not allow blood or exudate to remain on the wound. If in doubt as to whether a bit of tissue is viable, wait until nature demarcates the living from the dead tissue. (4) Choose a method of immobilizing and elevating the part in such a way that the

wound is readily accessible for inspection and dressing. (5) Do not hasten to achieve a definitive result. Procedures applied to the wound as needed are safer, yield better salvage, and do not prolong the recuperation unduly.

The initial aspects of any injury to soft tissue are just about the same as the initial phases of the skeletal response, i.e., hemorrhage, swelling, and then inflammation. As discussed earlier (see Ch. 4), the extent of the injury varies with the kinetic energy of the injury and the degree of contamination.

An extensive open wound caused by a high velocity injury is more likely to become infected than is one caused by a low velocity injury. Wound severity has been classified in four grades, which are related to outcome as well as to infection rate. In general, the less severe the grade, the lower is the infection rate.[31a,31b] The first goal of good débridement, as has been well described by Gregory,[30a] is to achieve as clean a wound as possible. That measure minimizes the risk of infection, the first important complication to be feared with an open wound once hemorrhage has ceased. The other two goals depend on the severity of the wound. A soft tissue covering of the bone should be devised if bone is exposed, but no important structures of the soft tissue that are necessary for functional purposes should be sacrificed.

Concomitant with débridement, it is essential to thoroughly assess the extent of the damage not only to identify obviously nonviable tissue and the type and severity of foreign body contamination, but also to see if major neurovascular structures have been lacerated. To achieve this most important diagnostic step, the limb is prepared as for an operation, and a copious amount of irrigating fluid is used prior to and during the entire procedure.

An additional incision may be needed for the assessment; if so, it should be carefully planned with respect to viability of the skin and subcutaneous tissues.[30a] Whenever possible, venous drainage of the limb and the injured tissues should not be interfered with by transverse incisions. Any excision of skin margins should be minimal. Sometimes an additional incision should be made when there is a high kinetic energy injury to assess how much nonviable muscle, caused by the fluid wave, is present. Nonviable muscle is dark and friable, rather than red and firm, and it will have lost contractility as revealed by a pinch test; it also does not bleed when scratched. As was noted for case 4-2, demarcation of the living from the necrotic tissue may not be distinct. In that event, one should remove only what surely is necrotic, wait a few days, and débride again. During the intervals between débridements the wound should be dressed at least daily because necrotic tissue, like exudate and extravasated blood, is an excellent culture medium for bacteria. In such cases no attempt is made to bring the wound edges together. In general, any fragment of bone with a soft tissue attachment, especially a large piece, is cleaned and preserved with the soft tissue attachment intact. All identifiable foreign bodies are removed. Lavage is performed intermittently through each step of the débridement. As in case 4-3, the open fracture of the tibia, a severe open wound often requires multiple procedures.

The decision to try to preserve a limb is based on the judgment that the limb is not badly mangled and that it does not demonstrate extensive damage to the neurovascular structures. When those structures are destroyed, after measures are taken to salvage whatever can be salvaged, the patient would have an ischemic, nonfunctional anesthetic limb. The decision for immediate or early amputation rests on the judgment that all reasonable salvage measures probably would fail.

When salvage is decided on, treatment of the open wound after débridement varies according to the case. The question is "When should the soft tissue wound be closed?," the answer to which is 'Only when there has been no gross contamination and no major necrosis'. The option of primary closure should be chosen with great reluctance, as the potential for an infection by bacterial contamination in nearly every wound, however minor, exists even after the most meticulous surgical débridement and irrigation.

Extensive but explicit discussion of the therapeutic option of primary closure of an open wound is necessary for three reasons. (1) It is the option that exposes the patient to the highest risk, which means that it is the option that fails more often than other methods of treatment. (2) The pathophysiological rationale for this option, as generally envisioned by those who exercise the option too often, confuses the open wound situation (a laceration) with an incised wound. (3) Usually published accounts of how open wounds should be treated

rarely consider, as a special category, open wounds which are the province of orthopedic surgeons, i.e., wounds in patients who have had musculoskeletal injuries. *The discussion here relates only to those situations.* Even when the lowest end of the spectrum of open wounds is encountered— perhaps a clean puncture wound from within where a sharp fragment of bone pierced the skin without penetrating the overlying clothing—the anatomical components of the injury include muscle necrosis to some degree and an extensive hematoma, not necessarily obvious on physical examination. Unless one recognizes these two pathological elements, which differentiate minimal soft tissue injury in orthopedic patients from a minimal laceration (from without) in a patient who does not have a fracture, mistakes are made and usually the mistake is performance of a primary closure when there is a need for venting a hematoma or an exudate.

Delayed closure within 3 to 10 days ordinarily is preferable when it becomes obvious that there is viability of all exposed tissue and no infection is evident. Sutures may be placed at the completion of primary or secondary débridement, with the prospect of closure at the time of any dressing change if the wound appears clean.

When the two primary objectives are achieved, i.e., that all nonviable and foreign material has been removed and all dead spaces have been eliminated, the next objective is that the wound edges be approximated without tension. This step may be achieved by either delayed suture or spontaneous healing by secondary intention during repeated dressing changes. Continued wound care to improve the granulation tissue coverage of exposed bone or soft tissues is necessary; but if the exposed area is too large for epithelialization within a reasonable period of time (about 2 to 3 weeks), epithelial coverage may be surgically indicated. One may opt to use split-thickness grafts, pedicle grafts (local or distant), or even vascularized grafts. If reconstructive procedures will be needed, split-thickness grafts may be used as a temporizing measure. What is important initially is the removal of nonviable tissue, so that the recipient bed is composed of living tissue that will support a graft.

Three of the four phases or stages described for bone repair are applicable to the repair of soft tissues, except that the repair matrix is collagen produced by fibroblasts instead of bone or fibrocartilaginous callus. The three stages are (1) hemorrhage and necrosis, (2) inflammation and resorption of nonviable tissue elements followed by fibrous tissue formation or scarring, and (3) maturation and remodeling of the scar. The duration of the initial stage depends not only on the dimensions of the wound but also on the extent of vascular injury. These two variables also constitute the main influences on the time required for cleanup of the extravasated blood clot and necrotic tissue before repair begins. If the initial inflammatory reaction to the injury is severe, the repair sequences (see Ch. 2) may be delayed.

At this point and to digress a bit, a few remarks are appropriate on the soft tissue injury that accompanies fractures in children. Most textbooks strongly advocate closed treatment of fractures in children whenever possible, particularly in younger children. There are empirical (rather than pathophysiological) reasons for this advocacy: (1) Most of those fractures are closed, and open treatment introduces the possibility of infection. (2) Fractures in children rarely fail to unite, even when the method of immobilization (usually a cast) does not immobilize the fracture fragments — it merely limits their motion. (3) Even after the fracture heals, there rarely is much of a long-standing problem with the function of the part, even when the cast is used for 2 to 3 months. (4) Even if the reduction of the fracture fragments is imperfect, the potential for remodeling of the bone usually allows spontaneous correction of minor (and sometimes major) degrees of malalignment or overriding. Although all four of these considerations can be supported by physiological data, both clinical and experimental, and are undoubtedly valid, it should be noted that they do not specifically concern the role of the soft tissues in regard to not only injury but also repair. That role may be as important as any of the mentioned considerations that pertain to the skeleton. Even if the injury to soft tissue usually is not great, as might be expected because most orthopedic injuries in children are derived from falls or sports and not from motor vehicle accidents or other high energy trauma, the amount of scar that forms in response to hematoma or slight motion of fracture fragments in the cast may be considerable; however, the cyclic stresses of muscle tension and the micromotions of the soft tissues that occur once the initial painful post-trauma period has passed tend to orient the collagen fibers of the scar in an anatomical fashion. Moreover, as remodeling of callus and bone is expected to be rapid in the child, one may speculate that the same would apply to the soft tissues, and in the present context that means the scar.

From the material considered above, it is apparent that mobilization of an injured part can be safely, albeit cautiously, begun only when the injured skeletal structures are sufficiently healed (or possibly immobilized by traction or by internal or external fixation devices), thereby allowing safe motion of the soft tissues. The timetable for soft tissue repair (on the order of 2 to 3 weeks) contrasts strongly with that for skeletal repair, which for major complete fractures often is on the order of months. This consideration is one of the primary arguments stated by proponents for internal fixation of fractures, but it should be used in children with great reluctance because the risks that are introduced are considerable, e.g., those of anesthesia and contamination, and are potentially catastrophic; the advantages, compared to those in adults, are rarely important.

We may now return to the subject of repair by scar in more detail, inasmuch as it has not been more than alluded to in the discussion of inflammation (see Ch. 2) and because it has major implications regarding rehabilitation regimens and timetables.

The process of fibroplasia, which is most active for about a month after injury, involves not only the synthesis of the matrix but the migration of cells and the orientation and differentiation of collagen and mucopolysaccharides into specialized functional tissues such as fascia, ligaments, and tendons (see Fig. 6-3, below).

Wound differentiation, as used here, does not reflect merely cellular changes; it also means maturation and increase in tensile strength of the collagen by increased cross-linking between the collagen molecules. As the collagen matures, the fibroblast changes its morphology to that of a fibrocyte. It can revert and become active again if there is another injury (or possibly inflammation), as shown experimentally in the intrinsic repair of the flexor tendons of rabbits or in tissue culture.[29]

In any case, restoration of tensile strength in a wound is mediated by collagen maturation. One cannot hasten the healing process to gain tensile strength more rapidly is soft tissue anymore than one can in bone. It can be delayed by depriving the process of its mechanical components, i.e., the appropriate patterns of stress, strain, and functional activity. The rate of gain in tensile strength of scar varies with the tissue and the species. In humans there is an initial delay, or lag, of 4 to 6 days post injury, followed by a rapid increase up to the 12th day, and then a gradual gain for a year or more. In most animals the process is much quicker.

Closure of clean traumatic wounds is performed as atraumatically as possible, with minimal damage being inflicted on each layer of tissue. If a skin edge is to be débrided, it is done smoothly so that the result resembles an incised wound and not a laceration. Crushing by clamping, tugging, or compression with retractors is minimized during the procedure to minimize the amount of hemorrhage and necrosis. The result should be a wound that heals with minimal scar tissue between all tissue planes. The objective is a wound with minimal inflammation.

Another question concerns the timing of delayed suture. Once it has been decided that no further débridement is needed, the decision to close the wound, because all the tissues look healthy, should not be made precipitously. One must take into consideration the tension that will be placed on the suture line — tension that will reflect not only the volume of lost skin, subcutaneous tissue, and muscle but also the residual edema in the part. An increase in the tension also will be caused by the tendency of the remaining tissues to contract, causing the wound edges to gape; that tendency is potentiated by any fibrosis that may have resulted from the injury.

Arguments can therefore be mounted for hurrying the moment of delayed closure: (1) The gap will be narrower if there is little scar formed. (2) Epithelialization from the margins will be needed to cover a minimal gap; and because that repair epithelium is so inferior to normal skin, lacking as it does the subcutaneous fat, hair follicles, and so on, it is advisable to minimize its width. (3) The shorter the period of healing needed for the open wound, the sooner rehabilitation can be started.

The arguments for delay also are strong. (1) The dangers of failure because one has underestimated the tension are great. A failed secondary or delayed primary suture, although not usually disastrous, prolongs the healing process and may compromise the final functional result. (2) Too optimistic an assessment as to the health of the tissues and the adequacy of previous débridements may also lead to failure, not because the tension is too high but because of infection.

Obviously, then, the decision as to when delayed primary or secondary suture should be done must be based on subsidence of the major components of the swelling of the part (hemorrhage and edema) and the observed health of the wound's surface. If one anticipates that a long interval will be needed for the swelling to subside or if much soft tissue has been lost, it may be wise to wait until the wound looks healthy and then use relaxing incisions on either side (later covered with split-thickness grafts), thereby allowing the wound to be closed without tension.

In general, most wounds can be closed by resuturing within 3 to 10 days of the original injury even when the initial wound is contaminated or potentially contaminated. With some types of wound, e.g., burns or radiation injuries, the most important consideration is contracture from scar, not the accompanying skeletal injuries. These contractures tend to span the skin folds of large joints, so the function of the joint is at risk. In some locations, e.g., the back, neck, buttocks, and abdomen, even large wounds contract considerably within 2 to 3 weeks, after which they require a small skin graft. However, large wounds in the limbs, particularly the legs (see Fig. 4-4), contract little, in which case split-thickness mesh grafts or grafts of other types may be used as soon as conditions permit. As a final note on the repair of wounds it should be mentioned that systemic factors also must be borne in mind. Wound healing is impaired by such factors as protein depletion as from dietary deprivation or systemic illness, vitamin C deficiency, prolonged corticosteroid therapy, and x-irradiation.

TENDON INJURIES

Damage to tendons, in the broadest sense, includes many traumatic as well as nontraumatic conditions. Examples are laceration with a sharp or jagged object, surgical transfer of a tendon's attachment, and even so-called tendinitis. The clinical problems associated with these lesions depend on the lesion's site, chronicity, and severity as well as the functional demands that may be characteristic of particular tendons.

As a specialized form of connective tissue, tendon is distinguished by long parallel bundles of collagen with flattened fibrocytes. Usually the tendon has a paratenon or a tendon sheath with a synovial lining consisting of inner and outer layers, called mesotenon or epitenon. Physiologically, the tendon in a sheath presents the unusual mechanical requirement that a vascularized fibrous band be able to slide for a distance of several centimeters within a fraction of a second. The mechanical situation therefore differs in one essential from that in a joint, where one tissue slides over another for distances on the same order during time intervals on the same order. This essential difference is that in the case of the tendon the design has to include blood vessels, whereas in the case of the articular cartilage it does not. It is not surprising therefore that the capacity of cartilage, when injured, to undergo repair is minimal. With tendons, the vascular design consists in entry of vessels at the attachments (to bone and muscle) as well as at intervals along the tendon's course through loose synovial bands, the vinculae, which are capable of excursions equivalent to those of the tendon. These bands and the vascular arrangement are important elements in the repair of injuries to the tendon as is the gliding sheath mechanism.

The *process* of the repair of a laceration of a tendon, but not its extent or chronology, is similar to that described for repair of a wound and soft tissue, and the same holds for surgical repair of tendons.[29,47,48,52,64] A few clinical examples can depict the variations in this repair.

The first example is a patient who has a sharp, clean laceration of both flexor tendons in a finger. The surgical procedure here must be as meticulous as possible. Even if the laceration has not occurred in "no-man's land," the ultimate result of the repair must allow the tendons to glide in the sheath for the requisite distance. Any scar that forms must not bind the tendons either to each other or to the sheath or surrounding structures. It also must not be so bulky as to have a limited excursion in the narrow sheath. The fact that a flexor tendon heals from cells derived predominantly from extrinsic

sources rather than from intrinsic cells (i.e., tenocytes) is important. The rationale for treatment of each element in the entire wound must be based on attention to the anatomical structures at the location, with consideration toward preserving undamaged blood supply to those tissues.[47,48,52,64]

Case 6-1   A 17-year-old boy had a laceration at the proximal interphalangeal joint that severed both the flexor profundus tendon and the superficialis tendon in the long finger of the left hand. The injury occurred as he attempted to catch a falling glass. The emergency treatment did not involve primary suture of the tendons. The physician chose only to close the skin and referred the patient for further treatment. A few days later, it was evident that there was no infection in the wound, and plans were made for definitive treatment; for nonmedical reasons, however, treatment had to be deferred for 6 weeks. At that point the option chosen was to remove both ends of the tendons from the sheath and to replace them with a long graft from a plantaris tendon. In that way there would be only one tendon-to-tendon suture line, and it would be located in the palm so there would be minimal risk of scarring of tendon to sheath and so on at the site of the original injury. The grafted tendon was designed to reestablish the function of the flexor profundus. The function of the superficialis was sacrificed to avoid the risk of losing all finger flexion because of scar.

The more complex option of in situ suture of the ends of the profundus and excision of the superficialis was rejected because it was expected that the length of profundus tendon proximal to the laceration that would be available would not be adequate. (Because of the 6-week postinjury interval that tendon would be markedly retracted.) The histological section of removed tendon showed granulation tissue and fibrous tissue proliferation of the tendon end as well as a moderate degree of perivascular inflammatory infiltration throughout the tenosynovial tissue (Fig. 6-1).

In the not too remote past, efforts to repair tendons in situ produced poor results — until the dissecting microscope and microvascular surgery were more advanced. With current techniques, repair of both tendons is being done even in areas formerly thought to be "no man's land," and the results are closer to the ideal of minimal scar formation at the site of union.[29,52] In the present case

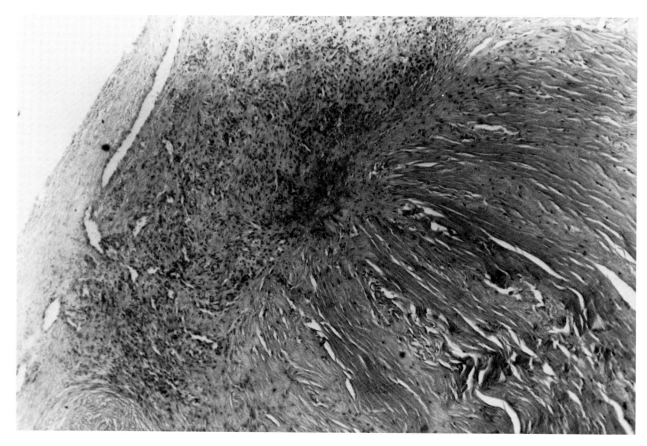

Fig. 6-1. Case 6-1. Photomicrograph of cut profundus tendon end 6 weeks after laceration on broken glass. Note the granulation tissue and fibrous tissue proliferation (×40).

such a repair would have had to be done soon after the injury, not following a 6-week delay. Maintaining function of each finger and tendon becomes especially important during the repair of lacerations of the wrist, palm, and digits, but it should not be attempted for wounds that are not clean and sharp.

During the postoperative rehabilitation, institution of motion as early as possible with gentle gliding of the tendon through the sheath for short distances under minimal tension is essential for good results. It is as important as good surgical technique. Motion stimulates epitenon cell proliferation in the appropriate orientation and hastens the recovery of tensile strength in the scar as it forms and remodels.[29,62]

Disruption of a tendon during the early stages of repair may occur at the site of the laceration up to 5 days after injury if the motion therapy is too vigorous. Later, rupture can occur between the newly formed collagen of the scar and the residual normal collagen that is being replaced. This process, as described, is similar to that for a healing fracture, i.e., creeping substitution.

It should be obvious that a contaminated wound on a finger or a hand, with laceration of one or more tendons but with associated injuries involving other structures, does not offer the surgeon either of the options just described. Although such severe injuries are not uncommon, their spectrum is so wide that the individual case is best assessed and treated according to the principles already de-

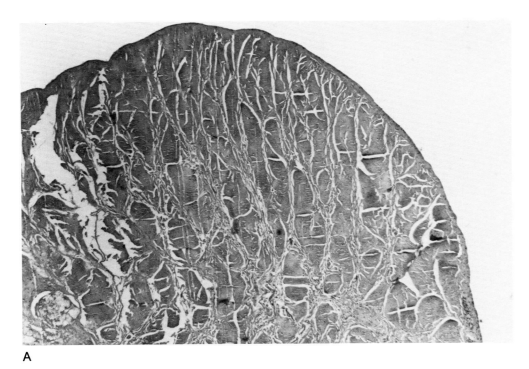

A

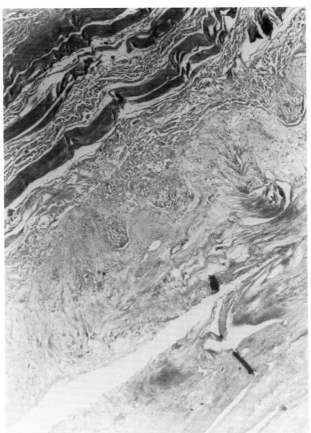

B

Fig. 6-2. Acute rupture of the long head of the biceps in a 38-year-old man. (**A**) Cross section of the tendon shows an area of normal collagen fibers with only a margin with disrupted fibers ($\times 25$). (**B**) Longitudinal section of the tendon with a few normal collagen fibers and degenerated frayed fibers ($\times 43$).

scribed earlier in this chapter that govern débridement, early immobilization, prevention of infection, and preservation of viable tissues.

There are tendons at other sites that pose different problems from those just described.[18] The *long head of the biceps*[32] (Fig. 6-2), proximally or distally, the triceps, the tendo Achilles,[10,56] and the proximal or distal tendon of the quadriceps[3,5,18] (Fig. 6-3) constitute one set, and the rotator cuff of the shoulder and the patellar ligament constitute another.[3,5] Even though repair by a similar process of scar formation occurs if any of these tendons are ruptured and repaired surgically, they do not require the same meticulous microsurgical repair as do those in the fingers or hand. These tendons have shorter anatomical paths of excursion than those of the wrist and hand, so the potential for tethering to adjacent tissues is less important; moreover, when tethering does occur, the functional impairment is not serious as a rule. With the first group of tendons (e.g., biceps),[32] the mechanism of injury often is rupture from overload, by unusual forces applied during activity during sports or work. In the second set (rotator cuff),[15,16,24,46,56] there may have been preexisting changes within the substance of the tendon predisposing it to rupture.

In the first set, the symptoms that are common to tendon rupture are immediate pain and loss of muscular strength. The lesion usually is a tear at the musculotendinous junction and not in the tendon itself. Often the tear is not complete; i.e., some fibers are spared. If the rupture is partial and the part is protected by immobilization for a few weeks, the continuity of fibers is reestablished by fibrosis. In some situations, perhaps with complete ruptures or in individuals such as professional athletes where rapid recovery is imperative and there has to be a better chance for complete and rapid restitution of strength, these considerations are important and surgical repair may be indicated. If surgery is attempted, the repair should be done as soon after the injury as possible so as to minimize the amount of scar and avoid shortening (contracture) of the muscle belly. Even while the scar is maturing, rehabilitation should be begun in the form of motion and mild muscular contractions. There rarely is permanent weakness after either conservative or operative treatment.

With the second set of tendon ruptures, it usually is difficult to document that a degenerative lesion was present before the rupture. When there are prodromal symptoms or there is a credible history of occupational (or sports) overuse, it is logical to presume that the tendon was weakened by degenerative processes, but it can be proved only when one can show that degeneration actually existed in the tendon adjacent to the tear (Fig. 6-2B). The problem is compounded by our ignorance of the process by which the degeneration is initiated and its natural history. An association between prolonged steroid therapy and tendon ruptures (biceps, quadriceps) has been reported, but these cases are uncommon. In contrast, partial tears of tendons associated with histologically demonstrable degenerative changes are common.[5] Two examples reveal some of the pathophysiological implications.

The first example is tears of the calcaneal tendon. The spectrum of these tears ranges widely. The acute, severe total rupture as may occur during isometric maximal stress (e.g., in weight lifters) or during maximal push-off (e.g., in ski-jumpers) is one end of the spectrum. Here one may discount any question of degenerative change, by the history. (In our examination of the histological changes in one case of a ski-jumper there were no such changes.)

The other end of the spectrum (total tears) is the case of the elderly individual who while walking normally suddenly has severe pain in the calf, with weakness. The diagnosis is easily made,[18] conservative treatment (a cast with the foot plantar-flexed) is usually pursued, and slow recovery is the rule.

For incomplete tears there also is a wide spectrum that ranges in severity to include the condition once called plantaris rupture but that is now accepted as an incomplete tear of the gastrosoleus (but rarely operated on). In these cases there is no histological proof of the location of the lesion or evidence of degeneration. An intermediate example is described below because it provided histological material.

Case 6-2 A 59-year-old woman noted a slowly enlarging mass of the right heel cord that had been present for 7 months. Pain occurred only with walking. The firm fibrous mass, palpable in the posterior aspect of the calcaneal tendon, was excised, and the tendon deficit was repaired in situ. The cut

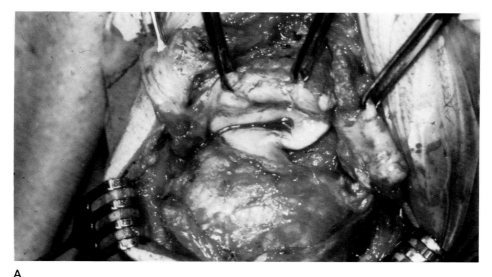

A

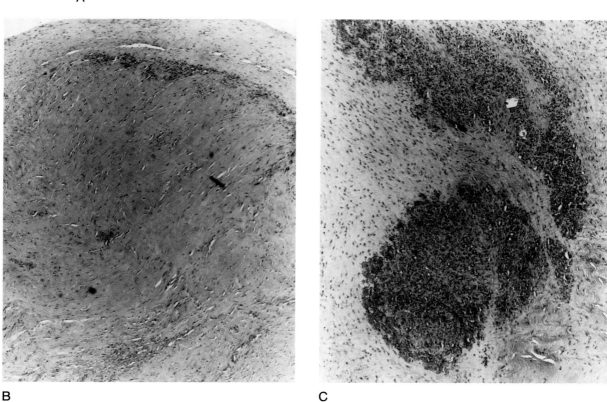

B   C

Fig. 6-3. A 54-year-old man had a sudden onset of pain in the left thigh near the knee as he was walking up stairs. The knee gave way, and he then walked with a limp and had to use a cane for the next 3 weeks. Because of the weakness of the knee and a gap in the thigh muscle above the patella the patient was referred for surgical repair of a ruptured quadriceps tendon. (**A**) At surgery the defect in the tendon was smooth and 5 cm across. Repair was performed by direct suture after mobilizing both ends. (**B**) Photomicrograph of the proximal tendon end shows fibrous tissue repair perpendicular to the tendon fibers. (**C**) Granulation tissue and fibrous tissue are present within the substance of the tendon (×90).

specimen was firm, white tissue infiltrating the residual calcaneal tendon. The histological findings were those of scar with abundant capillaries among well aligned bundles of collagen (Fig. 6-4), but some of those bundles showed fragmentation and fraying of fibers, and some hemosiderin was evident in the histiocytes. The patient had been ill and relatively inactive for the year preceding the onset of symptoms, so a return to the application of normal stresses probably resulted in a tear of the portion of the calcaneal tendon that manifested degeneration and repair. More than a year was required for consolidation and reorientation of the collagen

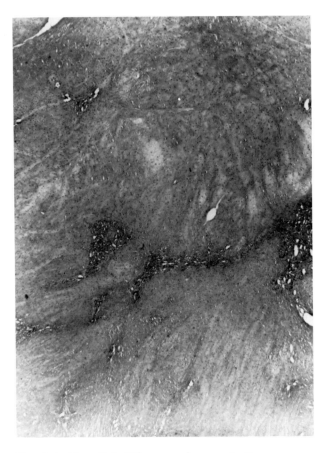

Fig. 6-4. Case 6-2. Fibrovascular repair tissue among frayed collagen fibers of the partial tear of the calcaneal tendon (× 27).

fibers, and the only treatment prescribed was limitation of activity within the bounds of comfort.

The endpoint of repair is defined by the point at which nearly all the collagen fibers are normally aligned and have a normal appearance and physical properties. The cells also must be properly aligned. The tendon then is adequate for unrestricted activities of daily living even during the year of rehabilitation — but competitive sports activities must be set aside for 18 to 24 months. When such a long interval is not practical, as for most athletes, who return to sports as soon as they have minimal or no symptoms, the individual risks reinjury with even a minor overload or series of overloads.[3]

Before proceeding to the second example of tendon injury, where degenerative changes are more evident, the category of condition now popularly called *tendinitis* deserves comment as it affects the calcaneal tendon. It most commonly occurs in individuals who run either for sport or for physical fitness, and it causes pain in the posterior aspect of the affected calf (the lower third) or just above the attachment of the tendon to the calcaneus. It often occurs after the patient has run a goodly distance, after which he or she presents with spot tenderness that may not be elicited by the examining physician but that can be by the patient. Obviously, the transient nature of the abnormal physical finding speaks against a gross tendon tear. In all probability, microscopic or even submicroscopic tears with small foci of edema could explain the symptom complex. With such small tears, not involving even the smallest of blood vessels (and there are few vessels in the substance of tendons) there would be no hemorrhage, and the swelling could subside quickly. The explanation for the recurrent symptoms is a matter of speculation. It may be postulated that the tendon has microscopic (or submicroscopic) foci of degeneration or that there is a cyclic loading and unloading, which causes the disruption of the fibers. It is a popular notion that the result is similar to a fatigue fracture in metal that is bent backward and forward, but that analogy is faulty for the following reason. In the metal the configuration of the lattice of atoms is demonstrably altered, whereas in the tendon the collagen (a polymer) would not undergo that type of structural change; however, what change it does undergo (if any) is not known.

Surgical repair of ruptured tendons seems to decrease the length of time needed for external immobilization of the knee and ankle and allows more rapid resumption of motion in those joints, but it should be reserved for complete or nearly complete ruptures. Activity can be resumed, but not as soon as after repair of flexor tendons of the hand, for instance, where active use can be undertaken within weeks. A frayed and degenerated tendon end is a poor tissue for firm suturing, however, as well as for active repair processes; and often use of a substitute tissue, such as the plantaris tendon or strips of fascia lata, is needed for reinforcement of the repair site. In such cases an additional aspect of repair process, i.e., resorption of the partially necrotic autogenous graft tissue, which must undergo replacement by cells and new collagen, must be kept in mind.

MUSCULOTENDINOUS INSERTION INJURY

The next example of tendon injury and repair is that of the musculotendinous cuff of the rotator muscles of the shoulder[16,24,32,57] (Fig. 6-5). It deserves special attention because commonly there are pathological changes that occur at that site, and many symptom complexes have been described during the healing of cuff tears. For a proper perspective, the reader should refer to Codman's classic book[15] on the shoulder before considering such a concept as impingement[56] and then evaluate treatment of the rotator cuff tear with such a concept in mind.

Pathologists have long been aware that routine postmortem examinations frequently reveal tears of the rotator cuff of the shoulder; and even more frequently, older individuals have degenerative changes in that structure. Often those changes are severe. Given the great difficulty of correlating antemortem historical details with postmortem findings, there is no credible body of evidence that points to a conclusion that such postmortem changes were associated with long-standing symptoms. It may also be argued that the postmortem specimens that have been examined are derived, for the most part, from elderly individuals—not the age group in whom, during life, rotator cuff injuries and tears come to light.

Nevertheless, the propensity of the cuff tissue to degeneration and to tears should be an accepted concept, even if not proved beyond reasonable doubt. Moreover, that concept should be kept in mind when pursuing a diagnosis and, more importantly, when planning treatment. The fact that degenerative changes are so much more commonly found without tears than those found with tears is evidence that the tear usually is a secondary lesion.

The *rotator cuff tear*, whether partial or complete, is associated with the pathological findings of degenerative fibrillated margins (Fig. 6-5D&E). It is evident in the case in Figure 6-5 that the degenerative changes are of much longer standing than would be attributed to the recent injury; but instances may be found where the changes are acute, and often the changes are a mixture of acute and chronic processes. The symptomatic manifestations of the lesions range from slight discomfort that interferes with work or sports to extreme pain, even despite immobilization. The pain may be so severe as to prevent sleep, and it may be refractory to narcotics and analgesics. The severity of the pathological findings ranges from a minor tear of one of the three tendons of the rotator cuff (supraspinatus, infraspinatus, and teres minor) to complete rupture of two or all three of those tendons. There often is little correlation between the severity of the lesion and the severity of the symptoms.

Even with minor tears (sometimes not even grossly demonstrable), there may be a secondary effusion in the subacromial (subdeltoid) bursa, whose floor consists of the tendons in question. The accumulation of fluid may cause exquisite, acute pain that can be relieved only by evacuation of the fluid. Over time the degenerative process may lead to calcification in the cuff,[4,69] and sometimes the foci of calcification are formed within, or are acutely extruded into the bursa along with this effusion to form a white paste,[15] which may be demonstrable radiographically. On occasion, it is evident on a radiograph of the chest in a patient who is without symptoms related to the shoulder. Therefore the mere fact that degeneration has occurred need not indicate that treatment is required.

One may postulate that the process on occasion begins as a tear followed by degenerative changes

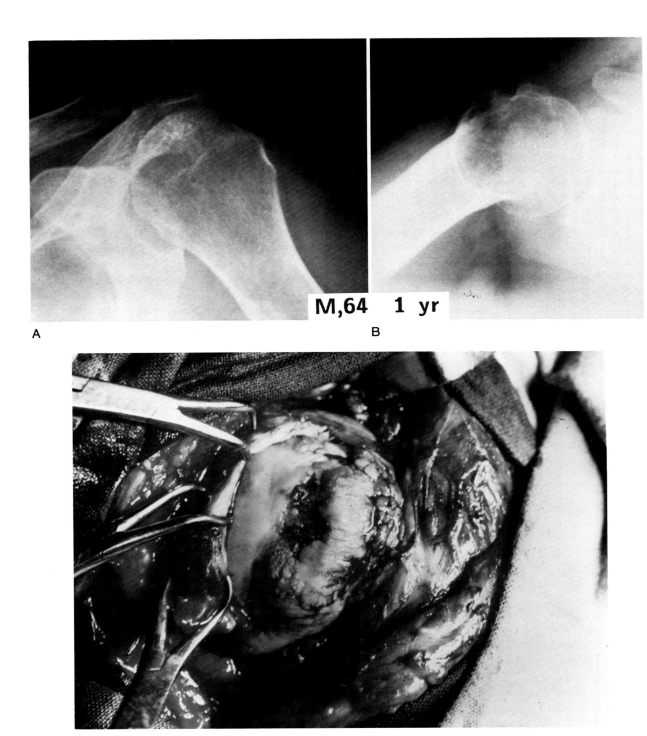

A

M,64   1 yr

B

C

Fig. 6-5. A 61-year-old farmer had had intermittent pain in his right shoulder for 1 year until an acute injury 2.5 months before presentation. Limited abduction and weakness resulted. AP (A) and lateral (B) radiographs of the shoulder show narrowing of the joint space and marginal osteophyte of the head of the humerus. The humeral head appears closer to the acromion than normal. (C) There is a complete tear of the rotator cuff. *(Figure continues.)*

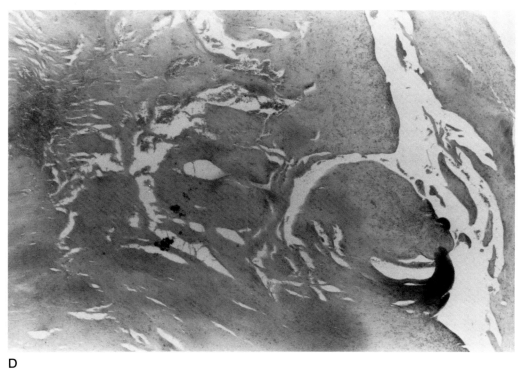

D

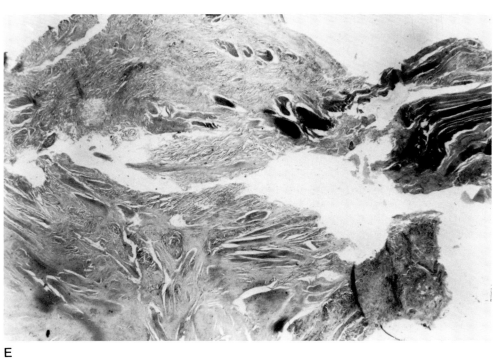

E

Fig. 6-5 *(Continued)*. **(D)** Fibrillation of the torn end is present ($\times$40). **(E)** Collagen fibers of the cuff within repair fibrosis ($\times$43). *(Figure continues.)*

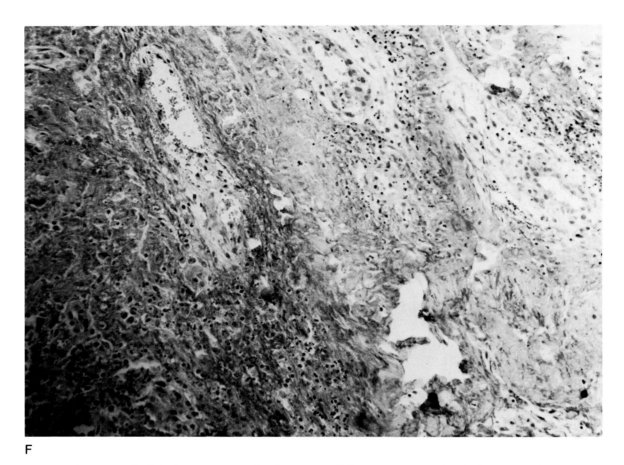

F

Fig. 6-5 *(Continued).* **(F)** Photomicrograph of rotator cuff degeneration with calcification and acute and chronic inflammation composed of polymorphonuclear leukocytes and round cells (×25).

in the tendon matrix and collagen fibers; but how often this sequence occurs is still unclear despite extensive studies by Codman,[15,16] Neer,[57] Mac-Nab,[46] and others. It is also not certain whether the acute or chronic inflammation (with polymorphonuclear cells, round cells, and calcification) (Fig. 6-5F) that accompanies the other pathological findings (degeneration, calcification) is primary or secondary to repetitive overuse as well as to structural deterioration. It is our view that most tears represent secondary phenomena, the degenerative process being primary. The symptoms, then, are such as might be seen after any injury, and the character of the repair would correspond to that occurring in degenerated tissues that are undergo-

ing continual minor trauma, which interrupts the repair process.

Several other names have been given to the lesions just described as they affect the rotator cuff of the shoulder; most imply a definite localized and specific pathological process, i.e., "bursitis" (of the subdeltoid bursa), "tendinitis" (of the rotator cuff or the biceps, calcified or noncalcified), or "periarthritis." Other names simply are descriptive, e.g., "frozen shoulder."

What one conceptualizes pathophysiologically when using the term "frozen shoulder" to convey the idea that there is a markedly restricted and painful range of motion should take into account the probability that the restriction of motion is usually not permanent.[46] The thaw, which may not occur until several weeks or months elapse, may be spontaneous. Usually it is ascribed to successful physical therapy. In any case, it is not reasonable to picture the restraint on the shoulder's movements as due to scar. It is not likely that a diffuse scar affecting the cuff and adjoining muscles can stretch either spontaneously or with mild physical therapy. One certainly should not, by forceful manipulation under anesthesia, conceptualize that the maneuver will rupture adhesions. Possibly the best pathophysiological explanation of the "frozen shoulder" is a chronic inflammation with copious edema, and resolution of the inflammatory process can then be postulated as the result of rest and the absence of the perpetuating trauma.

The popularity of the term "impingement syndrome," which attributes many tears to degenerative processes initiated by repetitive trauma in the form of compression of the cuff between the humeral head and the acromion, has led to a number of operations to relieve the "impingement." The anatomical and radiographic evidence that there really is impingement is not convincing, nor is the clinical evidence that relief of the compression in the form of removal of part of the acromion process relieves the symptoms. Nearly always the surgeon performs acromionectomy as part of a complex operation, and all too often an adequate trial of conservative therapy has not been pursued to allow the symptoms to resolve spontaneously.

What is emphasized here is that the surgeon's concept of the pathophysiological character of the lesion should dictate first what diagnostic measures should be pursued and then what the therapeutic regimen should be. When a patient presents with pain in the shoulder, the surgeon should determine to the best of his or her ability (via history taking and physical examination) the structure that is most likely to be involved in the pathological process, e.g., bursa, joint, bone, tendon sheath, or rotator cuff. At the same time the surgeon should conceptualize the process that is most likely to be at work, e.g., inflammation, degeneration, or acute rupture. There is no set sequence of diagnostic tests that would "cover" all the possibilities. There are several sets of circumstances that are best met, from the diagnostic point of view, by an immediate regi-

men of rest (e.g., use of a sling and swathe to restrict use of the shoulder), and this regimen supplemented by analgesics over a few days might then dictate what radiological measures would be helpful for diagnosis: radiographs (Fig. 6-6A&B), arthrography, computed tomography, or bone scans. Pertinent tests on the blood (e.g., erythrocyte sedimentation rate, hemogram, agglutination tests) might be considered at this point. Other sets of circumstances might best be met by immediate radiological investigation, perhaps followed by aspiration of the subacromial bursa or the joint. Circumstances may arise where an arthroscopic examination is the definitive determinant of the therapy to be pursued. That technique might be the optimal way, short of open arthrotomy, to reveal, for example, the extent of the degeneration of the rotator cuff tendons or the existence of a tear and if it would allow easy surgical repair.[22,23]

Lesions of the rotator cuff of the shoulder have been chosen here to illustrate the complexity of injury to tendons and their repair. The discussion emphasizes the natural sequences of repair. Surgical measures to optimize the natural sequences should be undertaken once it is evident that those sequences will not reach a satisfactory end result.[24] They consist in removal of frayed and degenerated borders of the torn tendon(s) and approximation of the edges of the tear if possible. If insufficient healthy tendon remains for approximating suture, various options are available, e.g., grafts (see Ch. 10).

The complex anatomical relations in the shoulder alluded to above do not resemble those that affect most other tendons. Only rarely can one associate a traumatic lesion of the tendon of the rotator cuff with secondary pathological changes in a bursa or the joint. The attempt has been made, however, to attribute changes in that tendon from "impingement" by osteophytes or roughened bone nearby on the cuff. The anatomical evidence of association between the lesions of bone and those of soft tissue, however, is not convincing; neither are the results of operations (partial acromionectomy) based on the above rationale as satisfactory as anticipated. Most other tendons, if not surrounded by tendon sheaths, course in a bed of loose connective tissue. Repair of injuries to or suc-

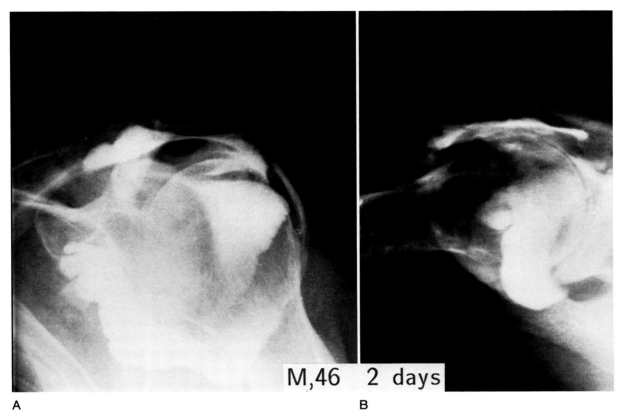

A   B

Fig. 6-6. (A&B) Arthrograms of the shoulder of a 46-year-old carpenter demonstrates an acute rupture of the rotator cuff. The radiopaque dye has escaped into the periarticular bursal structures.

cessful surgical procedures on those tendons, as has been discussed, depend on the restitution of continuity to the tendon and, of equal importance, formation of minimal scar restricting the excursion of the injured tendon relative to the sheath. In the shoulder, restitution of continuity is not as essential. In several studies it has been shown that not only can degenerative lesions exist, but tears can exist without causing symptoms or disability. However, if the scar of repair involves neighboring structures (e.g., the sheath of the biceps tendon or the synovial membrane of the joint), there will be symptoms and disability. The word "injury," as it pertains to lesions of the rotator cuff, therefore includes situations whose diversity requires a more specific conceptualization of exactly where the pathological process is at work and of what it consists. The trauma to the rotator cuff in a baseball pitcher who externally rotates his shoulder far beyond its normal range cannot be compared to that incurred by a young, loose-jointed woman who habitually dislocates the shoulder either spontaneously or during swimming. The middle-aged carpenter in whom a rotator cuff tear is demonstrated arthrographically (Fig. 6-6A&B) cannot be grouped either diagnostically or therapeutically with the elderly patient with obvious osteoarthritis (Fig. 6-5A&B) who also has a cuff tear (Fig. 6-5C). In all of these instances the pathophysiological assessment must take into account the many variables; and then, as the quintessential element of the assessment, the surgeon should identify the variable that not only is most likely to be at the root of the syndrome but that is amenable to appropriate therapy. Success of therapy depends on that identification and the choice of the appropriate operation as much as on the technical expertise of the surgeon.

The duration of symptoms and the severity of the functional impairment must always be evaluated with the likelihood in mind that with an acute onset of symptoms there will be spontaneous relief within a few weeks. In most instances, the patient is willing to accept some degree of discomfort, particularly when the activities of daily living and work can be performed, even though a complete rupture of the rotator cuff has been proved by arthrography. Surgical procedures should be considered or offered only when the indications are clear-cut.

LIGAMENT INJURY

Ligamentous injuries are so common that few individuals go through life without having had a series of them, although most are so minor they are discounted from the surgical point of view. The degree of disruption varies from a tear of a few fibers of one ligament to complete disruption of many ligaments about a joint. Much has been written about injuries to ligaments of the joints at risk, i.e., knee,[37,58,60] ankle,[54] shoulder, elbow, thumb,[55] and finger, but few reports[6,41] emphasize the pathophysiology of each injury or the therapy.

Ligamentous injuries, even when considered trivial, may assume significance because of continuing pain, swelling, or instability of the adjacent joint(s). Before these sequelae make their appearance the physician must decide what early treatment is best, a decision that presumes reasonable knowledge of how the repair process proceeds and the motions of the adjacent joint(s) that can be allowed, if any.[13,14,26,37,50]

Ligaments are short, tough bundles of collagen fibers that span a joint.[26] Some of the closely packed collagenous bundles adjacent to diarthrodial joints are oriented in such a way as to be at maximum stretch with the joint at one extreme of its motion in one axis (e.g., maximally flexed), whereas others are at maximal stretch with the joint at the extreme of motion in another position (e.g., maximally extended). Still others are maximally stretched at other positions, e.g., between flexion and extension. There is a distinct pattern of variation in the orientation of the collagen bundles in every ligament, especially one near a diarthrodial joint with an extensive range of motion. The variation is less diverse in a joint with a small range of motion. The pathophysiological implications of this variation are discussed later. The anatomical topology of any ligament with regard to the attachments of the several collagenous bundles also should be emphasized because they play an important role in pathophysiology. No bundle has an attachment that is narrowly circumscribed, and often the attachment involves several square centimeters of the surface of the bone. If only a part of that area has had fibers pulled off, presumably because the injury to the joint (a subluxation) occurred while those (detached) fibers were stretched, the position of the joint at the time of injury would be the best guide to identifying the nature of the injury. It would also have implications as to its severity i.e., what fraction of the ligament has been torn.

One of the implications of the above topological facts is that surgical repair of a ligament at one of its attachments (i.e., not in its substance) is at best a reconstitution of some, but not all, bundles of fibers. The concept that there will be no fiber bundles on the stretch after such a repair should be well understood. Restitution of the ligament to its normal state would be impossible, and all that can be expected is restoration of some but not all of the normal stability to the joint.

Ligaments are able to stretch more than are tendons, not only because their bundles are not parallel and thus resemble a fabric cut on the bias but also because the histological orientation of the fibers is wavy and suggests that in the relaxed position the fibers are "crimped."[26] When stretched to the point of rupture, ligaments follow a classical deformation curve once the crimping has been eliminated.[58]

Minor strains of ligaments about the ankle, knee, and finger represent tears of variable extent, usually in the substance of the ligament. The pathological sequence of repair, as described for soft tissues, proceeds to formation of scar, provided additional stretch is not exerted on the ligament so more fibers are torn and the newly formed fibers and capillaries are not disrupted. The course of repair is smooth if the joint is protected over the 2- to 4-week period after the injury, the variable time interval depending on the severity of the sprain and thus the volume of repair tissue that has to be deposited. It takes about 4 weeks until the new ligamentous tissue can function fairly well, but even so that tissue does not restore the injured bundles to their normal lengths. That goal requires maturation (contraction) of the scar, and several months may be needed to achieve that status; moreover, often as the joint is used, the injured tissue remains somewhat elongated compared to normal, so the joint is prone to repeated strains (i.e., subluxations).

The pathophysiological implications of the variation in orientation of collagen bundles in a ligament, previously mentioned, are that restitution of the pattern depends on permitting the scar tissue, as it forms, to be subjected to cyclic loading and motion to a degree insufficient to disrupt the young fibers but sufficient to have them organize in bundles in the pattern characteristic of the uninjured ligament. Without such cycle loading and motion, the scar forms as in any injured tissue, i.e., with its fibers interlacing in all directions. If too long an interval of immobilization of the joint is allowed while the injured ligament heals, the disorganized but tough mature scar cannot function as did the uninjured ligament, which results in, variably, some decrease in the range of motion of the joint as well as a decrease in the ability of the repaired ligament to bear normal loads. In addition, because the ligament is located so close to the synovial membrane, the scar may well extend to that structure, so that during subsequent motion pain and swelling due to traction on the synovium may occur.

When a ligament gives way in its entirety, it may do so at its bony attachment with or without an avulsed fragment of bone or within the substance of the ligament. Tears through the substance always are frayed and may be transverse or oblique, or the fibers may give way at different points in the substance of the ligament. If no surgery is done and repair and restoration of function occur spontaneously, the efficacy of the repair and its chronology depend on how far the ends of fibers are from each other when the joint is immobilized for the repair process. The frayed ends of the torn fibers will undoubtedly constitute tissue masses disrupted by interstitial hematoma, and hematoma also will fill the gap between the two masses of torn tissue. That gap can be minimized by proper positioning of the joint (or extremity); conversely, it can be increased by improper positioning. As mentioned in Chapters 3, 4, and 5, early motion of the part can induce secondary or cyclic hemorrhage, which increases the volume of cells and fluid that must be resorbed as well as increasing the volume of fibrous tissue that must be laid down. Good conservative treatment means minimizing these adverse influences; but whether surgical repair can further minimize them often comes into question (as with tendon repair, discussed above). When a ligament is torn at a bony attachment and a flake of bone is avulsed, and it can be reattached surgically, the process of repair is more rapid and results in a more favorable anatomical component because the topology of the ligament is restored to normal. The process of repair is similar to that for avulsion injuries described in Chapter 5.

When disruption occurs within the substance of the ligament, it gives rise to a process of repair that parallels that of tendon healing or fracture healing. The newly-elaborated connective tissue of ligament repair, as described by Moberg and Stener, is similar to that indicated earlier for tendon repair.[55] After the hemorrhagic phase is complete, within a few days to a week, there is a bulky mass of gelatinous nondifferentiated connective tissue at the site of repair. This tissue is gradually reorganized to a connective tissue scar, so that within 6 to 8 weeks after the injury the gray reparative connective tissue simulates the white, firm, fibrous mass of the ligament. The bulky component of the scar (callus) may persist as a swelling for a period of months or longer, particularly in the region of the interphalangeal collateral ligaments of the fingers or metacarpal phalangeal joint of the thumb. If the ruptured ends of the ligament cannot be drawn together, a demonstrable instability at the affected joint may be the result. Whether the instability becomes a functional impairment depends on many factors, some already mentioned, among which a complex neurosensory adjusting mechanism plays an important role.[6]

Earlier in this chapter special attention was directed to the rotator cuff of the shoulder to explore some of the complexities of tendon repair. Similarly, ligamentous repair in the knee is discussed for several important reasons. One is that the knee frequently is traumatized in such a way that the injury to one or more ligaments is the paramount feature of the joint's ultimate residual impairment. Another is that the injury to the ligament(s) has to be considered in relation to the intra-articular as well as the extra-articular anatomy, an uncommon situation for ligamentous injury. Finally, impairment of the knee is of such importance in certain individuals (i.e., athletes) that extraordinary methods of repair or reconstruction are advocated.[71] These methods illustrate certain pathophysiological situations that merit extended discussion.

Sprains of the medial collateral ligament comprise the most common injury to the knee. This injury rarely involves the entirety of the ligament, mainly because the traumatic event usually is not so severe as to involve a subluxation. As mentioned above, different sectors of the ligament are on the stretch according to the degree of flexion of the joint, and so only a relatively small part of the ligament usually is injured. That injury is a separation in the substance of the fibers, either at the joint line or, usually, distal to it, because the ligament's area of attachment proximal to the joint is much more extensive than that to the tibia. Accordingly, there is tenderness and swelling where fibers have been disrupted — signs indicative of hemorrhage and edema. When the trauma has not been severe and there has been no previous major trauma to the knee, the important factors that allow one to conceptualize the pathophysiology (and diagnosis) are the timing and development of the signs and symptoms, and their sequence and localization. If, within an hour or two of the injury there is still minimal swelling (and if the patient has been able to walk from the scene of the accident and thereafter without severe pain), there is little likelihood of a tear of more than a few ligamentous fibers; the possibility of a tear of synovial membrane and of the meniscal attachment is also remote, particularly when the swelling does not involve the joint as a whole (i.e., when no parapatellar bulging is apparent). Such a patient, when seen 6 to 24 hours after injury, should not be subjected to an unnecessary invasive procedure (arthroscopy) with the justification of learning if there is an injury to the meniscal attachment or to a cruciate ligament.

Those injuries would almost certainly cause the joint to swell with fluid, either blood or synovial effusion; the time factor would indicate which fluid is more probable. Thus, a large fluid collection, evident within several hours, probably represents blood and justifies an arthroscopic procedure to better delineate appropriate treatment.

The surgeon's conceptualization of the extent to which the medial collateral ligament itself was injured dictates the further diagnostic tests that are needed and then the most appropriate treatment. For the situation described, where the joint reveals no effusion and the absence of severe local tenderness and swelling implies that only a few fibers were torn, no further testing, even ordinary radiography, is needed. Only when there is significant worsening of the above signs during the day or days after the injury is there a need for tests, i.e., radiographs, stress tests of the knee, or arthroscopy. With a mild strain, the knee should be put to rest (i.e., using an immobilizer) and protection afforded from additional activity for the next 1 to 3 weeks during which time the scar in the ligament forms. So mild an injury would ordinarily not result in healing of the ligament with lengthening, so the knee's stability is not compromised.

That end result is not so easily attained if the ligament is torn over more than one-half of its width or if in much of the torn portion the fiber ends are widely separated. Regardless of whether there is additional injury to a cruciate ligament or the medial meniscus, it is likely that the part of the ligament that has *not* been torn would not restrict the separation of fiber ends in the torn part. With a major tear, as is conceptualized because of the rapid evolution of signs, the diagnostic tests of importance include those that indicate instability (e.g., drawer sign, Lachman test) and might include radiographic stress tests and perhaps arthroscopy. However, surgical repair of the torn medial collateral ligament might well be the best therapeutic option — in preference to a long-drawn-out regimen of conservative therapy. The surgical option would ensure more rapid restoration of stability to the knee and would allow any other repairs that might be needed.

The physiological timetable of repair of either the torn or sutured ligament dictates that an interval of at least a month, and perhaps two, is needed before the scar matures to the degree necessary to withstand the stresses to which the knee is normally subjected. Those stresses exceed manyfold the stresses that ordinarily apply to tendon repairs.

Repair to the meniscus, when it is torn at the periphery,[11] would be one such adjuvant procedure, as would excision of a torn internal meniscal edge. Although these procedures can now be done via the arthroscope, they are better done under direct vision as supplementary procedures when the medial collateral ligament is sutured. It should be obvious that a tear in the substance of the anterior cruciate ligament, if reparable by suture, should also be sutured; if there has been an avulsion of bone from the tibial spine, the avulsed attachment of the cruciate ligament is reattached in normal position.

MENISCAL INJURY

Acute meniscal injuries are commonly recognized now because of the development of arthroscopy.[68] The question thus arises: What should be done when such an injury is recognized? As mentioned, a peripheral tear where the meniscus is anchored to the medial collateral ligament should be sutured; otherwise, the meniscus may well suffer recurrent displacements as well as abnormal wear because of its abnormal mobility. The consequences, then, would be those described below. One of the most challenging questions, however, is if a "bucket handle" or more medial tear should be repaired. Although it is true that a knee functions better with an intact meniscus than after a meniscectomy or after removal of a small torn part of the meniscus so as to leave a smooth inner edge, either of those situations is better than having the torn meniscus present as a surface abrasive to the femoral and tibial articular cartilages. Tears deep into the meniscal substance seem to lend themselves to suture,[9,11] but the end result is not yet known.[33] The general principle demonstrated experimentally[43] and extrapolated from menisci removed from humans (see Fig. 6-7, below) is that avascular cartilage does not repair itself by scar unless a vascularized attachment is broached. There is no reason to suppose that this principle does not apply to lesions

in the human as well as in animals. However, suture of a clean tear in a meniscus may well allow the edges of the tear to remain opposed, even if not connected by scar, and the smooth surfaces so achieved would surely be less abrasive than if the tear were not treated and possibly less abrasive than the sharp, albeit smooth, edge of the meniscus when part of it has been excised.

The most important consequences of a ligamentous tear of the medial collateral ligament that has healed by scar but remains lengthened is, as mentioned, abnormal mobility of the medial meniscus. That structure then is exposed to the risk of tears and degeneration. The first tear may occur during the same injury as the tear of the medial collateral ligament or, more likely, during subsequent injuries. These injuries are common in athletes, whatever their level of performance, and the late sequelae are common in all active men; as more women indulge in sports, it is expected to be evident in them as well. However, most patients with ligamentous injuries that have healed without articular stability having been completely restored to function with minimal difficulty except in regard to sports.

Case 6-3 This patient was treated before the days of arthroscopy and is presented because of the studies on the removed meniscal specimen. A lateral meniscus with several tears was removed from the knee of a 24-year-old male athlete 3 months after a severe injury to the knee, after which the knee had locked. The problem was a forceful abduction (valgus) injury that was incurred during football. There was immediate effusion and incomplete extension of the knee, both of which persisted. There had been several previous injuries but none as severe as the present one. An arthrotomy was performed, and displaced torn meniscus was removed. A moderate roughening of the femoral articular surface of the lateral condyle was seen. Histological features demonstrated in the meniscus (Fig. 6-7A) were complete longitudinal tears that showed no evidence of healing except at the ends of the tears where the peripheral fibrous attachment was reached (Fig. 6-7B). The partial tears within the substance of the meniscus showed the remains of old hemorrhage, probably the residuals of the hemorrhagic effusion into the joint. There was increased cellularity of the cartilage at the edges of

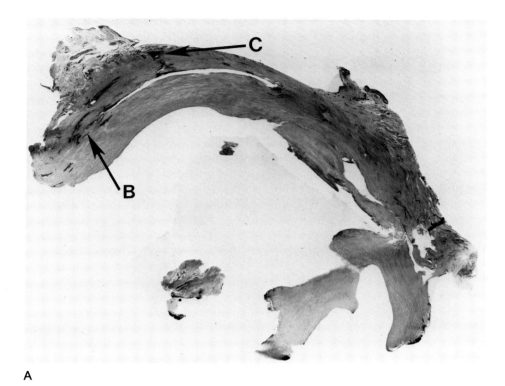

A

Fig. 6-7. Case 6-3. A 24-year-old man developed symptoms of locking of the right knee after an acute external rotation valgus injury 3 months earlier. The locking was localized to the lateral side of his knee. A lateral total meniscectomy was performed. (A) A section of the entire meniscus shows a main longitudinal tear and several lesser tears (×2). *(Figure continues.)*

these partial tears and some necrosis. Granulation tissue and fibroplasia were seen at the periphery (Fig. 6-7C). This finding suggested that healing by fibrous scar similar to that seen in tendon and ligament can occur near the peripheral margin of the meniscus, but the longitudinal tears near the inner border of the meniscus were not healed. The continual motion of the femoral condyle and the compression of the split meniscus against the tibial plateau probably kept the torn fragments somewhat distracted, and they abraded all the articulating surfaces.[39]

Injury to the anterior and/or posterior cruciate ligaments follows many of the same pathophysiological principles as have been discussed relative to the medial collateral ligament of the knee as well as a few others. In similar fashion, these two ligaments most often are not torn completely, but partially. In such cases the torn fibers tend to heal by scar without being lengthened, provided of course the conservative regimen of treatment is pursued for the several weeks needed for maturation of scar and no additional stretch injury is incurred. One difference between the cruciate ligaments and the collateral ligaments is the axes of motion they are primarily designed to limit. The cruciate ligaments primarily protect against anteroposterior translatory movements, whereas the collateral ligaments protect against other axes as well: varus-valgus and rotation. The type of dynamic splinting used should be chosen according to the ligament most severely injured, but for practical purposes the splint should protect against all motions other than flexion – extension because when a cruciate ligament is injured, even with a partial tear, the collateral ligaments most likely are also torn to some degree.

A difference that is more important is the fact that the cruciate ligaments are intra-articular and

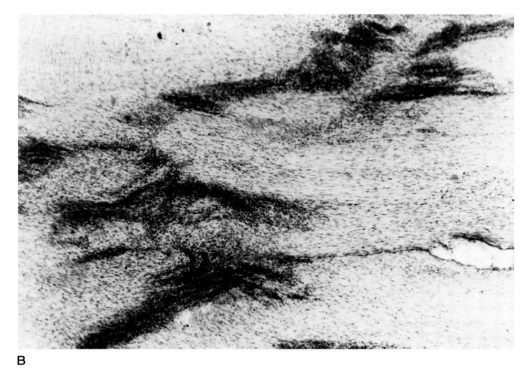

B

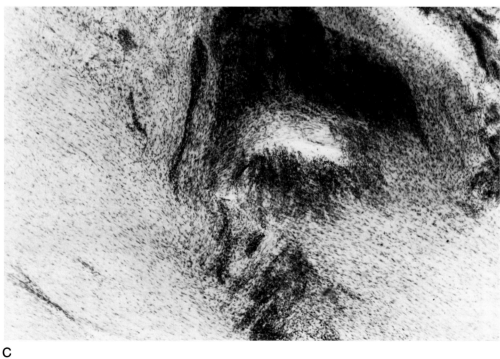

C

Fig. 6-7 *(Continued)*. **(B&C)** There is evidence of healing at either periphery near the vascular attachment of the meniscus ($\times$43). (Areas examined in **B** and **C** are denoted by "B" and "C" in **A**.)

therefore reliant on a circulation from either end, whereas the collateral ligaments can, during repair, receive a blood supply from the granulation tissue that arises anywhere along their course. The torn cruciate ligament more than likely has had some of its sparse blood vessels torn in the process, and therefore even if some fibers of the ligament remain intact the blood supply for the repair process is always compromised to some extent so that repair cannot be rapid. If conservative treatment (protection) is administered, it should be continued many weeks, and even then only incomplete restoration of stability may be the result. Such an outcome is adequate for nearly all occupations and activities, the exception being some sports.[6,41]

Because of the public's present preoccupation with sports and the demands on professional athletes, who frequently have had a series of injuries to the knee often resulting in a deficiency of the cruciate ligaments, this topic is controversial. Various pathophysiological theories may well be invoked to justify any one of a variety of reconstructions. All physicians would agree that seldom, if ever, can a partial tear in the substance of a cruciate ligament be sutured. Whether augmentation by a transposed tendon or a prosthetic material can restore sufficient stability to allow a professional athlete to return to the former level of performance is actively being debated. The longevity of any of the procedures advocated, or of any of the prosthetic materials, more than likely does not exceed a few years at best.

MUSCLE INJURIES

Although injury to muscle has been discussed as part of the soft tissue injury as it occurs in patients with fractures, how muscle undergoes spontaneous repair and how it regenerates[12,17] have not been considered nor have other processes affecting muscle commonly encountered in orthopedic practice, e.g., ischemic necrosis as part of a compartment syndrome,[49] reactions to repeated drug injections,[63] congenital torticollis,[27,44,53,67] or myositis ossificans.[1,25,30]

Following a contusion, crush, or tear, many of the muscle fibers are interrupted at the site of in-

jury as hemorrhage occurs at the site. Some muscle fibers retract, including their sarcoplasm, sarcolemma, perimysium, and epimysium. The epimysium of the remaining fibers may remain intact even when the perimysium appears disorganized and the sarcoplasm and sarcolemma become necrotic. The extent of the damage to any single muscle fiber, even with minimal gross evidence of damage, varies considerably. Initially, however, there is clumping of the sarcolemmal nuclei and granular, cloudy swelling of the sarcoplasm. If there is a loss of the sarcolemma, there usually is striation and splitting of the myofibril fibers; then, within 24 to 48 hours of the injury, macrophages invade the muscle fibers. The hemorrhagic exudate present at the site of the injury is resorbed by mechanisms described previously. If there is ischemia of muscle fibers, whether the foci are small or large, the crossbanding disappears indicating dissolution of the actin–myosin complex. Concomitantly, the undamaged muscle nearby, being immobilized, atrophies and may even degenerate.[40]

While the process of ischemic tissue and hematoma cleanup takes place, if the injured or ischemic focus is small the process of regeneration of muscle begins. This also proceeds in large lesions, but only at their periphery. There are mitoses of the regenerating muscle fibers (from the sarcolemma), and they differentiate to generate new muscle fibers. The process of healing occurs across small gaps. Healing by regeneration depends on the integrity of the endomysial sheaths, which guide the muscle sprouts much as endoneurium does during nerve repair. The endomysial connective tissue tubes therefore are important for regeneration of active muscle tissue. By the sixth day after an acute injury (e.g., an incision), the new myofibrils show distinct cross striations, and functional muscle develops within 2 to 3 weeks.[28] Some of the muscle fibers retain their complete endomysial sheaths, but many remain incomplete. They then are connected to the muscle's origin or insertion by scar tissue. If the nerve fibers from the motor point of the muscle are still intact down to the site of injury, the regenerated muscle regains its active function. If those nerve fibers have been cut, some innervation may be achieved by branching of nerve fibers from intact motor units, but some of the repaired muscle fibers remain inactive because of denervation.

More importantly, those muscle fibers trapped in scar do not achieve a normal extent of excursion; and as the scar contracts, those fibers are squeezed until they are ischemic and degenerate. Often such areas histologically include small foci of fat cells as well as scar and degenerated muscle.

The obvious practical lesson to be derived from this sequence of events is that the amount of scar in the injured area should be minimized by whatever means are at hand. If a surgical procedure involves muscle, the trauma of retraction, incision, and suturing should be minimal, as should the interference with circulation. Any effective prophylaxis against infections or inflammations or necrosis (as with a compartment syndrome) should be instituted.

Once repair is complete, the final functioning muscle becomes a complex of normal uninjured muscle, scar tissue, and partially regenerated muscle fibers. The muscle may not return to normal but may repair sufficiently well to allow the patient satisfactory function.[3,5]

Ischemic Necrosis

In case 5-7 a late, uncommon effect of ischemic necrosis of muscle occurred in the anterior compartment of the leg of a patient who had a laceration and some loss of the blood supply. The end result was scar with some calcification of the necrotic muscle (see Fig. 5-9G). This picture is also seen, on occasion, after the more common lesion known as the compartment syndrome.[49] It occurs mostly in the forearm and leg as a result of closed trauma.

Originally, the term compartment syndrome meant the clinical phenomenon of pain that appeared after a cyclic series of muscular exertions. In the leg it was known as *shin splints* and was attributed to swelling of the anterior compartment muscles, as typically occurs when running: Many patients have given a classical and diagnostic account of experiencing the pain after running a specific distance. The pathophysiological explanation, then, was slight edema in addition to venous engorgement within the compartment, and the condition was thought to occur only in those individuals whose fascial structures afforded less

opportunity for compensatory drainage or swelling. Obviously, release of the attachments of the fascia would allow unrestricted swelling, and in practice this treatment has effectively prevented pain.

Another application of the term was for the condition seen mostly in the forearm, *Volkmann's ischemic contracture*.[8,31,36] This condition, caused by an injury to or near the elbow, was attributed to a direct or indirect injury to a blood vessel followed by massive edema, which in turn resulted in ischemia to the muscle. The exact pathophysiological vascular lesion is still not defined — where no direct pressure on the brachial artery can be demonstrated. In some cases the artery can be shown to be temporarily occluded by spasm, which if unrelieved permits thrombosis to make the occlusion permanent. Allowed to progress or persist without relief, the edema causes necrosis of muscle followed by scarring and, in severe cases, major disability. The same sequence has been described in cases where a patient's extremity has been trapped for long periods, e.g., when a drug addict sleeps for hours with his arm pinned under his body or when an individual is pinned in a collapsed building, with an extremity trapped under the fallen girders or masonry.

Since methods have been devised for measuring interstitial fluid pressure within a muscular compartment, such cases can be shown to have elevated compartmental pressures.[49] The degree of elevation provides an indication for fascial release, and one can now identify which compartments need that procedure. Concomitant with the development of these methods there has been widened application of the concept to cases of acute trauma. In such cases an urgent or emergency situation exists once a muscle is ischemic because the pressure of the interstitial fluid is too high.

The following case illustrates the sequence of changes when treatment is delayed. This case occurred long before the techniques for measuring compartmental pressures were available and is presented to demonstrate the histological changes in the tissue.

Case 6-4 An 8-year-old boy sustained a supracondylar fracture of the right humerus. He underwent closed reduction and immobilization in a long arm plaster dressing. Five days after the fracture the

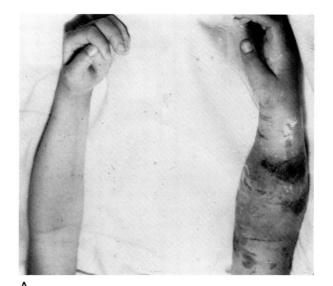

A

Fig. 6-8. Case 6-4. (**A**) Swelling, skin necrosis, ecchymosis, and blistering of the right forearm 5 days after a supracondylar fracture of the humerus in an 8-year-old boy. (**B**) Necrosis of muscle with interstitial hemorrhage and fibroblastic infiltrate ($\times 40$). *(Figure continues.)*

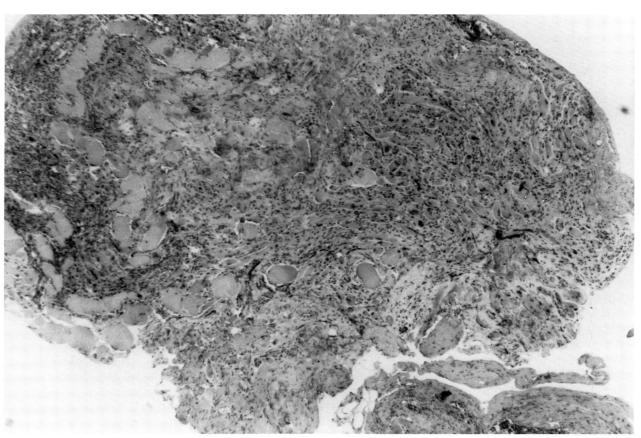

B

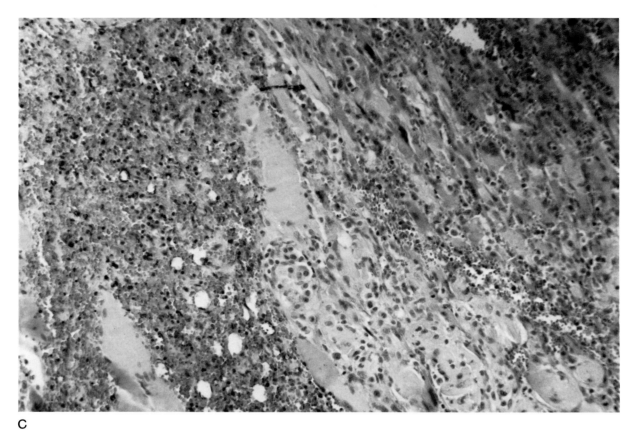

C

Fig. 6-8 *(Continued).* (C) Resorption of necrotic muscle cells by the cellular infiltrate including giant cells (×100).

patient began to lose function in the fingers: first sensation, then motion. The circulation was first recognized as impaired because the fingers became cold and pallid. Blisters were present upon removal of the plaster bandage, there was swelling of the forearm, and areas of skin necrosis were evident (Fig. 6-8A). Twelve days after the injury a fasciotomy was performed on the forearm. Areas of hemorrhage and pinkish gray fibrous tissue were present in the supinator and pronator muscles (Fig. 6-8B). A medium-sized artery was found to be thrombosed in the proximal part of the forearm. The histological findings of the biopsied muscle revealed necrosis. The nuclei of the fibers were absent and considerable interstitial hemorrhage and fibroblastic infiltration were evident (Fig.

6-8B). In other areas, there was degeneration of the ischemic muscle, some of which was undergoing resorption via numerous giant cells (Fig. 6-8C). A small artery showed occlusion by an organizing thrombus, and the arterial wall showed considerable hemorrhage and fibroblastic and lymphocytic infiltration.

These findings are characteristic effects of muscle ischemia of about 1 week's duration. The considerable secondary fibrosis of the muscle would prove to be progressive and irreversible and to give rise to the beginning contracture that is a hallmark of the late effects of the Volkmann's contracture.

It is obvious that this situation should have been anticipated and identified much earlier after the supracondylar fracture of the humerus. Muscle cells do not tolerate anoxia long, approximately 6 to 8 hours; and once the necrosis occurs, some fibrosis is inevitable. In the compartments of the forearm the muscles acting on the wrist and fingers are at risk, and the massive fibrotic replacement of the muscle always leads to some impairment of the hand. In the lower limb there may be similar necrosis in one or more compartments of the leg and even in the thigh, e.g., after Bryant traction applied for a femoral fracture in an older child, an error in treatment. Wherever it occurs, the contracture often develops slowly because it is a direct reflection on the progressivity of the fibrosis.

So many clinical situations can result in a compartment syndrome that only a few are mentioned here. One group comprises any injury to the skeleton near a major artery, e.g., dislocation of the knee. Another group includes extensive injury to soft tissue, e.g., a wringer injury to the arm[2] or (important from a medicolegal viewpoint) constriction of an extremity by a circular bandage or cast used to treat an injury (however minor) or as postoperative protection. Also the constriction can be mediated by a tourniquet that was applied too tightly or for too long. Whenever a suspicion arises that a compartment is in the process of compromise, the surgeon should act quickly; thus each patient must be monitored with diligence.

The following signs or symptoms are those to look for, especially if they persist after removal of the cast, tourniquet, or bandage: pain, pallor, paralysis, paresthesias, and diminished pulse or pulselessness. If any of these are present, one should do the appropriate tests, perhaps a Doppler test for the pulse or (most important) a measurement of the intracompartmental pressure. The manometric techniques for that determination are reasonably simple and reliable, and they may assist in making the decision whether a fasciotomy is needed to relieve the pressure.[49,70]

Chronic Hematoma

As noted earlier, an acute injury to muscle such as that associated with a closed fracture usually results in little functional impairment. The hemorrhagic exudate resorbs over a short period of time; and if uninfected it may, at worst, leave some residual fibrosis that is usually of little consequence. On occasion, however, the hemorrhage into the muscle may not be stanched by either natural means or treatment, and the part will continue to expand.[65] Depending on the timing of the accumulation of blood and its extent, tests may be indicated to determine if a vessel has been transected or perforated, or if a false or true aneurysm has formed, i.e., arteriography or computed tomography (CT). Even if a treatable vascular injury has been ruled out, a large mass of necrotic clotted blood may have accumulated, which may fail to be absorbed because the walls of the hematoma have become increasingly fibrotic. At times the hematoma calcifies or even ossifies (Fig. 6-9A). The expansion may be the result of minor trauma that has caused repeated hemorrhages into the residual hematoma or exudation into it. A mass may present with minimal discomfort, but often it simulates a soft tissue tumor (Fig. 6-9B) so clinically and radiologically the diagnosis may not be obvious. If there was an immediately antecedent injury or surgical procedure in the vicinity, it is apparent what tests should be done; but if more than 1 month has elapsed from the time of injury or operation, the possibility that the lesion is not related to those events is heightened. Hematomas of longer duration may be accompanied by a history, often cyclical, of increasing or decreasing size. Such cycles represent periods of resorption and of renewed bleeding within the encapsulated mass of fluid and granulation tissue. Routine radiographs may show a zone of radiolucency or radiodensity about the soft tissue mass. These zones represent the relative densities of the center and periphery, either of which may be calcified.

Modern diagnosis of such lesions might include a study with ultrasound or magnetic resonance imaging (MRI) instead of CT (but usually for economy, not with all three test modalities). Aspiration of the mass, if it is fluid, sometimes is the shortest route to the diagnosis, especially if the mass is fluctuant. Aspiration also may lead to spontaneous acceleration of the resorptive process. However, usually the lesion, if it is to be eradicated, must be excised. The specimen is composed of a central mass of blood and a fibrovascular wall of granula-

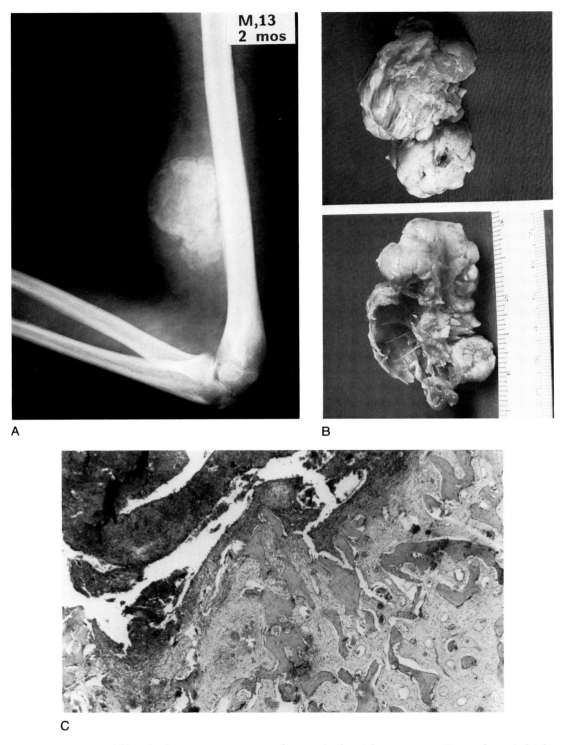

Fig. 6-9. A 13-year-old boy had spontaneous onset of a mass in the right arm over a 2-month period. There had been no known injury. (**A**) Radiograph shows an ossified mass in the biceps muscle. (**B**) Gross specimen shows the loculated shell of the excised mass. (**C**) Photomicrograph reveals an ossified hematoma (×3).

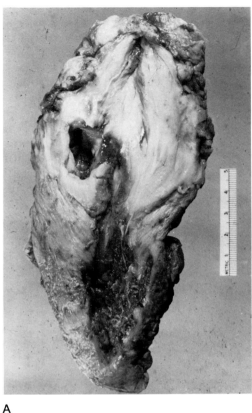

A

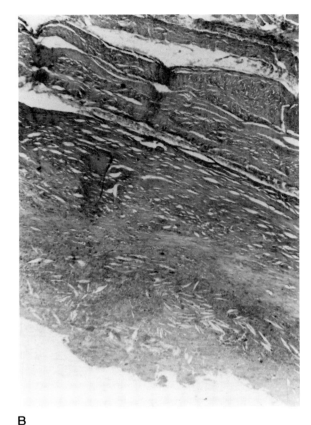

B

Fig. 6-10. (A) Split gross specimen of the chronic hematoma of the gluteus maximus muscle with a fibrotic wall and residual mass of blood. (B) Photomicrograph of the fibrovascular wall of the hematoma containing cholesterol crystal clefts.

tion tissue (Fig. 6-10A) with a dense fibrous tissue capsule containing collections of macrophages loaded with hemosiderin. There are also crystals of cholesterol at the periphery (Fig. 6-10B) of the lesion, when it is long-standing.[65]

Fibrosis

While on the subject of injury to soft tissue and to muscle in particular, a few lesions, some of which have been mentioned at the beginning of this section, can be discussed. One is the rather uncommon lesion of fibrosis in muscle, not as a residual of intermuscular hemorrhage from trauma but, rather, from irritants contained in injected substances. The typical story is that of an infant or child who has

had repeated injections into the *quadriceps muscle* or the *gluteus medius* or *maximus muscle*,[63] or less commonly into the triceps or deltoid muscle. The fibrosis is so extensive as to restrict the range of motion of the adjacent joint or joints. Many months or even years after the injections, the complaint is painless restriction of function of the affected joint, e.g., a contracture of the hip secondary to restriction of the tensor fascia lata and glutei or an inability to flex the knee if the injections were into the quadriceps.

Histologically, the muscles show so massive an increase in fibrous tissue around and between muscle fibers and so little evidence of the irritant or of the postulated inflammation that one may question the pathophysiological sequence implied above, i.e., that there is tethering of the excursion of the

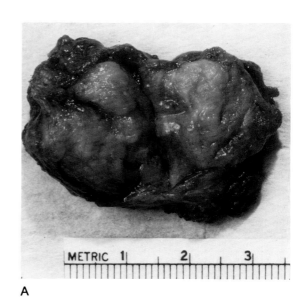

A

Fig. 6-11. (**A**) Sternocleidomastoid fibrostic tumor excised from an 11-month-old infant. (**B**) Muscle fibers are diffusely surrounded by collagen (×30). (**C**) Fibrosis is extensive between normal muscle fibers (×100).

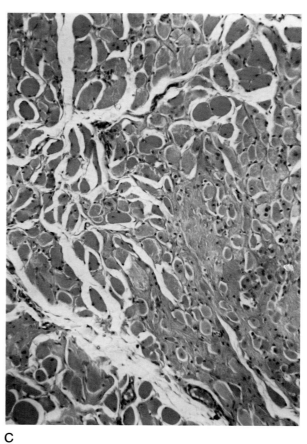

B

C

affected muscle and that the inflammation has long disappeared, leaving only the fibrosis. The fibrosis syndrome is treated surgically by removal of scar, appropriate release, Z-plasties of fascia and tendons, and resumption of early motion of the affected joints. It has been proposed that only certain individuals are predisposed to this syndrome, even as certain individuals are predisposed to keloid formation in the skin.

A second condition also mentioned earlier is a special form of intramuscular fibrosis that occurs in the *sternocleidomastoid muscle* of infants.[27,44,53,67] It is called *congenital torticollis* and typically is first appreciated when a "tumor" of the muscle is noted at or within a few weeks of birth. The mass may subside within a few days or weeks, and in such cases the resulting fibrosis may not be enough to restrict the motion of the cervical spine or to cause habitual wry positioning of the head and neck. These mild cases are often associated with a history of difficulties with the delivery and so can be confidently explained by stretching trauma to the sternocleidomastoid muscle. In the more severe cases, the motion of the cervical spine is impaired, often to the extent that the head is tilted. In those cases there is often asymmetry of the head and face that can be so severe as to raise the question whether the above pathophysiological sequence is a sufficient or even necessary precursor. When one eye is situated perhaps 1 cm below the other (also true of the ear) or when one side of the face is flat whereas the other is chubby in an infant not yet 1 year old, the postulated mechanical effect of abnormal pull by the fibrosed sternocleidomastoid muscle and its effect on the growth of the parts mentioned may well invoke other considerations: Did the fibrosis begin long before birth, perhaps as a consequence of ischemia? Is there a more basic anomaly of growth of the part?

Be that as it may, the histological features of the tumors and the fibrosis include degenerated muscle fibers replaced and surrounded by a fibrous tissue that is often dense (Fig. 6-11). The extensive disorganization of the endomysial and perimysial sheaths of the muscle fibers in a mass of fibroblastic tissue engulfing isolated fragments of muscle that show considerable variation in size may resemble the "desmoid tumors" of muscle. Whether these

lesions represent a residual of birth trauma, ischemia, or combinations of the two is still unresolved.

In any case, the residual contracture of the sternocleidomastoid muscle gives rise to the torticollis that brings the patient to the physician. Release of the sternocleidomastoid muscle at or near its insertion in the clavicle and, at times (with severe contracture), also from its origin at the mastoid process of the skull, followed by measures to keep the neck in the corrected position, usually results in resolution of the deformity of the neck. Frequently, however, the asymmetry of the face persists.

Myositis Ossificans

Another muscular lesion is myositis ossifications.[1,25,30] We have discussed several instances of injury to muscle in which the hemorrhagic exudate either resolves to leave little residual fibrosis or scar, or uncommonly persists to produce an expanding hematoma surrounded by a fibrous wall. Myositis ossificans is another type of lesion (as determined histologically) that has been termed heterotopic ossification. If manifests as five types of lesion.

The first type may present a diagnostic problem inasmuch as it may be confused with a tumor, and in this situation it presents a problem to the pathologist because the tissue specimen may resemble a sarcoma.[1] This manifestation of myositis ossificans is a solitary, apparently spontaneous lesion. Its importance is apparent in case 6-5.

Case 6-5 A 17-year-old boy slowly developed a painless, hard mass in the deltoid area adjacent to the humerus. A 2×2 cm area of ossification was evident radiographically. Only after repeated questioning did he recall that he had had a blow to the right arm 2 months earlier. The tissue was excised and consisted of well formed, bony trabeculae lined by rows of osteoblasts (Fig. 6-12A). There also was active osteoclastic activity. The intertrabecular tissue was vascular and loosely fibroblastic. A seam of cartilage crossed the bony mass, and there was enchondral ossification on either side it (Fig. 6-12B). A few muscle fibers could be seen in the peripheral area of the specimen, but the most

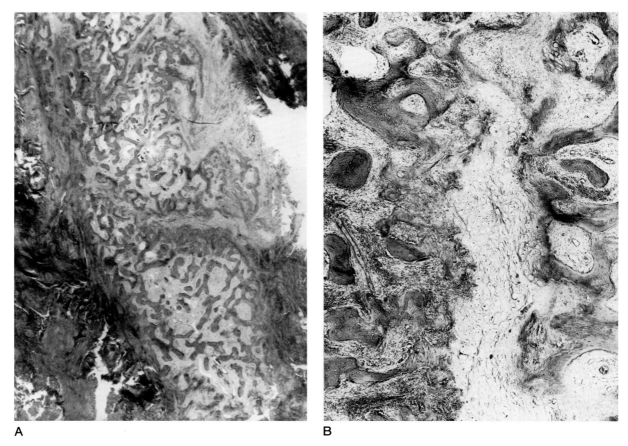

A B

Fig. 6-12. (**A**) Myositis ossificans composed of well formed trabeculae of bone within muscle. A zone of fibrocartilage is present near the middle of the ossicle ($\times 10$). (**B**) Enchondral ossification has occurred at the zone of fibrocartilage ($\times 100$).

important histological finding was that the central area of the lesion was less mature and aggressive than the peripheral area.

1. This process of bone formation may be so intense as to mimic the bone formation that occurs with osteogenic sarcoma. As in this case, there may be islands of cartilage and immature fibrous tissues as well as extensive new bone. Such new bone, during the early months of the myositis ossificans, is immature (i.e., woven, not trabecular or lamellar, bone) and is lined by multicellular rows of osteoblasts. Individual fields may be indistinguishable from osteosarcoma, so that the importance of the observation that the lesion's center is more active than its periphery now emerges. This "zonal phe-

nomenon" is not apparent after the lesion matures, but that maturation may take many months or even a year or two. Therefore another important point, in addition to those just mentioned (eludication of the problems of clinical diagnosis and histology) is that the lesion matures slowly and, if excised prior to its maturation, tends to recur.

2. An entirely different lesion is the rare form of this histologically identical process called *generalized myositis ossificans*. It is a disease of unknown etiology and on occasion displays a pattern of inheritance that is dominant with incomplete penetration. The reader is referred to McKusick's text for description of this rare syndrome.[51] The lesions of myositis ossificans are disseminated to a few or

many parts of the body, whereas the earlier-described form of myositis ossificans usually has only one or rarely two foci.

3. The manifestations of the third category of myositis ossificans suggest that repetitive trauma may be an etiological factor. This form is seen in patients in certain occupations, e.g., active young boys or men who are horseback riders or jockeys. They develop what is called "rider's bone" in the adductors of the thigh, i.e., myositis ossificans at the origins of those muscles (bilaterally). Baseball pitchers may develop this lesion in the biceps and brachialis anticus muscle. Similarly, it is seen where repeated stretching of shortened muscles is instituted in patients who have had poliomyelitis. In such cases the diagnosis and presumed pathophysiology are obvious even though the essential reasons for the ossification are obscure.

4. The fourth form of myositis ossificans is that seen in many, but not most, patients who have spastic paralysis due to cranial or spinal cord lesions. In traumatic cases it develops during the first 3 to 6 months after the accident. The most common site is the adductor region of the hips, and it may well be associated with the greater intensity of spasticity in that region. However, it may also affect other areas, as the elbow (Fig. 6-13). Note in Figure 6-13 that histologically the features are the same as those described above, but, importantly, the zonal phenomenon is not present. It should be mentioned that extensive studies on serum alkaline phosphatase in paraplegics have shown that the levels are high just prior to and during the active development of the lesion but not during its maturation. This finding probably represents "washout" of enzymes from the site of activity rather than a reflection of a generalized metabolic abnormality responsible for the lesion.

The clinical consequences of the lesion in paralyzed patients, at most, consists of restriction of the range of motion of the adjacent joints, the degree being variable. If excessive, thereby hampering nursing care, sitting, or ambulation, excision of the (mature) mass is indicated. However, its tendency to recur should be kept in mind as should the possibility that trauma plays a role in its formation. The excision should therefore be as atraumatic as possible.

5. The fifth form of myositis ossificans requires comment. It occurs as a complication of total hip arthroplasty and appears often enough that prophylactic measures (irradiation) are being taken in some centers. The prevalence of this complication seems to be declining with the recognition that some technical maneuvers increase and others decrease its likelihood. Surgical approaches without osteotomy of the greater trochanter are common, as are other ways to minimize the surgical trauma. Although histologically and probably pathophysiologically this "form" of myositis ossificans does not differ from that encountered in the spastic paraplegic (Fig. 6-13), it deserves mention because when it occurs as an extensive lesion, possibly involving the large part or all of the remaining circumarticular musculature, it restricts motion to such a degree as to make the arthroplasty a failure. Excision of the mass also poses the problem of the likelihood of recurrence, as for the solitary "spontaneous" lesion.

INTERVERTEBRAL DISC

Although many of the pathophysiological principles governing injury and repair of cartilage and ligaments apply to intervertebral discs, these structures deserve special consideration for several reasons, not least among which is their proximity to the spinal cord and nerve roots. Another reason is that such injuries are common and comprise a large fraction of industrial and motor vehicle accidents; therefore they play a key role in litigation, as well as disability evaluation and compensation. They also are special in that the mechanism of injury, in contrast to appendicular fracture, more often is one of compressive axial loading.

The most important consequences of the injury are the effects of mechanical derangement, i.e., the pressure of extruded disc substance on the neural structures just mentioned and the derangement of neighboring zygoapophyseal joints. Although degenerative changes in the intervertebral discs do play a large part in certain cases where there is an injury or so-called stenosis, that subject is discussed in the chapter on arthritis (see Ch. 8).

The most common injury to an intervertebral disc, compression, does not cause hemorrhage un-

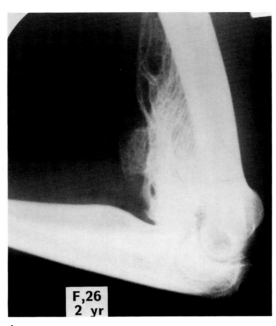

A

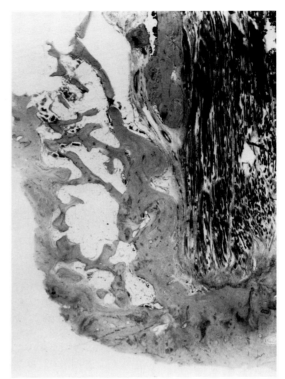

B

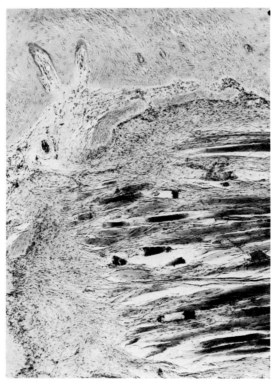

C

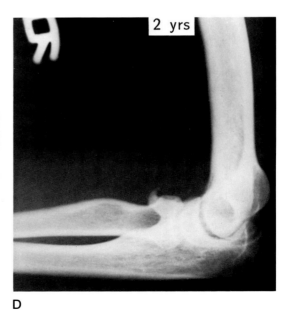

D

less it is so severe as to present as subluxation or dislocation. There are no vessels of consequence in the nucleus of the disc, the annulus, or the cartilage plates.[42] The nucleus (jelly-like in the young and consisting of variably degenerated fibrous tissue, mostly liquid, in the adult) is incompressible and with moderate compression breaks through either the annulus or one or both vertebral plates instead of ballooning out the restraining intervertebral ligaments. If there is a focus of weak subchondral bony support in a plate, a small hernia of cartilage may result, called Schmorl's node. If a small amount of fluid escapes through the annulus, the small or even large rent in that structure ordinarily heals, as described above for other ligaments. Consider, however, two critical geometric aspects of the anatomy.[34,35,38,42] One is that diminishing the thickness of the disc disaligns the zygoapophyseal joints and loosens the annulus. In addition, the physical character of the disc surely would be changed, and its effectiveness as a shock absorber would be lost for some time after the injury, the time needed for the intervertebral ligaments to shorten. Probably the thinned disc would never regain its original physical character, nor are there physiological mechanisms that cause it to thicken. However, the compensatory mechanisms in the remainder of the spinal joints ordinarily allow the spine as a unit to function well once the changes in position of the vertebrae adjoining the injured disc and the zygoapophyseal joints accommodate.

The second critical geometric aspect to the injury is what happens to and around the dislocated nuclear material. Because it is not foreign to the patient it elicits no inflammatory response in the surrounding (fibrous) tissue other than the relatively mild one, the response to abnormal pressure. The crucial feature of the geometry is the spatial relation between the extruded tissue and the neural structures. If the site of extrusion is near the intervertebral foramen, the nerve roots may be compressed. It it is in the spinal canal, the cord or

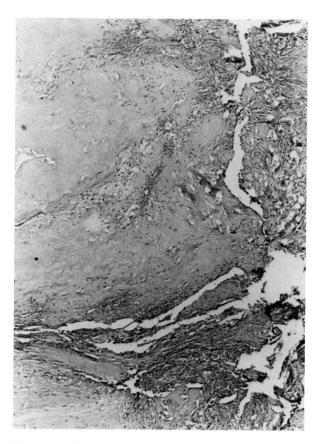

Fig. 6-14. Fibrovascular granulation tissue repair of extruded fragment of four intervertebral discs of a 44-year-old man removed 3 weeks after an acute episode (×100). The patient had had chronic low back pain for 5 years.

cauda equina may be compressed. Even the mild inflammatory response to the pressure may evoke enough edema to result in increasing (or fluctuating) pressure. In any case, the extruded material is not rapidly resorbed. It atrophies and is slowly replaced by fibrous tissue (as for other tissues not used); if the extruded material includes not only part of the nucleus but also some of the fibrous or

Fig. 6-13. A 26-year-old woman sustained a severe head injury with secondary spastic spasticity of the left upper limb. She recovered from the head injury and spasticity over a 2-year-period. **(A)** The left elbow developed veil-like ossification of the brachialis muscle, shown in this lateral radiograph of the humerus. The bony mass was excised. **(B)** Mature trabecular bone surrounds fiber of brachialis muscle (×10). **(C)** Fibrosis at the interval between muscle fibers and bone (×63). **(D)** Lateral radiograph of the elbow after excision. Partial function of the elbow gradually returned. The ossification did not.

cartilage substance of the disc, the rate of atrophy may be very slow indeed (Fig. 6-14). These pathophysiological considerations play an essential role in therapy. Thus the chronology of the symptoms of pain (e.g., sciatica, low back pain, or cervical pain) and of the signs that indicate pressure on one or more nerve roots or even on the cord itself should be used as a basis to conceptualize the process at hand, at the site of the extruded material. The edema plays a role in the development of pressure, thus it is advantageous to have the fluid resorbed quickly (within a matter of days) by putting the part at rest. Changes in the severity of pain or its location and changes in the neurological deficit require interpretation on the basis of the pathophysiological time frame, with the influence of physical activity as an additional item to be factored into the equation.

At present, a new chapter is being written on injuries to the intervertebral disc because of the advent of CT and MRI, which are changing much of the emphasis in diagnosis. It already is apparent that the diagnosis of "spinal stenosis" as a consequence of injury to the intervertebral disc is not nearly so common a lesion as previously recorded on the basis of pre-CT criteria. The capacity of CT and MRI to show dimensional and structural changes in the disc and neighboring structures, as well as in their relations, adds immeasurably to better pathophysiological interpretation of the lesions.

SUMMARY

We have considered injury to soft tissues, dividing those tissues into anatomical entities (tendons, ligaments, muscles). Whenever there is a disruption of any tissue, in addition to the responses they have in common — hemorrhage, exudation, necrosis, inflammation, and fibrosis — they each have a particular chronology and intensity of response. The injury depends on the structure of the anatomical entity. The solidity of tendons, ligaments, and cartilage is not conducive to accumulation of hemorrhage (intensity of response) compared to the loose character of muscle or areolar tissue. Similarly, the duration (chronology) varies. Such variation in

chronology is particularly evident in regard to fibrosis, as represented in the stages of reconstruction of the damaged structure.

Nevertheless, the initial aspects of any tissue injury are somewhat similar, depending on the nature of the wound. How it is incurred is obviously important. It is also obvious that an open injury takes on a different dimension than a closed one. We have already commented on these aspects of open wounds applicable to an open fracture (see Ch. 4) and need not repeat them here.

The process of wound repair has three phases: (1) inflammatory phase, (2) vascular phase, and (3) maturation phase. At first, there is an accumulation of hemorrhage and exudate until, within the first few hours, the injured cells and tissues give rise to an *inflammatory process*. This phase incites a release of substances that produce vascular changes, fluid exudation, and cellular exudation to help rid the tissue of any injurious agent (see Ch. 2). These released substances cause vasodilatation with increased blood flow. Exudation of white blood cells by a process known as chemotaxis is followed by a general slowing of flow, and a fibrin clot is formed to plug lymphatics and vessels. These processes help to localize the products of the injury. Once the accumulation of white blood cells and exudate ceases, cleanup can begin — the process of wound healing. This step is not a separate and distinct stage; each of these histologically distinct elements frequently coexist in separate foci distributed irregularly in the injured tissue at any one instant during the repair phase.

For repair to occur, the *vascular component* must regenerate a blood supply to oxygenate the tissue. After the initial trauma, the vascular response results in the disrupted arteries and capillaries regenerating with solid columns of cells at their ends, which then grow into the wound. These buds join adjacent proliferating buds or mature vessels and become recanalized, so blood flow is reestablished. Lymphatics follow a slower path to recanalization.

At about the same time, *fibroblasts* enter the wound and produce *collagen* for the matrix, through which the vessels and nerves (also regenerated if they were transected) course. On occasion these structures are strangulated by the contracting scar. The fascial planes, intermuscular connective tissue septa, and *fat* begin to repair with interlacing bundles of scar unless motion occurs to orient the fibrous tissue along, instead of across, the planes of motion. Although few severely damaged muscle cells regenerate to produce functional muscle and few muscle cells recover from hours of anoxia, the residual scar in muscle (as in tissues primarily fibrous) develops over time (months) and reorganizes along functional lines. (See case 4-1, the patient with a segmental fracture of the femur who required many years to overcome his muscular impairment.)

The principal problems associated with achieving full restitution of function when any soft tissue structure is damaged stem either from an excess of any one or more of the components of the injury or the responses to it (e.g., excessive hemorrhage, excessive inflammation, or excessive fibrosis) or from derangement of the response. Excessive fibrosis is illustrated by the contractures that have been discussed and derangement of the response by heterotopic ossification. In these instances, the pathophysiological approach to treatment envisages aborting the abnormal process (if possible) and then reconstituting the injured structure so far as possible. With contractures, the objective is reconstitution of the normal mobility (of a joint, muscle, or tendon), and that usually means excising or freeing scar, plasty of scar, or even replacement of scar by a prosthetic material. Of course, such surgical approaches must take into account, first, an obvious surgical principle — that if conservative measures are likely to work, applied over a reasonable time period, they should precede any operation. This principle applies, in the context of contractures, to the stretching that vigorous therapy can do to lengthen scars. Second, also obvious perhaps, is that a surgical procedure should never elicit scarring of such a degree (or in such a location) that it renders a procedure ineffective. Third, the secondary effects of the repair of injured tissues should never be trivialized. A scarred extremity whose blood supply is precarious may not tolerate a surgical procedure of consequence; an operation to relieve contractures, done many months or years after the contractures developed, may fail because the joints involved and perhaps those at a distance also developed contractures not amenable to surgical release. Finally is a principle that often is ignored: the need to evaluate the totality of influences that make a procedure succeed or fail. One of those influences is the cooperation of the patient in terms of the therapeutic program, especially if it requires persistent physical therapy over weeks or months, or careful protection of the injured part.

One of the important aspects of soft tissue reconstitution after injury — and in this respect it is analogous to reconstitution of the mechanical structural capability of bone — is the reorganization of the gliding planes between the various soft tissue components. It requires the removal of necrotic debris, realignment of connective tissue fibers, and regeneration of fat and loose areolar tissue between muscle groups and muscle bundles, which allows the return of flexibility and gliding qualities to muscles, fascia, and musculotendinous junctions. Severed tendons in particular locations require accurate approximation of their ends to restore their gliding function.

Thus after major injury of soft tissue repair results in a scar that represents a relatively inactive, minimally vascularized tissue. When the injury to soft tissue, including muscle, is extensive, that scar usually is extensive. Therefore the immediate objective of treatment after the injury is to minimize the amount of scar and to have its character such that it will cause minimal impairment. The later objective is restoration of function through the scarred part. To attain this objective, the surgeon must employ an array of treatment modalities, conservative as well as operative, depending on the many and varied factors of the individual cases.

REFERENCES

1. Ackerman LV: Extraosseous localized non-neoplastic bone and cartilage formation (so-called myositis ossificans): clinical pathological confusion over the neoplasms. J Bone Joint Surg [Am] 40:279, 1958
2. Adams JP, Fowler FD: Observations in wringer injuries. J Bone Joint Surg [Am] 43:1179, 1961
3. Albright JP: Musculotendinous problems about the knee. p. 195. In Evarts CMcC (ed): Surgery of the Musculoskeletal System. 2nd Ed. Churchill Livingstone, New York, 1989
4. Anderson HE: Calcific diseases — a concept. Arch Pathol Lab Med 7:341, 1983
5. Anzel S, Cobey K, Weiner A: Disruptions of muscles and tendons. Surgery 45:406, 1959

6. Brand RA: Knee ligaments: a new view. J Biomech Eng 108:106, 1986
7. Bowden REM, Gutman E: The fate of voluntary muscle after vascular injury in man. J Bone Joint Surg [Br] 31:356, 1949
8. Brooks B: Pathological changes in muscle as a result of disturbances in circulation: an experimental study of Volkman's ischemic paralysis. Arch Surg 5:188, 1922
9. Cabaude HE, Rodkey WG, Fitzwater JE: Medial meniscus repairs and experiment in morphologic study. Am J Sports Med 9:129, 1981
10. Carden DG, Noble J, Chalmers J, Lunn P, Ellis J: Rupture of the calcaneal tendon. J Bone Joint Surg [Br] 69:416, 1987
11. Cassidy RE, Shaffer AJ: The repair of peripheral meniscus tears. Am J Sports Med 9:209, 1981
12. Clark WE, LeGros: An experimental study of the regeneration of mammalian striped muscle. J Anat 80:24, 1946
13. Clayton ML, Miles JS, Adbulla M: Experimental investigation of ligamentous healing. Clin Orthop 61:146, 1968
14. Clayton ML, Weir G Jr: Experimental investigation of ligamentous healing. Am J Surg 98:373, 1959
15. Codman EA: The Shoulder. T Todd Co, 1934. Reprinted by Krieger, Malabar, FL, 1984
16. Codman EA: Rupture of the supraspinatus 1834–1934. J Bone Joint Surg [Am] 19A:643, 1937
17. Cooper RR: Alterations during immobilization and regeneration of skeletal muscle in cats. J Bone Joint Surg [Am] 54:919, 1972
18. Daffner RH, Riemer BL, Lupetin AR, Dash N: Magnetic resonance imaging in acute tendon ruptures. Skeletal Radiol 15:619, 1986
19. Dineen P, Hildick-Smith G: The Surgical Wound Symposium, The Biology and Management of Surgical Wounds. Lea & Febiger, Philadelphia, 1981
20. Dunphy JE: Wound healing. N Engl J Med 259:224, 1958
21. Dunphy JE: The fibroblast—a ubiquitous ally for the surgeon. N Eng J Med 268:1367, 1963
22. El-Khoury GY, Albright JP, McGlynn FJ: Arthrotomography of the glenoid labrum. J Bone Joint Surg [Am] 64:506, 1982
23. El-Khoury GY, Albright JP, Abu Yusef MM, Montgomery WJ, Tuck SL: Arthrotomography of the glenoid labrum. Radiology 131:333, 1979
24. Ellman H, Hanker G, Bayer M: Repair of the rotator cuff. J Bone Joint Surg [Am] 68:1135, 1986
25. Feagin J, Jackson D: Quadriceps contusion in young athletes—myositis ossificans. J Bone Joint Surg [Am] 55:95, 1973
26. Frank C, Amid D, Dip I, Woo SLY, Ateson W: Normal ligament properties and ligament healing. Clin Orthop 196:15, 1985
27. Garceau GJ: Congenital muscular torticollis hematoma, fact or myth. RI Med J 45:401, 1962
28. Gay AJ, Hunt TE: Reuniting of skeletal muscle fibers after transection. Anat Rec 120:853, 1954
29. Gelberman RH, Manoke PR, Menske PR, Akeson WH, Woo SLY, et al: Flexor tendon repair. J Orthop Res 4:119, 1986
30. Geschichter CF, Maseritz IH: Myositis ossificans. J Bone Joint Surg 20:661, 1938
30a. Edwards CC: Staged reconstruction of complex open tibial fractures using Hoffman external fixation: decisions and dilemmas. Clin Orthop 178:130, 1983
31. Griffiths DL: Volkman's ischemic contracture. Br J Surg 28:239, 1940
31a. Gustilo RB, Anderson JT: Prevention of infection in the treatment of 1025 open fractures of long bones. J Bone Joint Surg [Am] 58:453, 1976
31b. Gustilo RB, et al: Problems in the management of type III (severe) open fractures: a new classification of type III open fractures. J Trauma 24:742, 1984
32. Hawkins RJ: The rotator cuff and biceps tendon. In Evarts CMcC (ed): Surgery of the Musculoskeletal System. Vol. 2. Churchill Livingstone, New York, 1983
33. Heatley FW: The meniscus—can it be repaired? J Bone Joint Surg [Br] 62:397, 1980
34. Hirsch C, Paulson S, Sylvin B, Snellman O: Characteristics of human nucleus pulposi during aging. Acta Orthop Scand 22:175, 1952
35. Hirsch C, Schajowicz F: Studies on structural changes in the lumbar annulus fibrosis. Acta Orthop Scand 22:184, 1952
36. Holden CE: The pathology and prevention of Volkmann's ischemic contracture. J Bone Joint Surg [Br] 61:296, 1979
37. Jack EA: Experimental rupture of the medial collateral ligament of the knee. J Bone Joint Surg [Br] 32:396, 1950
38. Jaffe HL: Intervertebral disc changes in degenerative disc disease. p. 762. Metabolic Degenerative and Inflammatory Diseases of Bones and Joints. Lea & Febiger, Philadelphia, 1972
39. Johnson RJ, Kettelkamp DB, et al: Factors affecting late results after meniscectomy. J Bone Joint Surg [Am] 56:719, 1974
40. Kakulas BA: Muscle trauma. p. 592. In Mastraglia FE, Walton JN (eds): Skeletal Muscle Pathology. Churchill Livingstone, Edinburgh, 1982
41. Kannus P, Markku J: Conservatively treated tears of

the anterior cruciate ligament — long term results. J Bone Joint Surg [Am] 69:1007, 1987

42. Keyes DC, Compere EL: The normal and pathological physiology of the intervertebral disc. J Bone Joint Surg 14:897, 1932

43. King D: The healing of semilunar cartilages. J Bone Joint Surg 18:333, 1936

44. Lidge R, Bechtol RC, Lambert CN: Congenital muscular torticollis, etiology and pathology. J Bone Joint Surg [Am] 39:1165, 1957

45. Levin ML: The diabetic foot: pathophysiology, evaluation, and treatment. p. 12. In Levin ME, O'Neal LW (eds): The Diabetic Foot. CV Mosby, St. Louis, 1988

46. Macnab I: Rotator cuff tendinitis: the frozen shoulder. p. 35. In Evarts CMcC (ed): Surgery of the Musculoskeletal System. 2nd Ed. Churchill Livingstone, New York, 1989

47. Mason ML, Allen HS: The rate of healing of tendons. Ann Surg 113:424, 1941

48. Mason ML, Shearon CG: The process of tendon repair. Arch Surg 25:615, 1932

49. Matsen FA III, Weinquist RA, Krugmere RB, Jr: Diagnosis and management of compartment syndrome. J Bone Joint Surg [Am] 62:286, 1980

50. Maynard JA, Pedrini VA, et al: Morphological and biochemical effects of sodium morrhuate on tendons. J Orthop Res 3:235, 1985

51. McKusick V: Heritable Disorders of Connective Tissue. 4th Ed. CV Mosby, St. Louis, 1972

52. Meals RA: Flexor tendon injuries — current concepts review. J Bone Joint Surg [Am] 67:817, 1985

53. Mickelson MR, Cooper RR, Ponseti IV: The ultrastructure of the sternocleidomastoid muscle in muscular torticollis. Clin Orthop 110:11, 1975

54. Miltner LJ, Hu CH, Fang HC: Experimental joint sprain. Arch Surg 35:234, 1937

55. Moberg E, Stener B: Injuries to the ligaments of the thumb and fingers: diagnosis, treatment & prognosis. Acta Scand Chir 106:166, 1953

56. Nada A: Rupture of calcaneal tendon. J Bone Joint Surg [Br] 67:449, 1985

57. Neer CS: Cuff tear arthropathy. J Bone Joint Surg [Am] 63:1232, 1983

58. Noyes FR, DeLucas JL, Torvik PJ: Biomechanics of anterior cruciate ligament failures: an analysis of strain-rate sensitivity and mechanisms of failure in primates. J Bone Joint Surg [Am] 56:236, 1974

59. O'Donoghue DH, Rockwood LA, Frank GR, et al: Repair of the anterior cruciate ligament in dogs. J Bone Joint Surg [Am] 48:503, 1966

60. O'Donoghue DH, Rockwood CA, Zaricznyj B, Kenyon R: Repair of knee ligaments in dogs. J Bone Joint Surg [Am] 43:1167, 1961

61. Odland G, Foss R: I. Epidermal regeneration. II. Inflammatory cells epith-mesenchymal interrelations and fibrogenesis. J Cell Biol 39:135 and 152, 1968

62. Peacock EE Jr: Repair of tendons and restoration of gliding function. In Peacock EE Jr, Van Winkle W Jr (eds): Wound Repair, 2nd Ed. WB Saunders, Philadelphia, 1970

63. Peiro A, Fernandex I, Gomar F: Gluteal fibrosis. J Bone Joint Surg [Am] 57:987, 1975

64. Potenza AD: Effect of associated trauma on healing of divided tendons. J Trauma 2:175, 1962

65. Reid, JD, Kommareddi S, Lankerani M, Park M: Chronic expanding hematomas. JAMA 244:2441, 1980

66. Ross R: Wound healing. Sci Am 220:40, May 1969

67. Sanikern MG, Edwards P: Birth injury to the sternomastoid muscle. J Bone Joint Surg [Br] 48:441, 1966

68. Scott GA, Jolly BL, Henning CE: Combined posterior incision and arthroscopic intraarticular repair of the meniscus. J Bone Joint Surg [Am] 68:847, 1986

68a. Trueta J: The treatment of war fractures by the closed method. Proc Roy Soc Med 33:65, 1939

69. Uhtoff HK, Sarkar K: Calcifying tendinitis. Int Orthop 2:187, 1978

70. Whitesides TE Jr, Haney TC, Morimoto K, Harada H: Tissue pressure measurement as a determinant for the need of fasciotomy. Clin Orthop 113:43, 1975

71. Zarin B, Rowe CR: Combined anterior cruciate-ligament reconstruction using semitendinosus tendon and ilio tibial tract. J Bone Joint Surg [Am] 68:160, 1986

7

Aseptic Necrosis

Necrosis, or infarction of a delineated, usually small, volume of bone substance was alluded to in Chapters 2 and 6. Usually it is followed by the process of repair that has been described in those chapters mainly from the histological point of view but only as it refers to small, even microscopic, volumes of tissue. However, there are many instances where the necrosis constitutes the major and primary element in the pathological process. Some of these instances correspond to syndromes that belong in two etiological categories. One occurs after trauma to certain susceptible sites. The other is called nontraumatic, and in that category the necrosis often is associated with one of several systemic diseases. However, not all nontraumatic infarctions can be traced to a systemic disease, and some in fact are truly idiopathic or at least are so designated at present.

For both categories of the condition, traumatic and nontraumatic, we prefer to use the older term aseptic necrosis of bone, rather than the newer ones (avascular or ischemic necrosis, infarction, and osteonecrosis), but we use the newer ones also with no attempt at distinguishing shades of meaning. "Aseptic necrosis" has been, and is, a generally accepted term. For many years a distinction was needed for the necrosis that was associated with what was then the more important and frequent process, infection.[89] Now we realize that "pure" infarction or necrosis can be caused by a number of diseases, infection at present being one of the less common. Today infection is rarely confused with necrosis, as was the case in olden days. Our preference rests mostly on our comfort with the term we grew up with. Classicists may raise the objection that "avascular" is derived from a root meaning

absence of vessels, and "ischemia" from a root meaning deficiency of blood, but analogous objections could be marshaled against the word aseptic. We do not particularly like the term "osteonecrosis," a word newly coined, because it has been used to designate a specific, probably vascular, clinical entity involving the femoral condyles in older individuals. Perhaps it had best be restricted to that syndrome rather than be used to designate a *process* involving other pathophysiological patterns.

The subject of necrosis of bone *as a process* (not a syndrome) when caused by sepsis or fracture has been discussed briefly in Chapters 2 and 6. Devitalization of tissue, including bone, can develop from other causes such as mechanical trauma without fracture, or radiation injury, burns, frostbite, or even tumors (see Ch. 9). In all such cases, the reason for the loss of blood supply (ischemia) is obvious. Gangrene or massive necrosis of tissue (and that includes bone) is a process that is much more widespread than the process under discussion. There the vascular insufficiency is due to obstruction of major vessels of an organ, a limb, or digit, and so on. In contrast, the necrosis described under sepsis or injury usually involves small volumes of bone (and soft tissue) and is ascribable to thrombosis or interruption of localized networks of small vessels. In this chapter we restrict ourselves to lesions that involve aseptic necrosis of major segments of bone tissue not attributable to either of those two types of lesion. It may occur after trauma or associated with some specific diseases, or it may occur "idiopathically"; but in all cases it is characterized by involvement of a large volume of bone, always at one or more specific sites of predilection.

If one accepts the idea that necrosis of bone can

occur without histological or clinical evidence of lesions in the adjacent soft tissues, and in particular the blood vessels (marrow excepted), one is faced with many questions. When are histological changes first detected?[10] How do they correlate with symptoms? What clinical laboratory tests help diagnose the condition, and when are they reliable? When applying known histological data on the pathophysiology of necrosis and its repair to the clinical evidence derived from diagnostic (primarily radiographic) methods of evaluating those processes, one encounters major problems. Only too often there is a delay of several months between the fact, ascertained retrospectively, and the physician's recognition that aseptic necrosis has occurred. Once there is recognition, more often than not the extent of the lesion and its chronology are not well appreciated. The appropriate treatment, at each stage of the lesion, whether it is applied empirically or fashioned along pathophysiological principles, is often controversial. The histological changes, as described below, are not well documented for each stage of the process, which may explain some but not all of the difficulties just mentioned.

Obviously one would expect necrosis to occur in bone when its blood supply is suddenly disrupted. Some sites in bone, e.g., the head of the femur,[18,37,38,61,99,105,126,127] the body of the talus,[96] the carpal scaphoid,[120] or the lunate bone,[51,82,108] are especially susceptible to sudden ischemia because they have few arteries, and the arteries that are present, because of their position, are at risk. When a traumatic event curtails flow of blood to the part for a critical interval, obviously it dies. The susceptibility of the part is in large measure dependent on the absence or inadequacy of a collateral circulation, and for the sites mentioned that is the situation. Necrosis of bone, where no trauma has occurred, is also attributable to interference with the blood supply. Only a few of the large variety of circumstances that may be responsible for curtailment of blood flow to a localized focus of bone are discussed, and those lesions are relegated to the latter part of this chapter.

Three cases of traumatic aseptic necrosis suffice to illustrate the traumatic category. It should be emphasized that in these cases the volume of bone that has become necrotic is considerable, and it is this feature that distinguishes these cases from the complication of fracture healing involving aseptic necrosis that may be responsible for some nonunions of fractures. In the cases to be described, the problems from the pathophysiological point of view are less those of repair of a fracture and more the inadequacy of the necrotic bone to mechanically support the repair process during that process, as well as the limited capacity of the necrotic bone to perform ordinary mechanical functions.

The traumatic cases are to be distinguished from the nontraumatic because in them we believe the ischemia's onset dates directly to the injury. Whether this assumption indicates that the pathophysiology of aseptic necrosis in traumatic cases differs from that in some nontraumatic cases (see below under steroid treatment) can be of importance in one's perception of the pathophysiology.

It is important to recognize that varying patterns of structural failure occur in a wide range of volumes of necrotic bone — from that of a whole femoral head depicted in case 7-1, to an intermediate amount depicted in case 7-2, to that resembling the smaller volume depicted in case 7-3.

Case 7-1 A 61-year-old woman was seen 23 months after fracture of the right femoral neck. She had had gentle reduction of a minimally displaced fracture; fixation of the femoral neck fracture with three threaded pins had been accomplished without difficulty. She was allowed to bear weight 6 months later. She was pain-free for 3 months, at which time she began to experience mild pain in the hip, first felt with motion of her hip. Sixteen months after the fracture, one pin believed to be penetrating the joint was removed. There was minimal relief of symptoms. At 21 months the patient slipped on a step and had a sudden onset of pain in the hip. Two months later, i.e., 23 months after the fracture, a radiograph showed necrosis of most of the femoral head. Union of the fracture was evident at the superior margin, and a radiolucency proximal to that section of the femoral head was considered to represent a refracture (Fig. 7-1A).

The histological sections from two cores of bone removed at the time of tibial bone grafting and insertion of three threaded pins confirmed the radiographic interpretation. The articular cartilage appeared normal. One of the cores showed the break at the mid-area; but, most importantly, there

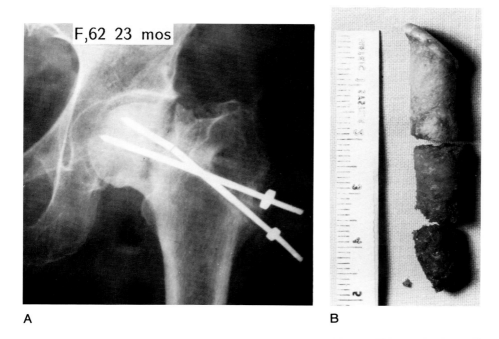

A

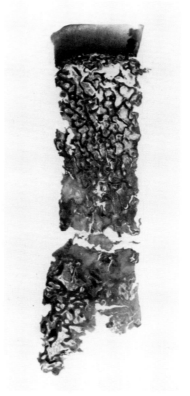

B

C

Fig. 7-1. Case 7-1. (A) AP radiograph of the hip shows increased density of necrosis of the entire femoral head after 23 months and fracture of the neck of the femur in a 62-year-old woman. (B) Core biopsy specimen shows the white necrotic area of the femoral head. (C) Necrosis of the area between the articular cartilage and the fibrocartilaginous fracture zone (×4). (A from Bonfiglio and Voke,[15] with permission.)

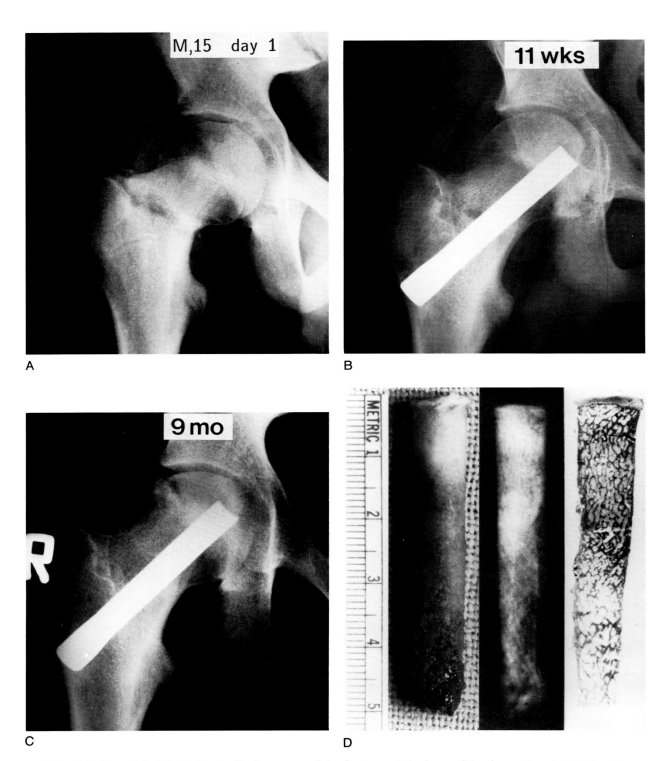

Fig. 7-2. Case 7-2. **(A)** Moderate displacement of the fracture at the base of the femoral neck. **(B)** Partial healing of fracture at 11 weeks. Note the disuse atrophy at the margin of the femoral head and the unchanged density of the remainder of the head. **(C)** At 9 months the necrotic area has collapsed from the margin of the head to the foveal center. **(D)** Composite of core. Gross specimen, radiograph, and photomicrograph show the necrotic area above the healed fracture of the femoral neck at 9 months. *(Figure continues.)*

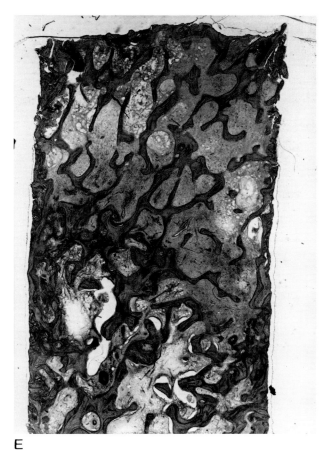

E

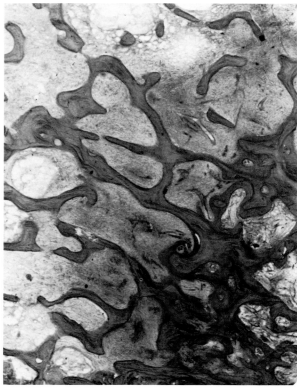

F

Fig. 7-2. *(Continued)* (**E**) New bone is layered on the necrotic trabeculae at the margins of the area of necrosis (×16). (**F**) Necrotic bone and marrow proximal to the zone of necrosis (×60). (**G**) Fracture at the cartilage of the subchondral cortex at the edge of the bone necrosis (×20). (**G** from Bonfiglio,[11] with permission.)

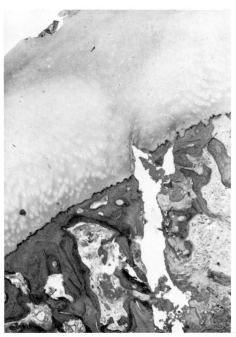

G

was total necrosis of the bone from the site of re-fracture to the subchondral cortex (Fig. 7-1B). The necrotic trabeculae were evident proximal to the refracture site and new bone with a fibrovascular connective tissue replacement distal to it (Fig. 7-1C).

Case 7-2 This case is an example of an interme-diate volume of aseptic necrosis. A mature 15-year-old boy sustained a fracture of the base of the right femoral neck with a moderate degree of dis-placement (Fig. 7-2A). Eleven weeks after a closed reduction, internal fixation with a Smith-Petersen nail, and immobilization in a hip spica cast, the fracture appeared to be healing (Fig. 7-2B). There was atrophy (relative radiolucency) of the femoral head at the margins of the head–neck junction. The density at the center of the femoral head was unchanged and was comparable to that of the ace-tabular wall. The patient had been walking with crutches and had no pain. He remained on crutches for 6 months. He was then pain-free until 9 months after the fracture, when he complained of a sponta-neous onset of pain with unprotected weight-bear-ing. When the hip was examined, the only finding was muscle spasm in the external rotators and flexors. The radiographs showed union of the frac-ture, but there was a slight collapse of the weight-bearing area of the femoral head, and a step-off is seen at the edge of the articular cartilage (Fig. 7-2C). A zone of increased density surrounded the area immediately distal to the step-off, i.e., at the lateral margin of the femoral articular cartilage. The capsular (soft tissue) shadow of the right hip showed a convex lateral and medial border, which was not evident on the 11-week radiograph and suggested a joint swelling that may represent fluid or synovitis.

Histological studies of cores of the femoral head (Fig. 7-2D) removed at the time of treatment showed that there was healing of the original frac-ture, and there was new bone layered on necrotic trabeculae and fibrovascular marrow at the mar-gins of the area of necrosis (Fig. 7-2E). The femoral head proximal to that site was necrotic, both mar-row and trabeculae being so affected (Fig. 7-2F). At the margin of the collapse, the subchondral bone showed partial repair and disruption extend-ing into the cartilage (Fig. 7-2G).

The large size of the necrotic area in this pa-tient's femoral head reflects the fact that most of the ordinary circulation to the head (mediated through the visceral capsule of the hip) and in par-ticular the superior capital vessels, had been inter-rupted, and the negligible collateral circulation to the femoral head via the ligamentum teres could not prevent much of the bone from becoming ne-crotic. The amount of repair that occurred prior and subsequent to the structural failure of the can-cellous bone was also seen. The histological find-ings suggested that the zone of repair extended for only a few millimeters under the necrotic bone.

Case 7-3 A 20-year-old man sustained a disloca-tion of the left hip, which was easily reduced on the day of injury. The patient was kept in traction in bed for 2 days and then was permitted to walk using crutches. Three weeks after the dislocation the ra-diographs of the hip show radiolucency of the fem-oral head in the lateral and medial cancellous por-tions, particularly when compared with the normal hip, but no changes centrally (Figs. 7-3A&B).

The patient was free of pain, but the radiographs taken about every 2 months persistently showed the areas of lucency and relative density. The den-sity of the relatively dense area remained the same as that seen contralaterally (Figs. 7-3C&D).

This radiological pattern (the radiolucency and density) constitute an important *early* sign for the identification of bone necrosis. It also was present in case 7-2 at 11 weeks after the injury. It occurs because the resorption process, akin to disuse atro-phy, can occur only in living bone, i.e., bone with a circulation capable of hyperemia, whereas in dead bone the original density is maintained. During the days immediately after the injury, if the resorptive process (i.e., the reduction in bone density) af-fected *all* of the femoral head, there would be no indication of necrosis. However, it is probable that the hyperemia in the injured part is intensified by the necrosis of adjoining tissue. Living bone at the margins of the area of necrosis therefore show in-tensification of the lucency, even after a short pe-riod, e.g., several weeks. Such a finding should alert the physician to the need for obtaining radio-graphs of the patient rather frequently. The poten-tial for necrosis is known to occur in 10 to 40 per-cent of patients following dislocation of the hip. The longer the time interval between the injury and reduction of the dislocation, the greater is the

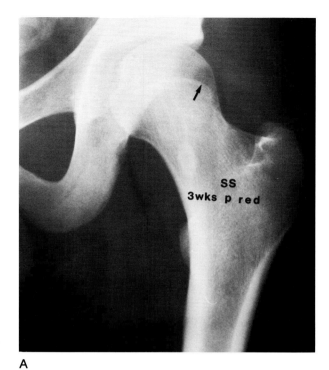

Fig. 7-3. Case 7-3. (A) AP radiograph showing atrophy of bone at the margin of the head 3 weeks after reduction of a dislocation of the left hip (arrow). (B) Lateral view of the change. *(Figure continues.)*

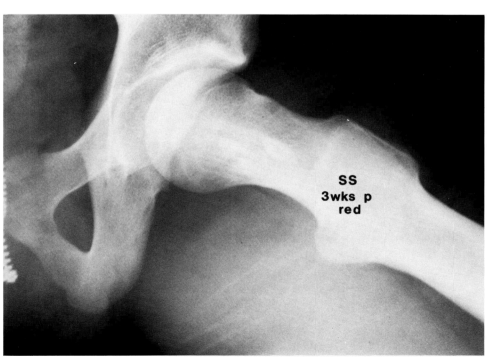

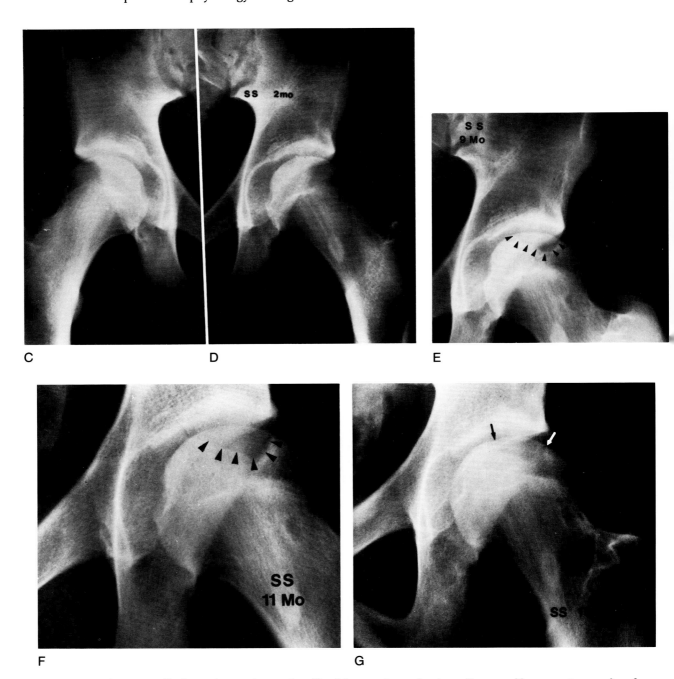

Fig. 7-3 *(Continued).* **(C&D)** AP radiographs of both hips at 2 months show disuse and hyperemic atrophy of the left femoral head neck margin (arrow). The density of the central area is unchanged compared to that of the right femoral head. **(E)** At 9 months the AP radiograph shows increased density (arrowheads) at the periphery of the central focus of radiodensity. **(F)** AP radiograph at 11 months. The necrotic zone is demarcated (arrowheads), but there is no clear evidence of collapse. **(G)** Radiograph at 15 months shows infraction of the subchondral cortex (white arrow) and collapse of the femoral head at the weight-bearing area black arrow). *(Figure continues.)*

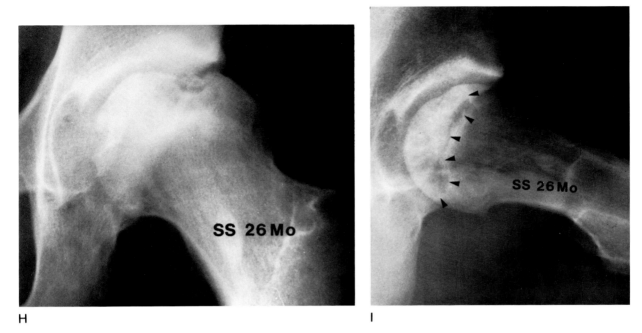

Fig. 7-3 *(Continued)*. **(H&I)** AP and lateral radiographs at 26 months show clear depression of the necrotic fragment (at the site of arrowheads in **I**) of the femoral head.

risk. With reduction of the hip during the first few hours, the incidence of necrosis is 10 percent or less, whereas intervals of more than 24 hours increase the incidence toward 40 percent.

After 9 months, the patient began to complain of pain in the hip brought on by running. Radiographic evaluation then showed a poorly demarcated zone of *increased* density in the periphery of the central focus of radiodensity (Fig. 7-3E). There also was a suggestion of a microfracture at the articular margin of this zone that previously did not undergo resorption. This radiographic increase in density corresponds to a zone of deposition of new bone. The increase represents deposition of new bone on old, dead trabeculae at the margins of the infarct. The central area of the dead bone is unchanged in structure and density, but its density may appear decreased relative to the surrounding increase in density.

However, a critical incident has occurred that is responsible for the pain this patient perceived so long after the injury. That incident is a fracture, a structural failure, perhaps so small as to be termed a microfracture.

It is important to understand that the presence of a "microfracture" in a case of suspected aseptic necrosis indicates that there is a pathophysiological change in the entire part[30,35,112] — in this case, the entire hip joint. It is the fracture that is responsible for the pain, which nearly always is minimal or absent at rest and mostly related to motion of the joint. There is synovitis within the joint and a restricted range of motion because of that synovitis. The synovitis occurs secondarily, and therefore the symptoms generally become worse with prolongation or intensification of activity. The microfractures in question are compactions of the cancellous bone in the area of resorption that, however subtly, alter the biomechanics of the joint and stimulate the synovial membrane to become inflamed.

Although there may be no evidence of collapse radiographically from the injury, as in case 7-3 at 11 months (Fig. 7-3F) and again at 15 months (Fig. 7-3G), it always should be expected. Radiographs at 15 months in this case were interpreted as showing "slight cystic changes," quasi-jargon used by the radiologist to interpret as a central focus of lucency the original density of the necrotic bone surrounded by increased radiodensity of repair bone. It should be noted that, in the other two cases, one showed collapse of the cancellous bone at 9 months, whereas it was not recognized radiographically in the other until 23 months (Fig. 7-1A). It probably did occur in the first case at 9 months when the patient first complained of pain when running.

In case 7-3, because the patient had persistent pain with activity at 26 months after the dislocation, new radiographs were taken. They showed partial collapse of the cartilage of the femoral head, which then measured 3 to 5 mm in thickness and 15 mm in width (Figs. 7-3H&I). This change is similar to but more extensive than the crescent sign noted in a patient to be described below with nontraumatic necrosis (Fig. 7-11A, below).

The films in case 7-3 illustrate a *second* important *radiographic sign* that the aseptic necrosis has actually occurred *before* the collapse, i.e., the presence of *increased density* along an advancing front bordering the zone of radiolucency. This front, which bordered the infarct, represents a zone of new repair bone deposited on the trabeculae of dead bone. From the therapeutic point of view, it is critical that necrosis be recognized at or before this point in the evolution of the process. Protective use of crutches for a protracted period or drilling and bone grafting prior to the crush-down of the femoral head probably would have prevented what eventually happened in this patient.

The additional radiographic sign associated uniquely with aseptic necrosis, but more often absent than present, is the "crescent sign." It did not occur in any of the three cases illustrated, but it should be mentioned because of its importance in the pathophysiological interpretation of structural failure. The sign is a subchondral radiolucency extending for a considerable fraction of the arc of subchondral bone.

A general principle to be emphasized is that when there is necrosis of the femoral head a point nearly always is reached at which there is segmental or complete collapse of the cancellous bone. That collapse represents a fracture or compaction of the necrotic bone during the repair process. This structural failure, when it occurs subchondrally, is evidenced by the crescent sign (see Fig. 7-11, below). When the collapse occurs somewhat dis-

tally, as in the three illustrated cases, the radiological signs already described can be recognized, but *all* of these signs are *late* rather than early manifestations of the process. Both types of structural failure, subchondral and segmental compaction, are discussed in more detail later in the chapter.

Possibly if computed tomography (CT)[84] or magnetic resonance imaging (MRI)[122] were available for case 7-3, the area of necrosis or segmental collapse could have been delineated early. Data are accumulating that CT with multiplanar reconstruction and MRI can detect aseptic necrosis in its early stages before structural failure has occurred (see Fig. 7-6, below). MRI has the advantage of not using x-rays, so repetition of the test for diagnostic purposes or monitoring the course of the necrosis does not pose the risk of radiation damage. These studies suggest that MRI will become the most sensitive method once the parameters and correlations are established. There now is more widespread application of MRI by institutions with the expensive MRI apparatus, and data are being accumulated from patients with aseptic necrosis in several centers.

Each of the three cases just described illustrate today's customary diagnostic routine as applied to traumatic cases. We use ordinary radiological indicators to reveal if the process of necrosis has supervened that will complicate the repair process. Newly developed, more sensitive techniques such as radioisotopic scans and, as mentioned, CT and MRI have been advocated, but if they can facilitate better treatment is still uncertain. Certainly these techniques are not uniformly available to most practitioners; moreover, they are costly diagnostic measures. They cannot be advocated lightly without strong evidence, not yet at hand, as to their effectiveness. The importance of early recognition of necrosis should be obvious, but unfortunately the clinical features of necrosis present major obstacles to the establishment of better diagnostic routines.

The fact that aseptic necrosis of bone is *painless* for months after its onset needs to be underscored.[3,12,99,101] Following a known episode in which there is disruption of the circulation of a part of a bone, as in each of the first two cases, the complications came to light only some months after the fracture was healed and long after the patients resumed weight-bearing. In the third case, the hip that had been dislocated did not become painful until 9 months after the dislocation (and reduction). Internal and stable fixation of the fracture fragments in cases 7-1 and 7-2 had resulted in mechanical stability, so there was no pain from the fracture site despite the fact that necrosis occurred presumably within a day or two after the injury.

It may be important to recognize that the pain began to be perceived not as bone pain referred from the direct spot where the necrosis was occurring but, rather, as pain in the joint adjacent to the area of necrosis. How one interprets the delay in onset of pain is important if a suitable pathogenesis of the pain is to be conceived. The delay means that there were no stimuli provoked by the necrosis per se and that there were no stimuli from the fracture in cases 7-1 and 7-2 or from the dislocation in case 7-3. Soon after the injury the joint surfaces had been restored to normal in terms of alignment and motion, most if not all of the synovial collection of blood or fluid had been resorbed, and the tear in the synovial membrane had healed. The fractures or dislocations had been stabilized, so minimal or no pain would be expected from the fragments during the first 2 to 3 weeks post injury even if healing had not been complete.

The first reason that the necrosis initially is painless is that within the affected bone there are no sensory nerve endings to mediate painful stimuli. Even if there were cellular reactions to the necrosis at its periphery, or edema or inflammation, and histologically no such evidence exists, they could not evoke afferent stimuli to the brain. The second reason is that even though the chemical stimuli that occur later at the periphery of the necrotic area, i.e., an outpouring of proteolytic and other enzymes and the other products of deterioration of cells, they are not irritating. Because cancellous bone is the tissue involved, the necrotic cells are mostly those of the fatty marrow. Necrotic products form at a site removed from the nerve endings in bone, which are nearly all at the periosteal surface or in the walls of blood vessels.

Therefore the late onset of the pain must be explained by a phenomenon other than necrosis per se. One clue to the explanation is that the pain in each case was associated with functioning of the adjacent joint, and therefore the pain should relate to some change in that joint. That change in case 7-3 obviously was attributable to an effusion, which was demonstrated radiographically. Probably there also was an effusion in case 7-1 and case 7-2, although the amount was probably too small to show up on radiographs. Why might an effusion develop so long after the trauma? One possibility is that microfractures developed in the necrotic bone as a result of normal stresses. The fractures then would cause some change in the coaptation of the nearby articular surface. The joint membrane would then become irritated because the articular surface no longer would be congruous. It should be noted that the collapse of the understructure of the articular cartilage would tend to be more extensive in certain sections, depending on the distribution of the load and the location and number of the broken trabeculae, but in all cases the articular distortion would be too small to be recognized radiographically. Nevertheless, the articular cartilage, with its subchondral plate, would be deformed cyclically with motion of the joint's surfaces. At best, the deformation at the site of microfractures would not cause a break in the cartilage initially, but the motion would, by a milking action, force the products of necrosis (edema fluid, enzymes) into the subsynovial region and probably into the joint, where the synovial membrane, exposed to the irritants, would become inflamed.

The situation in case 7-3 with regard to the late onset of pain supports the above pathophysiological explanation. Soon after the reduction of the dislocation, motion of the hip was painless; and the joint was soon functioning normally. Only months later did the physical findings show a limitation of the range of motion of the hip, particularly with internal rotation. These findings are characteristic for any irritative process in the joint and are usually explained by reflex muscular spasm, particularly in the small external rotators, which are close to the synovial membrane. The findings support the contention that the pain was primarily articular in origin. The painful maneuvers of the physical examination are expressions of one physical phenomenon: distention of the joint when it is placed in positions that limit the volume of the joint cavity.

The above putative pathophysiology has some therapeutic implications that deserve mention.

One is that there would be no need for treatment of the necrosis of the cancellous bone per se or for the collapse (because they are not symptomatic) were it not for the secondary but symptomatic effects on the joint. This concept suggests, first, that early unloading of the joint might allow, in time, replacement of the volume of necrotic bone and restitution of the understructure of the articular surface. It would be proper prophylaxis. A second suggestion is that an effective therapeutic maneuver might be any surgical measure that supports that understructure and prevents the cyclical distortion. A third suggestion is that a crucial feature of symptomatic necrosis is that it involves cancellous, not cortical, bone. When segments of cortical bone lose their blood supply (which also pertains to massive autografts or allografts that are primarily cortical), they do not undergo the compaction described above because of their great compressive strength and their greater resistance to resorption, which then occurs slowly. In addition, such composite cortical grafts or segments usually are juxtaposed anatomically to joints when they are used to replace segments excised for tumors. The articular cartilage, devoid of vessels, cannot generate a vascular supply for creeping substitution of the cortical bone.[20]

It has already been mentioned that the structural integrity of the necrotic cancellous bone was at risk because of its lack of vascularity. The fact that the physical characteristics of necrotic bone differ from live bone in important ways has been considered one explanation for the phenomenon under discussion.[19] Necrotic bone is less elastic than live bone, and its brittleness may well render it susceptible to microfracture. Microfractures also occur in live bone, but there the process of repair is initiated immediately, and there is a well coordinated substitution of repair bone that takes up the stresses throughout the sector of the microfractures. With aseptic necrosis there is no potentiality for such pervasive repair. One can readily conceive of a *series* of microfractures in the repairing zone induced cyclically by ordinary walking. When in fracture cases these microfractures are located in the subchondral layer of the femoral head, as in case 7-2 (Fig. 7-2G), the support framework for the articular cartilage is compromised, and the cycle of degeneration of the cartilage can begin.

Note that the above conceptual pathophysiological sequence is based in large part on a history of symptoms and an interpretation of physical findings; unfortunately, it is not based on evidence from clinical radiological examinations, presumably because the microfractures are too small to be detectable radiographically. However, they can be deduced from histological evidence.

All too frequently a patient with a dislocation of the hip or a fracture of the femoral neck has the acute lesion treated appropriately only to have the catastrophic complications appear months or even years later, as if out of the blue.[3,10,12,17,30,50,60,99,101,112] As is evident later in the chapter, the same pattern can occur in nontraumatic situations, e.g., congenital dislocation of the hip and slipped epiphysis. Monitoring the situation by all appropriate methods available, as was done for case 7-3, may not effectively ascertain if a patient at risk has developed necrosis. Recognition of the complication, at present, is possible unfortunately only after much damage is done. When there is a substantial risk (as represented by subcapital fractures, dislocations, and fracture of the femoral neck with extensive displacement), strong indications exist for prophylactic protection of the joint over a prolonged period. How long that period should be is unfortunately impossible to assess at present. Cases are on record in which the secondary, symptomatic consequences of the necrosis make their appearance 2 years after the traumatic event.[3,12,15,21,30,99,101,112] Do those cases justify so long a period of protection to the hip? With the often crippling nature of the complication as a stimulus, some prophylaxis surely is justified. In cases similar to those illustrated, even in the absence of radiological evidence of aseptic necrosis, 9 to 12 months of protection is advocated, and longer if there are positive or even equivocally positive abnormalities on the radiographs. When this somewhat arbitrary period of protection is about to end, there is good reason to apply one or more of the newer radiological modalities[5,84,122] already mentioned to help decide if the patient is safe from complication.

There are many cases, however, where one's hope to avoid the catastrophic complication of aseptic necrosis after a fracture of the hip has to be put aside because of overriding considerations.

The prophylaxis (non-weight-bearing on the affected extremity after the reduction and internal fixation of the fracture) is out of the question in many elderly patients (those with even moderately severe osteoporosis or with neurological deficits) and in patients with Parkinson's disease, for instance, who have to be allowed to walk as soon as possible after the injury and who are unable to use crutches or a walker in such a way as to avoid weight-bearing on the affected limb. For such patients the monitoring radiological routine may well be an academic exercise.

These examples indicate that the available methods of diagnostic study are not a reliable substitute for a high index of suspicion of pathophysiological possibilities. Continual reevaluation of any patient in a high-risk situation is mandatory, and the available methods should be used to aid that reevaluation. The strategy for monitoring the patient must be based on the correlation of knowledge of the histological sequences and the possible radiographic changes that characterize aseptic necrosis.

The histological changes that are described here for the femoral head also occur with some variations in other sites of aseptic necrosis, e.g., the head of the humerus, carpal scaphoid or lunate,[87] and the body of the talus. In general, they have the same implications with respect to methods used to recognize necrosis. Because of anatomical and functional differences, treatment of course varies for each site. However, the pathophysiological sequences must be understood if any treatment applied is to be effective. The overriding principle of prophylaxis is that the site be kept structurally intact so that fragmentation of the adjacent articular cartilage and secondary degenerative changes are avoided. The overriding principle of treatment is to maintain the articular cartilage of the femoral head whenever possible or to reconstitute it so that it is congruous to that of the acetabulum and so that it has a mechanically sound understructure. When these goals cannot be achieved, other types of reconstruction (e.g., total hip replacement arthroplasty) may be best. Much of the following histological data come from studies of femoral heads removed during total hip replacement. Necrosis is more common at that site than at any other.

First we portray the early stages of the situations in the three cases discussed earlier. One of our objectives is to correlate the three principal radiographic signs with the pathophysiological process as revealed by the histology:[10,11,14,15,21,29,30,99,101,112] (1) the relatively (but not actually) increased density; (2) the subsequent absolute increase in density; and (3) other structural alterations, which include the "classical" radiolucent crescent sign and segmental collapse.[27,30,35,99,112] It must be understood that these three radiological abnormalities do not invariably characterize each affected hip; moreover, although the pattern of radiolucency in the first category is usually the earliest of the signs, it does not occur at all in some cases (i.e., those in which the repair process fails to achieve even minimal effectiveness—in other words, where repair is practically nonexistent). Moreover, each of the other two categories of signs may be the only one noted at the time the patient is first seen, so one cannot surmise if previous to that time there indeed were detectable radiological abnormalities.

The description offered here is a synthesis of observations derived from many specimens of femoral heads, either core specimens or specimens removed from patients who have had a prosthetic hip replacement after fracture of the femoral neck.[2,9,10,11,15,21,29,30,35,99,101,112] They reveal the following changes.

At the moment of irreversible ischemia in a large segment of the bone, all cellular elements obviously die, including the osteocytes, hematopoietic cells, and fat cells in the marrow. Perhaps, depending on how much of the peripheral circulation remains, some of the periosteal cells survive. The trabecular and cortical components retain their architecture until the time when the dead bone is invaded by granulation tissue.

The amount (volume) of the necrosis in each femoral head varies greatly. There may be necrosis of the entire head, or, at the other end of the spectrum, a focus of necrosis in the anterior superior portion of the head. At first, before 3 days have elapsed, little evidence of necrosis is visible histologically because it takes that period of time for the disintegration of nuclear proteins (chromatin in particular) to reach the point where ordinary histological stains reveal cell death.

It is in the marrow that the ischemic changes are

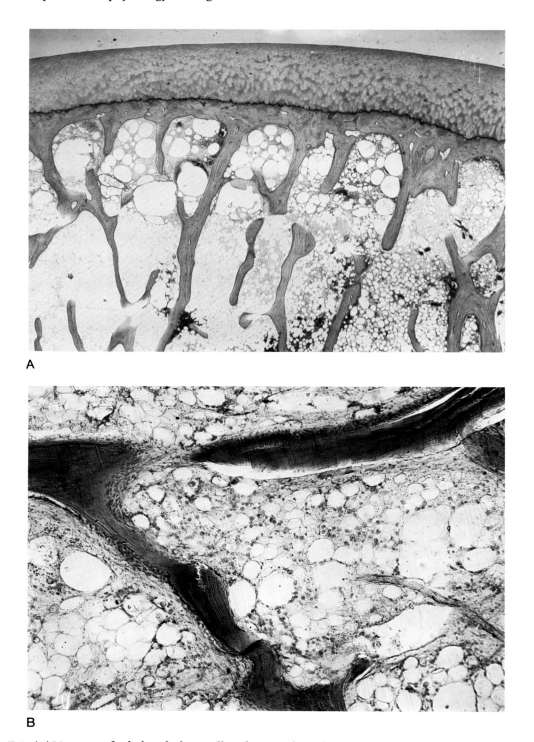

A

B

Fig. 7-4. (A) Necrosis of subchondral cancellous bone with agglomeration of fat cells and loss of staining of osteocytes (×100). **(B)** Pools of free fat in fibrovascular marrow of repairing aseptic necrosis of a femoral head (×250). *(Figure continues.)*

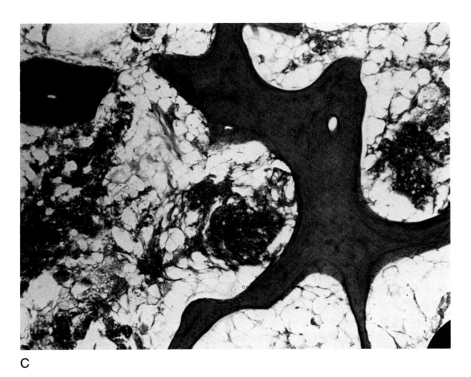

C

Fig. 7-4 *(Continued)*. (C) Amorphous calcification of necrotic fatty marrow (×200). (D) Loss of osteocyte cell staining with empty lacunae in the subchondral cortex with vascular channels and new bone along the necrotic trabeculae (×250). (C from Bonfiglio,[11] with permission.)

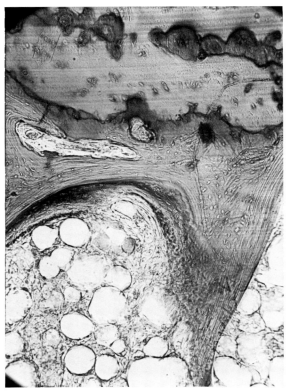

D

first recognizable. First there is a clumping and agglomeration of some of the fat cells and some loss of staining definition in the nuclei of the other cells (Fig. 7-4A). Some macrophages appear at the margins of the infarction, and they become more numerous from the fourth day onward. They phagocytize dead fat cells and hematopoietic cells (Fig. 7-4B). When the cell walls of the fat cells are digested, pools of free fat appear in the marrow (Fig. 7-4B); and this phenomenon becomes more evident over the next few days and then proceeds for several weeks or longer. Incidentally, during this interval, bone scans with bone-seeking isotopes may indicate that the area under study is "cold," but often such a scan shows no abnormality and the radiograph also appears normal.

Necrosis of the marrow fat may be followed by calcification or fibrosis of the marrow, and either of these states may occur within the area during the following weeks. The calcification rarely is sufficiently intense to cause an increase in bone density that can be seen on ordinary radiographs. The calcification is thought to be the result of crystallization of fatty acids with saponification and formation of calcium soaps, and it has been noted particularly in the ischemic margin of the necrosis of decompression syndrome[70] (Fig. 7-4C).

During the 3 weeks after the ischemic episode, the osteocytes disappear from the lacunae (Fig. 7-4D), but not all the osteocytes autolyse at the same rate. Some may be lost during preparation of the histological slide. Even though a cell may be dead, there is a delay in the disappearance of the nuclear material, varying from days to about 1 month. Often the cells stain normally for even a week or two until the vascularization process approaches the necrotic trabeculae; then new proteolytic enzymes from blood-borne cells and plasma are made available to complete the lysis of the nuclear material. Thus for 2 weeks or so from the moment of injury one cannot delineate with certainty the limits of the dead bone on the basis of microscopic sections.

There is an additional factor to consider when one sees no osteocytes in groups of lacunae. It has been shown in several studies,[29] notably the one by Sherman et al.,[112,113] that in normal adult bone there is a variable amount of focal necrosis as part of the normal aging process. The foci increase in size and number with age. When the patient has atherosclerosis, there may be a considerable volume of bone devoid of osteocytes. Certain sites (femoral head, tibial shaft) are more prone to show this phenomenon than others.[29,112,113] Foci where some of the osteocytes are absent are noted in several diseases, e.g., sickle cell disease, and with some pathological processes such as radiation injury to bone.

The invasion of fibrovascular granulation tissue (as part of the inflammatory response to an injury) into the necrotic marrow of the osteoporotic cancellous bone begins within 1 to 2 weeks after a fracture of the femoral neck (Fig. 7-4D). The destroyed marrow circulation is then quickly replaced by vessels from the granulation tissue, and the hematopoietic and fatty marrow can then be reconstituted. By 4 weeks after the fractures in cases 7-1 and 7-2, granulation tissue would extend up to some areas of the subchondral cortex of the femoral head. The dead trabeculae then begin to be removed piecemeal by osteoclasts. This osteoclastic removal of material with mineral radiodensity would be the first histological event that might have a radiological counterpart — radiolucency. For that abnormality to be detectable, however, a considerable volume, perhaps as much as one-fourth (as derived from the studies of osteoporosis in vertebrae) of the total in the plane of the x-irradiation, would have to be removed. Comparison may also be pertinent to the similar resorptive process that occurs with disuse atrophy, e.g., when a cast is applied to the foot and leg. Then a tibial lucency develops above the ankle, after about 2 weeks. The mechanism is the same but much more rapid, because the circulation not only is not at risk but also is not obstructed in any way.

At the same time that the osteoclasts do their job, new bone derived from osteogenic cells accompanying the capillary invasion is laid down on the remaining trabeculae of necrotic bone. The originally necrotic cancellous bone is replaced in that way, i.e., by creeping substitution with new appositional bone. As the repair proceeds, the new trabeculae develop in a pattern that is a response to stress. This pattern is subject to change, as an expression of the remodeling process. Some degree of repair continues for as long as any dead bone remains. Often the repair continues to be active, but on a declining level, for years.

During the process of replacement of dead bone by living bone, particularly at the edge of the necrotic zone where resorption is most active, the transforming bone structure is weak, and collapse is most likely to occur there. When it does, the same cycle that has just been described begins all over again because usually some additional necrosis has occurred. Alternatively, the sequence described in Chapter 3 begins, i.e., hemorrhage, exudation, callus formation, and so on.

Only two methods of studying aseptic necrosis, radiological and histological, have been emphasized. A word may be appropriate concerning other methods. Several isotopic techniques are now being studied to determine to what extent the vascular supply to the femoral head at the time of fracture or at intervals thereafter has been compromised.[5,21,54,80,107,116] None of these techniques is sufficiently reliable to be used to identify patients at risk. Methods devised to measure the

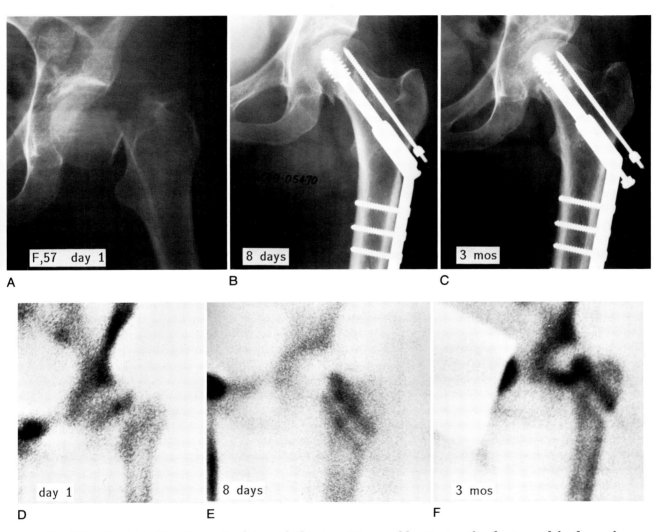

Fig. 7-5. (A) Initial AP radiograph of the right hip in a 57-year-old patient with a fracture of the femoral neck. (B) Eight days after internal fixation. (C) Three months after internal fixation. (D) Initial bone scan with ⁹⁹ᵐTc polyphosphate shows a cold area of most of the femoral head. (E) It appears cold at 8 days. (F) Note the cold wedge area of the head and the increased uptake in the margin at 3 months.

amount of blood in the site of interest, at the time of initial treatment of the fracture, or within a week or two afterward are plagued not only by too many false-positive or false-negative results to justify their routine use but also by other major difficulties. The interpretation of results may be difficult because the overlying tissues obscure the happenings in the femoral head. Other methods also have been devised for use weeks to months after the injury. In most of them, bone-seeking isotopes are used with the following rationale. The volume of radioisotope uptake depends on the activity of the repair, i.e., the volume of new bone deposited. The dead bone should appear as a "cold" area, whereas the reactive bone would appear "hot" (Figs. 7-5D – F). With this rationale and with the use of the pinpoint collimator, several isotopes (^{99m}Tc polyphosphate[54] and ^{18}F[107]) are under investigation. Each is administered systemically to a patient after fracture of the neck of the femur. In some cases they permit early detection of an area of necrosis that might not be evident by routine radiography[5] (Fig. 7-5). These methods are not in general use because they are not of proved value and the equipment needed is complex.

Another proposed technique still in the investigational stage makes use of the fact that the marrow macrophages pick up some radioactive isotopes, e.g., gallium- or technetium-99m-tagged colloidal sulfur.[116] The pickup occurs only in living bone, and it is maximal during the invasion of marrow in the early stages of repair, when macrophages abound. Another substance suggested is indium 111 chloride-tagging the white blood cells. Necrotic marrow cells would not pick up the isotopes. If refinements of these and possibly newer radioisotopic techniques prove to be reliable and sensitive, they might allow one to detect or suspect that there is necrotic bone soon after the ischemic event, but none of the techniques qualifies in either respect.[116] These techniques utilize whole-body or whole-bone external radiography to register the areas of high pickup.

One other approach has also been studied extensively. It utilizes a probe inserted into the femoral head after systemic injection of a radioactive substance to measure such parameters as intramedullary pressure and oxygen content. The results of all these methods indicate that although each offers some promise none is recommended for general use. The techniques must therefore be characterized as "under study."

Magnetic resonance imaging, a technique for imaging tissues and tissue elements, is a noninvasive method using spin echo magnetic resonance to provide an image of the anatomical structures.[103,122] The following case serves as an example of its potential value. As yet, the correlative parameters have not been clearly delineated.

Case 7-4   A 16-year-old boy sustained a fracture dislocation of the left hip in a motorcycle accident (Fig. 7-6A). The post-closed-reduction film shows widening of the articular cartilage radiolucency because of a retained interposed fragment of the femoral head (Fig. 7-6B). An open reduction was done and the fragment removed (Fig. 7-6C); the patient was kept in bed 2 weeks and allowed to walk with crutches (touch-weight-bearing) at 6 weeks. Because of the high risk for aseptic necrosis, MRI was performed at 2 months, and the T_2-weighted image shows the bright signal of a living head on the right and a marked decrease in signal of the medial two-thirds of the left (presumed partially necrotic) femoral head (Fig. 7-6D). Radiographs 2 weeks later showed marginal disuse atrophy and a relatively dense center of the head (Fig. 7-6E). At 5 months (Fig. 7-6F) it is more apparent that the relative density change pathognomonic of necrosis is present. Because of the patient's age and the necrosis of only part, not all, of the femoral head a decision was made to use tibial bone grafts to prevent collapse of the head and to preserve its contour. Cup or surface replacement arthroplasty was considered the next best choice but was excluded because the area of necrosis was too large. Total hip arthroplasty was excluded because of the high rate of loosening and failure in the young adult patient. The histological studies of the cores removed to allow placement of the grafts show aseptic necrosis of the femoral head (Fig. 7-6G). The MRI in this patient gave an indication of necrosis by the altered signal in the dead bone versus that in the living bone. The potential to alter the signal response may help delineate not only living from necrotic tissue but also to identify granulation tissue repair.[122]

Clinically, the ordinary *radiographic evaluation* remains the standard method for recognizing asep-

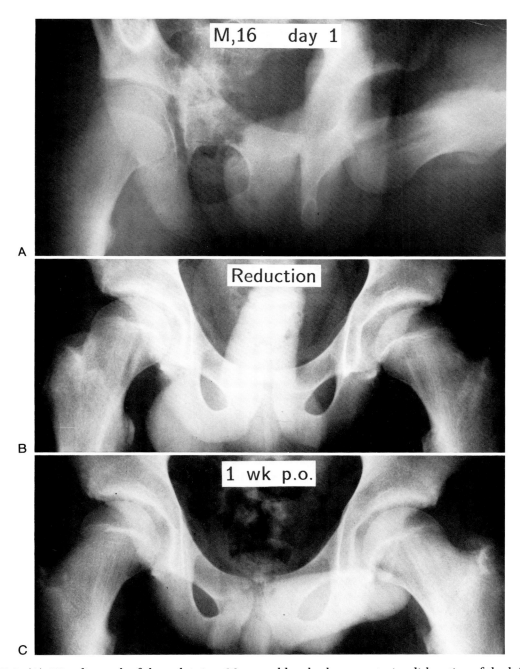

Fig. 7-6. **(A)** AP radiograph of the pelvis in a 16-year-old male shows posterior dislocation of the left hip with fracture of the femoral head. **(B)** AP radiograph of the pelvis with a wide medial joint space of the hip after reduction of the dislocation. **(C)** Normal joint space after open reduction and removal of the free fracture fragment. *(Figure continues.)*

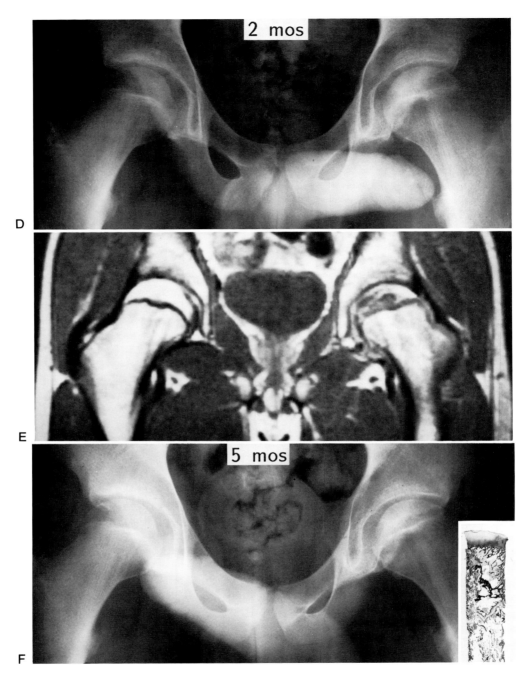

Fig. 7-6 *(Continued).* **(D)** MRI at 2 months shows absence of T_2 density in the medial portion of the femoral head, which is considered evidence of necrosis when compared to the bright signal of the normal right femoral head. **(E)** At 2 months the AP radiograph shows disuse atrophy of the margins of the head and a slight increase in density of the left femoral head centrally. **(F)** At 5 months the radiograph changes. The increase in density correlates with the thicker trabeculae of the microscopic section of the core biopsy ($\times$ 2). *(Figure continues.)*

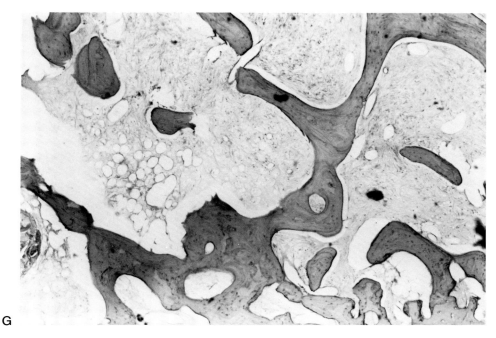

G

Fig. 7-6 *(Continued).* (G) Photomicrograph of the proximal area of a core biopsy near the subchondral cortex shows necrotic marrow fat and trabeculae ($\times$63).

tic necrosis. Longitudinal utilization of the routine radiographic techniques done at frequent intervals is needed to diagnose the condition and then to monitor its course in all patients who are at risk, except when contraindicated of course. The patient who has scintigraphic evidence (but not radiographic verification) that there is an area of involvement would still require confirmatory unequivocal radiographic evidence from examinations repeated at intervals of 3 months or less to justify either invasive diagnostic testing or trials of any but the most conservative therapy.

In the three cases just presented, the elements of radiographic evidence have been described. It should be emphasized that the chronology of the changes varies considerably. The cases demonstrate that the variability seems not to depend entirely on the volume of bone that may be necrotic. The time interval that may elapse before the onset of symptoms or appearance of a characteristic pattern of radiographic features seems to depend more on unknown factors, but the characteristic *pattern* of changes that develops long after the trau-

matic ischemic event, whatever the interval, must always be searched for.

It has already been mentioned that the feature of the pattern that appears earliest in the traumatic category of cases of aseptic necrosis is atrophy, or a relative radiolucency. That feature usually can be ascertained only by comparing the involved hip with the contralateral hip (Fig. 7-7). Atrophy is possible, as mentioned, only in living bone and represents disuse of the part. It must be reemphasized, however, that what is sought as an indication of aseptic necrosis is the *absence* of atrophy in a localized focus where there should be atrophy. The focus shows a normal density and is surrounded by the atrophy.

Unfortunately, for patient and surgeon there is apparently one insurmountable obstacle to an early diagnosis of aseptic necrosis, not only immediately as treatment after the trauma is undertaken but during the first weeks or months thereafter, i.e., before the atrophy can be recognized radiographically. That obstacle is the absence of any symptoms or signs to invite the surgeon to perform tests for

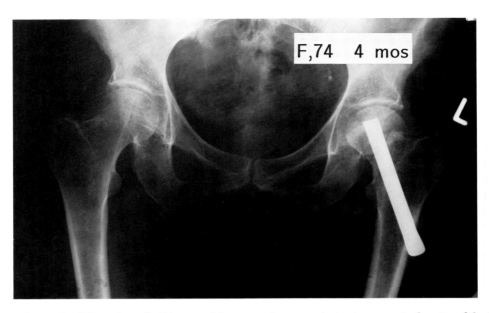

Fig. 7-7. Radiograph of the pelvis of a 74-year-old woman shows a relative increase in density of the head of the right femur 4 months after fixation with a Smith-Petersen nail.

identifying the complication. Furthermore, there are no reliable tests to provide such identification. Ideally, the diagnosis, definitive or presumptive, should be made prior to treatment of the fracture of the femoral neck (or dislocation, as in case 7-3) because then the treatment of the necrosis would be as important or more important than treatment of the fracture. The obstacle to definitive early diagnosis of necrosis at present seems insurmountable — witness the unsuccessful radioisotopic and other experimental attempts at early diagnosis. A patient defined as being "at high risk" would be one in whom two factors are present that are known empirical predilections to aseptic necrosis, i.e., certain fracture patterns (e.g., subcapital femoral) and extensive displacement of fracture fragments. These two factors can be recognized preoperatively. There are also two factors that can be recognized either intraoperatively or postoperatively, and both relate to whether the operation for internal fixation has proceeded without incident. Intraoperatively, for instance, it may be that the reduction was achieved only after several manipulations of the extremity, that the final (accepted) reduction position was not ideal or was unstable, or that during the internal fixation the screw

or nail of the fixation device did not enter the capital fragment smoothly but tended to separate it from the distal fragment. Postoperatively, also, instability of fixation or poor position of fragments might be considered "at risk" factors. When one or more of those "at risk" factors occurs in a patient for whom prophylactic protection would be difficult, e.g., an elderly individual, the complication of necrosis can be absolutely prevented by treating the fracture with total hip arthroplasty or hemiarthroplasty.

Additional deterrents to radiological diagnosis of aseptic necrosis may also plague the clinician. When a metal device is inserted for fixation of the fracture, whatever the device may be, it occupies the area of potential or actual necrosis. The result, generally, is that the pattern of atrophy versus relative density is obscured by the metal; moreover, changes due to the operative trauma incurred by inserting the metal device(s) must be taken into account. They undoubtedly increase the danger of ischemia of previously viable cancellous bone. Operative damage to the trabeculae, even if it is minimal and unavoidable, must be considered an added risk for significant aseptic necrosis.

In case 7-3, the patient with a dislocation of the

hip, the only risk factor should have been the nature and severity of the injury with no radiographic obscuring of the bone. In such a case, radiographs of the pelvis or hips should have been made at 1-month intervals during the first 6 months while the patient's hip was protected (i.e., non-weight-bearing). The relative density difference then might well have been detected early. Given the patient's youth and the serious impairment that usually supervenes if there is aseptic necrosis and compac-

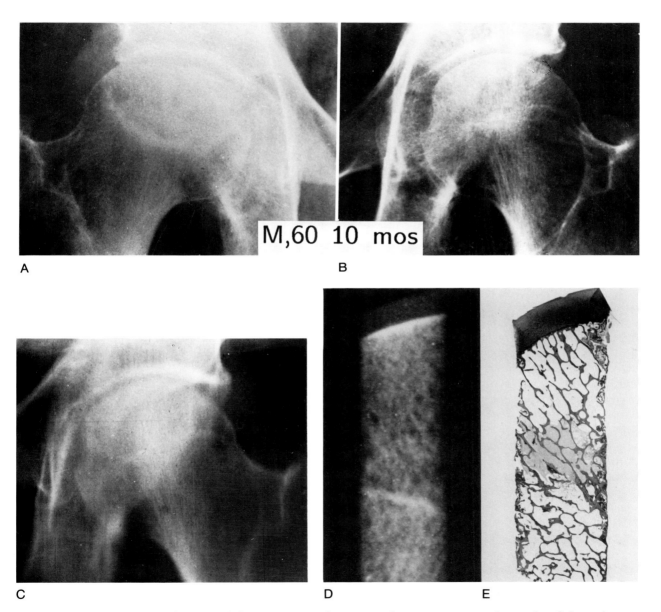

A

B

M,60 10 mos

C

D

E

Fig. 7-8. (A&B) Zone of increased density surrounds an area of necrosis in AP radiographs of the right (symptomatic) and left femoral heads (silent). (C) tomogram of the left "silent" hip of a 60-year-old man with nontraumatic aseptic necrosis. Radiograph (D) and photomicrograph (E) of the coring specimen show the trabeculae thickened by new bone at the margin of the necrotic bone and marrow (×2). (B, C, & E from Bonfiglio,[11] with permission.)

tion of the bone, one might even have been justified in prescribing as initial treatment absolute bed rest with traction for several weeks and then non-weight-bearing ambulation or touch-weight-bearing crutches for the first 6 months, assuming the patient would comply with the regimen. By 6 months it should be possible to definitely determine if there is a *relative density difference*. The same observation was made after treatment of two patients with a fracture dislocation of the neck of the talus after a period of plaster immobilization of the ankle following closed reduction (see later in the Chapter). Despite non-weight-bearing, the body of the talus appeared dense, because the surrounding living bone had undergone severe disuse osteoporosis (see Figs. 7-29 and 7-30, below).

When there is an *actual increase* in radiographic density, in contrast to the apparent and relative density difference just discussed, its pathophysiology is different. It results from the deposition of new bone on old trabeculae. Therefore it will also not be evident within the first weeks after trauma. Its pattern of distribution, however, will differ from that of the necrosis in that it tends to be linear, following the pattern of the borders of viable bone. New bone can be formed only on the edges of the necrotic marrow when there has been cellular proliferation and capillary invasion (Figs. 7-2D&E). The pattern of new bone formation may be a spherical or irregular zone about a focal area of necrosis. The new bone then is responsible for the use by radiologists of the descriptive term "cyst-like" because the added density forms a sphere surrounding a less dense center (Figs. 7-8B&C). The main objection to the term is the fact that a cyst, by definition, is a sac containing liquid or semisolid material.

As noted earlier (Fig. 7-4C), calcification in the marrow may also be responsible for a slight increase in density in a bone that has undergone necrosis of the marrow. The increased density involves the center of a necrotic focus rather than the periphery, and it tends to appear early in the postinjury period, i.e., within the first 3 months. No evidence, using isotopes, is available to show that the calcification is metabolically active. In contrast, the areas of increased density that surround an infarct, e.g., that depicted in the tomogram of the right hip (Fig. 7-8C) always shows increased uptake of radioactive isotope. It always occurs in areas of new bone formation and is shown radiographically and in a photomicrograph of a coring specimen (Figs. 7-8D&E). In many instances of aseptic necrosis, absent or reduced uptake (a "cold spot") is seen in the central area of necrosis (Fig. 7-5).

There is evidence obtained in a study of old lesions in caisson disease by radiography and bone scintigraphy that increased activity may be present for 10 years or more in areas that appear radiographically normal; moreover, it was shown that structural failure may occur as late as 10 years after the necrosis first appears.[54] This finding means that the active process of replacement of necrotic bone tends to continue over periods that are much longer than those generally associated with repair processes.

The new bone that is deposited on the necrotic trabeculae soon after the revascularization of marrow is the essential element in the process of repair by creeping substitution. In fracture cases, that new bone and the callus of the fracture are continuous. In the repair of aseptic necrosis, as a rule, there is no external callus, and the internal architecture of the cancellous bone may be reconstituted with minimal or no change in the gross anatomical configuration, especially in cases where collapse of trabeculae does not occur. Minor secondary degenerative changes with few or no clinical symptoms may then be the end result. In such cases the process of repair takes between 2 months and 2 years. These sequences have been well documented in studies on necrosis after fracture of the femoral neck or dislocation of the femoral head as well as in some nontraumatic causes.

There are two radiographic signs (in addition to the changes in density) that indicate that the cancellous bone has undergone *structural failure* (i.e., refracture): (1) radiolucency underneath the sub-

Fig. 7-9. A 51-year-old woman had had left hip pain for 1 year. AP radiographs show minimal collapse (stage 3) in the superior (**A**) and anterolateral (**B**) aspects of the head of the femur. (**C**) ^{99m}Tc bone scan is positive. (**D**) Several cuts of the CT scan show an increase in density and collapse of the necrotic head of the femur (arrows).

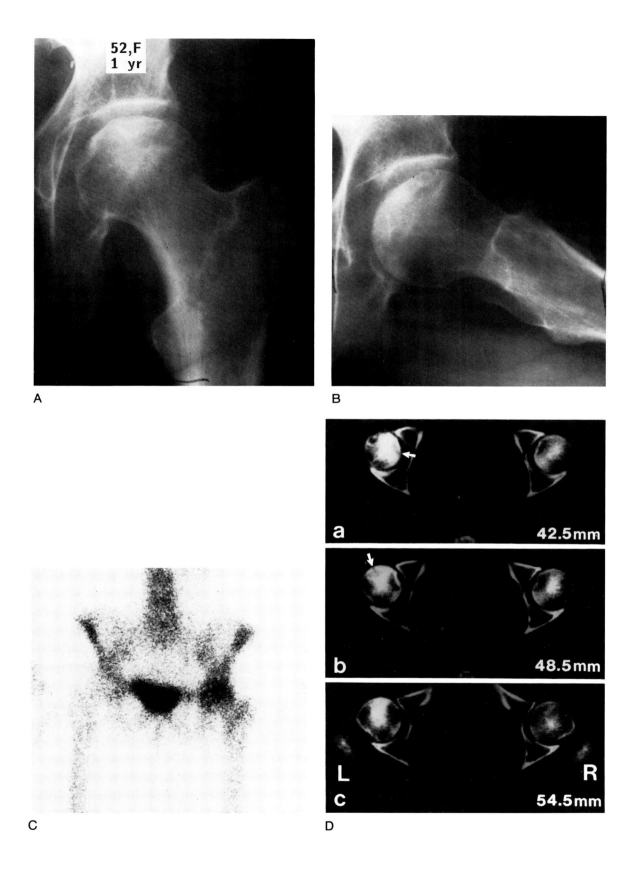

A

B

C

D

chondral cortex, or the *crescent sign;* and (2) the increased radiodensity of *segmental necrosis* with *collapse* (as shown by radiographs, bone scans, and CT scan (Fig. 7-9). The chronology of these signs is important. A composite drawing from many femoral heads illustrates a few of the configurations that may be encountered (Fig. 7-10). It has been demonstrated in cases 7-1, 7-2, and 7-3 that several months (9 months or more) usually elapse between the injury and the appearance of these structural alterations. Both the *crescent sign* (Fig. 7-11A) and *segmental collapse* (Fig. 7-12) occur at interfaces between living and dead bone, and they tend to occur at the advancing resorptive edge of bone repair. They occupy that area because the subchondral (subarticular) bone has been weakened before there is sufficient new bone formed to compensate for the resorbed trabeculae (Fig. 7-12E). It is not certain whether the initial or any subsequent fracture of one or more trabeculae allows other trabeculae progressively to fail or a single application of a large load is responsible for failure of the cartilage's understructure. Probably there are repeated disruptions of trabeculae and fragmentation of some before the patient has enough symptoms to be a suspect for aseptic necrosis.

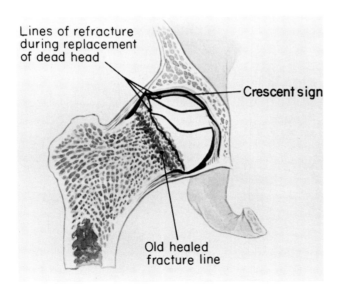

Lines of refracture during replacement of dead head

Crescent sign

Old healed fracture line

Fig. 7-10. Aseptic necrosis of the femoral head stress fracture patterns in traumatic and nontraumatic aseptic necrosis. (Modified from Phemister,[100a] with permission.)

When there is *segmental* collapse of the cancellous bone, it occurs at a distance from the articular cartilage, and a crescent sign does not usually appear. Instead, a linear zone of decreased density develops, clearly separated from the subchondral cortex (Fig. 7-13A). It has the histological features of fibrocartilaginous fracture repair (Fig. 7-13B).

The surgeon who has treated the original fracture usually is the first to be consulted by a patient when symptoms appear that have been caused by one of these structural alterations. Thus what clinically is considered an "early" manifestation of aseptic necrosis really is *late*, relative to the time of the fracture and the probable onset of the ischemia.

The preceding part of this chapter, devoted as it is mostly to aseptic necrosis of the femoral head, is largely based on a logical assumption, i.e., that at some moment the ischemia to a large segment of bone becomes "irreversible." When aseptic necrosis follows a fracture, that assumption does not invite reasonable challenge. In nontraumatic cases the absence of good evidence of the time of the "crime" has led to much speculation on that aspect of the process. One theory has it that there are repeated episodes of ischemia that progressively allow the larger volume of bone to become necrotic. That and other theories as they apply to nontraumatic situations are discussed below, but here one problem, raised by the traumatic cases, has to be discussed.

If there is a moment when the ischemia becomes irreversible, what is the evidence of the circumstances leading to the irreversibility? The importance of how one answers this question is that it strongly affects pathophysiological interpretation of what constitutes ideal treatment of the acute fracture. Given the vulnerability of the small arteries and veins that nourish the femoral head and the structure of the periosteum on the femoral neck, any displacement of fragments, particularly in subcapital cases, would be expected to tear every vessel. There is good experimental evidence that osteocytes cannot survive ischemia of 12 hours. One therefore would expect that *all* subcapital fractures, regardless of whether they have been reduced, and if reduced, regardless of whether the reduction was perfect, would undergo necrosis of part or all of the proximal fragment. It would be highly improbable if not impossible for

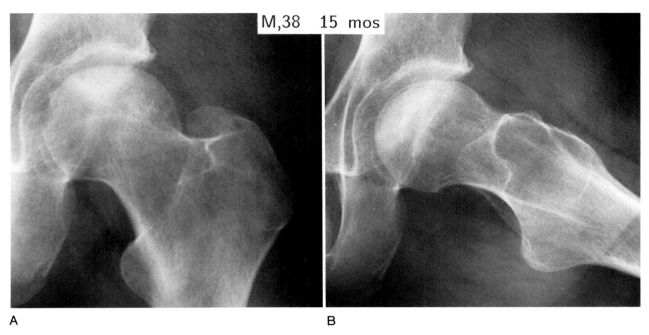

M,38 15 mos

A   B

Fig. 7-11. AP **(A)** and lateral **(B)** radiographs of a 38-year-old man who had had symptoms in the right hip for 15 months. A cresent sign is visible in the lateral view. **(C)** Photomicrograph of the core biopsy shows the fracture between the subchondral cortex and the necrotic bone of the head of the femur. The marrow spaces show amorphous calcification. *(Figure continues.)*

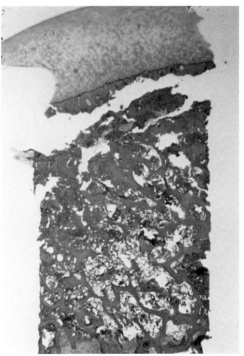

C

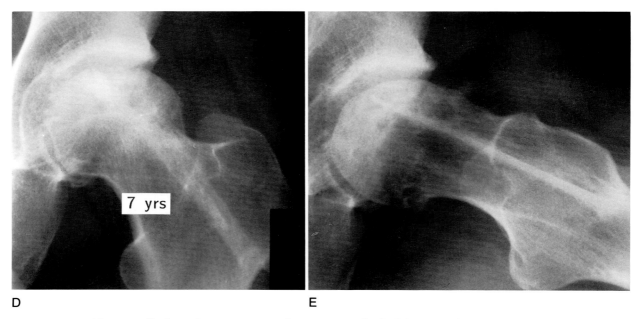

D   E

Fig. 7-11 *(Continued).* **(D&E)** Seven years after coring and tibial bone grafting the necrotic bone has repaired and the crescent sign is absent.

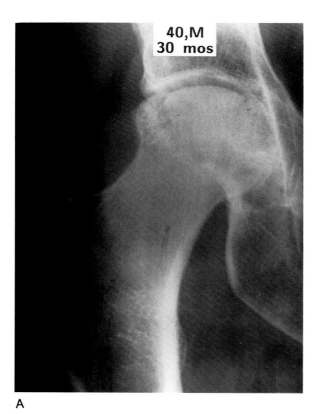

A

Fig. 7-12. **(A)** AP radiograph of the right hip of a 40-year-old male alcoholic shows a large segmental collapse of the right femoral head. A prosthetic replacement procedure was performed. *(Figure continues.)*

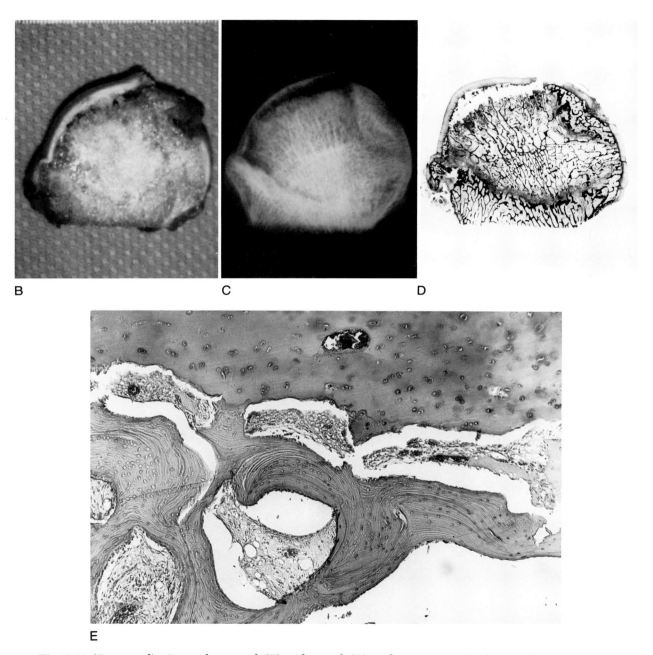

B   C   D

E

Fig. 7-12 *(Continued)*. Gross photograph (**B**), radiograph (**C**), and microscopic (×1) coronal section (**D**) of the specimen. Note the separation of the cartilage and subchondral cortex from the infarct and the zone of reaction bone at the periphery distally. (**E**) Photomicrograph of the cartilage and subchondral cortex shows vascular invasion and resorption of dead bone at the site where the "crescent sign" develops (×63). New bone has been deposited on the underlying trabeculae, a sign of repair.

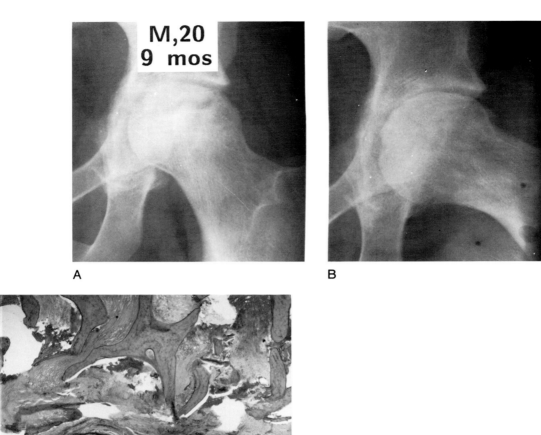

A

B

C

Fig. 7-13. AP (**A**) and lateral (**B**) radiographs of a 20-year-old man 9 months after reduction of a dislocation of the left hip shows segmental collapse of the femoral head. The joint space is narrow centrally. (**C**) Photomicrograph of the junction between a fragment of necrotic bone above and living bone below shows fibrocartilage of fracture repair (×100).

vessels of microscopic size that have been torn to have their ends so positioned as to allow them to establish an anastomosis, given the probability that there would be substantial hemorrhage at the site. Furthermore, if those vessel ends did indeed anastomose over time (perhaps days or weeks) the osteocytes would have died in the interval. A paradox arises that requires some explanation. It stems from the clinical fact that so many of the fractures as described *do not* progress to aseptic necrosis.

Many patients with subcapital femoral fractures that are markedly displaced have a reduction procedure days after the injury and yet exhibit no clinical evidence of aseptic necrosis at subsequent follow-up. Naturally, therefore, many surgeons may be curious as to how those lucky patients could be identified and distinguished from the others. There are a few studies already alluded to concerning that question (e.g., isotopic injections,[5,21,54,79,107,116] intramedullary pressure methods,[63,92] extended bleeding from the femoral head at operation).[34] The failure of all these tests to yield reliable results suggests that the wrong question is being asked. If, as we suggested above, *all* the femoral heads in question are ischemic after the injury, the question to be asked should be the following: Why do certain femoral heads, in fact most, recover from the ischemia without loss of structural integrity, and what is it that makes the others unlucky? Asking the question in that way focuses attention away from the immediate vascular status and more on the repair sequences.

The available data to help answer the question are largely statistical, as follows. There are identifiable populations at special risk for aseptic necrosis, as has been mentioned, e.g., elderly subjects, patients who are markedly inactive due to systemic conditions, and patients with osteoporosis or neurological diseases such as parkinsonism. There may also be local factors, also previously mentioned, that impose special risk, i.e., marked displacement or communition of the fracture fragments, insecure fixation after reduction of the fracture, inadequate reduction, and a traumatic reduction. These systemic and local factors are not capable of definition or quantitation. Nevertheless, they invite the speculative concept that during the repair sequences, i.e., resorption of ischemic bone and creeping substitution, the local pattern of trabeculae presents a

lesser margin of safety for load-bearing than is present in the lucky patients.

However speculative our argument is, the pathophysiological implications are important. The first is that so far as prevention of aseptic necrosis is concerned (unless the fracture can be reduced and pinned within 12 hours), there need be no great rush to reduce the fracture. Because the femoral head is ischemic anyway and the process of restoration of circulation will take many days or weeks, the emphasis on treatment of the fracture, if the femoral head is to be retained, is to immobilize the fracture fragments somewhat to limit the hemorrhage and prevent further damage to the local vessels. Because every patient with a subcapital femoral fracture is at risk for aseptic necrosis, those known statistically to be at special risk should be considered for prosthetic replacement. For the others, when definitive treatment is administered, the local factors predisposing to aseptic necrosis must be addressed: atraumatic and accurate reduction of fracture fragments, firm fixation, prolonged protection from excessive loading, and so on. From the investigative point of view, the above pathogenetic view of aseptic necrosis in fracture patients invites one to explore new avenues of research focused on the period of repair shortly after treatment of the acute fracture.

The course of the aseptic necrosis after fracture (or other trauma) has now been described clinically, radiologically, and histologically up to the stage where the compression fractures become the most important feature that governs the clinical course of the patient. For the purpose of description, the early stage of the aseptic necrosis may be viewed as the interval between injury and occurrence of the compression fracture(s); and in that regard, the early stage usually encompasses an interval of a few months. We define the intermediate stage chronologically as the months (up to a year or two) between the occurrence of those fractures and the onset of degenerative changes in the adjacent joint, the latter changes constituting the "late phase." The degenerative changes may not proceed rapidly if there are only minor distortions of the articular surface or if the loads on and activity of the joint are limited. Inasmuch as the late stage of the condition is considered identical for the two etiological categories of aseptic necrosis, the traumatic and the nontraumatic, that stage is described later.

The time it takes to repair the necrotic cancellous bone when it is not attributable to major trauma can only be estimated — not only because of the indeterminacy of the starting point but also because it varies depending on the volume of the dead bone. That may range from microscopic to several cubic centimeters. Intervals on the order of weeks, at a minimum, are needed for repair to occur that is visible microscopically. Even longer intervals are needed for it to be visible by radiological methods, and still longer times are required for the structural reconstruction to be mechanically functional.

It should be emphasized that there are only a few documented instances of long-term histological observations from specimens in adults who had segmental areas of necrosis of the femoral head after union of a femoral neck fracture as described in the three case histories above. In some of those patients it took 4 to 7 years to repair the necrotic lesion (Fig. 7-14). In the case in Figure 7-14 it measured 2.5×3.5 cm in cross section (depth not known), and in that case the hip was protected for years by the use of crutches. The calculated rate of creeping substitution was estimated at 0.5 cu mm/ month.

Several authors have devised elaborate gradations of the extent of structural alteration in the femoral head in order to formulate an algorithm for appropriate treatment and to predict the outcome, but we prefer four simple terms for those gradations: no collapse, minimal collapse (<2 mm), moderate collapse (2 to 3 mm) or severe collapse (4+ mm)[8,14,15]. Stages of the process, i.e., sequences have been delineated, i.e., 0 to 6 as described by Marcus et al.[85] and its modification[118a] and Ficat and Arlet,[47a,b] but these stages seem contrived and may constitute an impediment rather than an aid to understanding the situation. In general, the greater the degree of structural alteration or secondary degenerative arthritis, the more difficult and hazardous are attempts to preserve the femoral head with any method of treatment. In a young person or a vigorous adult, one may nevertheless attain unexpectedly good results with a treatment that includes retention of the femoral head compared to the expected outcome in older

individuals with lesions of roughly equal severity. In young patients, every effort should be made to avoid salvage procedures, such as total hip arthroplasty.

Major emphasis has been placed above on the femoral head, primarily because specimens of that area are readily available from patients who have had fractures of the femoral neck and who, after a variable period, have had a total hip replacement. However, the identical pathophysiological process occurs at other anatomical sites of predilection for traumatic necrosis or vascular insult. They are now considered briefly. Such sites are the carpal scaphoid, the lunate, the head of the humerus, and the talus. The chronology may differ for each because of anatomical differences.

The lunate is a particularly interesting example because of its multiple surfaces of articular cartilage and the complex forces acting on them.[6,7,41,73,82,108] The fragmentation of the bone during repair of the necrosis is attributable to those forces, and the radiograph presents a striking example of structural alterations of the trabecular pattern of bone after a considerable fraction of its volume has undergone necrosis. The resulting secondary degenerative arthritis may be severe, even though there may not be a severe alteration in the bone's topography.

Circulation to the lunate enters at the dorsal and volar aspects of the bone in most specimens, but the blood supply entering the volar aspect is the major source.[42,69] The proximal dorsal pole of the lunate based on intraosseous anastomoses seems most precarious so far as blood supply is concerned. In contrast to traumatic aseptic necrosis as it affects the femoral head, that in the lunate is not always (even rarely) associated with a single traumatic event, and it often is associated with a series of traumatic episodes. It may be truly idiopathic if minor trauma is discounted. If trauma is indeed implicated to account for the pathological radiographic changes, the most logical sequence of events would be a series of interruptions of the blood supply to the bone. There would be stretching or tearing of the precarious volar vessels, which are at risk when extreme dorsiflexion occurs or when there is compression, as in patients with cerebral palsy with severe spasticity during flexion.

The blood supply to the lunate therefore differs

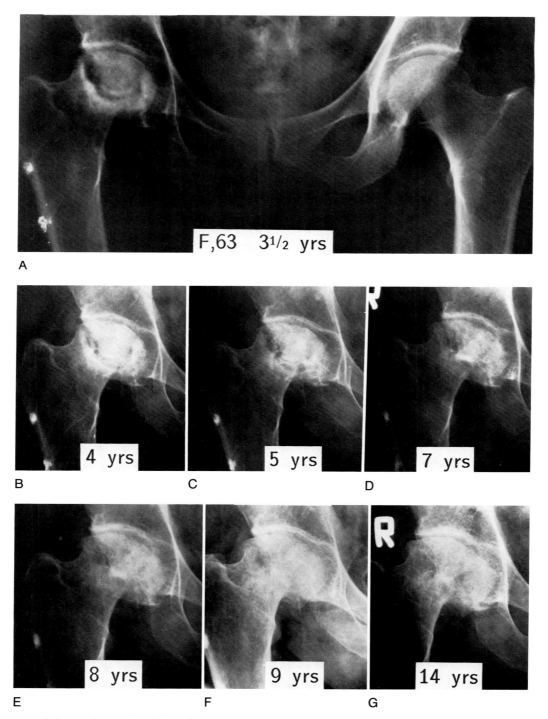

Fig. 7-14. (A) AP radiograph of the pelvis shows segmental collapse of the right femoral head 3.5 years after a 63-year-old woman sustained a fracture of the femoral neck. Threaded pins used initially to fix the fracture had been removed 3 weeks before these films were made. The patient refused further surgery. She was treated by walking with crutches, touch-weight-bearing for 2 years, and then walking with a cane. **(B–D)** AP radiographs show the gradual healing of the segmental collapse fracture gap by 7 years. **(E–G)** Radiographs show repair of the necrotic bone over the period of follow-up to 14 years. A moderate degree of minimally symptomatic degenerative arthritis developed.

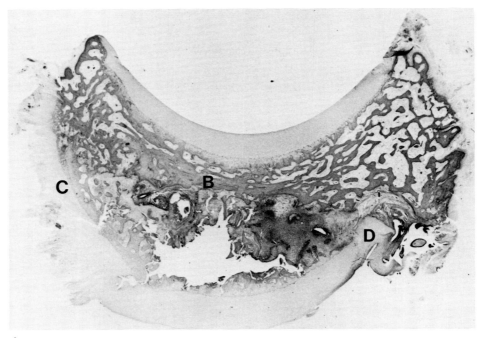

A

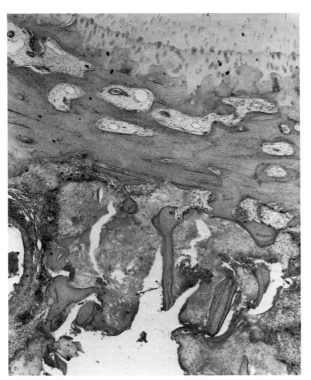

B

Fig. 7-15. A 24-year-old man with pain in his wrist for 22 months underwent excision of the lunate. (A) Photomicrograph of the whole specimen showed central collapse of the body at a fracture of the subchondral cortex and body (×5). (B, C, D refer to areas shown in **B, C, D**.) (B) Necrotic trabeculae and marrow at the site of fragmentation. The subchondral cortex is undergoing replacement by new bone, and the cartilage is viable (×90). *(Figure continues.)*

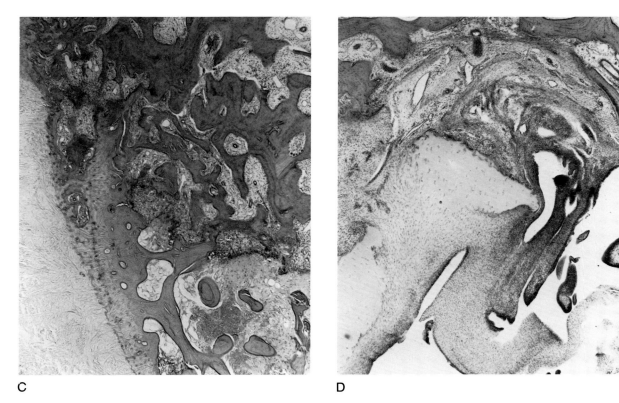

C   D

Fig. 7-15 *(Continued).* **(C)** Repair at the edge of necrotic bone osteophyte (×100). **(D)** Pseudarthrosis at the edge of the subchondral cortex fracture (×100).

considerably from the patterns of vessels to the femoral head, humeral head, and body of the talus. Those patterns have in common one feature, i.e., that a good portion of the circulation courses in relation to the visceral capsule and synovial membrane along the neck of the bone.

Once the lunate is rendered ischemic either partially or completely, as with lunate or perilunate dislocations, the following sequence would be compatible with aseptic necrosis of other sites at risk (e.g., head of femur, body of talus): (1) repair of the lunate without collapse or (2) repair with structural alteration by stress fractures such as subchondral cortex stress fractures or collapse and fragmentation. This fragmentation is known as Kienbock's disease.[6,42,73,108]

The histological features of aseptic necrosis of the carpal lunate are similar to those described above for the head of the femur, and they involve

the analogous structural collapse of the repairing bone (see Figs. 7-39 and 10-4). They are well represented in a specimen removed from a 24-year-old patient with Kienbock's disease (Fig. 7-15). That condition is generally attributed to repetitive fractures, but rarely, if ever, is there a good history of documented acute fracture. In our view, the repetitive fractures occur long after the early repetitive injuries to the soft tissues that cause thrombosis of the vessels. The thrombosis is followed by ischemia, which leads to necrosis of the bone; in the case in Figure 7-15 the entire bone is involved. Necrotic bone has a tendency to fracture, as has been mentioned. Sometimes a patient with necrosis of the carpal lunate presents long after the supposed ischemic event or events, and there is radiographic evidence of fragmentation of the bone in areas comparable in size to those demonstrated in other sites of fractures at repairing revascularized sites (Fig. 7-15). Fragmentation of bone, part of which is necrotic and the rest composed of viable trabeculae with fibrovascular connective tissue, is noted at the fracture site. It occurs between the living juxtacapite portion of the lunate (which has undergone creeping substitution) and the necrotic subchondral cortex. The bone underneath the cartilage of the radial articular surface also reveals some foci of necrosis, and there is necrosis in the cartilage at that site. This finding raises the question as to the pathway of nutrition of the articular cartilage. Nutrition usually is considered to be via the synovial fluid, but when there is impaired motion of a joint or when the cartilage is fragmented (Fig. 7-15) that pathway may be inadequate. In Figure 7-15 the necrotic bony tissue is undergoing replacement at one margin near the fragmented subchondral cortex (Fig. 7-15C). At the other end of the fracture, the articular cartilage is being replaced by fibrous tissue adjacent to the site of the pseudarthrosis (Fig. 7-15D). The condition now present is secondary degenerative joint disease manifested by the fibrillation of cartilage and the presence of marginal osteophytes (Fig. 7-15A).

SECONDARY DEGENERATIVE JOINT CHANGES: DEGENERATIVE ARTHRITIS AFTER ASEPTIC NECROSIS

Many of the arthritic changes that follow aseptic necrosis resemble those in the later changes in primary degenerative arthritis, but the major differences are in the chronology and tempo.

With primary degenerative arthritis the initial changes occur in the cartilage matrix, presumably with secondary loss of synovial fluid nutrition to the cartilage cells. These changes are followed within a matter of a few weeks by degradation of the mucopolysaccharide–chondroitin sulfate and glucosamine complexes. Clumping or aggregation of cartilage cells occurs first followed by disruption of the collagen fibers and fissuring or fibrillation of the cartilage. The cartilage then fragments, and the debris floats off in the joint fluid to become trapped

in synovial folds. Over the next few months or more, the loss of cartilage down to the subchondral cortex is followed by eburnation of one or both of the opposed weight-bearing or load-bearing surfaces. Concomitantly, there is progressive new bone formation in the subchondral cortex of the eburnated surfaces that continues thereafter for many years. This change does not occur in the necrotic areas until replacement has occurred.

Because of the continuing activity, which is reflected in an accumulation of a bone-seeking isotope (technetium or gallium) on bone scan or other isotopic indicators used in bone scans, such areas will always be positive. The inability of those scans to display quantitatively the tempo of bony deposition is responsible for our reluctant conclusion that scans do not provide any information of importance in regard to aseptic necrosis in its intermediate or late stage. Any volume of residual necrotic bone, expected to show up as a cold spot, nearly always is concealed by activity in the adjacent area.

The other changes of degenerative arthritis, such as marginal or plaque osteophytes and degenerative cysts, are late manifestations. Most of the articular cartilage over necrotic bone that has not been distorted by fracture usually is well preserved because its normal nourishment by synovial fluid has not been compromised (Figs. 7-11C and 7-12). Loss of chondrocytes may be evident, nevertheless, in the deeper layers next to the necrotic subchondral bone, especially where there has been buckling or fracture of cartilage (Fig. 7-15D). Its physiological nutrition by synovial fluid apparently is dependent on appositional pressures, the movement by articulating congruent surfaces, and perhaps maintenance of the normal composition of synovial fluid (i.e., free of exudate). The cartilage matrix retains its normal thickness and contour until the necrotic layer of subchondral cortex and margins of the joint are invaded by vascular buds. Then there is replacement of the cartilage, first by fibrous tissue, then by fibrocartilage, and finally by bone, as in primary degenerative arthritis. This replacement is first seen at the margins of an area of segmental collapse where the cartilage structure is disrupted, buckled, or fractured. The vascular invasion and replacement by fibrous tissue, fibrocartilage, and bone are initiated in close proximity to the cartilaginous lesion (Fig. 7-15A; see also Figs.

5-1G&H). The changes seen microscopically are the same as those described in Chapter 8 regarding osteoarthritis. The cartilage fragments, fissures, and fibrillates, and it is eroded until all cartilage is gone and the end-stage of eburnated bone is reached. The additional major difference between this osteoarthritis, which in essence is traumatic whether the aseptic necrosis is engendered by an acute fracture or by another process, and primary or senile osteoarthritis is the geographical distribution of the cartilaginous lesions. However, the marginal osteophytes that develop soon after subchondral cortex fracture are identical radiologically and histologically in the two conditions. With primary osteoarthritis, the peripheral areas of the articular cartilage suffer the most, whereas with this variety the area that has lost its infrastructure is the one most affected.

The synovitis that develops secondary to necrosis is nonspecific and cannot be distinguished from that which can arise from direct trauma to the joint membrane or to infection with organisms of low virulence. There is synovial proliferation and infiltrates of lymphocytes and the other cells of chronic inflammation, particularly in perivascular foci. Pannus formation is not an important component of the process (Fig. 7-15D).

NONTRAUMATIC (IDIOPATHIC) ASEPTIC NECROSIS

Certain diseases are prone to the complication of aseptic necrosis, i.e., the nontraumatic cases.[8,11,22,23,32,39,40,43,56,67,68,72,76,78,98,101,115] There are several known conditions that are associated, more or less frequently, with aseptic necrosis (e.g., decompression disease,[44-47,54,57,74,87,88] steroid therapy,[1,39,40,129] sickle cell disease[33], and it is paradoxical that their pathophysiology is so diverse and their pathological changes regarding aseptic necrosis are so similar.[64] Nevertheless, each particular disease entity does have an influence on the selection of appropriate treatment for the aseptic necrosis. The strongest influence on that treatment is the exact anatomical vascular pattern of each bone at risk and the extent to which it is involved.

In all cases of nontraumatic aseptic necrosis one or more of the following three mechanisms has been invoked as a pathogenetic mechanism: embolization, obstruction (from without), and coagulation (i.e., obstruction from within).

The exact way the bone lesions develop during decompression sickness in caisson workers or divers is somewhat uncertain. The lesions are usually bilateral; they involve cancellous bone; and they are generally multifocal, although they may be so widespread their foci seem confluent. Radiologically similar lesions, usually diagnosed bone infarcts, develop in patients with severe arteriosclerosis, and it has been suggested that the three etiological mechanisms (coagulation, extrinsic obstruction, and embolization) affect the vessels at risk. The three mechanisms are so intimately interconnected that it may be impossible to decide which occurs as the initial lesion.

With decompression sickness (caisson disease) only one of the three above mechanisms—embolization caused by bubbles of nitrogen gas—is usually considered the direct cause of the necrosis. In patients undergoing decompression too rapidly, gases bubble out of solution in the blood (and in all other fluid-rich tissues as well), and that is thought to be the basis for the circulatory obstructions, which then are responsible for the bone lesions. Sinusoids in the fatty marrow of cancellous bone are especially at risk for the following reason. In a study of rats undergoing decompression, Philp et al.[102] observed intravascular platelet adhesion and aggregation. It occurred on a layer of denatured plasma protein, consisting probably of fibrinogen and adherent plasma lipids that coated the gas bubbles. The affected bubbles presented a surface for adhesion of leukocytes and red blood cells. Those aggregated cells represented microthrombi, which possibly became emboli. The observation also offered an explanation for the postdecompression thrombocytopenia observed in experimental animals and man. Similar transient episodes of thrombocytopenia have been observed in alcoholics during bouts of alcohol ingestion.[8] A few days after the thrombocytopenia there is a rebound thrombocytosis. Therefore one may postulate a particular susceptibility of the vascular tree in the bony sites of predilection for lesions of aseptic necrosis in caisson disease. Some significance must attach to the fact that most of the viscera escape embolization, and the difference between the pattern of circulation in bone vis-à-vis viscera may be the crucial factor. The susceptibility of bone is explained by the presence of many thin-walled vessels with diameters much larger than those of capillaries. In conjunction with many fat cells, they constitute soft structures surrounded in a sponge-like architecture of rigid trabeculae of bone. Any swelling of the contents of the small, rigid chambers, the unique cancellous structure of the bone ordinarily affected, can inhibit or stem entirely the flow of blood in the chamber. The culprit may be a gas bubble, a collection of exuded fluid, or a coagulum in a sinusoid. The coagulum, when resolving, swells by imbibing fluid. A combination of these features is not found in other locations in the body. Except for the rigid microchambers, the features mentioned also are found in the brain, and it is of interest that the clinical feature of caisson disease, other than the bone lesions, that causes most permanent impairment is lesions of the brain.

Caisson disease is of clinical importance with regard to the lesions of aseptic necrosis primarily when those lesions are adjacent to major joints. This statement is true despite the fact that many more lesions are present in medullary locations that are not juxta-articular — the lower end of the femur, for instance. It is also noteworthy that those lesions are rarely symptomatic. It does not mean that they are unimportant because one peculiar phenomenon concerning those lesions is the increased association of a specific kind of malignancy (malignant fibrous histiocytoma) with such foci. There is no obvious explanation for this association, as aseptic necrosis from other causes is not associated with malignant tumors of any kind.

Fat Embolism

A number of investigators have postulated that fat embolism is a possible mechanism by which necrosis of bone is produced; especially in patients who have no obvious underlying disease process.[71,72,98] This concept has been disputed by Hartman,[58] who postulated that, from the sizes of the lesions commonly observed, occlusion of a vessel by a fat globule, cell, or group of cells would have to take place at a site more proximal in the circulation than in the sinusoids. He based his view on a study of 31 patients with various conditions unrelated to aseptic necrosis who underwent lymphangiography that involved injecting a poppy seed oil preparation into the lymphatics of the extremities. In those patients, the fat embolization, inherent in the injections, did not cause aseptic necrosis of any bone. There are no known reports of bone necrosis following the posttraumatic fat embolism syndrome (now termed the respiratory distress syndrome); and despite the high incidence of fat macroglobulinemia, according to Tedeschi and co-workers,[121] in a wide variety of clinical situations it never leads to aseptic necrosis.

Nevertheless, fat embolism cannot be entirely dismissed from our consideration of the relation between aseptic necrosis and associated diseases because it is the mechanism most commonly invoked as the pathophysiological pathway for development of that complication in patients who are receiving steroid medications. Aseptic necrosis of bone is generally seen in about 10 percent of those patients, especially patients with renal transplants or who have received steroid therapy over long periods and usually in high dosage. This situation illustrates, as does caisson disease, the difficulty of implicating any one factor in the development of aseptic necrosis. In patients receiving steroid medication, the pathophysiological proposal must first explain why fat emboli develop in some cases (but not all). The usual explanations involve fatty change in the liver, a rise in serum lipids, deposits of lipids in the walls of vessels, or all of these factors.

Mention has been made of a study of steroid-treated patients in whom aseptic necrosis involved one hip.[109] The contralateral hip, which was normal (asymptomatic, no radiographic changes) was subjected to a core biopsy that revealed, in most cases, hemorrhage in the marrow; most of those hips subsequently developed aseptic necrosis, whereas those without hemorrhage did not. The conclusion was that perhaps the initial event responsible for the aseptic necrosis, in the affected cases at least, was hemorrhage. Whether this conclusion can be applied to all cases of aseptic necrosis of the hip, traumatic as well as nontraumatic and in the nontraumatic cases in which no steroids are involved, is debatable. Two facts argue against it: One is that evidence of old and substantial hemorrhage in nearly all resected specimens is not found in any important percentage of cases. The second is that the evidence presented is that of fresh rather than old hemorrhage, and therefore the evidence becomes less compelling.

Obviously, a feature of the systemic disease of patients for which they were receiving protracted steroid therapy may be a risk factor for aseptic necrosis in that the osseous metabolism or vascular dynamics may be deranged (as in collagen disease and renal disease). Hematological abnormalities may be predilections not only for hemorrhage, as mentioned, but also for thrombosis.

The hematological and hepatic abnormalities in question bear a close resemblance to some abnormalities that occur in chronic alcoholics, in whom aseptic necrosis of the femoral head is not uncommonly encountered. In addition, steroids are known to induce a hypercoagulable state with demonstrable sludging of the cells of the blood and embolization of those cell aggregates. This phenomenon leads directly to the third postulated mechanism of aseptic necrosis, intravascular clotting. It should be mentioned that the osteoporosis due to steroids may also predispose the femoral head to trabecular fractures and an increase in the area of necrosis.

Abnormalities of Coagulation

Based on a study of 50 patients with nontraumatic necrosis of the femoral head, Boettcher et al.[8,56] postulated that a constellation of events alters the coagulation mechanism, resulting in sludging, thrombosis, or hemorrhage in an area that is susceptible because of the peculiarities of its blood supply. Femoral head necrosis is considered, in effect, a skeletal expression of one of a group of systemic diseases, each one of which may have a different disturbance of the coagulation mechanism.

Abnormalities such as high or low platelet counts or other bleeding or clotting defects have been found in a large number of patients who come for medical attention with aseptic necrosis as well as patients with alcoholism, hyperuricemia, gout, or hyperlipidemia. Diseases known to have a predilection for aseptic necrosis often are suspected of having transient abnormalities of bleeding or clotting.

It has been repeatedly demonstrated that with increasing serum concentration of ethyl alcohol there is a tendency for in vivo intravascular agglutination of red blood cells, preceded by sludging and followed by stasis and microhemorrhages. Acute thrombocytopenic purpura has also been described after heavy alcohol ingestion, followed by rebound thrombocytosis upon withdrawal of alcohol. A pronounced decrease in fibrinolytic activity has been described following ingestion of beer. Recall that many of the coagulation factors essential to the chain reaction of ordinary clotting are produced in the liver, and deficiency states of prothrombin or any of the other clotting factors, as well as thrombocytopenia and increased fibrinolytic activity, are seen in patients with the liver disorders that often accompany alcoholism.

Patients with gout are known to have increased platelet adhesiveness, increased platelet turnover, and increased thromboplastin activity. Sodium urate crystals enhance clotting by activation of the Hageman factor, one of the protein components of the coagulation mechanism. In addition to its direct effect, alcohol indirectly affects these mechanisms by decreasing urinary urate excretion, thereby causing secondary hyperuricemia.

With the aseptic necrosis attributable to steroid therapy, one must consider that there may be coagulation abnormalities associated with the underlying disorder requiring the use of steroids. Those disorders are, for example, thrombocytopenia, thrombocytosis, polycythemia, and systemic lupus erythematosus. All of these conditions have been associated with aseptic necrosis even in those patients who have not received steroid therapy. Some patients with renal failure on dialysis have had necrosis of the femoral head before they had a renal transplantation and before steroid therapy was started.

Nevertheless it must be admitted that there is a sizable group of patients who, after a meticulous and thorough investigation, must be diagnosed as having truly idiopathic aseptic necrosis. A few of them will have had steroid therapy but in such small doses over so short a period of time that one is loath to invoke an association between the therapy and the bony lesion. Moreover, in some cases the patients unquestionably do not have any of the conditions mentioned that are known to be associated with aseptic necrosis.

Although most authors consider that a distur-bance of the peripheral blood supply to a site may be responsible for necrosis in nontraumatic cases, it is worth mentioning that one rarely sees local thrombosed vessels in histological specimens of aseptic necrosis from nontraumatic cases. Studies

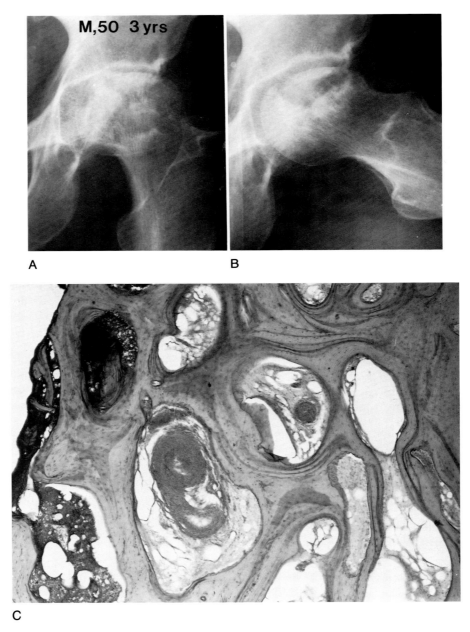

Fig. 7-16. **(A&B)** Radiographs show aseptic necrosis with segmental collapse of the left femoral head in a 50-year-old male alcoholic 3 years after onset (supportive). **(C)** Photomicrograph of a core section shows thrombosed vessels in the necrotic marrow (×100). **(From Bonfiglio,**[11] **with permission.)**

of the ligamentum teres by Chandler[32] and Catto[30] in such cases have revealed some obliterated vessels, however, and incidental observations of thrombosed vessels, particularly arterioles, have been noted in core biopsies of two patients with femoral head necrosis. One of these cases is illustrated in Figure 7-16.

ASEPTIC NECROSIS BY ANATOMICAL SITE

Some of the manifestations resulting from the lesion and the repair process at each of the various sites of predilection of aseptic necrosis are now discussed. The emphasis is on those factors that are involved in the clinical assessment and treatment of specific lesions. The blood supply at each site, the influence of the cause (trauma or disease) of the ischemia, the stage of the lesion, the age of the patient, and his or her level of activity may influence treatment.

Femoral Head

Much of what has already been stated in this chapter relates to aseptic necrosis of the femoral head. Clinically, when symptoms appear in the nontraumatic as well as the traumatic cases, the patient complains of pain while walking. The onset of pain either is sudden with gradual worsening or occurs intermittently, becoming constant over a period of weeks. Continued physical activity causes a synovitis to become evident with effusion into the joint that evokes pain in the groin or buttock, or is referred to the knee. Physical findings include a decrease in the range of motion of the hip, particularly during internal rotation or extension.

The blood supply to the femoral head has been extensively studied,[18,37,38,61,111,125-127] particularly as it relates to aseptic necrosis. The most pertinent studies are those of Tucker, Howe et al.,[61] Trueta and Harrison,[126] Sevitt,[110] Sevitt and Thompson,[111] Brodetti,[18] Crock,[38] and Consentino.[37] The femoral head receives its blood supply in small part from the ligament teres but mostly from a series of small retinacular arteries forming a circular anastomosis at the base of the femoral head (Fig. 7-17). Those retinacular vessels course along the neck from the retinacular attachments of the capsule to the anastomosis, and they are derived principally from the femoral circumflex vessels, primarily the medial vessel.

The retinacular vessels, arteries and veins, are unique in that for several centimeters they course just under the synovial membrane of the hip joint and just external to the thin bony cortex of the femoral neck. They may be squeezed shut by pressure from within the joint, torn by even a slight displacement of fragments if there is a fracture, or obstructed if the joint is held at its limit of internal rotation, at which point the small external rotators are tightly wrapped around the femoral neck. It should be noted that all three of these conditions usually limit, or even prevent, blood flow in all of the retinacular veins and perhaps in the arteries as well. Therefore despite the fact that there is a sizable number of retinacular vessels, their vulnerability is not mitigated by the presence of any important collateral circulation. The few vessels in the ligamentum teres are too small to provide a substantial collateral circulation to the osseous tissue at greatest risk, the subchondral cancellous bone of the femoral head.

The influence of the patient's age on aseptic necrosis as it affects the femoral head merits extensive discussion because important pathophysiological principles are exemplified, principles that also pertain to other destructive lesions in patients in various age groups.

The first group, infants, may be divided into two subgroups. During the first 3 to 6 months of life there is no ossification of the secondary center of ossification of the femoral head. Aseptic necrosis in that age group is usually ascribed to congenital dislocation of the hip,[36,49,66,105,123,124] to its (misguided) treatment, or to other destructive lesions (e.g., septic arthritis) and perhaps some other processes as well (e.g., dysplasia). It affects a tissue that is pure cartilage, and in that regard the concept that aseptic necrosis is a lesion that affects bone is violated. Because no histological studies have been reported on the cartilaginous anlage of the femoral head in such cases of congenital dislocation, the evidence that the process of necrosis has involved the tissue in question must be considered tentative.

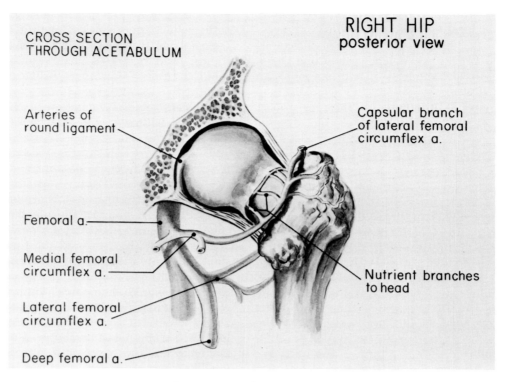

Fig. 7-17. Vascular anatomy of the right hip, posterior view.

That evidence, purely radiological, consists in a determination that in a group of otherwise normal infants, studied retrospectively, there was a selection of those with dislocation of the femoral head. In some of the group the dislocation was reduced, whereas in others the diagnosis was missed and no reduction attempted. In a sizable number in each of these subgroups, the development of the femoral head lagged behind that of the contralateral, normal hip. The center of ossification appeared later and was usually smaller for several years, if not permanently. Often the center of ossification first appeared as a multifocal radiodensity that took months or even years to coalesce. The density of the center frequently was greater than normal, a phenomenon already discussed as an important diagnostic feature of aseptic necrosis in documented cases.

It may be argued that these data, although susceptible to interpretation as aseptic necrosis, may also be interpreted as manifestations of dysplasia. Be that as it may, the defective growth of the femoral head in such cases, whether transient or permanent, fits well with a disturbance of the retinacular vessels, which supply not only the metaphyseal vessels but also the epiphyseal vessels responsible for the nutritive supply to all the proliferating cartilage cells in the femoral head. The inhibition of growth and development in such cases usually is not important with regard to femoral length (approximately 80 percent of which is derived from the lower epiphysis), but considerable distortion of the hemispherical structure of the femoral head may be a sequela. Happily, the recuperative power of the cartilage is usually adequate to the situation, and despite the necrosis (or dysplasia) the end result most often is restitution of the femoral head to normal or near-normal hemisphericity.

This same sequence of events may well follow a septic arthritis of the hip in the same age group (0 to 6 months). However, it may not be the outcome if the development of the acetabular roof has been inhibited either because of a vascular insult or a septic process. That deficiency is not ascribable to aseptic necrosis but, rather, to either the dysplasia or the distorted mechanics that attend a dislocation or a subluxation, or in septic cases to the actual septic destruction of the acetabular cartilage. The pathophysiological influence of the acetabular shape on the developing femoral head may cause the latter to be distorted, i.e., to become ovoid rather than hemispherical. In contrast, the effects described for the femoral head may well be ascribed to ischemia because the retinacular vessels are at risk not only with the hip dislocated (stretched laterally and shortened medially) but also during maneuvers of reduction, and finally when positioning the extremity in a plaster cast after reduction. In fact, the positioning has been shown to be hazardous not only for the hip that was dislocated but also for the contralateral hip. Several reports are available that reveal aseptic necrosis in the previously normal hip when it was immobilized in extreme internal rotation and abduction. That position stretches the capsule of the hip, compressing the retinacular vessels, and it winds the external rotators tightly around those vessels.

With older infants, after the secondary center of ossification has appeared, the sequence of events, once the aseptic necrosis has passed the initial stage of the vascular insult, is as described from the radiological point of view noted above. There is the additional important finding, however, that the ossification center may be distorted (flattened or irregular). This finding is best explained as a consequence of destruction or damage to the growing and multiplying chondrocytes in the articular cartilage. If the process is severe, the femoral head may never recover its potential for growth as a hemispherical articulating half of the hip joint. Instead, it may become irregular, flattened, or shaped like one-half of a football, capable of rotation on only one axis.

A disturbance to the circulation based on the studies of Trueta[125] suggested that interruption of the vessels of the lateral epiphysis by the stretched capsule, with a hip in the position of extreme abduction, and flexion of the hip result in total or partial necrosis of the secondary center of ossification. There are no human pathological specimens to confirm the radiographic features of this ischemia. However, experimental studies in pigs support the clinical observations just described. The incidence of posttreatment necrosis in congenital dislocation of the hip varies widely following closed reduction. In most early reports it is 30 to 40 percent. After there was general modification of treatment regimens so that positions of no more than 90° flexion and no more than 25° abduction were adopted, the incidence fell to about 15 percent.

The complication of necrosis has been reported to occur with greater frequency after open reduction than after closed reduction, presumably because cases requiring open reduction offer major difficulties not often encountered with cases amenable to closed reduction. The deformities of the femoral head and neck, when they occur, always are accompanied by an acetabular deformity, which in turn leads to a high incidence of degenerative joint disease. It is seen mostly in patients who have been followed for a long time[31,66] (see Fig. 7-36F, below),[36] but ordinarily it is not seen until long after adolescence has passed. This complication of congenital dislocation of the hip is rare and deserves mention here only because it can be prevented by paying attention to avoiding compromise of the circulation during treatment.[131]

When there is aseptic necrosis of the femoral head in an infant, the therapy aims at different goals than in an adult and uses different means. Because of the ease with which conservative therapy in young children or infants (recumbency, immobilization) can be carried out for many months, the hazards of continuing distortion of the femoral head by fracture of necrotic bone can be avoided. The likelihood of restitution of the part, because of the high recuperative potential of infants, must be recognized; and the months of conservative therapy necessary for that goal to be reached must not be curtailed. If any surgical procedures have a role to play under these circumstances they must be of proved efficacy and safety, and to date none fits those criteria.

Aseptic necrosis of the femoral head during childhood is a rare phenomenon, but it differs not only from that just described for infants but also from that previously described for adults. It is rare because the conditions (with one exception) that serve as predilections, are uncommon during childhood, those conditions being, fracture of the femoral neck and the various metabolic and hematological diseases already mentioned; the exception is sickle cell anemia. Aseptic necrosis may supervene as a complication when there has been a congenital dislocation of the hip, but the most common associated condition is slipped femoral capital epiphysis, and then primarily when there has been an attempt at manipulative or open reduction (see Fig. 5-17). In that situation and in patients who have the rare subcapital or midcervical fracture, the pathophysiological aspects of diagnosis (especially the lag in manifestations) and the likelihood of loss of structural integrity of the femoral side of the articulation resemble those in the adult. The high potential for repair of the articulation in the infant and young child is not evident after the individual reaches the age of 8 years.

Among the differences between children and adults, aside from the potential in young children to reconstitute the geometry of the hip joint if it has been altered and the absence of that potential, is the markedly reduced predilection of the altered joint to develop disabling degenerative changes. Possibly the potential in young children to reconstitute the joint (a potential that declines rapidly after age 2) is an expression of normal remodeling sequences of bones in the young, and that process may also explain the fact that even severely affected hips in children, and to a lesser degree in young adolescents, rarely manifest a disabling osteoarthritis. Not only do the alterations in tissues (osteophytes, loss of cartilage, eburnation) develop much more slowly than do those in adults but the symptoms and signs do as well. The child or adolescent gets along surprisingly well even with a major involvement of the hip. These empirical facts — empirical because so little is understood concerning the pathophysiology of remodeling — have obvious implications with regard to surgical therapy. Surgery is to be considered primarily when the likelihood that nonsurgical therapy probably will not yield adequate improvement and when the risk – benefit ratio of surgery is not high. The surgical rationale nearly always is one that (for the hip) aims at maximizing mechanical influences that affect remodeling, i.e., varus osteotomy of the femoral neck or Chiari or other osteotomy of the ilium. The notorious lack of success of prosthetic replacement, arthroplasty, in the young (up to the age of 25 at least) is not well understood, so that in the young adult (and possibly in adolescents and older children) arthrodesis for a badly damaged hip may well be the best procedure.

Treatment

The pathophysiological approach to treatment of the lesion in the femoral head in adults has as its goal replacement, if possible, of the necrotic tissue by structurally competent live bone. Because the volume to be replaced is relatively large, it takes a long time for complete creeping substitution, if indeed it is ever complete. Certainly several months are needed, at a minimum, but one cannot be sure that complete substitution can be achieved even if years elapse and conditions are ideal (absence of excessive stress). The maximal stimuli for repair occur during the first weeks after the necrosis has begun, as already described for the repair of fractures. The removal of necrotic tissue does not constitute removal of an impediment to that repair. The necrotic bone may persist without being a stimulus for inflammation, and absorption of the necrotic bone while the living bone is being deposited occurs routinely; there is little evidence pro or con that it affects the rate of the creeping substitution. Certainly the idea that deposition of new bone might be accelerated is attractive if resorption is considered to be a slow process; but in the absence of such evidence, the surgical trauma and the certainty that during surgical removal of the dead bone some live bone is also removed and vessels thrombosed leads us to conclude that the disadvantages of removing the dead bone outweigh the theoretical advantage. If done purely for the purpose mentioned, replacing the necrotic bone either with a clot after coring[31,63] or a bone graft[8,9,12,14,15,18] (which except for its surface cells also is necrotic) has no justification. However, any operative procedure at the site affords the reparative mechanism a new stimulus, and that factor is desirable. Whether that stimulus can be applied noninvasively, e.g., by application of an electrical current, is now under study. However, the crucial element of treatment is prevention of the mechanical complications that are so apt to occur when the brittle, repairing, necrotic bone fractures and the understructure of the articular cartilage fails. If appropriate prophylactic measures are not undertaken prior to that complication, the involved joint inevitably suffers the accelerated osteoarthritic changes already described.

The prophylactic measure that has proved most effective for aseptic necrosis of the femoral head is insertion of autogenous grafts of cortical bone to support the necrotic segment of cancellous bone and the articular cartilage along the walls of the channels in that segment when its understructure is materially threatened.[8,9,11,12,14,15] The grafts, securely and accurately placed within the segment of the necrotic bone and attached cartilage, are invaded by vascular connective tissue and repair bone from living bone in the head, neck, and trochanteric area and thus unite the necrotic bone to the graft within each channel (see Fig. 5-31). Although graft bone is not living, it helps support the necrotic area and overlying articular cartilage for at least a few weeks or months; and the operation per se is a stimulus to accelerated, uninterrupted creeping substitution of the remaining necrotic bone as well as of the graft. It is crucial to the success of the procedure that it be done before the cartilage has been damaged to a substantial degree. If the crescent sign is detectable, probably the ideal time for prophylaxis has passed.

The surgeon must realize that the possibility of salvage of the articular cartilage is worth pursuing even though the effort may be futile (not necessarily because it was started too late). The volume of necrotic bone may be so large that the added support of the graft may not suffice, and the remaining necrotic bone fractures. Moreover, the conditions that existed prior to the advent of aseptic necrosis, which prompted that complication, are in general incurable; and their persistence constitutes negative influences on healing. In fact, they may be responsible for renewed episodes of aseptic necrosis. It is not known whether in nontraumatic aseptic necrosis the process occurs as a single episode, as a continuum, or as repetitive episodes. As is obvious from the discussion above, the diagnostic methods available are not able to provide any information on that point.

Treatment of the patient with aseptic necrosis of the hip that has progressed to the late stage of os-teoarthritis, or that is well along in that direction, should be treated as if the osteoarthritis were the lesion requiring treatment, the aseptic necrosis being "unimportant." If conservative therapy is indicated because the symptoms and impairment are not severe, that regimen may be continued for as long as the patient wishes; in the older child or the young adult particularly, that course may be advisable, given the unsatisfactory results of total hip arthroplasty and especially resurfacing arthroplasty in those age groups. When surgical therapy is indicated, e.g., total hip arthroplasty or arthrodesis, the regimen is exactly as for the osteoarthritic patient. If sites other than the femoral head are involved with aseptic necrosis, the option of bone grafting to lend support to the articular cartilage rarely is available because at the other sites the articulation tends to have been compromised by the time the patient presents for treatment. When the smaller bones are involved, the option of arthrodesis is often preferable to other surgical procedures, and only rarely is the option of replacement arthroplasty (e.g., for the lunate or scaphoid) more attractive.[41,117]

Once bone necrosis is identified, effective treatment depends on a number of factors, including the cause, associated disease, and systemic conditions affecting the patient, the age of the patient, the location and volume of the necrosis, and the state of repair of the necrosis at the time the patient presents to the physician. To arrive at a decision on what advice to offer the patient, one must consider the natural history based on knowledge of the repair process at each site and what if anything can be done to assist the repair process to achieve a predictable and reasonable end result.

Approaches to treatment fall under two categories: (1) preservation of the involved area by nonsurgical means and (2) reconstructive surgery. Preservation of the affected bone should first be attempted by nonsurgical means, which includes protected weight-bearing pursued over a period of a few months during which time radiological evidence of improvement should be apparent (Fig. 7-14). If this treatment is not adequate, coring and bone grafting is done to permit repair before secondary structural change occurs. Once structural alteration has supervened, the treatment depends

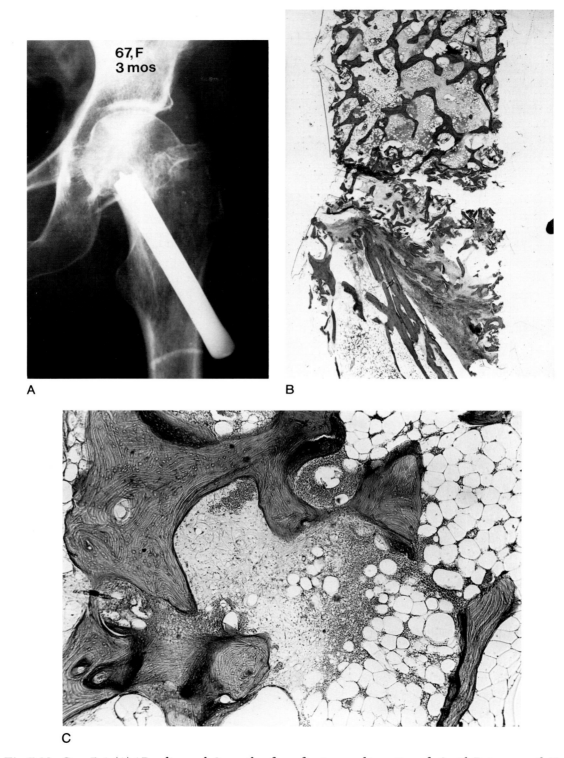

Fig. 7-18. Case 7-4. (**A**) AP radiograph 3 months after a fracture and insertion of a Smith Petersen nail. Note the area of decreased density in the lateral aspect of femoral head and the slight relative increase in density in the area above the nail to the subchondral cortex. The nail has backed out. (**B**) Core of the fracture site and femoral head shows no union of the fracture. The necrotic marrow is now invaded by granulation tissue (×30). (**C**) Photomicrograph of necrotic marrow fat and bone (×100). *(Figure continues.)*

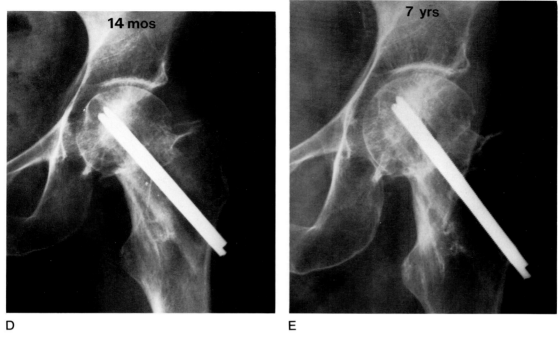

Fig. 7-18 *(Continued).* **(D&E)** AP radiographs of the hip at 14 months and 7 years after insertion of two tibial grafts and three threaded pins show union. (**A–E** from Bonfiglio,[12] with permission.)

on its degree; if there is minimal or moderate collapse, stages 1 to 3, tibial bone grafting, osteotomy, or reconstructive surgery could be considered.

The pathophysiological aspects of treatment can be illustrated by two examples.

Case 7-5 A 67-year-old woman had had a fracture of the femoral neck, and 3 months later an AP radiograph showed an area of diminished density above the fracture line (Fig. 7-18A). The diminished density occurred in the anterolateral area with a border of slightly increased density slightly medial to that because of the presence of new bone on old (Fig. 7-18B). A Smith-Peterson nail, which had been introduced to treat the fracture initially, had backed out. A Phemister procedure was performed (see Fig. 7-23A, below). A core biopsy showed minimal repair of the fracture site (Fig. 7-18B) and necrosis of part of the femoral head with evidence of marrow fibrosis and minimal deposition of new bone on old necrotic trabeculae (Fig. 7-18C). The prospect was satisfactory for union of the fracture and repair of the necrotic area without collapse. The patient used crutches for 9 months

after the procedure. At 14 months union had occurred, and the patient was walking with a cane (Fig. 7-18D). At 7 years the fracture remained united, the hip joint was normal radiologically, and the patient had normal function and used no external support (Fig. 7-18E).

Case 7-6 A 29-year-old carpenter fell 10 feet from a tree and sustained a fracture of the left femoral neck. It was internally fixed with a compression screw and two threaded pins. The patient used crutches for 7 weeks and then was allowed to walk with a cane. The fracture healed within 3 months, and the patient returned to work. Follow-up films at 7 months were read as showing no evidence of aseptic necrosis, but at 15 months (Fig. 7-19A) the films were considered equivocal for aseptic necrosis; yet by the criteria discussed earlier, necrosis was evident. There was disuse atrophy of the acetabular and trochanteric bone as well as increased density of repair, both of which contrasted with the unchanged density of the necrotic femoral head. At that time, no collapse of the necrotic or atrophic bone was evident, and the opportunity to take

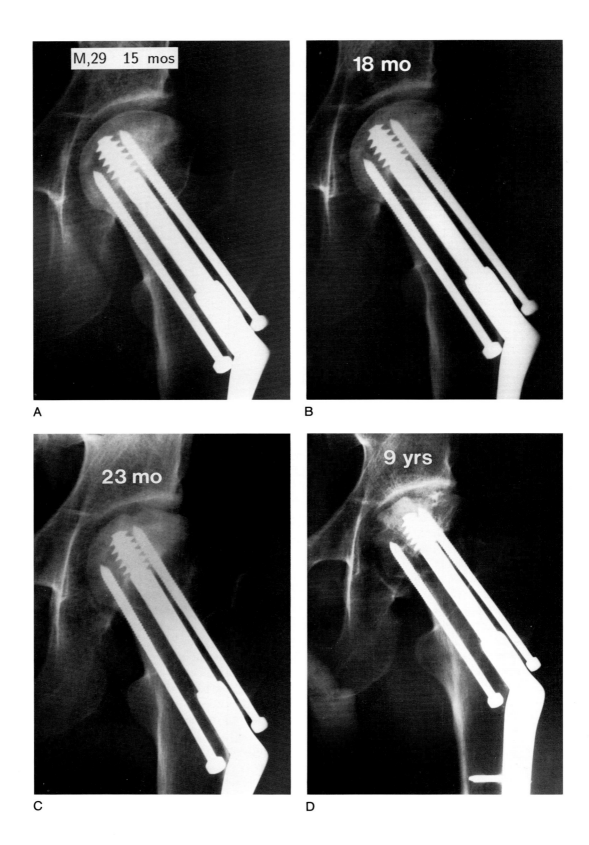

A

B

C

D

measures to prevent it was missed. Subsequent radiographs showed the evolution of the collapse. At 18 months the patient reported no pain, and there were no signs of a complication; but radiographically there now was evidence of a slight depression and resorption of the subchondral cortex at the margin of the necrotic area (Fig. 7-19B). At 23 months there was an evident depression and segmental collapse of the area of aseptic necrosis (Fig. 7-19C). The patient's hip became symptomatic shortly after the 18-month checkup.

The use of a compression fixation device, as in this patient, made the risk of nonunion of the fracture negligable, but it had no effect on the risk for aseptic necrosis; it may even have increased that risk slightly. (Compression of cancellous bone might lead to impaction, i.e., microfractures, and that undoubtedly devitalized additional trabeculae.) Three risk factors were present from the start of treatment and should have been, but were not, appreciated: severe trauma, extensive displacement of the fracture fragments, and the pattern of the fracture (subcapital). These risk factors were potentiated by the fact that recognition of the early stage of necrosis would be obscured radiographically by the large compression screw. Therefore the chance for successful prophylaxis, i.e., deferring weight-bearing on the affected limb for at least 6 months after fracture, was missed because of the surgeon's failure to recognize the risk and his anxiety to return the patient to work. Few alternatives existed for the initial treatment of the fracture in this patient, i.e., reduction of the fracture and internal fixation, even though a multitude of devices are available for the latter purpose. Probably none of them would diminish the risk of aseptic necrosis because, as mentioned, that risk, so far as therapy is concerned, depends primarily on the circumstances that obtain during the *healing,* not the initial postinjury stage. Emphasis therefore should be focused on the prophylactic regimen.

Once the collapse has occurred, the surgeon is faced with the dilemma of treatment. The residual volume of necrotic bone still plays a role, albeit not a principal one, in that regard. The removal of that necrotic bone and of the now incongruent articular surface of the femoral head is part of the hemiarthroplasty or total prosthetic replacement, neither of which were satisfactory choices in a young man, a skilled artisan who may well have to do heavy work, and who incidentally had a heavy build. He therefore had four known risk factors (age, sex, weight, activity) that would predispose a prosthetic replacement to early failure and the need for revision surgery.

It is of interest to point out that in case 7-5, the 67-year-old woman, all of these risk factors were absent so that the indications for prosthetic arthroplasty were good, although those for the more conservative grafting procedure were perhaps more compelling. Previous text has emphasized that once there is collapse of the atrophic or necrotic bone, support of the articular cartilage by a graft of cortical bone is not as successful as when that measure is applied before the collapse. It should be mentioned, however, that as an alternative to arthroplasty the grafting procedure may well succeed. It serves as an alternative that "burns no bridges," particularly if the collapse is not severe. Other options of treatment depend primarily on the surgeon's and patient's goals in regard to the joint, not the aseptic necrosis. Experience with the long-term follow-up of patients who have had a collapse of the femoral head treated by the grafting procedure is limited. The chance of maintaining and restoring the contour of a viable femoral head probably is better than even. The patient of case 7-6, apprised of the certainty that he would develop osteoarthritis in time, chose not to have any operation and after 9 years showed good evidence of repair of the necrotic femoral head (Fig. 7-19D).

The patient spent little time on crutches (7 weeks) and walked with a cane thereafter for a year. During that time he continued to work as a carpenter but modified his activities to accommodate the hip by sitting when possible or avoiding

Fig. 7-19. Case 7-5. (A) Radiograph of the hip 15 months after fracture of the left femoral neck shows increased density of the femoral head relative to the atrophy of disuse in the acetabulum and trochanter. (B) At 18 months there is collapse of the femoral head and resorption of the subchondral cortex at the margin of the necrotic area. (C) Segmental collapse of the area of aseptic necrosis at 23 months. (D) At 9 years repair of the necrotic area is evident. Moderate arthritis is present.

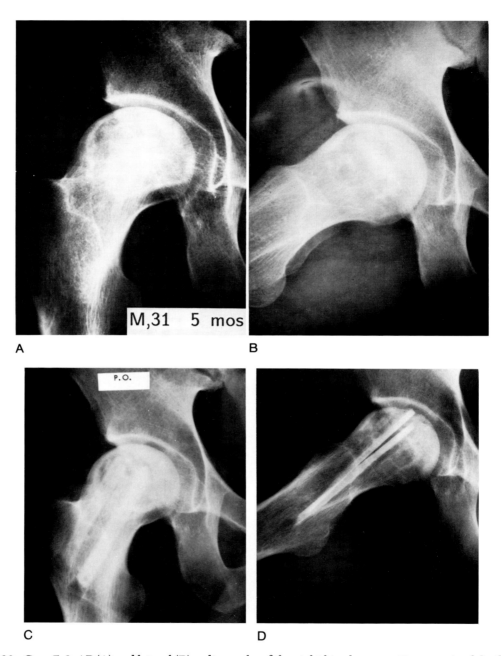

Fig. 7-20. Case 7-6. AP (**A**) and lateral (**B**) radiographs of the right hip show aseptic necrosis of the femoral head with minimal collapse (lateral view) 5 months after onset of pain. (**C&D**) Postoperative radiographs show placement of channels and tibial bone grafts. (**A–D** from Bonfiglio and Voke,[15] with permission.) *(Figure continues.)*

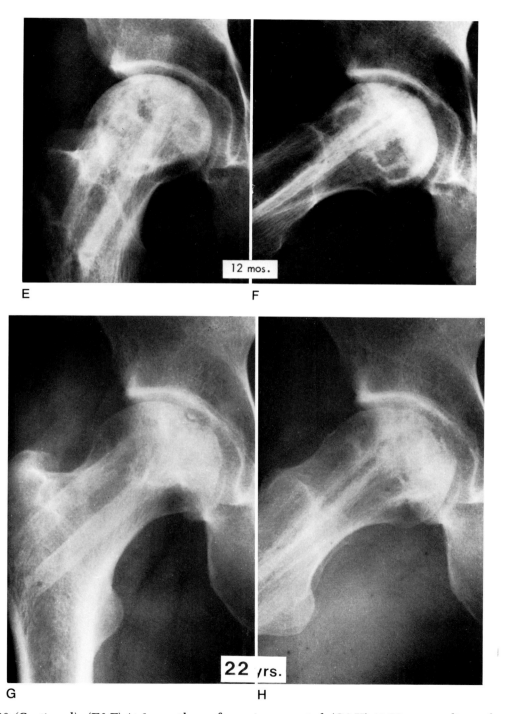

Fig. 7-20 *(Continued).* **(E&F)** At 1 year the grafts are incorporated. **(G&H)** At 22 years radiographs show repair of the necrosis except for a small central fragment at the fovea. The cartilage shadow is normal. *(Figure continues.)*

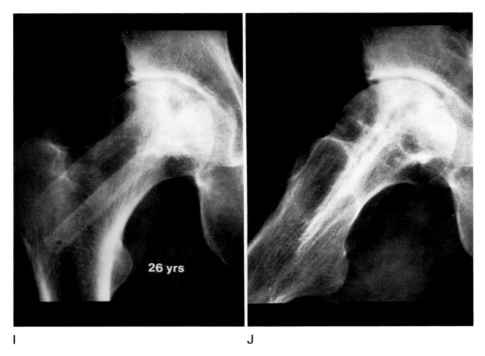

26 yrs

I   J

Fig. 7-20 *(Continued).* **(I&J)** At 26 years the joint cartilage space is narrower. The hip is now symptomatic, and the patient underwent total hip arthroplasty.

lifting for about a year. At 18 months, when his hip began to hurt again, he used crutches for 3 months and then returned to the use of a cane and resumed work. At 9 years he was not protecting his hip; he worked full time as a carpenter and noted pain only with hard work.

This result brings up an alternative to surgical intervention for aseptic necrosis, i.e., the natural history of the process of repair after femoral neck fracture and internal fixation with union commented on earlier (Fig. 7-14).

The range of clinical problems with *nontraumatic* aseptic necrosis and the treatment of each are best illustrated by three examples.

Case 7-7 A 31-year-old man had pancytopenia in the form of a hypersensitivity reaction. He developed right hip pain 13 months after this reaction. This known latent period for nontraumatic aseptic necrosis is of the same temporal order of magnitude as the posttraumatic interval before there is collapse of the femoral head after fracture or dislocation. The necrosis was confirmed histologically and treated by the Phemister method (coring and bone

grafting) (see Fig. 5A&D) about 18 months after the drug hypersensitivity reaction. Pre- and postoperative radiographs (Fig. 7-20) showed that there was typical aseptic necrosis, minimal collapse, and well positioned bone grafts. The bone grafts were incorporated by 12 months postoperatively, without further collapse of the femoral head, during which interval only minimal weight-bearing was permitted (Fig. 7-20E&F). At follow-up 22 years later the contour of the femoral head was spherical, and only minimal degenerative changes were evident (Fig. 7-20G&H). The patient had minimal symptoms and no functional disability. Only minimal degenerative changes were evident on the radiograph. During the next 4 years the symptomatic periods increased in severity, and at 26 years loss of articular cartilage was evident (Fig. 7-20I&J).

Review of a similar case may be helpful in regard to the severity of lesions and their treatment.

Case 7-8 A 45-year-old man with ulcerative colitis was treated with steroids. He developed aseptic necrosis of the left femoral head with collapse (Fig.

7-21A). A total hip replacement arthroplasty was performed with satisfactory results (Fig. 7-21B). By the time involvement of the left hip had become evident, it also was recognized that there was (silent) necrosis on the right side. That condition was monitored closely for 18 months and did not change. Because the operation on the left had proved successful and the condition on the right remained unchanged and placed the patient at risk for collapse, a Phemister procedure was done on the right hip; it too was successful. On follow-up 7 years later the result was excellent (Fig. 7-21C&D).

This case, in which bilateral lesions were recognized at the time of presentation, brings up the question of bilaterality, which rarely pertains to cases of traumatic aseptic necrosis but which all too commonly does pertain to the category of nontraumatic aseptic necrosis. When bilateral involvement of the hip is present, the principles of treatment, illustrated in part in the case just considered, should also include the likelihood of successful results with each treatment method as influenced by the associated disease. When bilaterality is not evident but is known to be a likely event within some months or a few years of the onset of involvement, the treatment of each side is more complicated in terms of whether to intervene surgically, when to do so, and what to do.

Case 7-9 A 28-year-old man had subacute systemic lupus erythematosus of 5 years' duration. He had undergone a long period of treatment with steroids during which time he presented with pain that had been in his right hip for 23 months and that was now in his left hip. The radiographs of the right hip showed minimal collapse and those of the left hip moderate collapse. A Phemister procedure with tibial bone grafts was performed, giving him a comfortable right hip. That situation continued for 5 years until he developed degenerative arthritis, which gradually limited function of that hip. The left hip, untreated because of an inability to protect it with crutches, developed increasing collapse and degenerative arthritis over the 5-year observation period. The patient also developed involvement of the left humeral head with collapse secondary to necrosis during those 5 years. A Neer prosthesis was inserted to replace the left humeral head. Bilateral total hip replacements were then performed.

The patient was relieved of pain in his hips after this surgery, but he had to modify his activity by using a wheelchair between periods of walking with crutches during the postsurgical period. Five years later pain with exercise and walking developed because of loosening of the left hip prosthesis. A left total hip revision was performed a year later. The right hip was not loose radiographically. The pain was less, and he walked without crutches. The patient's lupus erythematosus is now in remission so steroid therapy is no longer required.

This patient clearly highlights the difficulty of treating bilateral necrosis of the femoral heads; his case was further complicated by involvement of the humerus. Under these circumstances few options other than joint replacement therapy could be considered, even though it would be impossible to protect an operated hip because of the involved shoulder.

Because of our special involvement with the development and application of the Phemister procedure, additional discussion of that technique may be appropriate. This procedure has been used by us, in most cases, where involvement of the hip was unilateral. We had poorer results with coring and bone grafting in the few bilateral operations we have done than when treating a unilateral lesion. With bilateral involvement, however, the operations are staged; and the patient uses crutches and a four-point gait postoperatively for long periods. There is less protection of each hip during weight-bearing using that regimen than when crutches and a three-point gait are used (the routine for patients with unilateral disease).

Repair of the femoral head in the patient with bilateral lesions is at substantial risk for two reasons. The first is that the postoperative regimen does not adequately ensure relief of weight-bearing loads and protect the developing repair tissue. The second is that the associated disease process (including metabolic side effects of the treatment) often includes systemic inhibition of repair processes, e.g., the effects of steroids on inflammation.

Only a few patients have had Phemister procedures done bilaterally (Fig. 7-8), and in nearly all those cases either minimal or no collapse had occurred preoperatively. It should be emphasized that, despite the fact that indications for the procedure in those cases were adhered to strictly, the

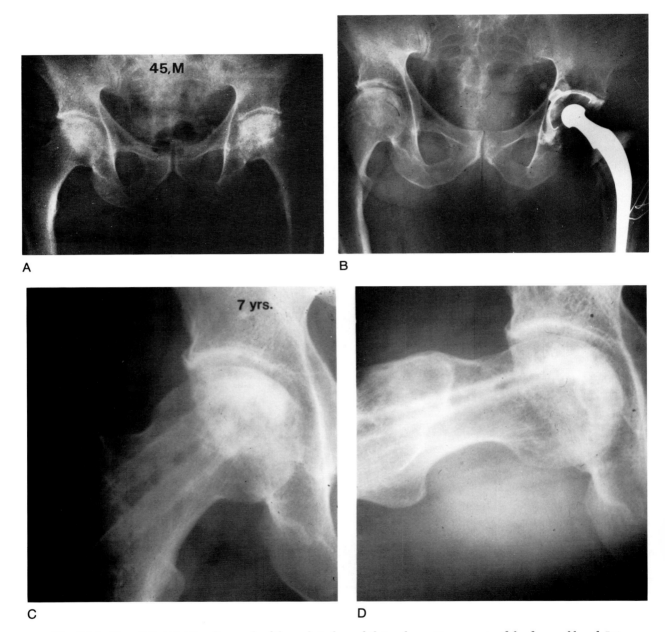

Fig. 7-21. Case 7-7. **(A)** AP radiograph of the pelvis shows bilateral aseptic necrosis of the femoral head. It is "silent" (stage 0,1) on the right, and there is moderate segmental collapse on the left (stage 2). **(B)** AP radiograph of the pelvis showing a "silent" hip on the right and total hip replacement on the left. AP **(C)** and lateral **(D)** radiographs 7 years after the bone grafts.

results were not as successful as in unilateral cases, probably because of the heightened risks just mentioned.

The natural history of repair of aseptic necrosis of the femoral head with some segmental collapse, secondary to a fracture of the neck and the femur, is by creeping substitution regardless of whether a Phemister procedure is done (Fig. 7-14). Further collapse after the procedure occurs infrequently (<8 percent) and usually is of minimal degree (<2 mm). The experience with nontraumatic necrosis without collapse is limited. No instances have been reported of a patient with a crescent sign or a subchondral fracture whose lesions healed spontaneously (i.e., with protected weight-bearing). The results of Phemister procedures in pa-

tients with either unilateral or bilateral segmental collapse have been variable, but there is more than an even chance of their healing without additional collapse. A small area of necrosis has a better potential for repair without surgery (Fig. 7-22) than a larger lesion without collapse. With larger lesions, further collapse occurs in more than one-half of the hips of patients who have not had the Phemister procedure. In one report coring alone did not prevent collapse in 60 percent of the femoral heads in which decompression surgery was performed before collapse of the femoral head.[31]

The alternatives for treatment in patients who have had some collapse include continued protection with crutches, although further collapse should then be anticipated. The use of a total hip

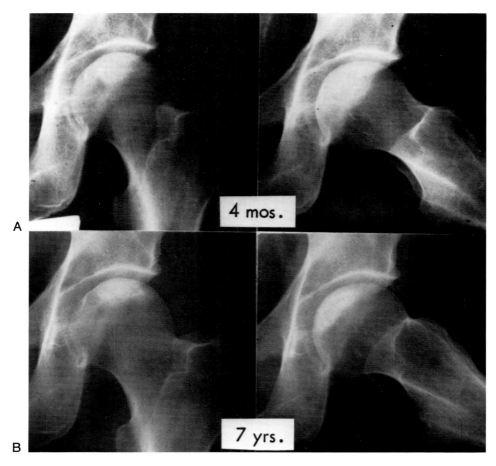

Fig. 7-22. A 45-year-old man with mild pain for 4 months. A central area of aseptic necrosis of the left hip was not treated. At 7 years, however, no collapse has occurred. (From Boettcher et al.,[8] with permission.)

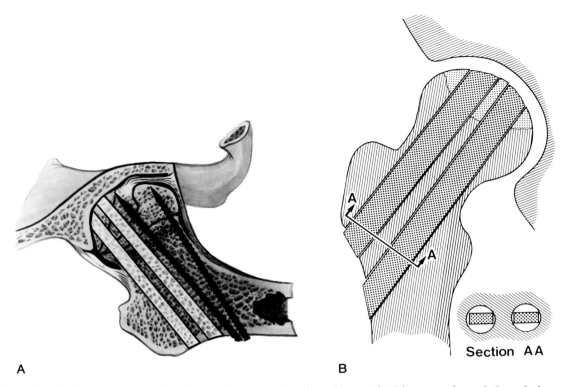

A   B

Fig. 7-23. (A) Sagittal view of the femoral head and neck with two tibial bone grafts and threaded pins (Phemister procedure) for fracture of the neck of the femur with aseptic necrosis of the head of the femur. (B) Sagittal view of the femoral head and neck with two tibial bone grafts inserted into cored channels for aseptic necrosis of the head of the femur. Note channels (grafts) are taped slightly toward each other. (A) Grafts have been trimmed to allow granulation tissue to grow into the cored channels.

arthroplasty or a hemiarthroplasty would probably not have held up for a sufficiently long time before revision would be required. An osteotomy could also be considered, but the experience reported by D'Aubigne et al.[41] was not satisfactory or sufficiently predictable. The long-term results of the Sugioka osteotomy are not yet known. Furthermore, the opportunity for revascularization and repair of the necrotic bone is not increased by an osteotomy.

Whether alternatives to treatment other than total hip replacement arthroplasty or arthrodesis (already mentioned) would be appropriate (e.g., various types of femoral osteotomy) is not discussed here. No accepted pathophysiological prin-

ciples support osteotomy as specifically addressing the aseptic necrosis.

The principles on which the Phemister procedure is based are as follows. (1) Removal of two cores of bone provides two channels through which the vascular granulation tissue can easily traverse the junction between living and dead bone. (2) They offer an increased surface area for revascularization and repair of those junctions by a factor of at least 2 over the area of the preexisting interface between the living and dead bone. That increased area, now in the form of two cylinders, replaces the periphery of the necrosis, i.e., the area of the surface of dead bone (Fig. 7-23A). (3) The rationale for inserting two grafts (tibial or fibular cortex) is that they support and stabilize the subchondral cancellous bone during the process of repair.

Whether that bone is necrotic does not enter into the rationale of inserting grafts. Neither does removal of necrotic bone during the coring process constitute an essential objective, beneficial as it may be. The method has been tested and validated in the experimental animal. Moreover, in a follow-up study of femoral heads from patients who had had successful Phemister procedures and who years later had degenerative joint disease treated by total hip arthroplasty, the above rationale has been shown to pertain.[115]

Talus

Aseptic necrosis of the body of the talus that complicates fractures of the neck of the talus and fracture dislocation depends on the degree of disruption of the blood supply to the talus. Recognition of the presence of aseptic necrosis before collapse occurs is mandatory so that protection by non-weight-bearing can be instituted. The blood supply to the body of the talus is supplied by branches of the anterior tibial, peroneal, and posterior tibial arteries as they pass the ankle joint.[96] The head of the talus receives small perforating branches from the dorsalis pedis artery and from small branches of the artery of the tarsal sinus, which is a branch of either the dorsalis pedis or the peroneal artery. The posterior tibial artery supplies an artery of the tarsal canal, which passes below the ankle joint, entering the tarsal canal where there are numerous perforating branches. The arteries of the tarsal canal and the tarsal sinus and their many branches form a sling around the neck of the talus from which numerous intraosseous vessels arise to supply the body. Following trauma, the vessels of the tarsal canal and sinus seem to be most vulnerable to injury. The incidence of aseptic necrosis varies from approximately 15 percent in those with fracture of the neck of the talus with minimal displacement or no displacement to 90 percent in cases of fracture dislocation. Total dislocation of the talus obviously results in total necrosis of the talus.

Recognition of the presence of aseptic necrosis is primarily radiographic. After the fracture or frac-ture dislocation is reduced and immobilized in plaster, the resulting disuse atrophy of living or vascularized bone becomes evident after a period of 3 to 6 weeks of immobilization.

Case 7-10 A 43-year-old man with a fracture dislocation of the talus, a fracture along the posterior third of the body, and subtalar joint dislocation of the body (Fig. 7-24A&B) shows that after reduction within 2 months a zone of radiolucency appears underneath the subchondral cortex and the subchondral cortex, particularly on the anteroposterior view (Fig. 7-24C–F) (Hawkins' sign).[59] This atrophy within the living subchondral cortex and adjacent trabeculae must be distinguished from the radiolucency underneath the necrotic subchondral cortex with fracture or segmental collapse. Other sites, such as the necrotic head of the femur or the humerus, have been described to show the result of invasion of the margin of the reparative vascular connective tissue in the description of the crescent sign or the subcortical radiolucency at those sites. The presence of a blood supply to the subchondral cortex manifests radiographically as disuse atrophy of the bone. As noted in Figure 7-24C–H, over time the density returns to normal, whereas the segmental collapse or fracture of the subchondral cortex follows a different course, i.e., progressive collapse and secondary degenerative arthritis in most instances when it is not actively treated.

Case 7-11 A 15-year-old girl sustained a fracture dislocation of the talus (Fig. 7-25A). At 6 weeks the body of the talus retains its original density and therefore is relatively more dense than the adjacent living tibia and fibula, indicating that the body is necrotic (Fig. 7-25B&E). At 20 months, a segmental collapse of the body of the talus occurred (Fig. 7-25C&F), which at 6 years (Fig. 7-25D&G), despite drilling and bone grafting 4 years earlier, resulted in late degenerative joint disease of the ankle.

This problem would then be treated by an ankle orthosis or ankle fusion and at times if necessary by a pantalar fusion. There are some reports that an early subtalar fusion helps to increase the blood supply to the necrotic body of the talus and therefore prevents late collapse. The results of that procedure are variable and it can not often be recommended. The long-term results of weight-bearing relief with crutches, cane, and patellar-tendon-

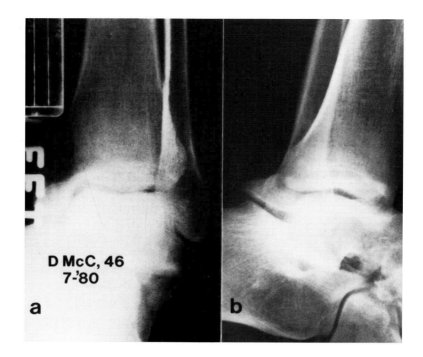

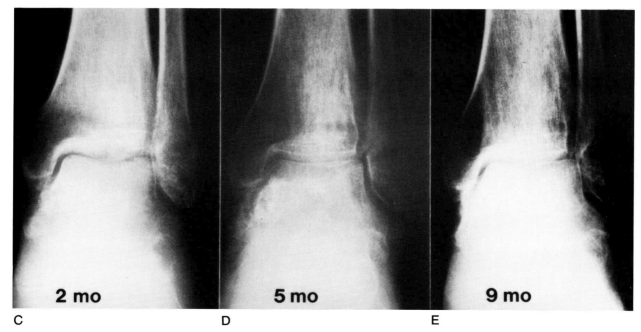

Fig. 7-24. A 46-year-old man sustained a fracture dislocation of left talus shown here in the AP (A) and lateral (B) radiographs. (C–E) AP radiographs. At 2 months there is reduced density of the subchondral cortex, "Hawkins sign," suggesting a viable blood supply to the talus. At 5 and 9 months there is generalized disease atrophy due to immobilization. *(Figure continues.)*

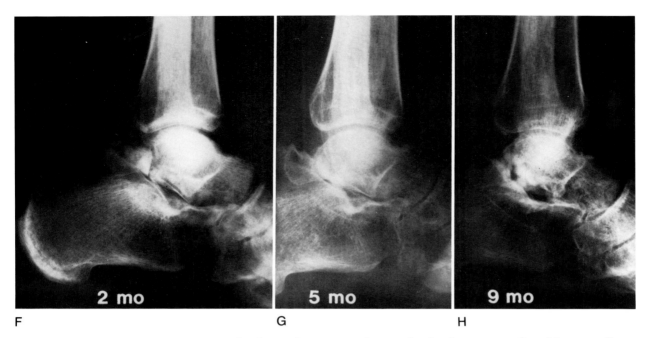

F   G   H

Fig. 7-24 *(Continued).* **(F–H)** Lateral radiographs at 2, 5, and 9 months also show an unreduced fracture of the posterior aspect of the talus. (Courtesy of IV Ponseti, M.D., University of Iowa, Iowa City.)

bearing casts or braces offers a reasonable approach until secondary degenerative arthritis is severe enough to warrant ankle fusion.

Head of the Humerus

The evolution of the changes described for other sites apply to the head of the humerus as well. Except for aseptic necrosis of the head of the humerus in decompression sickness, sickle cell disease, and steroid therapy in renal transplant patients, the site is not commonly involved by the usual nontraumatic associated conditions. However, more frequently, certain fractures of the proximal humerus commonly result in necrosis of the head of the humerus as a result of disruption of visceral branches of the anterior humeral circumflex artery or the posterior humeral circumflex artery.[79] Embolization of the ascending branch (the arcuate artery) of the anterior humeral circumflex artery would most likely account for infarction of the humeral head from nontraumatic causes. The following cases de-

lineate a few of the clinical and radiographic and pathological features of the problem at this site.

Case 7-12 A 40-year-old patient had had a fracture (Neer type 10[97a,97b]) of the anatomical neck of the humerus had disrupted the ascending branches of the anterior humeral circumflex artery 2 years before presentation. The fracture had healed in malposition. Twenty-four months after the fracture the patient developed pain from a segmental collapse of the medial portion of the head of the humerus (Fig. 7-26). This problem can be anticipated in a high proportion of such cases. They may then require prosthetic replacement, shoulder fusion, or resection of the head of the humerus for relief of symptoms.

It is obvious that a few three-part and most four-part fractures of the head of the humerus as classified by Neer[97a,97b] produce necrosis of the free segments of the head. In older patients a primary replacement prosthesis would expedite function as is frequently done for subcapital fractures of the neck of the femur.

That the repair of the necrosis follows patterns

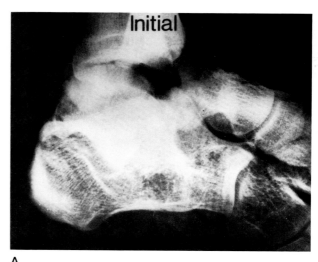

Fig. 7-25. (A) A 16-year-old girl sustained a fracture dislocation of the right talus. An open reduction was performed. (B–D) AP radiographs. (E–G) Lateral radiographs. The neck of the talus healed, but the body of the fracture shows the relative density of necrosis best seen on the lateral view at 6 weeks. At 20 months there was collapse of the lateral corner of the talus, which is best seen on the AP view. At 6 years both views show posttraumatic arthritis of the ankle joint, narrowing of the cartilage space, and osteophytes.

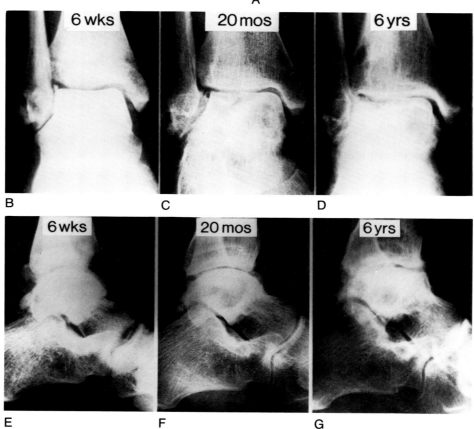

similar to that described earlier at other sites is illustrated by the next two cases.

Case 7-13 A 46-year-old renal transplant patient showed evolution of a lesion with radiological evidence of a subchondral cortex radiolucency at 12 and 14 months followed by structural change of a subchondral cortex crescent sign at 14 months and at 2 years (Fig. 7-27A–C). The segmental collapse

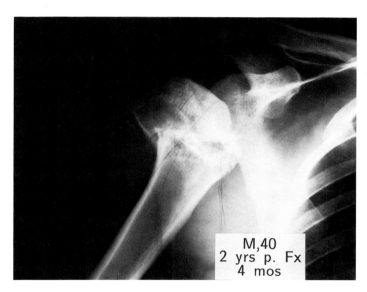

Fig. 7-26. A 40-year-old man with a three-part fracture of the neck and head of the right humerus developed pain 2 years after the injury and had aseptic necrosis and collapse of the central fragment of the head as well as union of the greater tuberosity to the shaft at 28 months after the fracture.

that began at 14 months is more clearly evident at 2 and 2.5 years (Fig. 7-27D&E). At 11 years the head is flattened, and secondary degenerative joint disease is now evident (Fig. 7-27F).

Case 7-14 A 31-year-old man had a Neer prosthesis inserted to replace the head of the humerus, which had undergone necrosis 7 years earlier after he had had 23 days of steroid therapy for a head injury. The patient developed pain in both hips and shoulders 6 months to 2 years after the steroid therapy. A Neer prosthesis was inserted in the left shoulder 5 years after treatment because of segmental collapse of the head of the humerus. The right shoulder became painful 8 months before replacement surgery because of segmental collapse of a humeral head infarct (Fig. 7-28A). A photomicrograph of the excised specimen shows residual necrosis with an osteochondritis-like lesion (Fig. 7-28B). Areas of calcified necrotic marrow account for the increased radiographic density of the infarct as described for the head of the femur.

This case illustrates that in a non-weight-bearing joint muscle forces acting across the joint are capable of producing the stress fracture of repair in the head of the humerus similar to what was described for the femoral head. The time sequence for the appearance of these structural alterations are comparable. The latter point is particularly true in patients who have had prolonged steroid therapy for whatever reason whose bones are rendered osteoporotic by such treatment and whose repair processes are altered as well.

Although we discussed the etiology of decompression sickness earlier, it is appropriate to refer to the radiographic surveys by the Medical Research Council (MRC) Decompression Sickness Panel[57] and that by Ohta and Matsunaga[96a] of Japanese divers, which indicate that the head of the humerus is more commonly affected than the head of the femur.

The kinds of lesions noted are in two major groups: (1) juxta-articular and (2) others, i.e., head and neck and shaft lesions. The radiographic classification of bone lesions described by the MRC Decompression Sickness Panel is one worth the interested reader's attention. The lesions in the articular and head sites are more likely to develop structural failure during repair and become symptomatic, whereas those that remain as circumscribed, walled-off, heavily calcified infarcts do not as a rule become symptomatic unless a sarcoma develops at the site, a rare complication.

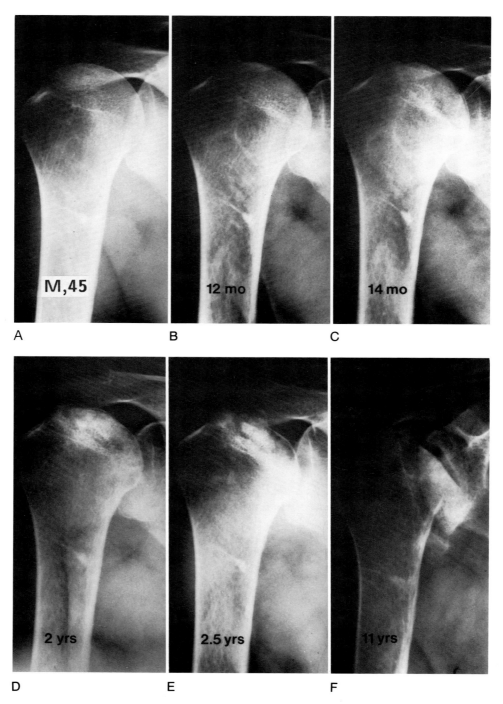

Fig. 7-27. A 45-year-old man with renal failure developed symptoms of aseptic necrosis of the right femoral head and both humeral heads 6 months and 11 months, respectively, after a renal transplant was performed. **(A–F)** AP radiographs of the right shoulder shows the evolution of the necrosis over 11 years from the pretransplant radiograph to collapse, healing, and arthritis. Note the presence of a "crescent" sign in the 14-month radiograph, before collapse occurred.

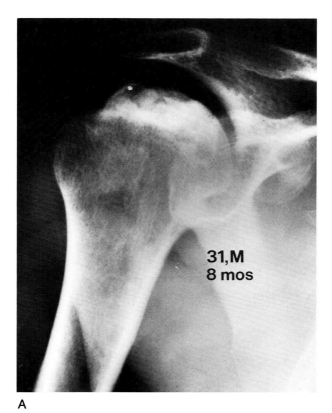

A

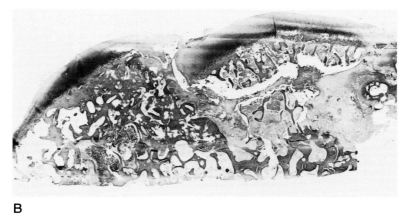

B

Fig. 7-28. (A) A 31-year-old male alcoholic had had pain in his right shoulders for 8 months. A radiograph showed segmental collapse and aseptic necrosis of the head of the humerus surrounded by a marked increase in bone density. A replacement prosthesis procedure was performed. (B) Photomicrograph of the resected segment of the head of the humerus shows an ununited fragment of necrotic bone surrounded by fibrous tissue and a repair zone of thickened trabeculae at the base, which accounted for the marked increase in density ($\times 4$).

Scaphoid

Aseptic necrosis of the carpal scaphoid occurs after injury to the wrist — usually a fracture of the scaphoid alone or a fracture dislocation of the wrist, when the lateral volar and dorsal branches from the radial artery and its superficial palmar branch are disrupted. There is a ligamentous ridge that runs obliquely around the dorsal surface from the tuberosity of the lateral side to the base of the scaphoid medially. The arterial foramina are commonest in this region. The constricted portion of the waist at the proximal end has fewer foramina, so fractures in this area are more likely to result in necrosis of the proximal pole. As is the case in other sites at risk, an associated nonunion of the fracture occurs in about one-third of these fractures. Union may be delayed in such instances. During the process of repair, replacement may be incomplete, resulting in cyst-like cavities or collapse of the proximal fragment.

As in other instances of aseptic necrosis, recognition of the necrosis depends on relative density secondary to disuse atrophy of living bone, as illustrated in the wrist of a 19-year-old man 14 months after a fracture of the carpal scaphoid with a nonunion and aseptic necrosis of the proximal half of the scaphoid (Fig. 7-29A). Insertion of a tibial cortical peg bone graft across the nonunion site into the necrotic fragment (Fig. 7-29B) resulted in union of the fracture and repair of the necrosis without collapse.

Murray, Russe, Mulder,[95] and others have reported a 90 to 96 percent union rate with bone grafting. Murray[52] used a dorsal inlay cortical peg graft and Russe[56] a volar inlay cancellous bone graft. Apparent aseptic necrosis of the proximal fragment did not seem to influence the outcome so

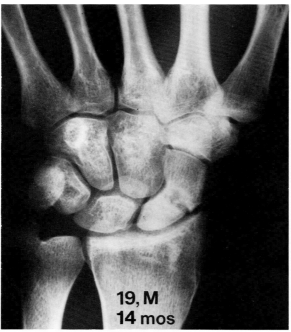
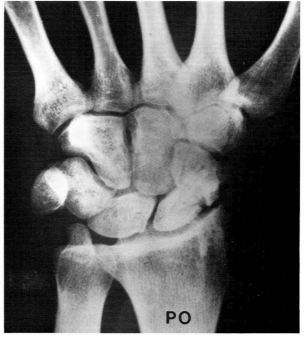

A   B

Fig. 7-29. (A) AP radiograph of the left wrist of a 19-year-old man shows aseptic necrosis of the proximal pole of the scaphoid and a nonunion of the waist of the bone 14 months after a fall on the left hand. (B) Radiograph obtained 1 year after insertion of a dorsal inlay cortical bone graft in the scaphoid. The fracture healed, and the necrosis repaired.

long as arthritic changes or collapse and fragmentation had not occurred. Mulder observed a return to normal density of the proximal fragment in more than one-half of the cases treated by the volar approach. Those fractures with a delayed union healed with a period of immobilization in a thumb spica cast in a high percentage of cases within 16 to 20 weeks. Removal of the proximal necrotic fragment of the scaphoid often led to a shift of carpal bones and secondary degenerative changes, so it is not indicated.

Lunate (Kienbock's Disease)

Whether fracture of the body of the lunate occurs as a primary event, resulting in necrosis of the lunate, or, as noted earlier (Fig. 7-15), as a secondary stress fracture during repair of the necrosis has not been clearly established. Lunate or perilunate dislocations do disrupt the blood supply[42,132] to the body with aseptic necrosis the expected outcome. The subject of wrist injuries has received an extensive amount of attention in recent years, which requires the readers to refer to texts and articles on the subject.[6,73,76,108] It serves our purpose to review the radiographic and pathological features of a few examples to show the similar evolution of the problem to that of necrosis at other sites.

Although most patients with established aseptic necrosis of the wrist give a history of antecedent injury to the wrist, a wide range of reported cases (less than 2 percent in one report and 61 percent in another) that showed evidence of a fresh fracture of the lunate indicate the uncertainty of this cause. Nevertheless, most authors consider aseptic necrosis of the lunate (Kienbock's disease) uniquely as it is secondary to a fracture, whether caused by the primary injury or secondary, occurring during the repair of necrosis.[7,24,41,42]

Case 7-15 A 23-year-old man injured his wrist in an auto accident. Two years later, because of pain, swelling, and tenderness of the wrist, he presented and was noted to have fragmentation and obvious increased density of the lunate (Fig. 7-30A). Resection of the lunate (Fig. 7-30B) showed a nonunion through the body of the lunate with fragmentation of the proximal radial border of the bone (Fig.

7-30C). There was evidence of extensive replacement of necrotic bone by living bone, as described for other sites subject to bone necrosis (Fig. 7-30D). A fracture of the cortex along the distal border of the lunate and cartilage degeneration are also present (Fig. 7-30E).

The diagnosis is made by radiographic recognition of a density change in the carpal lunate. After dislocation, the disuse atrophy of the distal radius and other carpal bones gives the relative appearance of increased lunate density. When a stress fracture is present, radiolucent lines appear underneath the subchondral cortex (Fig. 7-15)* or through the body of the lunate (Fig. 7-30). The diagnosis may not be apparent initially, so either tomograms or serial radiographs after a period of immobilization of the wrist help identify the necrosis. Bone scans are of limited value for identifying or depicting the extent of collapse or secondary degenerative joint disease. The ultimate result of the process is a slowly evolving degenerative joint disease compatible with function for many years.

The treatment varies from protective immobilization of the wrist to resection of the lunate with or without prosthetic replacement or of the proximal carpal row as well as various intercarpal or radiocarpal arthrodeses.[41,117] One of the methods that has yet to yield sufficiently definitive results is either lengthening of the ulna or shortening of the radius to correct an anatomical disparity between the length of the ulna and the radius (negative or positive ulnar variance).[41] Although the shape of the bone may not be altered, the operation halts the progressive collapse of the necrosis, seems to improve the lunate vascularity, and relieves the pain and limitation of wrist mobility. It is possible that the enforced immobilization of the wrist to allow healing of the ulna (or radius) gives the repair process time to replace the necrotic bone with living bone and to allow union of the stress fracture within the lunate. Comparable patients without surgery but with similar periods of immobilization have not been reported.

---

* See also Figure 7-58A in Rockwood and Green: Fractures in Adults. 2nd Ed. [Lippincott, Philadelphia, 1984].

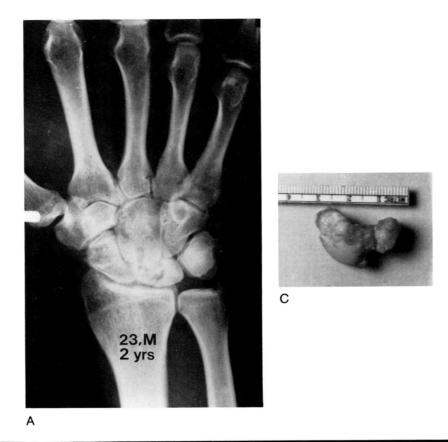

A

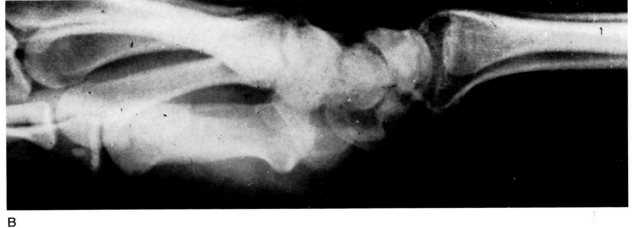

C

B

Fig. 7-30. A 23-year-old man had pain and swelling of his left wrist for 2 years after an injury. AP (A) and lateral (B) radiographs of the wrist show necrosis and fragmentation of the lunate with collapse (Kienböck's disease) and secondary degenerative arthritis. (C) Gross specimen shows erosion of the articular surface at the distal (captitate) margin of the lunate bone. *(Figure continues.)*

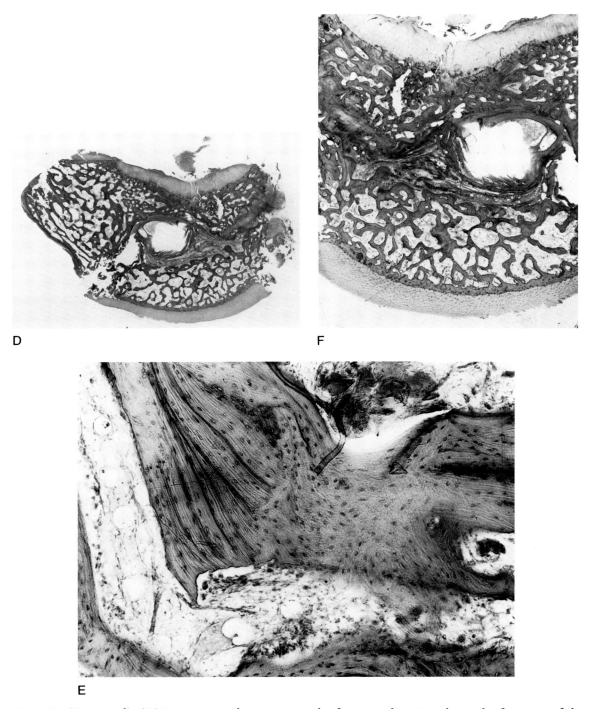

Fig. 7-30 *(Continued).* (**D**) Low power photomicrograph of a coronal section shows the fractures of the cartilage and cortex. The trabeculae are fragmented (×3). (**E**) Creeping substitution is occurring (×100). (**F**) Cartilage fibrillation is seen adjacent to a fracture of the lunate (×6).

Other Sites

The body of the talus, parts of the femoral condyles, the tarsal navicular, and the head of the second metatarsal are not uncommon sites for aseptic necrosis in the lower extremity. In the upper extremity the head of the humerus, the lunate, part of the scaphoid, and the distal parts of a metacarpal are often affected. Nearly all of these sites have in common an association with trauma. It either is definite (as in lesions of the talus, lunate, and humerus) or presumed, as with lesions of the metacarpals and metatarsals. The history of trauma rarely is one of a single accident. The history of repetitive trauma, usually from occupational pursuits, also can be of questionable etiological relevance because the lesion is relatively rare for any specific occupation.

The exceptional site, the femoral condyle, is one affected primarily in the elderly. For this reason, perhaps we should restrict the term osteonecrosis to lesions in that site and perhaps to those of the proximal part of the tibia as well, and only in elderly patients. This reasoning implies that the causation is arteriosclerosis. Such lesions pursue a somewhat different course than do other lesions of aseptic necrosis, the principal difference being a pronounced tendency to slow spontaneous restitution to normal architecture of the involved cancellous bone. This situation is the rule unless the articular cartilage is seriously undermined, and in such cases the degenerative arthritis supervenes unless surgical measures are undertaken (curettage and bone grafting) to prevent collapse of the cartilage.

The lesions that have been described (extensively) as occurring in the femoral head present certain important contrasts to the lesions that occur in the other sites. Not only are they more common, they also cause a greater degree of morbidity. It seems curious that lesions in sites other than the femoral head rarely occur in patients with the diseases that often are associated with aseptic necrosis. One exception is the head of the humerus, a common site for aseptic necrosis in patients with decompression sickness or hematological disorders. Sometimes the lesion, if it affects a small volume of bone, as in a lunate or scaphoid, is asymptomatic. Moreover, cases are on record that have been discovered incidentally: Only by taking a careful history was an injury discovered that occurred years before the radiological evidence became evident.

The inadequacies of purely anatomical studies in ascertaining the pathophysiology of aseptic necrosis and its repair should be evident. Given the fact that aseptic necrosis is such a common problem, many investigators have tried more physiological approaches toward a better understanding of the clinical aspects of the lesion.[62] The mere listing of some of the investigative approaches, none of which proved effective enough to be deserving of clinical trial, may serve to indicate that the problem is difficult and deserves study by whatever new techniques, methods, or approaches seem promising.

1. One somewhat simplistic method of investigation is observing if there is fresh bleeding from the fracture surface of the femoral head as observed in patients undergoing open reduction and fixation within 24 hours of a fracture. If there is none, an important correlation with aseptic necrosis would be expected.[34]

2. Analysis of carbon dioxide and oxygen concentrations has been done with probes inserted into the femoral head. The rationale was that dead tissue would not release carbon dioxide or use up oxygen in the same way as does live tissue.[133]

3. Radioactive or radiopaque substances have been injected systemically or directly into the femoral head; then, with a probe in that structure the washout of the test substance was recorded over time.[21,80] The rationale here was the same as above, the test substance being easier to monitor than tissue gases.

4. Measurement of the bone marrow pressure in bone substance via a probe has been advocated, the rationale being the idea that dead bone would display a different pattern of pressure fluctuations than would live bone.[53,63,83,92,124]

5. Thermal and electrical studies of the bone of the head have been attempted and compared with the same determinations on a known vascularized area, e.g., the trochanter.

6. Standard laboratory techniques have been employed extensively to study the incidence of aseptic necrosis of the femoral head following fracture. Histological data suggest that necrosis be-

Table 1. Incidence of Femoral Head Aseptic Necrosis Following Fracture

Investigator	Technique	No. of Heads	% Aseptic Nectrosis
Phemister (1934)	Radiographic	49	65 (complete & partial)
	Histological		84 (complete & partial)
Charnley (1957)	Nail extrusion	33	66 (some)
Coleman & Compere (1961)	Radiological	60	100 (partial)
	Histological		
Boyd & Calandrucio (1963)	^{32}P autoradiography	82	66 (some)
Bonfiglio (1964)	Radiological	250	100 (partial to complete)
	Histological		
Sevitt (1964)	BaSO$_4$ radiography	25	28 (complete; $n = 7$)
	Histological		58 (partial; $n = 14$)
			16 (live; $n = 4$)
Catto (1965)	Histological	47	11 (complete; $n = 5$)
			55 (partial; $n = 26$)
			34 (live; $n = 16$)

comes of clinical significance in about two-thirds of the patients who have had a subcapital fracture; in about 15 percent (8 to 28 percent) it is complete, and in the rest it varies from subtotal to inconsequential (Table 7-1).[10,21,29,35,101,111] Those patients who are at risk for the possibility of collapse of the femoral head after fracture during the process of repair of necrotic bone are the ones to whom the methods we have just discussed pertain.

Perhaps MRI studies,[103,114] as in Figure 7-6, now under way in several centers, will allow early and noninvasive determinations of aseptic necrosis. However, it seems doubtful that the present method, which largely measures water content in the tissues, will be an effective technique. After all, live and dead tissues do not differ importantly in their water content, but MRI has the potential for measuring other chemicals, and perhaps the development of a technique targeted at the degenerative products in an area of aseptic necrosis will prove effective.

ASEPTIC NECROSIS IN CHILDREN

Some aspects of aseptic necrosis, as it affects children, have already been discussed but only in regard to a few conditions (e.g., congenital disloca-tion of the hip, sickle cell disease) and with particular reference to the effects of the aseptic necrosis on the growth and architecture of the femoral head. Further consideration of the lesion in children requires that the principles expounded in the femoral head be applied to other causes for the necrosis. The first is fracture of the neck of the femur.[26,94,106] It should be noted that the sites in the skeleton of children that are at risk for aseptic necrosis are the same as those in adults (Fig. 7-31).

Some features of the arteries to the femoral head have already been described. Studies of the blood supply to the femoral head during growth reported by Trueta[125] indicated that the small arteries in the ligament teres do not contribute to the nutrition of the femoral head in infants and children up to 4 years of age. The metaphyseal vessels contribute little afterward but may be important up to the age of 4. In children and adolescents, only the lateral epiphyseal vessels supply the secondary center of ossification (Fig. 7-32). At the time of fusion of the epiphyseal plate there is a resumption of some supply from the metaphyseal vessels, and afterward the adult pattern of blood supply prevails.

In children, the neck of the femur is an unusual site for a fracture, and so incidentally are the other sites that in adults have a predilection for aseptic necrosis, e.g., the talus. Nevertheless, when they occur fractures of the femoral neck in children are associated with a higher incidence of aseptic ne-

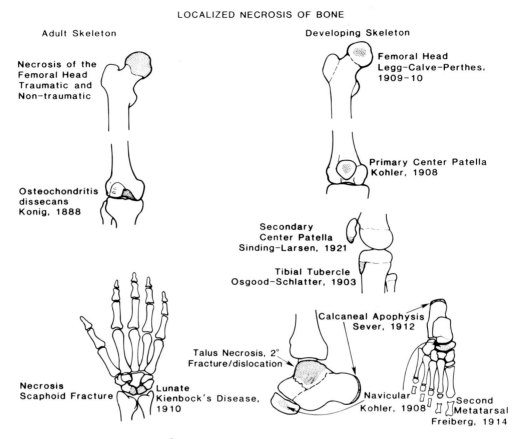

Fig. 7-31. Sites of aseptic necrosis in the adult or immature skeleton.

crosis of the femoral head than occurs in the adult. A disturbance of growth in length of the femoral neck and of the continuing maintenance of contour (hemisphericity) (Fig. 7-33) are complications not seen in the adult.

The prognosis for fractures of the neck of the femur in children of various ages regarding the likelihood of aseptic necrosis requires that the above pattern of blood supply be appreciated. Although it is a pathophysiological principle that, in general, fractures in children do not require as accurate a reduction as do those in adults and do not ordinarily require internal fixation, fractures of the neck of the femur are exceptions because of the unique and changing vascularity. Even when such a fracture is accurately reduced, and fixation is firm, after union of the fracture is evident, aseptic necrosis may occur. When it does occur, its consequences are more serious than in adults. The reason

it is more common in children may be that in developing bones the blood flow that is required is greater than in the adult; and therefore during repair of the fracture the bone is at higher risk for aseptic necrosis. The reasons it is more serious in children are as follows: (1) Therapy is more difficult in children. Although the initial treatment of the fracture is no different than in adults, keeping the child from bearing weight on the involved extremity for several weeks or months may be impossible. Once the complication is recognized, only three options of therapy are now available: conservative treatment, the Phemister procedure, and arthrodesis. Each entails the same problem of compliance just mentioned. Arthroplasty, as mentioned elsewhere, is unsatisfactory in children. (2) The limitations on the physical activity of children can blight their formative years, with serious damage to personality and education, because it can

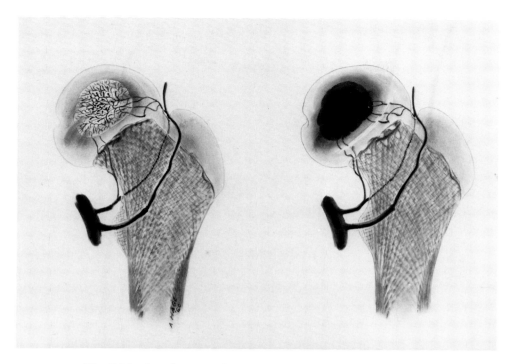

Fig. 7-32. Circulation to femoral neck and head in children.

markedly limit their options for play, social activity, and choice of vocation.

Union of the fracture usually occurs. Once femoral head necrosis is recognized, the patient should be maintained on a prolonged non-weight-bearing regimen until the area of aseptic necrosis is replaced by viable bone (Fig. 7-34). This period may last 2 to 4 years; if ambulation is premature, segmental collapse with structural alteration of the hip joint results. In the older child or adolescent, Phemister procedures do work sometimes, but in general the results are not as satisfactory as in adults for the reasons cited.

Necrosis of the head of the femur has been discussed in patients who have had congenital dislocation of the hip and fracture of the femoral neck. It also merits discussion when it complicates slipped capital femoral epiphysis or constitutes the primary lesion (LCP disease) (see Ch. 5).

In the case of slipped epiphysis (see Fig. 5-17), aseptic necrosis occurs primarily as a result of therapy, i.e., an attempt at closed (or open) reduction, whether successful or unsuccessful.[90] Its consequences and evolution are, in all respects, similar to the lesion seen in adults after fracture, and they need not be repeated here. Mention should be made of the fact that black children are much more at risk than are other children for reasons that have yet to be discovered. It also should be mentioned that the complication of acute chondrolysis, which occasionally occurs in cases of slipped epiphysis, may be difficult to differentiate from aseptic necrosis clinically, but radiological study easily reveals which complication exists. Incidentally, chondrolysis also occurs more often in blacks than in other races.

The primary etiology of *Legg-Calvé-Perthes disease* (coxa plana) is unknown, but large pools of clinical material (including little histological evidence, however) and experimental material have accumulated that may help to characterize its pathophysiology.[4,25,52,53,65,77,81,119,128,130] The moment of insult (or possibly insults) is not known. Recognition of the condition depends on the time at which the joint becomes involved; as in adults, the aseptic necrosis per se does not evoke symptoms. It is the sequelae of the necrosis (crush-down, synovial exudation) that are determinative in terms of recog-

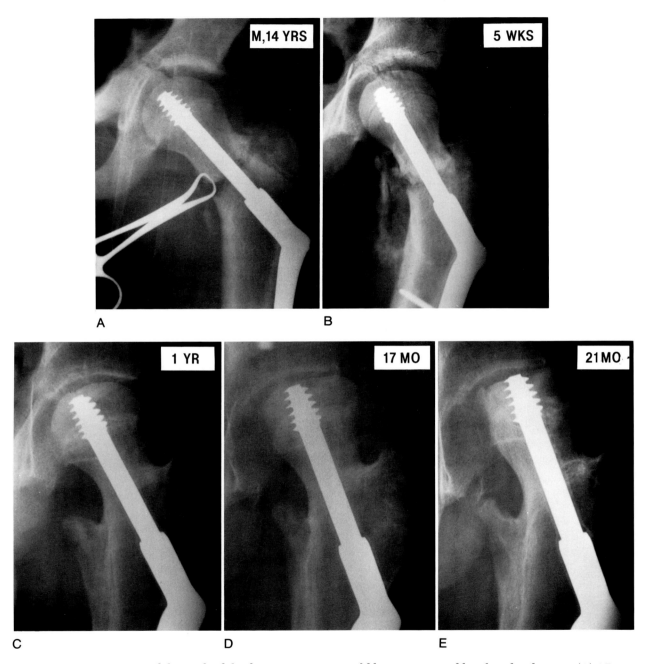

Fig. 7-33. Fracture of the neck of the femur in a 14-year-old boy was treated by closed reduction. **(A)** AP radiograph postoperatively shows good reduction and placement of fixation device. **(B)** At 5 weeks abundant callus is present. There is radiolucency within the neck of the femur and the acetabulum but not within the head. **(C)** At 1 year the fracture has united. The head of the femur is less dense laterally. **(D)** At 17 months, central collapse of femoral head is present. The epiphyseal plate is closed. **(E)** At 21 months collapse is more extensive around the end of the compression screw, and growth arrest is complete.

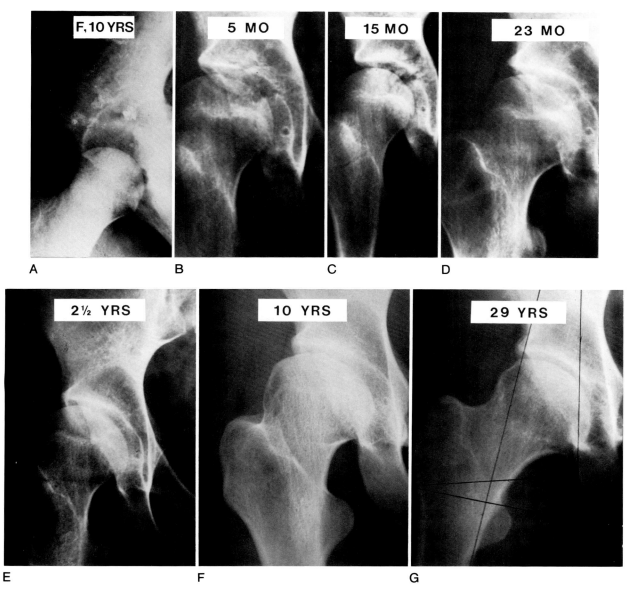

Fig. 7-34. (A) A 10-year-old girl sustained a dislocation of her right hip in a fall from a horse. (B) At 5 months a central area of aseptic necrosis with slight collapse is present. (C) She was kept on crutches with touch-weight-bearing for 2 years. (D) At 23 months the minimal central collapse is healing. (E) At 30 months the area has healed. (F) At 10 years the femoral head is larger, and the joint cartilage space is narrowed marginally. (G) At 29 years the patient's hip is painful with overactivity. The AP radiograph shows a narrowed joint space and marginal osteophytes. A Varus osteotomy had been considered but was not performed.

nizing the condition and determining the approximate time it started. It must always be remembered that the lesion predates the symptoms by weeks if not months. The extent of initial involvement may influence that interval, as may the effects secondary to repair and replacement of dead bone by vascular connective tissue such as those described for the femoral head and lunate in adults.

With Legg-Calvé-Perthes disease, a major difference from adult cases of aseptic necrosis occurs radiographically as a result of the effect of ischemia on epiphyseal and metaphyseal growth: There is a temporary cessation of growth that is most apparent in the very young child and infant. Recall that in the infant with congenital dislocation of the hip whose secondary centers of ossification in the femoral heads have not yet ossified, and who have aseptic necrosis, there is a delay in ossification. Moreover, when ossification does begin, the process may be irregular, particulate, or both. The development of the center lags in terms of size compared to the center on the unaffected side. However, the infants so involved are younger than children with coxa plana. With the latter condition the usual radiographic picture, if the affected child is age 2 to 8, shows the center of ossification to be denser than on the unaffected side, although in the earliest recognizable stages it usually is not irregular or smaller than on the unaffected side. Only somewhat later does evidence of crush-down appear, but it is not seen routinely. It may be evident by flattening of the center proximally and medially or by fragmentation of the center. Fragmentation does not represent the same sequence of changes as is seen with acute fractures but, rather, the process by which repair is taking place, i.e., invasion of the necrotic bone by granulation tissue and its evolution into a replacement for the cancellous bone. It is noteworthy that this process occasionally takes several months or even a year or two. Although histological samples are not available to explain the chronicity, the best explanation is that the radiolucent tissue between bony fragments is fibrocartilage, which often comprises an important part of callus in children.

One further difference between the aseptic necrosis of the femoral head in Legg-Calvé-Perthes disease and that occurring in nontraumatic cases in adults is that in children the process, instead of including breaks in the articular cartilage followed much later by the sequelae of osteoarthritis, seems to involve restructuring of the cartilage. There is flattening of the osseous nucleus, but apparently the overlying articular cartilage thickens and is more resilient than in adults and can be remodeled. The result is that, although the gross contour of the femoral head can deviate from the hemispherical, its surface remains smooth; and the joint therefore remains asymptomatic during the long period of treatment. A basic pathophysiological process in operation during the months (or years) of treatment is the capability of articular cartilage to be considerably remodeled during childhood.[75] This principle applies to both the femoral head and the apposing acetabular cartilage. A corollary of this principle is that the remodeling is largely structural, to conform to the distribution of loading of the joint and to its motion during the long period of the remodeling. It is this rationale on which conservative treatment of Legg-Calvé-Perthes disease is predicated. The idea is "containment," i.e., ensuring that the hip while at rest is kept in the position in which as much femoral cartilage as possible is in contact with the acetabular cartilage. This cartilage is presumably undergoing normal development and therefore remains hemispherical; it is not stimulated to abnormal remodeling as would be the case if it were opposed to an abnormally shaped femoral head.

In addition, after the plate is crossed by fibrovascular tissue during repair, partial or complete growth arrest occurs depending on the age of the patient and the severity of the ischemic necrosis. The end result varies with the degree of growth disturbance plus the completeness and rate of repair of the affected cartilage and bone.

That there may be changes in the structure of the matrix of the epiphyseal and articular cartilage in patients with Legg-Calvé-Perthes disease that precede the ischemic event has not been clearly established, but it appears to have some basis from the histochemical and ultrastructural studies of Ponseti et al.[105] The initial changes in the epiphyseal cartilage matrix weaken the matrix, resulting in occlusion of the retinacular vessels as they cross the deranged cartilage at the margin of the disrupted epiphyseal plate (Fig. 7-35). The theory is supported by observations that children with this dis-

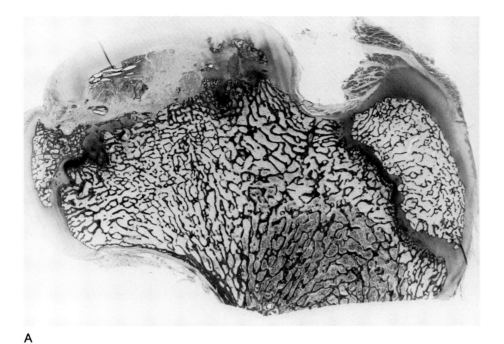

A

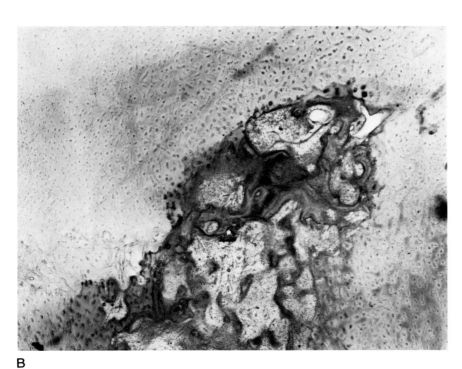

B

Fig. 7-35. (A) Autopsy specimen of a coronal section of the whole head and neck on the left femur of an 8-year-old boy with Legg-Calvé-Perthes disease shows thickening of the articular cartilage, central interruption of the physis, and structural alteration of the epiphysis (×3.5). (B) Lateral edge of the junction of the physis and epiphysis with marked evidence of repair of necrotic bone (×10). *(Figure continues.)*

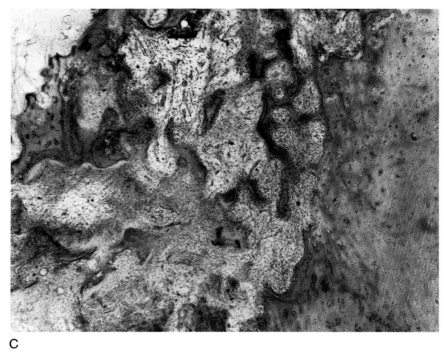

C

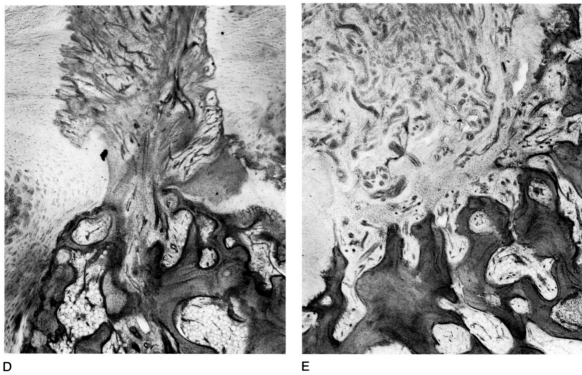

D

E

Fig. 7-35 *(Continued)*. **(C)** Lateral epiphysis repair (×23). Articular cartilage growth plate has been replaced by new bone and granulation tissue. **(D)** Granulation tissue extends from the metaphysis into the physis (×23). **(E)** Replacement of physis by fibrovascular connective tissue in a central area of the physis (×23). *(Figure continues.)*

Fig. 7-35 *(Continued)*. (**F**) Granulation tissue surrounds and is invading the necrotic trabeculae of the epiphysis (×23). (**G**) Articular cartilage and necrotic subchondral cortex have the appearance of osteochondritis dissecans. Note the clefts with layers of collagenous tissue resembling a nonunion (×20).

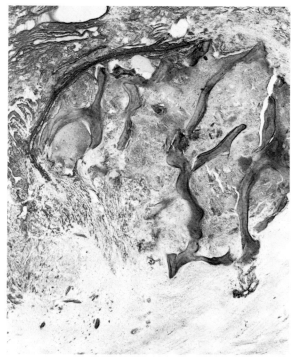

F

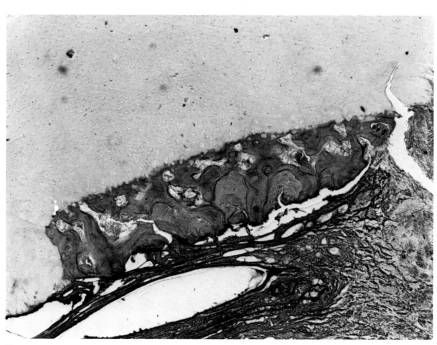

G

order have delayed skeletal maturation and abnormalities of proportionate growth in various regions of the body. More than one site of bony abnormalities has been described in the same patient.

The identification of *ischemic necrosis* after treatment of *congenital dislocation of the hip is based* on radiographic features rather than on pathological material. Because the necrosis occurs after treatment the etiology is considered iatrogenic, related to the position of the reduced femoral head in the acetabulum. A disturbance to the circulation based on the aforementioned studies of Trueta suggests that interruption of the lateral epiphysis vessels by compressive forces in the position of extreme abduction and flexion of the hip result in total or partial necrosis of the secondary center of ossification. There are no human pathological specimens to confirm the radiographic features of this ischemia. However, the incidence of posttreatment necrosis varies from 2 to 68 percent following closed reduction[48] with most reports in the 30 to 40 percent range before modification of treatment regimens and 13 to 15 percent after modification of hip position from the extremes to no more than 90° flexion and no more than 25° of abduction.[16] The presence of necrosis has been reported after open reduction as well.

The radiographic findings of this ischemic event are manifested by failure of the center of ossification to appear at the normal time, with a delay in growth of the secondary center. This stage is followed by fragmentation of the ossification center when it does appear and repair of the fragmented femoral head with residual deformity in the form of coxa magna, flattening of the secondary center, and valgus deformity of the neck secondary to arrest of the lateral aspect of the femoral epiphysis. These femoral head and neck deformities are accompanied by acetabular dysplasia, which in turn leads to a high incidence of degenerative joint disease in patients who have been followed for some time.[36,66]

The treatment of this complication of congenital dislocation of the hip is primarily one of prevention, as it is a rare occurrence in patients treated at birth or when they are less than 4 months of age. Ponseti[104] stated, "The problems of congenital dislocation of the hip must be solved in nurseries and not in the operating rooms." Delayed reduction

may require traction and adductor tenomyotomy with plaster immobilization in the position noted above. A concentric reduction in the acetabulum is essential to minimize the potential for late degenerative arthritis of the hip. It is suggested that monitoring the situation during the postreduction period is important and that osteotomies, either acetabular or femoral, may be necessary to maintain a concentric reduction.

Descriptions of the pathological changes in the femoral head of the child with *Legg-Calvé-Perthes disease* have accumulated slowly over time. They have been described in considerable detail by Catterall et al.[27,28] Similar changes have been observed as a naturally occurring lesion in dogs and experimentally in dogs and pigs.

What seems clear is that until failure of femoral head epiphyseal growth alteration secondary to the ischemic event or events is noted, there are few clinical or radiographic signs to help identify the process. All the classification schemes, groups, or stages depend on combinations of clinical or radiographic features at initial encounter with the patient during the evolution of the process at its endpoint. Unfortunately, none is totally satisfactory for predicting the outcome based on first findings.[86] The evaluation and treatment of each patient must be carefully individualized and weighed against the knowledge of the natural history of the condition. One expects a satisfactory, if not perfect, outcome in most children who received material or token symptomatic treatment.

A microscopic section of a whole left femoral head removed at autopsy from an 8-year-old patient who died of an unrelated cause is used to depict some of the histological features of Legg-Calvé-Perthes disease (Fig. 7-35). The loss of height of the physis (coxa plana) and the incomplete span of the epiphyseal plate centrally are obvious. The medial portion of the physis appears normal and is covered by normal articular cartilage. The lateral one-third of the femoral head has irregular ossification and changes within the epiphyseal plate and metaphysis. A tongue of epiphyseal plate extends into the metaphysis. Histologically, the femoral head physis shows pronounced structural alteration with necrosis composed of calcific debris within the marrow spaces of fragmented necrotic trabeculae (Fig. 7-35A&G). The joint cartilage is viable, but along parts of its basal layer the cartilage may show disturbed growth cells in the affected areas along with disturbance of endochondral ossification (Fig. 7-28C). At times, tongues of epiphyseal plate cartilage are seen in the substance of the metaphysis; whether they are secondary to fragmentation or a primary disturbance within cartilage is not yet clear (Fig. 7-35E).

The range of manifestations and their pathophysiology traditionally are portrayed according to phases, as has been done for fractures: early, intermediate, or late.[130] The early phase (because no one knows the latent period between the ischemic event and onset of symptoms) is that which exists prior to all evidence of radiographic abnormality. The intermediate interval includes stages represented by densification and decreased growth of the femoral head. That is the time during which fragmentation occurs. It represents an intermediate stage of repair and regeneration. The final phase, which is not well delineated from the intermediate phase, is called the reparative stage.

As a rule, subjective symptoms are not manifest during the initial phase until necrosis is fairly pronounced, both histologically and radiographically. Anteroposterior and Lauenstein (frog-leg) lateral views of both hips are needed for radiographic evaluation. The earliest radiographic signs are an increased medial joint cartilage space and a widened joint capsular shadow due to synovitis. There is failure of the *ossific* nucleus to grow so that there is secondary articular *cartilage* hypertrophy at the same time structural alteration of the ossific nucleus may occur. It ranges from a subchondral cortex radiolucent zone to a variable degree of segmental collapse of the femoral head (Figs. 7-36, 7-37, 7-38).

In the intermediate or fragmentation stage, multiple stress fractures of trabeculae within the ossified center or center nuclei are noted. The subchondral cortex fragments, and part of the necrotic subchondral cortex composed of dead and new bone remain attached the deeper layers of articular cartilage (Fig. 7-3G). This finding correlates well with the features of osteochondritis dissecans. It is surrounded by vascular connective tissue. The increased density and zones of radiolucency are radiographic representations of these two findings. In addition, irregularity of the epiphyseal plate and zones of radiolucency within the metaphysis (Fig. 7-35E) corresponding to the areas of cartilage and fibrovascular tissue extensions within the metaphysis, areas of repair with new bone on old lamellar bone, and fibrovascular connective tissue are present during the fragmentation stage (Fig. 7-35E). Some children go through a phase of rapid repair of the necrosis with little loss of physical contour of the femoral head because of the large cartilaginous protective layers (Fig. 7-35), as do some experimental animals and spontaneously occurring Legg-Perthes disease in dogs. These changes may occur spontaneously as part of the natural history of some of the affected hips or as a result of intervention by protective weight-bearing, immobilization in plaster, bed rest, or other forms of treatment, minimizing the repetitive effects of compression on the necrotic and repairing portions of the femoral head.

The final, or reparative, stage is in essence an extension of what preceded. Histologically, the new bone forms at the margins of the center of ossification and gradually spreads toward the center from the periphery, where the new circulation has been reestablished (Fig. 7-35E). The necrotic bone is usually gradually replaced by this vascular granulation tissue but at times persists as a small area of necrosis similar to an osteochondritis ossificans. This end result has been noted in humans (Fig. 7-28C) as well as in animals.[55,91,93] In some instances the disruption of the epiphyseal plate leads to premature closure of the plate with both shortening of the femoral neck and widening because of continued appositional new bone underneath the visceral capsule without concomitant longitudinal growth from the epiphyseal plate. In some areas the epiphyseal cartilage resumes endochondral bone formation, as does the subchondral cortex growth plate. The end result is likely to be a variable degree of remodeling from minimal distortion of the femoral head (Fig. 7-36) to a mushroom-shaped femoral head (Fig. 7-37) or severe deformity (Fig. 7-38) with variations from a coxa plana or coxa magna. The prognosis therefore depends on the extent of involvement that Catterall classified into four stages, including a group with at-risk characteristics that make the prognosis worse. They include obesity, adduction contracture, decreased range of motion at the onset, radio-

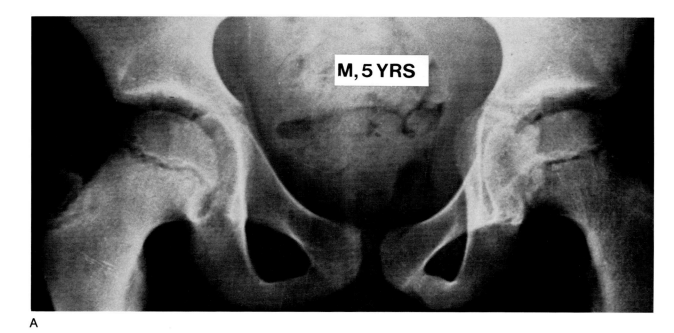

A

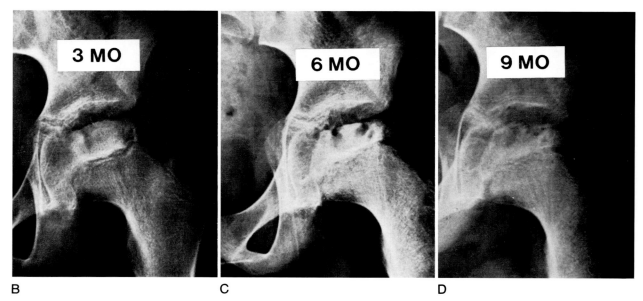

B   C   D

Fig. 7-36. (A–D) A 5-year-old boy with minimal collapse of Legg-Calvé-Perthes (LCP) of the left head of the femur shows the evolution the repair of the necrosis from the early through the intermediate phases. *(Figure continues.)*

graphic evidence of the presence of a lytic area in the lateral epiphysis and adjacent metaphysis calcification (ossification) lateral to the epiphysis, and a diffuse metaphyseal lesion plus lateral subluxation of the head and a horizontal growth plate. It is also known in most studies that the earlier the age of onset, the better is the end result. Conversely, the later the age of onset, the worse is the end result. The goal of treatment is to maintain a spherical and congruent femoral head well centered in

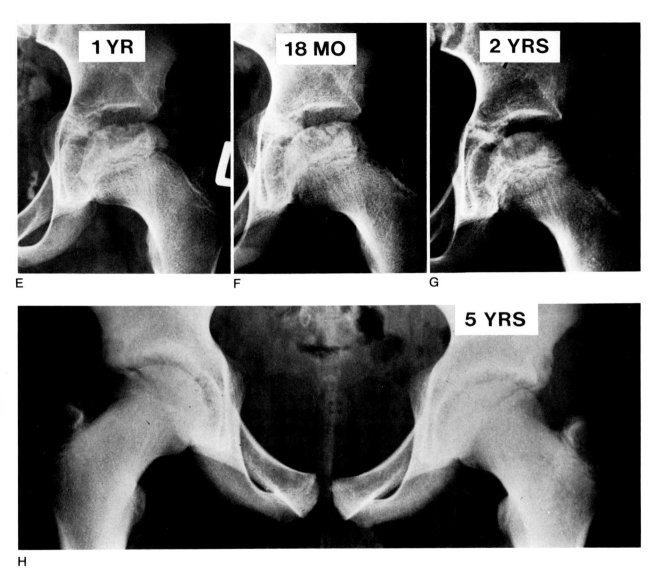

Fig. 7-36 *(Continued).* (**E–G**) Radiographs obtained during the intermediate and late repair stages. (**H**) At 5 years the result is excellent.

the acetabulum. Many of the treatment concepts are based on that goal. Nonsurgical treatment directed toward minimizing the effects of compression on the femoral head include non-weight-bearing in bed or on a cart for 1 to 2 years, non-weight-bearing walking with crutches or a brace, and symptomatic or no other treatment.

Long-term follow-up studies[36,52] suggest that the early radiographic results correlate reasonably well with the type of treatment. The best results

are in patients treated by prolonged bed rest with traction. Progressively fewer spherical femoral heads resulted from bed rest without traction, non-weight-bearing walking, and symptomatic or no treatment. A good radiographic appearance at the time of primary healing correlates well with a low incidence of degenerative arthritis in later years. A few studies have suggested that these methods do not alter the radiological course of the disease and that reasonable results could be obtained by

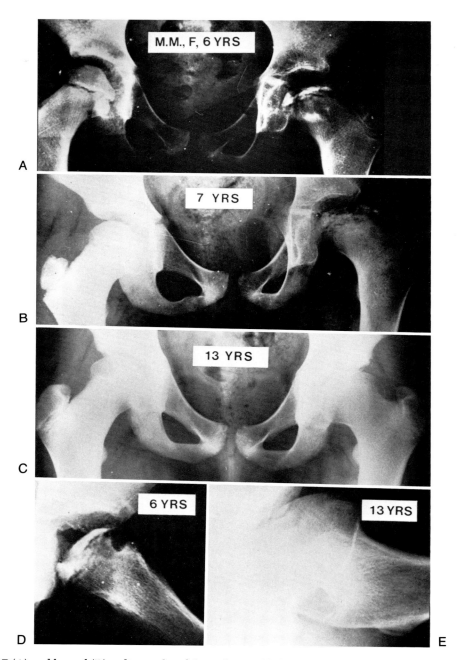

Fig. 7-37. AP (**A**) and lateral (**B**) radiographs of the pelvis and left hip of a 6-year-old girl with a moderately severe collapse of the left upper femoral epiphysis. Note the evolution of repair at age 7 (**C**) to a mushroom-shaped femoral head at age 13 (**D&E**).

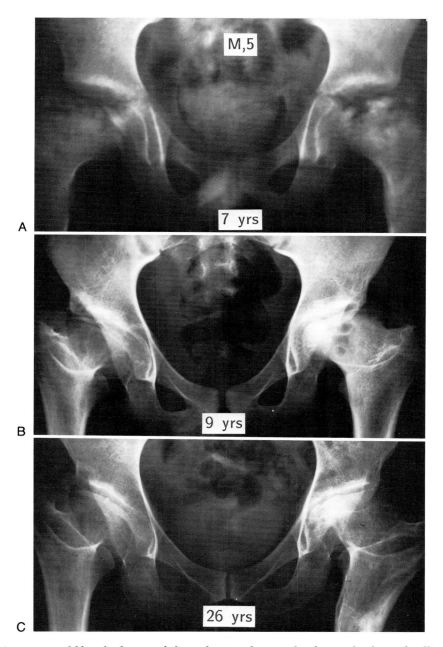

Fig. 7-38. (A) A 7-year-old boy had severe bilateral LCP. The initial radiographs showed collapse fragmentation, physis, and metaphyseal resorption. (B) At 9 years of age the radiograph showed growth arrest of the proximal femoral epiphyses, "pistol grip" deformities of the femoral head and neck, and degenerative cysts of the left femoral head. An osteotomy was done on the left with improvement in gait but little improvement in the range of motion. (C) At 26 years of age, the radiograph of the hips showed severe degenerative joint disease. The patient had pain in both hips, worse on the left, and markedly impaired function. Cup arthroplasties were performed.

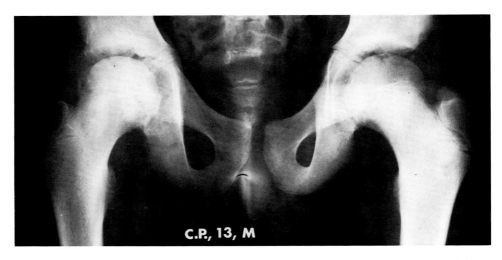

Fig. 7-39. AP radiograph of the pelvis of a 13-year-old-boy with leukemia shows increased density of the right femoral head with collapse due to necrosis of the epiphysis.

methods such as braces that allow walking. These findings suggest that surgical treatment is rarely indicated for this disease.

Surgical treatment includes femoral neck osteotomy, various types of pelvic, acetabular, or extra-acetabular osteotomies, or combinations of the two. No one treatment has proved to be universally successful. Perhaps any surgical treatment to preserve the hip in either adults or children may reactivate a stagnant repair and remodeling process.

Uncommonly, aseptic necrosis of the femoral head occurs in patients with *sickle cell disease*[33] after occlusion of the vessels by thromboses of sickled red blood cells; it also occurs due to tumor cells in patients with leukemia (Fig. 7-39). The hip symptoms result from two mechanisms, i.e., bone necrosis with the usual structural breakdown during repair of the necrotic bone and the arthritic changes resulting from the synovitis and pannus due to small vessel involvement of the synovial membrane and focal hemorrhage.

The radiographic appearance of increased density of the calcified infarcts or various configurations follow the classical sequence of necrosis, partial repair with continued weight-bearing, stress fracture, and the weakened repair margin. Subchondral cortex granulation tissue leads to loosening of the articular cartilage in joints of patients with sickle cell disease.

Clinical recognition presents no problems to the physician, but treatment is difficult at best. In a few instances, infarction localized at the femoral head has been treated by the Phemister procedure. Most affected joints are treated symptomatically until a fusion or resection can be performed.

REFERENCES

1. Anderton JM, Helm R: Multiple joint osteonecrosis following short term steroid therapy. J Bone Joint Surg [Am] 64A:139, 1982
2. Banks HH: Tissue response at the fracture site in femoral neck fractures. Clin Orthop 61:116, 1968
3. Banks SW: Aseptic necrosis of the femoral head following traumatic dislocation of the hip: a report of nine cases. J Bone Joint Surg 23:3, 1941
4. Barnes JM: Premature epiphyseal closure in Perthes disease. J Bone Joint Surg [Br] 62B:432, 1980
5. Bauer G, et al: Dynamics of technetium 99m methylene diphosphonate imaging of the femoral head after hip fracture. Clin Orthop 152:85, 1980
6. Beckenbaugh RD, et al: Kienböck's disease: the natural history of Kienböck's disease and consideration of lunate fractures. Clin Orthop 149:98, 1980
7. Bilos ZJ, Hui PWT: Dorsal dislocation of lunate with carpal collapse. J Bone Joint Surg [Am] 63A: 1484, 1981

8. Boettcher WG, Bonfiglio M, Hamilton H, et al: Non-traumatic necrosis of the femoral head: relation of altered hemostasis to etiology: experiences in treatment. J Bone Joint Surg [Br] 52:312, 1970

9. Bonfiglio M: Aseptic necrosis of the femoral head in dogs: effect of drilling and bone grafting. Surg Gynecol Obstet 98:591, 1954

10. Bonfiglio M: Aseptic necrosis of the femoral head, intact blood supply is of prognostic significance. p. 155. In: Proceedings of the Conference on Aseptic Necrosis of the Femoral Head, Surgery Study Section, NIH, USPHS, 1964

11. Bonfiglio M: Development of bone necrosis lesion. p. 117. In Lambertson CJ (ed): Proceedings of Fifth Symposium on Underwater Physiology. F.A.S.E.B., Bethesda, 1976

12. Bonfiglio M: Fracture of the femoral neck: early recognition and treatment of complications. J Iowa Med Soc p. 309, 1969

13. Bonfiglio M: Osteonecrosis. J Bone Joint Surg [Am] 69A:1107, 1987 (letter)

14. Bonfiglio M, Bardenstein MD: Treatment of bone grafting of aseptic necrosis of the femoral head and non-union of the femoral neck (Phemister technique). J Bone Joint Surg 40A:1329, 1958

15. Bonfiglio M, Voke EM: Effect of treatment by drilling and bone grafting (Phemister technique): aseptic necrosis of the femoral head and non-union of the femoral neck. J Bone Joint Surg 50A:48, 1968

16. Bradley J, Wetherill M, Benson MK: Splintage for congenital dislocation of the hip: is it safe and reliable? J Bone Joint Surg 69B:257, 1987

17. Brav E: Traumatic dislocation of the hip. J Bone Joint Surg 44A:1115, 1962

18. Brodetti A: The blood supply of the femoral neck and head in relation to the damaging effects of nails and screws. J Bone Joint Surg [Br] 42B:794, 1960

19. Brown TD, Vrahas MS: The apparent elastic modulus of the juxtarticular subchondral bone of the femoral head. J Orthop Res 2:32, 1984

20. Bullough PG, Jagannath A: The morphology of the calcification front in articular cartilage: its significance in joint function. J Bone Joint Surg 65B:72, 1983

21. Calandruccio RA, Anderson WE III: Post-fracture avascular necrosis of the femoral head: correlation of experimental and clinical studies. Clin Orthop 152:49, 1980

22. Campbell CJ: Aseptic necrosis of the hip as complication of disease not associated with trauma. p. 109. In: Proceedings of the Conference on Aseptic Necrosis of the Femoral Head, 1964

23. Campbell CJ: Aseptic Necrosis of Bone. AAOS Instructional Course 15. 1966, p. 234

24. Campbell RD, Lance EM, Yeah CB: Lunate and perilunate dislocations. J Bone Joint Surg [Br] 46:55, 1964

25. Canario AT, Williams L, Wientroub S, Catterall A, Lloyd-Roberts GC: A controlled study of femoral osteotomy in severe Perthes disease. J Bone Joint Surg [Br] 62B:438, 1980

26. Casale ST, Bourland WL: Fracture intertrochanteric neck in children. J Bone Joint Surg [Am] 59:431, 1977

27. Catterall AJ, Pringle J, Byers PD, et al: Review of the morphology of Perthes disease. J Bone Joint Surg [Br] 64:269, 1982

28. Catterall AJ, Pringle J, Byers PD, et al: Perthes disease: is the epiphyseal infarction complete? A study of the morphology of two cases. J Bone Joint Surg [Br] 64:276, 1982

29. Catto ML: A histological study of avascular necrosis of the femoral head after transcervical fracture. J Bone Joint Surg [Br] 47:749, 1965

30. Catto ML: The histological appearances of late segmental collapse of the femoral head after transcervical fracture. J Bone Joint Surg [Br] 47:177, 1965

31. Camp JF, Colwell CW Jr: Core decompression of the femoral head for osteonecrosis. J Bone Joint Surg [Am] 68:1313, 1986

32. Chandler FA: Aseptic necrosis of the head of the femur. Wisc Med J 35:609, 1936

33. Chung SMK, Ralston E: Necrosis of the femoral head associated with sickle cell anemia and its genetic variants. J Bone Joint Surg [Am] 51:33, 1968

34. Cleveland M, Bosworth DM: A critical analysis of fifty consecutive cases of fracture of the neck of the femur. Surg Gynecol Obstet 66:646, 1938

35. Coleman SS, Compere CL: Femoral neck fractures —pathogenesis of avascular necrosis, non-union and late degenerative changes. Clin Orthop 20:247, 1961

36. Cooperman DR, Wallenstein R, Stulberg SD: Post reduction avascular necrosis in congenital dislocation of the hip. J Bone Joint Surg [Am] 62:247, 1980

37. Cosentino R: Circulacion proximal del femur—relacion con las fracturas mediales del cuello del femur. In: 25th Congresso Argentined Cirurgia Actas Fasc, 1964, p. 336

38. Crock HV: An atlas of the arterial supply of the head and neck of the femur in man. Clin Orthop 152:17, 1980

39. Cruess RL: Cortisone induced avascular necrosis of the femoral head. J Bone Joint Surg [Br] 59:308, 1977

40. Cruess RL, Cross D, Cranshaw E: The etiology of

steroid induced avascular necrosis of bone: a laboratory and clinical study. Clin Orthop 113:178, 1975

40a. Davidson JK: A septic necrosis of bone, p. 194. Dysbaric osteonecrosis. Excerpta Medica, Amsterdam, 1976

41. D'Aubigne MR, Postel M, Mafzabraud A, et al: Idiopathic necrosis of the femoral head in adults. J Bone Joint Surg [Br] 47:612, 1965

42. Dobyns JH, Linscheid RL: Fractures and dislocation of the wrist. p. 411. In Rockwood and Green (eds): Fractures in Adults. Vol. 1. Ed. 2. Lippincott, Philadelphia, 1984

43. Dorman A: The results of treatment of Kienböcks disease. J Bone Joint Surg [Br] 31:518, 1949

44. Elliott DH, Harrison JAB: Bone necrosis in occupational hazard of diving. J R Naval Med Service 56:140, 1970

45. Elliott DH, Harrison JAB: Aseptic bone necrosis in Royal Naval divers. In Lambertson CJ (ed): Proceedings for Symposium Underwater Physiology. Philadelphia, 1971

46. Elliott DH: The role of decompression inadequacy and bone necrosis of naval divers. Proc R Med 64:1278, 1971

47. Epstein HC: Traumatic dislocation of the hip. Clin Orthop 92:115, 1973

47a. Ficat RP, Arlet J: Necrosis of the femoral head. In Hungerford D (ed): Ischemic Necrosis of the Bone. Williams & Wilkins, Baltimore, 1980

47b. Idiopathic bone necrosis of the femoral head. J Bone Joint Surg [Br] 67:3, 1985

48. Gage JR, Winter RB: Avascular necrosis of the capital femoral epiphysis as complication of closed reduction of congenital dislocation of the hip. J Bone Joint Surg [Am] 54:373, 1972

49. Garden RS: Stability and union in subcapital fractures of the femur. J Bone Joint Surg [Br] 46:630, 1964

50. Garden RS: Malreduction and avascular necrosis in subcapital fractures of the femur. J Bone Joint Surg [Br] 53:183, 1971

51. Gelberman RH, Baumer TD, Menon J, Akeson WA: The vascularity of the lunate bone and Kienböck's disease. J Hand Surg 5:272, 1980

52. Gower WE, Johnston RC: Legg-Perthes disease: long-term follow-up of thirty-six patients. J Bone Joint Surg [Am] 53:759, 1971

53. Green NE, Griffin PP: Intra-osseous venous pressure in Legg-Perthes disease. J Bone Joint Surg [Am] 64:666, 1982

54. Gregg PJ, Walder DN: Scintigraphy versus radiography in the early diagnosis of experimental bone necrosis. J Bone Joint Surg [Br] 62:214, 1980

55. Hallel T, Salvati EA: Osteochrondritis dissecans following Legg-Calve-Perthes. J Bone Joint Surg [Am] 63:906, 1981

56. Hamilton HH, Bonfiglio M, Sheets RF, Connor WE: Relation of altered hemostasis to idiopathic aseptic necrosis of the femoral head. J Clin Invest 44:1058, 1965 (abstract)

57. Harrison JAB: Aseptic bone necrosis of naval clearance divers, radiographic findings. R Soc Med 64:1276, 1971

58. Hartman J: The possible role of fat metabolism. p. 140. In Zinn WM (ed): Idiopathic Ischemic Necrosis of the Femoral Head in Adults. George Thieme, Stuttgart, 1971

59. Hawkins LG: Fractures of the neck of the talus. J Bone Joint Surg [Am] 52:991, 1970

60. Hougaard M, Thomsen P: Traumatic posterior dislocation of the hip with fracture of the femoral neck or both. J Bone Joint Surg [Am] 70:223, 1988

61. Howe WW Jr, Lacy II T, Schwartz RP: A study of the gross anatomy of bone. J Bone Joint Surg [Am] 32:856, 1950

62. Hulth A: Femoral head phlebography. J Bone Joint Surg [Am] 40:844, 1958

63. Hungerford DS: Bone marrow pressure, venography and core decompression in ischemic necrosis of the femoral head. p. 218. In Proceedings of the Hip Society, CV Mosby, St. Louis, 1978

64. Inoue A, Ono K: A histological study of idiopathic avascular necrosis of the head of the femur. J Bone Joint Surg [Br] 61:138, 1979

65. Ippolito E, Tudisco C, Farsetti P: The long-term prognosis of unilateral Perthes disease. J Bone Joint Surg [Br] 69:257, 1987

66. Ishii Y, Ponseti IV: Long-term results of closed reduction of complete congenital dislocation of the hip in children under one year of age. Clin Orthop 137:167, 1978

67. Jacqueline F, Rutishauser R: Idiopathic necrosis of the femoral head. p. 34. In Zinn WM (ed): Idiopathic Ischemic Necrosis of the Femoral Head in Adults. George Thieme, Stuttgart, 1971

68. Jaffe HL: Ischemic necrosis of bone. Med Radiogr Photogr 45:58, 1969

69. Jaffe HL: Metabolic, Degenerative and Inflammatory Diseases of Bones and Joints. Lea & Febiger, Philadelphia, 1972

70. Johnson L: Histogenesis of avascular necrosis. p. 55. In: Proceedings, Conference on Septic Necrosis of the Femoral Head. National Institute of Health, Surgery Study Section, Bethesda, 1964

71. Jones Jr JP: Alcoholism, hypercortisone, fat embolism and osseous avascular necrosis. p. 112. In Zinn

WM (ed): Idiopathic Necrosis of the Femoral Head in Adults. George Thieme, Stuttgart, 1971

72. Jones Jr JP, Engleman EP: Osseous avascular necrosis associated with systemic abnormalities. Arthritis Rheum 9:728, 1966

73. Kahlstrom SC, Burton CC, Phemister DB: Aseptic necrosis of bone. Surg Gynecol Obstet 68:129, 1939

74. Kawashima M, Torisu T, Hayashi K, Kitano M: Pathologic review of osteonecrosis in divers. Clin Orthop 130:107, 1978

75. Keret D, Harrison MHM, Clarke NM, Hall DJ: Coxa plana—the fate of physis. J Bone Joint Surg [Am] 66:870, 1984

76. Kienböck R: Concerning traumatic malacia of the lunate and its consequence: degeneration and compression fractures. Reprinted in Clin Orthop 149:4, 1980. Translated from Uber traumatische malazie des mondbeins und ihre Folgezustande: Entartungs formen und Kompression fraktures. Fortschr Geb Roentgenstr 16:78, 1910

77. Kutz J: Legg-Calve-Perthes disease—a symposium. Clin Orthop 150:1, 1980

78. Lagier R: Idiopathic aseptic necrosis of the femoral head: an anatompathological concept. p. 49. In Zinn WM (ed): Ischemic Necrosis of the Femoral Head in Adults. George Thieme, Stuttgart, 1971

79. Laing PG: The arterial supply of the adult humerus. J Bone Joint Surg [Am] 38:1105, 1956

80. Laing PG, Ferguson AB: Radiosodium clearance rates as indications of femoral head vascularity. J Bone Joint Surg [Am] 41:1409, 1959

81. Landin LA, Danielsson LG, Wattsgard C: Transient synovitis of the hip: its incidence, epidemiology and relation to Perthes disease. J Bone Joint Surg [Br] 69:238, 1987

82. Lee MLH: The intraosseous arterial pattern of the carpal lunate bone and its relation to avascular necrosis. Acta Orthop Scand 33:43, 1963

83. Lemperg RK, Arnoldi CC: The significance of intraosseous pressure in normal and disease states with special reference to intraosseous engorgement pain syndrome. Clin Orthop 136:143, 1978

84. Magid D: Femoral head avascular necrosis: CT assessment with multipower radiation. Radiology 157:751, 1985

85. Marcus ND, Enneking WF, Massam RA: The silent hip in idiopathic aseptic necrosis: treatment by bone grafting. J Bone Joint Surg [Am] 55:1351, 1973

86. McAndrew MP, Weinstein SL: Long term followup of Legg-Calve-Perthes disease. J Bone Joint Surg [Am] 66:860, 1984

87. McCallum RI: Aseptic necrosis of bone in compressed air workers. Decompression of Compressed Air Workers in Civil Engineering. p. 328. In McCallum, RI (ed): Oriel Press, Newcastle-upon-Tyne, 1965

88. McCallum RI, Walter DN, Barnes R, et al: Bone lesions in compressed air workers. J Bone Joint Surg [Br] 48:207, 1966

89. McCarthy EF: Aseptic necrosis of bone: a historic perspective. Clin Orthop 168:216, 1982

90. Mickelson MR, El-Khoury GY, Cass JR, Case KJ: Aseptic necrosis following slipped capital femoral epiphysis. Skeletal Radiol 4:129, 1979

91. Mickelson MR, McCurnin DM, Awbrey BJ, et al: Legg-Calve-Perthes disease in dogs: a comparison to human Legg-Calve-Perthes disease. Clin Orthop 157:287, 1981

92. Miles JS: The use of intramedullary bone pressure in the early determination of aseptic necrosis of the femoral head. J Bone Joint Surg [Am] 37:622, 1955

93. Mital M, Cohen J: So-called unresolved Osgood Schlatter lesion. J Bone Joint Surg [Am] 62A:732, 1980

94. Morrissey R: Hip fractures in children. Clin Orthop 152:202, 1980

95. Mulder J: The results of 100 cases of pseudoarthrosis in the scaphoid treated by Matti-Russe operation. J Bone Joint Surg [Br] 50:110, 1968

96. Mulfinger GL, Trueta J: The blood supply of the talus. J Bone Joint Surg [Br] 50:160, 1970

96a. Ohta Y, Matsunaga H: Bone lesions in divers. J Bone J Surg [Br] 56:3, 1974

97. Osterman K, Lindholm TS: Osteochondritis dissecans following Perthes disease. Clin Orthop 152:247, 1980

97a. Neer CS II: Displaced proximal humerus fractures, Pt 1. J Bone Joint Surg [Am] 52:1077, 1970

97b. Neer CS: Displaced proximal humerus fractures, Pt 2. J Bone Joint Surg [Am] 52:1090, 1970

98. Patterson RJ, Bickel WH, Dahlin DC: Idiopathic avascular necrosis of the head of the femur: a study of fifty-two cases. J Bone Joint Surg [Am] 46:267, 1964

99. Phemister DB: Changes in bones and joints resulting from interruption of circulation. I. General considerations in changes resulting from injuries. Arch Surg 41:436, 1934

100. Phemister DB: Changes in bones and joints resulting in interruption of circulation. II. Non-traumatic lesions in adults with bone infarction, arthritis deformans. Arch Surg 14:55, 1940

100a. Phemister DB: Treatment of the necrotic head of the femer in adults. J Bone J Surg [Am] 31A:55, 1949

101. Phemister DB: Fractures of neck of the femur, dislocations of hip and obscure disturbances producing aseptic necrosis of the head of the femur. Surg Gynecol Obstet 59:415, 1934

102. Philp RB, Inwood MJ, Warren BA: Interactions between gas bubbles and components of the blood: implications in decompression sickness. Aerospace Med 43:946, 1972

103. Pollack MS, Dalinka MK, Kressel HY: Magnetic resonance imaging in the evaluation of suspected osteonecrosis of the knee. Skeletal Radiol 16:121, 1987

104. Ponseti IV: Legg-Perthes disease. J Bone Joint Surg [Am] 38:739, 1956

105. Ponseti IV, Maynard JA, Weinstein SL, et al: Legg-Calve-Perthes disease: histochemical and ultrastructural observations of the epiphyseal cartilage and physis. J Bone Joint Surg [Am] 65:797, 1983

106. Ratliff AHC: Fractures of the neck of the femur in children. J Bone Joint Surg [Br] 44:528, 1962

107. Riggins RS, DeNardo GL, D'Ambrosia R, Goldman M: Assessment of circulation in the femoral head by F^{18} scintigraphy. J Nucl Med 15:183, 1974

108. Rodholm AK, Phemister DB: Cyst-like lesions of carpal bones, associated with ununited fractures, aseptic necrosis and traumatic arthritis. J Bone Joint Surg [Am] 30:1, 1948

109. Saito S, Inoue A, Ono K: Intramedullary hemorrhage as a possible cause of avascular necrosis of the femoral head. J Bone Joint Surg [Br] 69:346, 1987

110. Sevitt S: Avascular necrosis and revascularization of femoral head after intracapsular fractures. J Bone Joint Surg [Br] 46:270, 1964

111. Sevitt S, Thompson RB: Distribution and anastomosis of vessels supplying the head of the femur. J Bone Joint Surg [Br] 47:560, 1965

112. Sherman MS, Phemister DB: The pathology of ununited fractures of the neck of the femur. J Bone Joint Surg 29:19, 1947

113. Sherman MS, Selakovich W: Bone changes in chronic circulatory insufficiency. J Bone Joint Surg [Am] 39:892, 1957

114. Sierra A, Potchen EJ, Moore J, Smith HG: High field magnetic resonance imaging of septic necrosis of the talus. J Bone Joint Surg [Am] 68:927, 1986

115. Smith K, Bonfiglio M, Montgomery WJ: Non-traumatic necrosis of the femoral head treated with tibial bone grafting: a follow-up note. J Bone Joint Surg [Am] 62:845, 1980

116. Spencer RP, Lee YS, Sziklos JJ, et al: Failure of uptake of radiocolloid by the femoral heads: a diagnostic problem. J Nucl Med 24:116, 1983

117. Sprague B, Justis Jr EJ: Non-union of the carpal navicular — modes of treatment. Arch Surg 108:692, 1974

118. Springfield DS, Enneking WF: Surgery for aseptic necrosis. Clin Orthop 130:175, 1978

118a. Steinberg ME, Brighton CT, Steinberg DR, Tooze SE, Hayden GD: Treatment of a vascular necrosis of the femoral head by a combination of bone grafting, decompression, and electrical stimulation. Clin Orthop 186:137, 1984

119. Sutro CJ, Pomeranz MD: Perthes disease. Arch Surg 34:360, 1937

120. Taleisnik J, Kelly PJ: The extraosseous and intraosseous blood supply of the scaphoid bone. J Bone Joint Surg [Am] 48:1125, 1966

121. Tedeschi GD, Castelli W, Kropp G, Tedescho LG: Fat macroglobulinemia and fat embolism. Surg Gynecol Obstet 84:83, 1968

122. Thickman D, Axel L, Kressel HY, et al: Magnetic resonance imaging of avascular necrosis of the femoral head. Skeletal Radiol 15:133, 1986

123. Thomas CL, Gage JR, Ogden JA: Treatment concepts for proximal femur ischemic necrosis complicating congenital hip disease. J Bone Joint Surg [Am] 64:817, 1982

124. Thomas IH, Gregg PJ, Walder DN: Intra-osseous phlebography and intramedullary pressure in the rabbit femur. J Bone Joint Surg [Br] 64:239, 1982

125. Trueta J: The normal vascular anatomy of the human femoral head during growth. J Bone Joint Surg [Br] 39:358, 1957

126. Trueta J, Harrison MHM: The normal vascular anatomy of the femoral head in adult man. J Bone Joint Surg [Br] 35:442, 1953

127. Tucker FR: Arterial supply to the femoral head and its clinical importance. J Bone Joint Surg [Br] 31:82, 1949

128. Van Dam BE, Crider EJ, Noyes JD, Larsen LJ: Determination of the Catterall classification in Legg-Calve-Perthes. J Bone Joint Surg [Am] 63:906, 1981

129. Velayos EE, Leidholt J, Smyth CJ: Arthropathy associated with steroid therapy. Ann Intern Med 64:759, 1966

130. Weinstein S: Legg-Perthes disease. AAOS. Instructional Course Series 32. CV Mosby, St. Louis, 1983, p. 272

131. Weinstein SL, Ponseti IV: Congenital dislocation of the hip: open reduction through a medial approach. J Bone Joint Surg [Am] 61:119, 1979

132. White Jr RE, Omer Jr GE: Transient vascular compromise of the lunate after fracture dislocation of the carpus. J Hand Surg 9A(6):181, 1984

133. Woodhouse CF: Anoxia of the femoral head. Surgery 52:55, 1962

8

Arthritis

The subject of arthritis is so wide-ranging that in one chapter we of necessity must confine its focus if the material is to be useful. There are a few unfortunately but necessarily large books that attempt to "cover" the subject in the standard fashion of textbooks. Yet there are so many aspects of arthritis it is nearly impossible to provide a comprehensive exposition of each one even in a book of encyclopedic proportion. The text of the books listed in Chapter 11 is mostly devoted to medical (as opposed to surgical) considerations. In contrast, this chapter concentrates on the pathophysiology only of the surgical therapy. However, it should be understood that the surgeon perforce must have adequate appreciation of the nonsurgical considerations that pertain to each one of the arthritides if surgical therapy is to be properly applied. It is beyond the purview of this chapter to supply the reader with even the fundamentals, but it is expected that he or she has or will become familiar with them.

DEFINITIONS

Arthritis is strictly defined as inflammation of a joint, but the term is often used to designate conditions where the inflammation is not the essential process. Indeed, in some conditions where no inflammation is present it is used incorrectly. Nevertheless, it remains the accepted rubric under which the preponderance of joint lesions are classified. Attempts to avoid the suffix "itis" where the inflammation is secondary or negligible (e.g., arthrosis) have been unsuccessful. "Arthritis" in-

cludes many conditions that are so diverse as to require a separation of diagnostic categories.

In this chapter, we exclude much that relates to all forms of septic arthritis or tubercular arthritis, much of which was discussed in Chapter 2. It should be pointed out that many cases cured of the causative infection present conditions closely resembling osteoarthritis. We also exclude a large group of systemic diseases in which symptoms and sometimes signs indicate multiarticular irritation. These syndromes, e.g., palindromic rheumatism, polymyalgia rheumatica and Lyme disease, constitute a large fraction of the text of the books on arthritis listed in Chapter 11, and they are excluded here primarily because they require medical management nearly exclusively. Some of them could well be included in the first group of disorders under consideration, i.e., nonspecific arthritis.

We consider arthritides in the following groups: nonspecific,[63] rheumatoid,[21,27,44,48] traumatic,[23,36,38,40,53,59] osteoarthritic,[1,15,16,20-22,26,28,32,33,40,48,51,56,60,65] metabolic,[17] and miscellaneous.[13,14,18] In any one of these groups of conditions there may be a chronic or acute inflammatory process that is the most important pathological component, or the inflammation may be of secondary importance. Osteoarthritis and gout in particular illustrate this diversity. When the inflammation is secondary, the treatment must not be targeted primarily at the inflammation; rather, it should be directed at the etiological mechanism if possible. Obviously, treatment of the inflammation should never be neglected, even when it is of secondary importance.

333

NONSPECIFIC CONDITIONS

The surgeon often has the role of primary diagnostician. Patients who have symptoms and signs of an inflammatory condition in one or several joints may consult the surgeon without the ordinary triage provided by internists or generalists. The surgeon must determine if indeed there is significant inflammation in the joint, and if so what is causing the inflammatory or pseudoinflammatory reaction. Inflammation, as demonstrated in Chapter 2, can be caused by many agents, but one of the commonest diagnostic mistakes, as related to signs and symptoms localized to a single joint, is to miss a lesion in the neighboring tissues. Such a lesion may cause an irritation in the joint, whether it is a lesion in the bone (e.g., femoral neck), in an articular ligament (see case 2-2), or in the muscles or other soft tissues. The synovial membrane may be involved in the hyperemia or edema caused by the lesion. Indeed, if the lesion is osseous, there may be microfractures, and associated with them there may be a synovitis, in which case the synovitis could properly be called traumatic (see below).

In any case, the differential diagnosis of the monoarticular lesion is a demanding task. It may require not only routine radiographic examinations but also modalities such as computed tomography (CT), bone scans, or magnetic resonance imaging (MRI). Many, if not most, patients attribute the trouble to a vague or inconsequential injury that coincided with the onset of symptoms. This "association" should not deter the surgeon from considering, until proved otherwise, that the injury is a distraction. Evidence that there is a nonarticular lesion responsible for the articular symptoms and signs should always be sought. For example, traumatic synovitis and arthritis are valid, common entities, but they always are associated with a definite traumatic episode, immediately followed by symptoms and signs of sufficient severity as to leave no doubt of the etiological association.[53]

In the group of "nonspecific" arthritides and synovitises may be included those mentioned above: lesions adjacent to a joint that cause irritation of the synovial membrane — inflammation — which may prompt a thorough investigation that reveals no other cause for the irritation. Often, however, not even such a local lesion is demonstrable. When more than one joint is so affected, the synovitis may be associated with one of a rather large group of systemic conditions, e.g., systemic lupus erythematosus, or it may be one of a group of systemic conditions, none of which has surgical implications. Another lesion is para-articular or monoarticular idiopathic osteoporosis of the hip.[13] The synovitis may also be associated with one of several syndromes in which there are deformities of joints, e.g., acromegaly, or Hurler's disease.

All these multiarticular varieties of nonspecific synovitis or arthritis are of interest to the orthopedic surgeon, mostly because they test diagnostic acumen and require the development of testing regimens[12] to ferret out the true diagnosis; the assistance of an internist may be helpful when conducting that evaluation.

Aside from the ad hoc, and nearly always nonsurgical, symptomatic treatment of the joints affected with nonspecific inflammations, the orthopedic surgeon's conduct of the therapy should be confined to therapy nearly always of a conservative type, targeted at the local lesion(s) and therefore limited. The main limitation deserves strong emphasis. It pertains to the administration of drugs targeted at the affected joints. Aside from prescribing anodynes for pain as necessary, the orthopedic surgeon rarely should assume the responsibility for conducting a pharmacological regimen of therapy. That is an internist's responsibility, even as it pertains to such common drugs as steroids. Often a patient who has one of the diseases or syndromes evocative of nonspecific synovitis requires drugs with which orthopedic surgeons are unfamiliar; and when numerous medications, for perhaps a variety of medical conditions, are being taken by a single patient, one doctor (and it should be the internist) should be in charge of the medications lest drugs that cause harmful interactions are unwittingly prescribed.

It is evident that the synovitis in these cases represents a final common pathway, and the histological elements of the inflammation therefore are only the ultimate phenomena of a pathophysiological sequence that may have several disparate trains of events, all leading to the common cellular pattern of inflammation.[59,60] Perhaps there are pharmacological ways to inhibit or prevent the progression of these trains of events, but such matters should not be under consideration here, where mostly surgical considerations are under review.

Differential diagnosis is most difficult in cases in which only one joint is affected. Classifying a monoarticular synovitis or arthritis as "nonspecific" implies that some diagnostic measures have already been completed but have not revealed a *specific* etiological agent or pathogenetic mechanism. For example, the joint may have shown all the symptoms, signs, and chronology of a red-hot, acute inflammation, but the hemogram and erythrocyte sedimentation rate (ESR) were not indicative of sepsis, and the radiographs revealed little other than fluid in the joint. As another example, the symptoms, signs, and chronology may have been indicative of a chronic process, and the above diagnostic laboratory tests similarly were not indicative of a "specific" lesion. The diagnostic routine for each of these two instances may occupy a relatively short time, but during that interval the surgeon's thoughts should include an interpretation of the pathophysiology of the lesion. In the first case it is acute inflammation, whose progress may be rapid (see Ch. 2). Therefore additional diagnostic measures should not be delayed inordinately. In the second case, where the inflammation is chronic, delay for whatever reason is more acceptable.

Most patients with symptoms of arthritis (except pyogenic arthritis) do not require the surgical skills of an orthopedist until the chronic or late phase of the process is present. The orthopedist should be aware of the range of manifestations of the diseases that affect joints in order to assist in the evaluation and treatment by both nonsurgical and surgical means to preserve or restore function. These measures include, in addition to drug therapy, exercises to preserve function and strengthen muscles and aids in the form of splints or devices to minimize pain and to assist walking (canes, crutches, walker). Advice to the patient and the collaborating physicians on the expected course of the process is a critical component of the treatment during the early or intermediate phases of arthritis.

We need not spend much time exploring the theories of causation of the many varieties of nonspecific arthritis or synovitis, as the depth of knowledge is limited despite the voluminous literature on the subject. The reader is encouraged to consult one of the several texts on the subject (see Ch. 11) and the references at the end of this chapter.

We have mentioned the symptoms and signs of nonspecific inflammation in the discussion of interpretive skills in Chapter 1 when we cited the example of the patient with pain and effusion after a sprain of the knee. Again in Chapter 2 the subject is referred to in the discussion of pyogenic arthritis and other specific infections (tuberculous and fungal); and in Chapter 5 we touched on it with reference to posttraumatic arthritis of the radial head after an intra-articular fracture (Fig. 5-1). Finally, in Chapter 7 the subject arose in several instances of degenerative arthritis associated with aseptic necrosis of bone at various sites (see Figs. 7-15, 7-26, 7-29, 7-30, 7-34, 7-37, 7-38).

The orthopedic aspects of a patient with any one of the types of arthritis requires assessment of the degree of pain, the deformity, the restrictions of range of motion in each joint, and how each of these factors affects function. For comparison with end results after specific treatment, other diagnostic studies are emphasized in the cases used to illustrate the various kinds of arthritis.

As an introduction to the process, we have chosen three examples that illustrate the nonspecific conditions simulating arthritis and comment on those cited in previous chapters. We later emphasize the pathophysiological aspects of evaluation and surgical treatment of the more common forms of arthritis, i.e., rheumatoid and degenerative arthritis (primary and secondary). Only a few of the variations in either category that create problems for the orthopedist can be discussed in detail because of their nearly infinite variability.

It is not commonly appreciated that synovitis accompanies a number of benign lesion located near joints, e.g., osteoid osteoma and chondroblastoma, as well that which accompanies intra-articular conditions such as slipped capital femoral epiphysis, Legg-Calvé-Perthes disease, or osteochondritis dissecans.

Case 8-1 A 15-year-old boy for 8 months had had pain in the anterior aspect of the hip radiating to the thigh and knee. The pain, which was worse at night, was relieved by aspirin. The patient walked with an antalgic gait on the right. The thigh showed atrophy of the musculature. Tenderness was localized anteriorly and medially in the hip. Flexion,

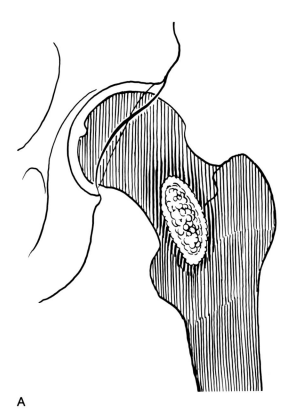

A

Fig. 8-1. Case 8-1. **(A)** Diagram of an AP radiograph of the right hip with a lesion in the base of the neck having features of an osteoid osteoma. **(B)** Gross specimens of the inflamed synovial membrane (right) and the excised osteoid osteoma (left). *(Figure continues.)*

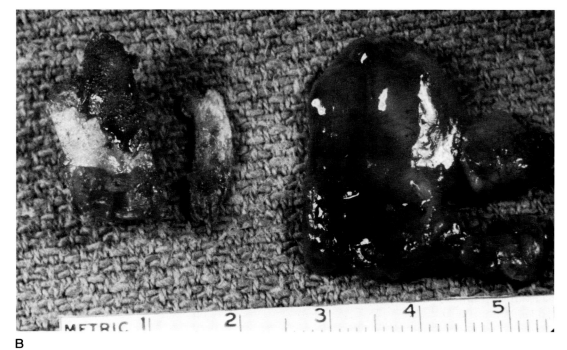

B

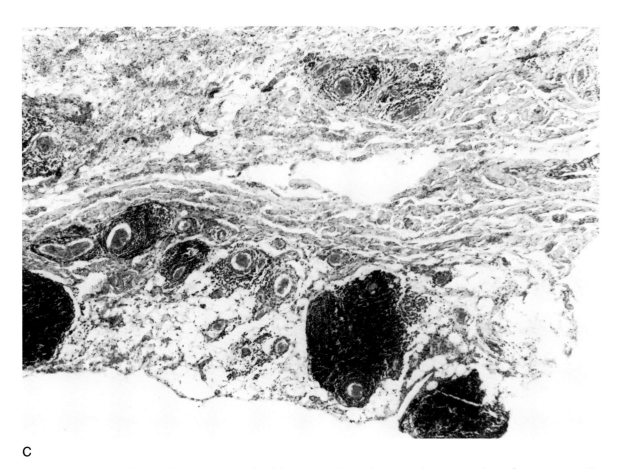

C

Fig. 8-1 *(Continued).* (C) Photomicrograph of the synovial membrane with perivascular inflammatory cells and a diffuse cellular infiltrate of the subsynovial layers.

abduction, and external rotation of the hip (**FABER** test or Patrick test) were painful. A radiograph of the right hip showed a lesion in the neck of the femur (Fig. 8-1A). The clinical and radiographic features are characteristic of an osteoid osteoma.

A gross photograph of the specimen shows a 1.5-cm lesion surrounded by the neck cortex on the left. On the right is an inflamed synovial membrane and visceral capsule (Fig. 8-1B). This acute synovitis is responsible for the symptoms of pain in the hip joint referred to the thigh and knee as well as the limitation of motion, particularly internal rotation because of the spasm of the small external rotators and the flexors of the hip.

The synovial membrane shows marked inflammation of the subsynovial layers with numerous follicular collections of lymphocytes in addition to the diffuse cellular infiltrate within the tissue (Fig. 8-1C). There are numerous capillaries throughout the membrane with a perivascular infiltrate of round cells. These findings are nonspecific.

Case 8-2 A 10-year-old girl had pain and limitation of motion of the shoulder of 1 year's duration. Radiographs of the shoulder showed a radiolucent lesion affecting the proximal humeral epiphysis (Fig. 8-2A). Histologically, it proved to be a chondroblastoma with an associated aneurysmal bone cyst.

A biopsy of the synovial membrane showed the increased vascularity and edematous nature of the reaction (Fig. 8-2B). There are small focal collections of inflammatory cells in perivascular areas as

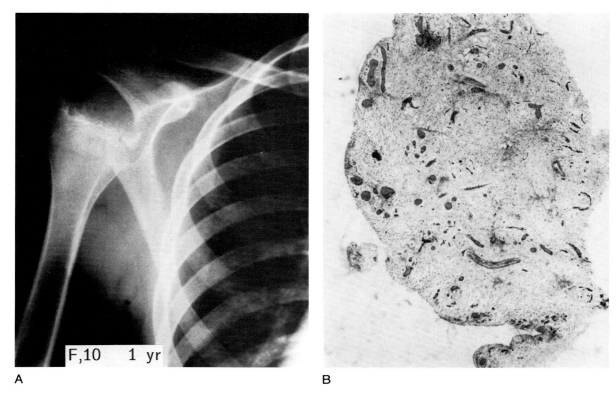

A   B

Fig. 8-2. Case 8-2. (A) Radiolucent lesion of the epiphysis of the right humerus (chondroblastoma). (B) Synovial membrane with focal collections of inflammatory cells (×27).

well as a diffuse but considerably less intense infiltrate of inflammatory cells in the rest of the tissue. The intensity of the inflammation is not nearly as marked as that in case 8-1, but it certainly accounts for some of the pain in this patient. The patient had persistent limitation of motion of the shoulder at the extremes of the range. Not infrequently, patients with epiphyseal chondroblastoma have difficulty recovering a full range of joint motion after curettage of the lesion, particularly those with lesions affecting the head of the humerus.

Case 8-3 A 10-year-old girl had complained of mild pain in the left hip and thigh for 2 months after a minor injury. She was unable to walk without a limp. One day before admission, she developed acute pain in the groin and thigh and could no longer walk. A radiograph of the pelvis demonstrated an acute slipped capital femoral epiphysis on the left (Fig. 8-3A). Because it was thought to be an acute injury, open reduction and pinning with

threaded pins was performed. At the time of arthrotomy the synovial membrane appeared to be inflamed and markedly engorged, so a biopsy was performed.

The microscopic section showed hyperemia, perivascular collections of lymphocytes, and synovitis with a diffuse lymphocytic infiltrate (Fig. 8-3B). The patient developed a chondrolysis syndrome of the left hip and had restricted function of that hip. Two years later, when spontaneous onset of right hip pain occurred because of a mild slip (Fig. 8-3C), in situ pinning of that hip was performed.

The presence of synovitis in slipped capital epiphysis may not only precede the radiological evidence of slip, it may contribute to the development of the chondrolysis that occurs in some of these patients by interfering with nutrition to the cartilage.

In each of these three examples of nonspecific

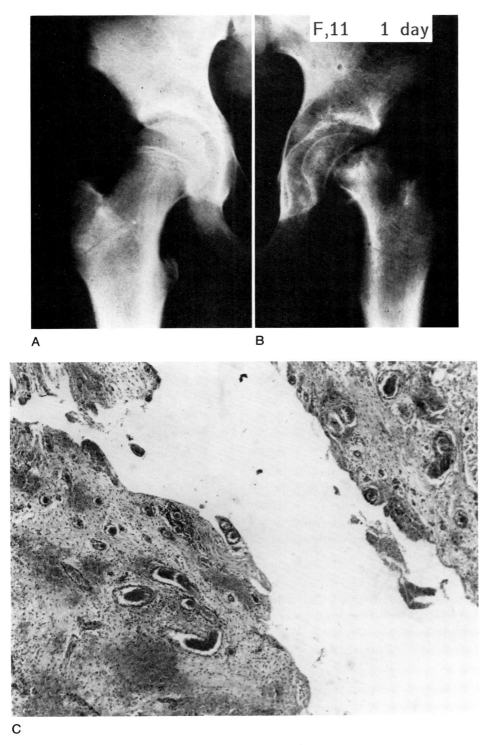

A

B

C

Fig. 8-3. Case 8-3. **(A)** AP radiograph of an acute slipped capital femoral epiphysis. **(B)** Radiograph of the right hip with a mild slipped capital femoral epiphysis. **(C)** Synovitis with hyperemia. Note the perivascular collections of lymphocytes (×25). **(A&B** from Ponseti and McClintock,[53a] with permission.)

synovitis simulating arthritis, the orthopedist's role is clearly that of determining the condition causing the irritation and then treating it by appropriate surgical treatment of the lesion.

Rheumatoid Arthritis

We now turn our attention to the more familiar form of primary arthritis, i.e., rheumatoid arthritis.[21,44,48] Consider a patient who presented with a diagnostic problem. Initially the differential diagnosis rested between a nonspecific arthritis and a specific form of infectious arthritis such as tuberculous arthritis. (At one time tuberculosis was a more common disease than at present.)

Case 8-4   A 25-year-old woman presented with an insidious onset of pain and swelling of the left knee of 6 months' duration. The patient began to limp and to restrict her activities. The pain, which was moderately severe and required aspirin for partial relief, was aggravated by activity, particularly walking, standing, or going up and down stairs. The knee showed parapatellar swelling (Fig. 8-4A), and there was atrophy of the left thigh and restriction of knee flexion and extension because of pain and swelling. The patella was ballottable in the extended position of the knee. The joint was warm to touch, and the margins of the articular surfaces were tender to palpation. The synovial lining felt somewhat thickened particularly at the joint margins and the suprapatellar pouch. Synovitis of undetermined origin was the working diagnosis.

Because of the tenderness at the joint margins, rigorous manipulation to test for ligamentous instability or meniscal injury was not performed. The knee, however, was stable in all planes on gentle testing. The hemogram and ESR were not indicative of sepsis. An AP radiograph of the knee (Fig. 8-4B) was remarkable for the presence of reduced bone density that was both generalized and intensified in the subchondral cortex in particular; other views confirmed this feature.

At this point a consideration of possible causes for these findings should direct our further evaluation and essential treatment. The absence of a history of injury would exclude some form of internal derangement of the knee related to trauma, as would the lack of obvious instability of the knee. A

meniscal injury could cause pain and swelling of the knee as a persistent or late manifestation but would be excluded by the lack of a history of prior injury. One should consider infection of the knee as a possibility and inquire concerning the possible sources of entry of bacteria or other organisms into the body from the skin, respiratory tract, or genitourinary tract or from contact with an infected person. Prior infections or prior treatment of any inflammation would be evaluated as discussed earlier (see Ch. 2). Maintenance of the integrity of the articular cartilage would likely exclude an untreated pyogenic infection but not necessarily a tuberculous, fungal, or inadequately treated pyogenic arthritis (including a gonococcal infection). The findings could fit an early rheumatoid arthritis equally well. Aspiration of the synovial fluid and its analysis might be considered by some as the next diagnostic maneuver to give a clue about the process within the joint, but more than likely it would not be diagnostic.[57a] Nevertheless, aspiration and cultures were performed.

The patient's tuberculin test applied at the time of initial examination after a week proved to be positive. The source of the infection probably was contact with a relative with tuberculosis. The joint aspirate had been inoculated into a guinea pig, which test was negative for tuberculous infection. Because of the uncertainty of the diagnosis, an open biopsy was performed. At the time of arthrotomy there was an obvious granulation tissue pannus over the margin of the joint (Fig. 8-4C). The articular cartilage was smooth and shiny in the nonmarginal areas. The synovial membrane was markedly hyperemic. The subchondral bone was noted to be porotic when a segment of the margin of the joint and a piece of the synovial membrane were biopsied.

A microscopic section of the pannus and the margin of the joint showed normal joint cartilage for the most part except at the edge, where there was an overgrowth of the vascular cellular fibrous tissue into the cartilage surface (Fig. 8-4D). The pannus did not penetrate deeply into the joint cartilage. The underlying bone was being resorbed by nonspecific granulation tissue containing an infiltrate of lymphocytes (Fig. 8-4E). The subchondral cortex resorption by granulation tissue accounts for the radiographic radiolucency in that area. The synovial membrane showed marked inflammatory infiltrates and in particular an increase in lymphocytes and increased vascularity (Fig. 8-4F). Fibrin accumulations were present in folds of the membrane. The findings were interpreted to indicate the presence of nonspecific synovitis and arthritis but not tuberculosis despite the positive tuberculin test. The absence of the characteristic granulomas of tuberculosis and the inability to find acid-fast bacteria in the sections supported that interpretation.

It should be noted that the acute and subacute stages of a number of arthritides present with a similar pathophysiological process.[44] They include rheumatoid arthritis, tuberculosis, and an acute posttraumatic arthritis. Other conditions that can simulate this picture are the chemical arthritides, e.g., chondrocalcinosis and gout. These conditions have in common an acute or subacute synovitis that produces an effusion and restricts joint function. It is a response to changes in the tissues — an inflammatory response within the synovial membrane and a hyperemia within the bony structures — that account for the loss of the subchondral cortex by resorption as noted radiologically and histologically (Figs. 8-4C&E).

Within a few months the patient in case 8-4 developed pain, stiffness, and swelling of other joints (ankles and wrists). She therefore met all of the American Rheumatism Association requirements for the diagnosis of rheumatoid arthritis. She was treated initially with exercise and nonsteroidal analgesics and later with courses of gold therapy, which failed, as did all the other forms of medical treatment that were prescribed. The effusion and thickening of the synovial membrane of her knee remained painful and was the most restricting feature of the disease.

When a patient has a poor response to local and systemic treatment and has minimal to moderate radiographic changes in one or two major joints (i.e., the presence of the joint cartilage and few secondary degenerative changes), the surgeon should consider synovectomy, a procedure designed to reduce the effects of the rheumatoid inflammation. Removal of as much inflamed synovial tissue and pannus as can be conveniently exposed reduces the volume of degradative enzymes being elaborated. It also removes some of the mechanical impediment to motion of the joint. Lastly, it minimizes the number of those cells that are precursors to fibroblasts: i.e., it reduces the scarring that would evolve if and when the inflammation subsides. The results are variable in the short term.[27] Synovectomy can provide relief of symptoms and signs as an interim procedure for young patients and for some older patients in the early stages of the disease. If and when that fails, a total joint replacement can be done.

The more extensive destruction of the knee in the next patient made synovectomy an inappropriate procedure.

Case 8-5   The radiographs of an 18-year-old woman who had multiple joints affected by the disease over a 12-year period show extreme atrophy of the bones of the hand, notching at the metacarpal heads, and subluxations at the metacarpophalangeal (MP) joint of the index finger and at the proximal interphalangeal (PIP) joint of the thumb (Fig. 8-5A). There is soft tissue swelling at the wrist and at the distal end of the ulna.

This patient, because of multiple sites of involvement, presented a problem for the surgeon, i.e., how to plan the treatment and when to execute each surgical procedure when a sequence is in order. Consultation with the rheumatologist concerning the patient's general medical status and response to drug treatment is an essential component of that planning. Those functions necessary for activities of daily living (eating, dressing, toilet care, sleeping) take priority over those of walking or sitting. Over a 12-year period this patient had been confined to a bed and chair existence and had developed contractures in the knees, hips, and elbows. Because of the progressive nature of her disease and a poor response to drug therapy despite attempts to splint the affected joints in a functional position, surgical treatment was necessary. The surgical plan was to correct the worse of the knee contractures by a fusion preceded by resection of the distal end of the ulna. (This patient was being treated before total joint arthroplasty was developed.) These two operations were designed to address two major problems: the patient's inability to lie in bed comfortably and to pronate and supinate the forearm. For better upper limb function, it was necessary to improve thumb function. The hyperextended thumb at the interphalangeal

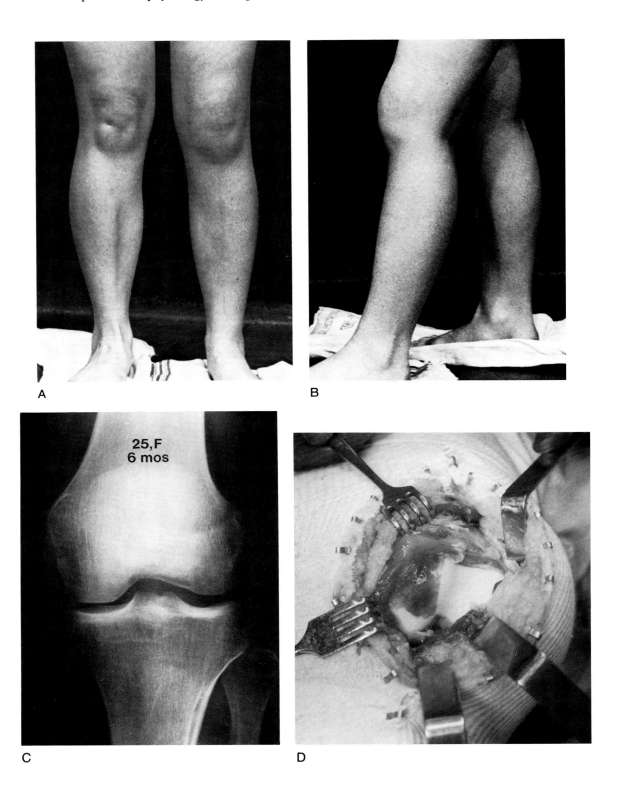

A

B

C

D

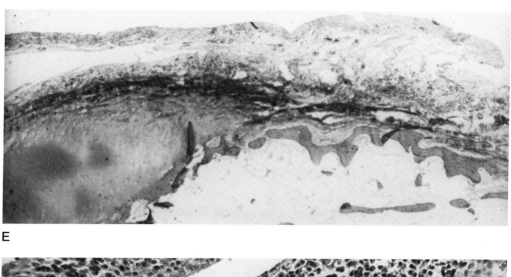

E

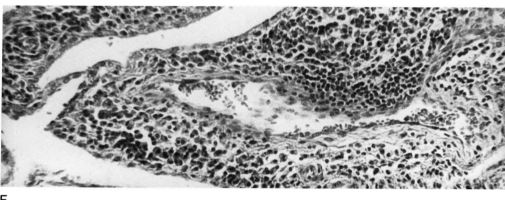

F

Fig. 8-4. Case 8-4. **(A&B)** Swelling of the left knee with atrophy of the left thigh and calf. **(C)** AP radiograph of the left knee with reduced bone density of the subchondral cortex in particular. **(D)** Pannus of the femoral condyle. **(E)** Margin of the articular cartilage with the overlying pannus and thinning of the subchondral cortex ($\times$4). **(F)** Synovial membrane shows marked inflammatory infiltration, mostly lymphocytes ($\times$40).

joint was to be fused in 5° to 10° of flexion. A more stable pinch between the thumb and index finger would then be possible. This patient had developed a destructive painful deformity of the wrists, the well known ulnar deviation and palmar flexion. An arthrodesis of that joint on the right was planned because it is often preferable to arthroplasty. The unpredictable results of an arthroplasty have been documented.

Because both wrists were affected and fusion of both was contraindicated because then they could neither flex or extend, the fusion was done on the right as the first procedure in the surgical se-

quence; the other procedure, fusion of the interphalangeal joint of the thumb, on the right upper extremity followed. After they had been completed and postoperative rehabilitation was well under way, attention was directed at the lower extremities.

The character and sequence of operations in this case is a fine illustration of the intimate relation between the timing of the procedures and the objectives. At the time the patient was under treatment, any objective that included achievement of independent ambulation would have been impossible because of the patient's years at bed rest and

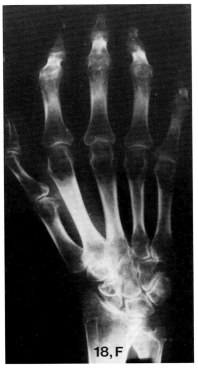

A

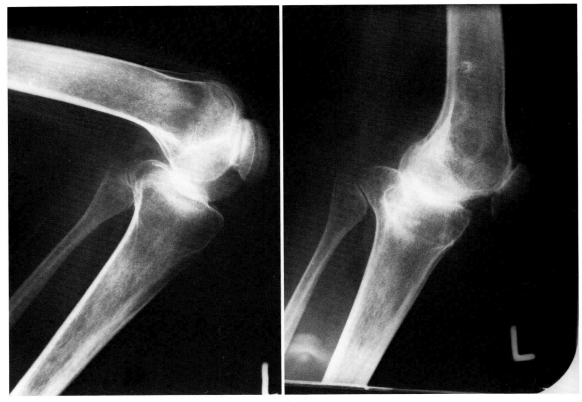

B   C

Fig. 8-5. Case 8-5. (A) AP radiograph of the hand with extreme disuse atrophy of periarticular bone. The MP joints show notching of the metacarpal heads. (B) Lateral radiograph of the left knee with flexion contracture. (C) Lateral radiograph of the left knee after skeletal traction. (*Figure continues.*)

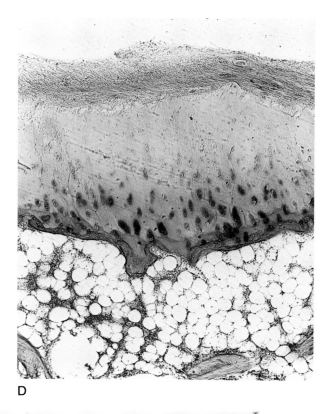

Fig. 8-5 *(Continued)*. **(D)** Photomicrograph of the articular surface of the left knee removed at the time of fusion with a fibrous pannus over the articular surface. The subchondral cortex is thin (×40). **(E)** Another area shows loss of articular cartilage, eburnation, and partial replacement by granulation tissue. Trabeculae have been resorbed in the cancellous bone. **A** diffuse lymphocytic infiltrate is present within the fatty marrow (×40).

D

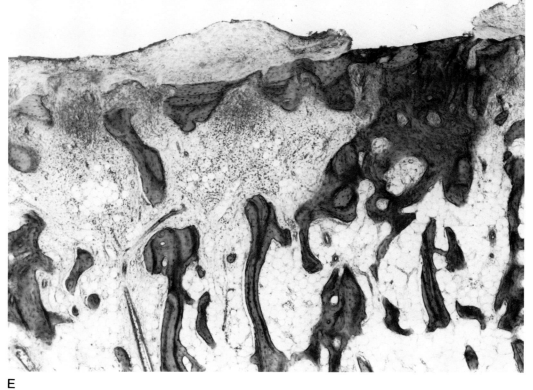

E

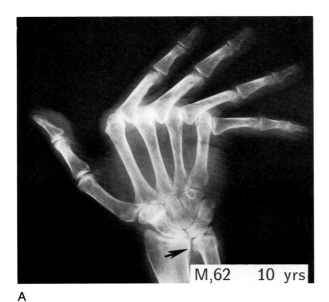

A

Fig. 8-6. Case 8-6. **(A)** AP radiograph of the hand and wrist shows notching of the distal end of the ulna and narrowing of the radial ulnar joint (arrow). **(B)** Photomicrograph of a resected distal ulna from another patient shows marked proliferation of the synovial membrane and erosion and notching between the articular cartilage and the ulnar styloid ($\times 2$). *(Figure continues.)*

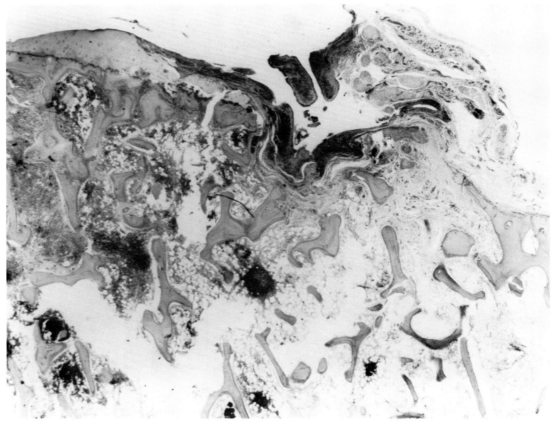

B

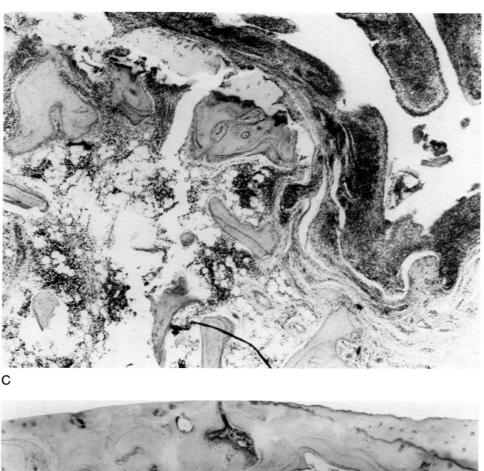

C

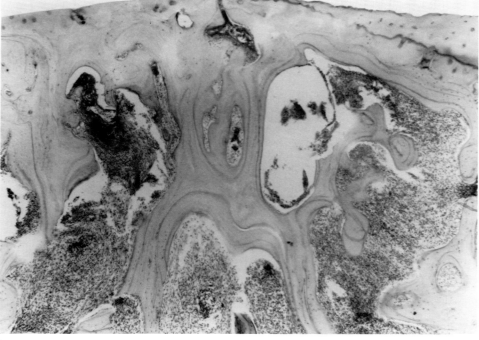

D

Fig. 8-6 *(Continued).* (C) Pannus over the margin of the articular cartilage (×20). (D) Eroded articular cartilage replaced by eburnated bone and subchondral marrow spaces with marked follicular collections of lymphocytes and plasma cells (×40).

the involvement of many major joints of the lower extremities. Therefore one objective was to increase the patient's comfort in bed, and even that was not as important as making her more self-sufficient by improving the function of her upper extremities. With today's state of the art and, in particular, the development of total joint arthroplasty, achievement of ambulation would not be easily dismissed. If it were contemplated, the operations on the upper extremities would still take precedence chronologically, but their character well might be targeted, not only at the activities of daily living that have been mentioned but also at use of crutches or canes.

The flexion contractures of both knees were treated by traction; and as gradual correction became evident, short periods of plaster cast immobilization were used to maintain the correction. The right knee ultimately had a useful range of motion; the left knee did not. Lateral radiographs of the left knee before traction shows a flexion contracture of 90° (Fig. 8-5B), and after traction there is loss of the articular cartilage (Fig. 8-5C).

A fusion of the left knee was then performed. At surgery the articular surfaces showed marked destruction. The articular cartilage was completely resorbed in some areas, and photomicrographs of one of those areas (Fig. 8-5D) show the complete loss of the articular cartilage and replacement of the subchondral cortex and cartilage by fibrous and granulation tissue (Fig. 8-5E).

In this case of rheumatoid arthritis, and in most cases that are of even moderate severity, it is apparent that the process progressed and aggressively affected all aspects of the joint. The proliferating synovial membrane, inhibiting motion of the joint in addition to growing over the cartilage as a pannus, allowed ligaments to shorten and scarring to develop deforming forces. The next three cases illustrate these deformities, as well as associated pathophysiological phenomena of surgical importance.

Case 8-6   A 62-year-old man had had rheumatoid arthritis of 10 years' duration. Changes in the metacarpals and other bones manifested as notching (Fig. 8-6A) from pressure erosion at the margins by the synovial tissue (Fig. 8-6B) and destruction of cartilage by the overlying pannus at the MP and PIP joints of the hand and the distal end of the ulna (Fig. 8-6C). Other radiographic changes included re-

sorption of the underlying subarticular cortex of the radius and similar changes at the distal radioulnar joint.

Case 8-7   A 59-year-old woman had had rheumatoid arthritis for 10 years at the time a total hip replacement was done for pain and loss of function in the right hip. A radiograph (Fig. 8-7A) and photomicrograph (Fig. 8-7B) of a specimen of the removed femoral head showed the chronic effects of that disease on the femoral head. There were marginal osteophytes but not extensive ones. Loss of articular cartilage in a number of areas was obvious, as was diffuse atrophy of the bony trabeculae.

A photomicrograph of one of the areas where articular cartilage remained shows inflammatory pannus on the surface of that cartilage with marked thinning of the subchondral cortex and narrow trabeculae (Fig. 8-7C).

The marked bony atrophy created special problems in the surgical treatment. The presence of central acetabular protrusion of the femoral head required that the surgeon use either a large amount of methylmethacrylate to support the acetabular cup, a large cup, a bone graft (autograft or allograft), or some combination of these three techniques. Each technique presents different pathophysiological considerations and biomechanical advantages or disadvantages. Only a few may be mentioned: the limited useful life of methylmethacrylate, the limited availability of autografts of suitable size and shape, the questionable survival of allografts, and the increased frictional force when a large cup is used. The evolution of the best combination requires well controlled studies with long-term follow-up. At least 5 years of follow-up are needed to demonstrate survival of the methacrylate or the graft.

Case 8-8   An unusual manifestation of proliferative synovitis associated with rheumatoid arthritis is illustrated by this patient. A 41-year-old man with known chronic rheumatoid polyarthritis had had pain and limitation of motion related to the right hip for almost 2 years. The radiolucent (i.e., "cystic") defect in the right femoral neck and head resulted from elaboration of large volumes of intra-articular fluid that exerted pressure on the rheumatoid synovial membrane of the joint. At some point on the femoral head, the rheumatoid inflamed tissue caused resorption of the thin cortex; then intermittently, as the disease exacerbated,

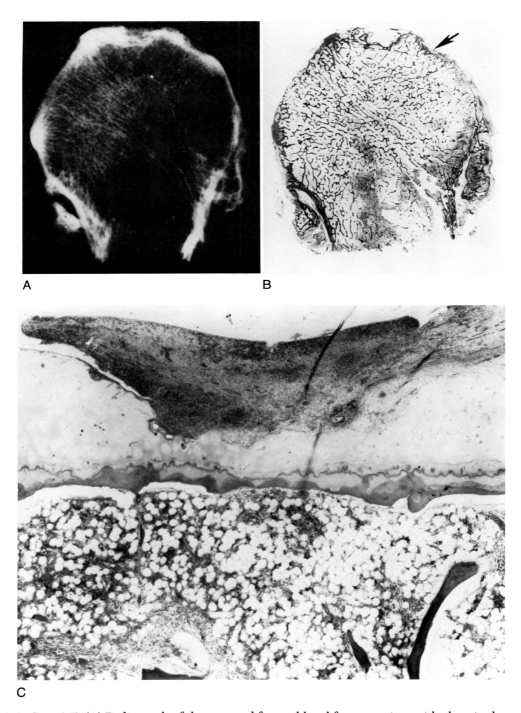

A

B

C

Fig. 8-7. Case 8-7. (**A**) Radiograph of the resected femoral head from a patient with chronic rheumatoid arthritis. (**B**) Specimen of the femoral head with marked atrophy of the trabecular structure and loss of articular cartilage with pannus in a number of areas (arrow). (**C**) Inflammatory pannus along the surface of one of the areas (arrow) adjacent to remaining articular cartilage (×40).

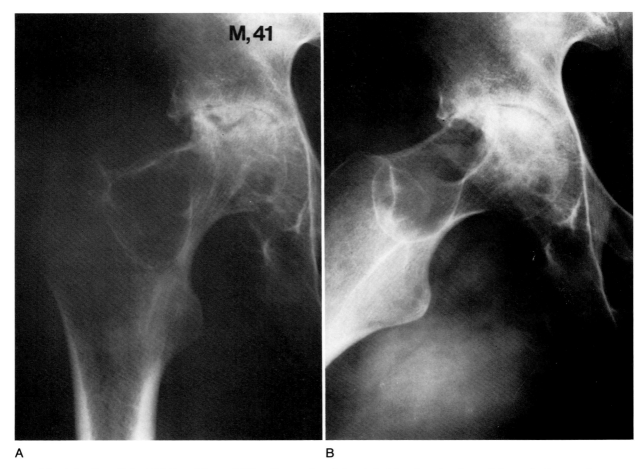

Fig. 8-8. Case 8-8. AP (**A**) and lateral (**B**) radiographs of the right hip, showing loss of the articular cartilage space and erosions of the neck of the femur. *(Figure continues.)*

fluid formed in the joint and pressure was exerted on the decorticated spot, causing more resorption and formation of a cyst that communicated with the joint. This situation is an unusual osseous manifestation of the disease (Figs. 8-8A,B). The loss of articular cartilage and the increase in acetabular and femoral head density reflect secondary degenerative changes. Grossly, the cyst extended from the articular margin of the synovial membrane to the base of the femoral neck. A photomicrograph of the wall of the cyst showed the characteristic rheumatoid changes in the synovial lining with a rheumatoid nodule within it (Fig. 8-8C). The synovial membrane was hyperemic and contained many inflammatory cells and evidence of bone fragments as part of wear debris (Fig. 8-8D). Rheumatoid cysts may involve soft tissues to a large extent (e.g., extension of a popliteal rheumatoid cyst down the calf to the ankle) but rarely produce the extensive bony change.

It is apparent that the clinical manifestations of rheumatoid arthritis in each patient at any point in time depend on the particular time in the process that the surgeon first sees the patient. The orthopedist would therefore be likely to be involved as a diagnostician in the evaluation of those instances of rheumatoid arthritis that do not have the classical clinical and radiological picture that makes the diagnosis easy for the rheumatologist or the generalist. Those clinicians might ask the orthopedic surgeon to consider a biopsy for diagnosis as well as for advice on treatment. The surgical treatment

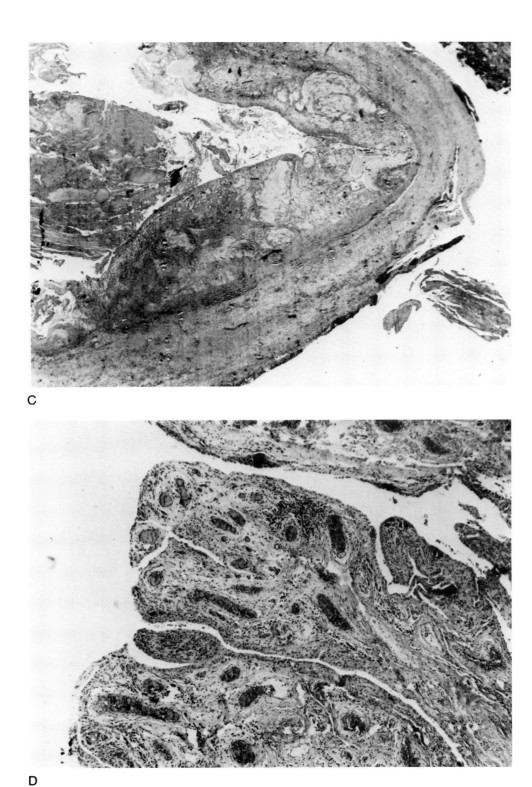

C

D

Fig. 8-8 *(Continued).* (**C**) Rheumatoid cyst membrane (×10). (**D**) Synovial membrane with wear debris, hyperemia, and a diffuse inflammatory infiltrate (×40).

elected in some instances might be one that prevents further destructive effects of the synovial membrane,[27] e.g., synovectomy as illustrated in case 8-4 above, procedures to correct contractures or deformities by arthrodesis, tendon transfers, or yet other procedures to restore function by an arthroplasty appropriate to the situation. In some patients any or all of these methods may be used. In case 8-8, excision of the "cyst" and grafts of the defect with autologous bone was the procedure followed.

Rheumatoid arthritis affects the hands and the feet all too commonly and often such involvement constitutes the major cause for functional impairment. The surgical rehabilitation of those anatomical sites requires attention to the site as a whole, rather than to individual joints; and for that reason the procedures targeted at those sites are multiarticular, e.g., excision of several metatarsophalangeal joints to allow more comfortable weightbearing or wearing of shoes, or excision of metacarpophalangeal joints to correct deformities and improve grasp. The pathophysiological principles do not differ from those applicable to the larger joints, as illustrated in the cases presented.

Degenerative Arthritis

The number of diagnoses of primary degenerative arthritis[1,3,6,7,12,15,16,20,22,26,28,31,32,33,34,35,39,48,51,55,56,64] is decreasing as knowledge about arthritis secondary to preexisting conditions increases.[17,18,23,26,43,53,58,62,65,67,68,69] Most patients seen by orthopaedic surgeons have arthritis of the secondary type. We have already commented on arthritis due to trauma or aseptic necrosis, and rheumatoid arthritis. The following examples illustrate the wide range of manifestations of this group of conditions and depict its pathophysiology.

Case 8-9 A 57-year-old farmer had a 1-year history of pain in the right hip of insidious onset; the pain was intermittent and worse with activity. He could not recall a specific injury to the hip. The pain was relieved by nonsteroidal anti-inflammatory medication. He walked with a limp and had discomfort at the extremes of the range of motion of the right hip, but motion was limited only a few degrees. At the time of the initial examination the

left hip was not painful and had a full range of motion. The radiograph showed only minimal narrowing of the articular cartilage space of the right hip. The left hip appeared normal (Fig. 8-9A). He was continued on medication and the use of a cane for protection of the right hip. Nine months later progressive degenerative changes had developed in the right hip manifested by more narrowing of the articular cartilage space. There also was lateral subluxation of the right hip and an increase in the subchondral cortical density. Minimal marginal osteophytes had become evident (Fig. 8-9B). The left hip also had developed increased density of the acetabular cortex but was still asymptomatic, despite narrowing of the cartilage space and slight lateral displacement of the femoral head.

Eighteen months later, the patient was unable to work and used crutches or a cane to walk short distances. His pain was not controlled by medication. The radiographs showed marked narrowing of the articular cartilage space in both hips (Fig. 8-9C). The density of the femoral head and acetabular bone was increased. The femoral head was flattened, and marginal osteophytes had developed on it. In addition, large medial acetabular osteophytes were evident bilaterally. Both of the femoral heads were subluxated laterally and had degenerative cysts (Fig. 8-9C). A total hip replacement was first performed on the right and 2 months later on the left. Grossly, the right femoral head showed severe eburnation with marginal osteophytes. A cut section of the gross specimen showed the flattened eburnated articular surface, degenerative cysts, and marginal osteophytes (Fig. 8-9D), and the specimen radiograph (Fig. 8-9E) amplified those findings (Fig. 8-9F). The content of the cyst was mucoid material (Fig. 8-9G); bony repair was evident at the margins of the cyst, the reaction being similar to that underneath the area of eburnation of the articular surface that was undergoing bone repair at its margin (Fig. 8-9H). The large marginal osteophytes were composed of bone with a fibrocartilaginous surface. Underneath the surface was cancellous new bone and marrow (Fig. 8-9I). In some of the areas where remnants of the articular cartilage existed, there was fissuring and fibrillation of that cartilage (Fig. 8-9J) and clumping (cloning) of the chondrocytes. There also was focal subchondral erosion by vascular granulation tissue (Fig. 8-9K). The capsule and synovial mem-

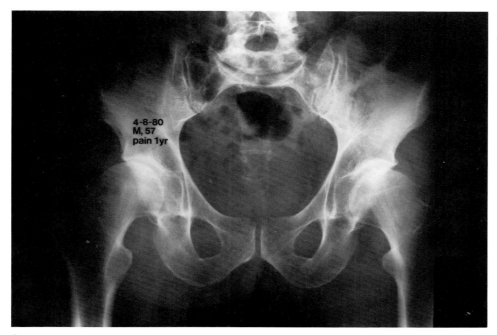

A

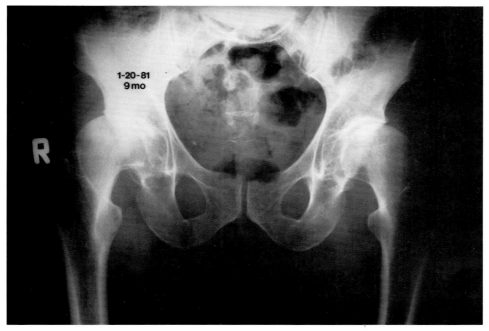

B

Fig. 8-9. Case 8-9. (A) Radiograph of the pelvis showing minimal loss of articular cartilage space in the right hip after the patient had had pain for 1 year. (B) Note the marked loss of articular cartilage space in the right hip 9 months later. *(Figure continues.)*

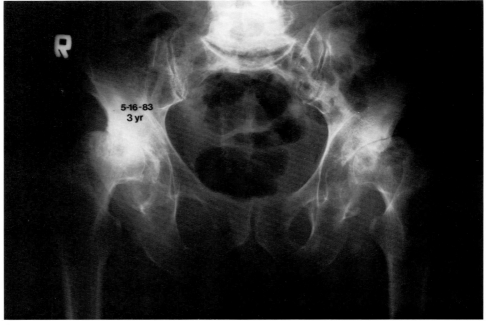

C

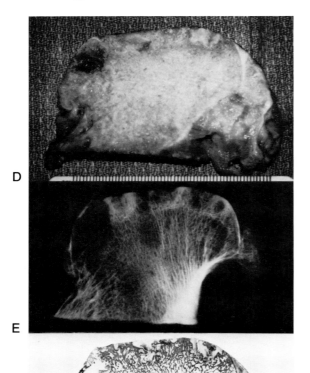

D

E

F

Fig. 8-9 *(Continued)*. (C) Three years later both hips display loss of articular cartilage space and secondary marginal osteophytes. (D–F) Gross specimen (D), radiograph of a split femoral head (E), and photomicrograph (F) demonstrate the correlation of osteophytes, eburnated surface, and subchondral degenerative cysts (×1). *(Figure continues.)*

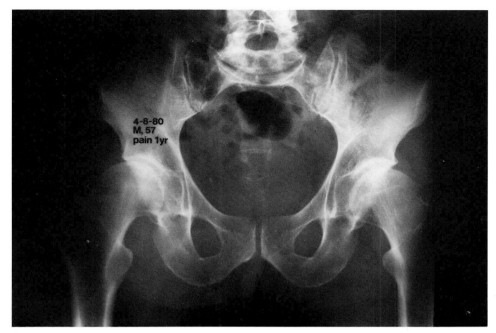

A

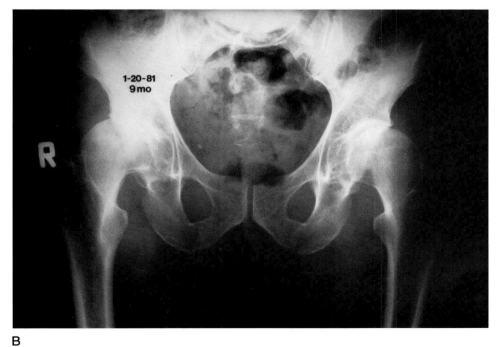

B

Fig. 8-9. Case 8-9. **(A)** Radiograph of the pelvis showing minimal loss of articular cartilage space in the right hip after the patient had had pain for 1 year. **(B)** Note the marked loss of articular cartilage space in the right hip 9 months later. *(Figure continues.)*

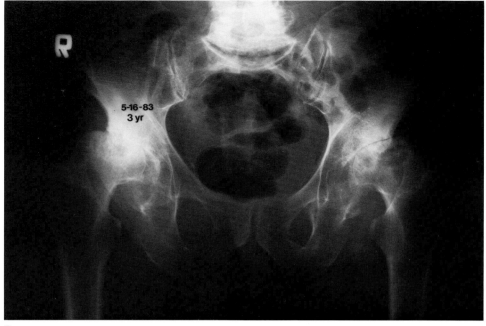

C

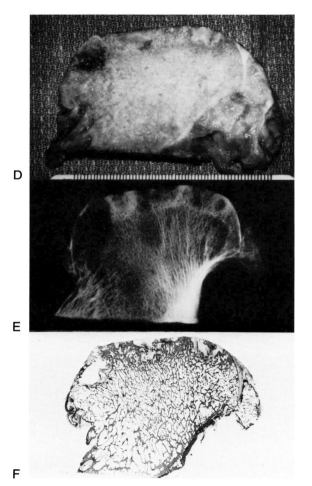

D

E

F

Fig. 8-9 *(Continued)*. (C) Three years later both hips display loss of articular cartilage space and secondary marginal osteophytes. (D–F) Gross specimen (D), radiograph of a split femoral head (E), and photomicrograph (F) demonstrate the correlation of osteophytes, eburnated surface, and subchondral degenerative cysts (×1). *(Figure continues.)*

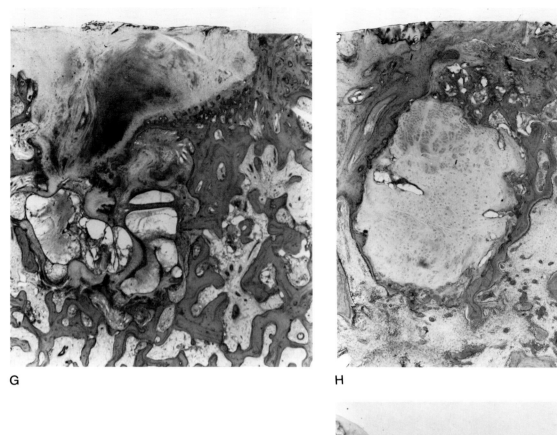

G

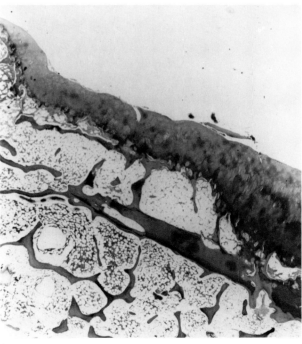

H

I

Fig. 8-9 *(Continued).* (**G**) Mucoid degenerative cyst (×14). (**H**) Degenerative cyst undergoing marginal ossification and repair (×14). (**I**) Marginal osteophyte with extensive fibrocartilaginous repair on the surface and underlying cancellous new bone and marrow (×27). *(Figure continues.)*

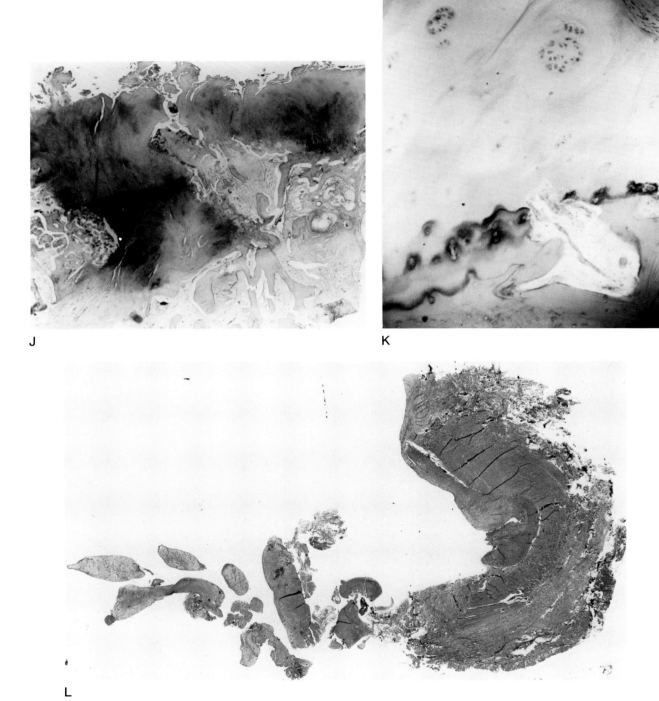

Fig. 8-9 *(Continued)*. **(J)** Fissuring and fibrillation of articular cartilage (×20). **(K)** Note the erosion of subchondral cortex by vascular granulation tissue (×100). **(L)** Proliferation of synovial membrane and capsule into the villous fronds (×4).

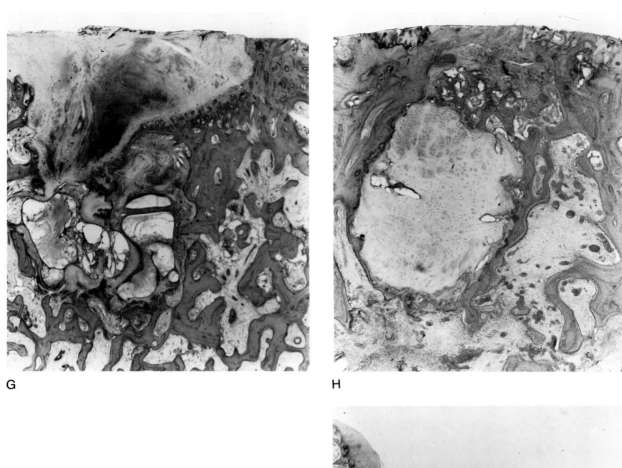

G

H

Fig. 8-9 *(Continued).* **(G)** Mucoid degenerative cyst (×14). **(H)** Degenerative cyst undergoing marginal ossification and repair (×14). **(I)** Marginal osteophyte with extensive fibrocartilaginous repair on the surface and underlying cancellous new bone and marrow (×27). *(Figure continues.)*

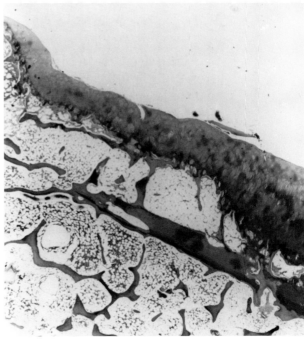

I

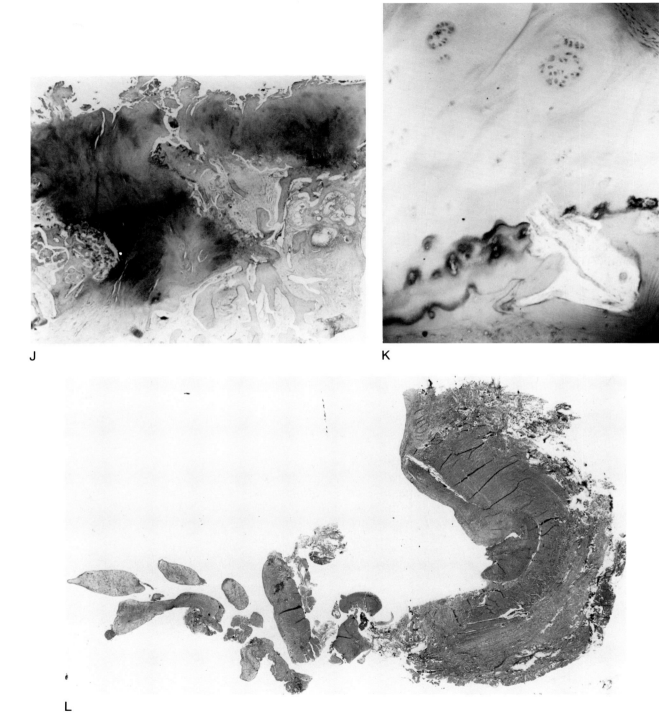

Fig. 8-9 *(Continued)*. **(J)** Fissuring and fibrillation of articular cartilage (×20). **(K)** Note the erosion of subchondral cortex by vascular granulation tissue (×100). **(L)** Proliferation of synovial membrane and capsule into the villous fronds (×4).

brane showed extensive villous formation (Fig. 8-9L) with some proliferation of the synovial cells but much less than was evident in the cases of rheumatoid arthritis.

Features of Osteoarthritis

All the features of the osteoarthritis described in case 8-9 and illustrated in Figure 8-9 merit discussion as a pathophysiological continuum. They can be conveniently considered under seven headings: (1) radiographic narrowing of the cartilage space; (2) increased bony density; (3) flattened femoral head; (4) marginal osteophytes; (5) subluxation; (6) cysts; and (7) reaction in the synovial membrane. It should be emphasized that these seven features do not occur as a sequence over time but interact as the lesion develops.

Radiographic Narrowing of Cartilage Space
Narrowing of the cartilage "space" is a diminution of the width of radiolucency between the femoral head and the acetabular wall. It represents a loss of cartilage matrix and histologically would reveal those changes that were evident on the remains of cartilage (Fig. 8-9J), i.e., fissuring, fibrillation, and chondrocytic changes (clumping). Undoubtedly, these morphological changes would have been preceded by chemical change in the cartilage matrix and, because of the chemical change, changes in the physical properties of the matrix such that it would undergo abnormal wear.[35] The fibrillation undoubtedly would cause sloughing of small bits of cartilage, which might well be responsible for some synovial irritation (see below) and the intermittent pain the patient experienced.

Increased Bony Density
Once the fissures in the cartilage reach the bony subchondral plate, they generate a repair reaction, i.e., produce more bone. One theory has it that even before the fissure develops to the depth mentioned the change in physical properties of the cartilage and its narrowing allow excessive loads to be transmitted to the bone, causing microfractures. The reaction to those processes is the production of callus. The radiological consequence in either event is increased subchondral density. As the fis-

suring and wear progress, the cartilage erodes and the bone underneath it becomes more dense. Thus when the cartilage is gone, in spots, the exposed bone resembles ivory; i.e., it is eburnated (Fig. 8-9H).

Flattened Femoral Head
The change in the shape of the femoral head in case 8-9 (and in nearly all cases in which that change develops) requires months or even years, and it is attributable to the fact that the wear of the cartilage is always uneven.[36,38,39] Once wear begins, the hemispherical contour of the femoral head and its acetabular counterpart are altered. The surfaces not only lose their congruence, they also become roughened so that wear is accelerated.[20,33,56] The bony repair response occurs at the sites of greatest wear, and the result is a gradual change in shape of the femoral head. This change, in turn, potentiates the wear phenomena on the acetabular wall, which also changes shape. The biomechanical effects, naturally, follow the pattern established by the predominant arcs of motion, which in the hip are flexion and extension. Thus the "flattened" head has that appearance on radiographs, whereas in reality the contour is more cylindrical. The main limitations of motion are therefore abduction–adduction and rotation. Because some degree of abduction–adduction motion, albeit limited, is indulged in during walking, the result of that motion is a tendency for subluxation of the hip to occur (see below).

Marginal Osteophytes
There is controversy concerning the exact way osteophytes form. One theory has it that at the margins of the articular cartilage the tissue to which the synovial membrane attaches thickens, and there is metaplasia of the elaborated repair tissue into cartilage and, in turn, into bone. Another theory postulates a transverse split in the cartilage at the synovial attachment, followed by development of bone and marrow in the gap. Still another theory postulates that there is a pull on the synovial attachment, the response to which is an elaboration of cartilage and bone. In any case, the marginal osteophyte tends to increase the expanse of articular cartilage and thereby to decrease the biomechanical integrity of the joint. The osteophytes at the

margin of the hemisphere of the femoral head might interfere only slightly with its motion; but were similar osteophytes to form at the fovea or in the notch of the acetabulum to which the ligamentum teres attaches, the result would be a lateralization of the femoral head.

Subluxation

Two mechanisms for subluxation of the femoral head have now been mentioned: (1) lateralization and (2) adduction-adduction of a flattened head. Yet another mechanism is intermittent hydroarthrosis. When the synovial membrane is irritated, be it by particles worn off the cartilage or by abnormal motion, there is always an increase in the volume of synovial fluid—as an exudate, as increased secretion, or both. Intermittent episodes, perhaps coincident with the patient's pain, would stretch the joint capsule, which would facilitate displacement of the femoral head from a socket, now incongruent with the misshapen femoral head.

Cysts

The explanation for pathogenesis of degenerative cysts is also controversial. When the cysts communicate with the joint, their formation can easily correspond in some measure to that described for the rheumatoid cyst, although in the patient in case 8-8 the perforation in the femoral cortex was mediated by an inflamed synovial membrane causing bony resorption. In contrast, in case 8-9, the perforation(s) would be caused by unroofing of a compartment of the marrow by fissuring of the cartilage down to the bony subchondral plate and seepage of synovial fluid through the perforations in that plate. Then the intermittent pressure of increased volumes of synovial fluid would progressively enlarge the cavity; the walls, originally composed of cancellous bone and normal marrow, would be converted to repair bone and loose fibrous reactive marrow. Another "explanation," which is especially attractive when there is no communication between cyst and joint, is that there is degeneration of foci in the marrow[22] and the same reaction at the periphery as described elsewhere for necrosis: resorption of this necrotic material and formation of a fibrous and bony shell around it.

Reaction in the Synovial Membrane

The synovial reaction is one of inflammation, but it is rarely acute, as in septic cases. Usually it is chronic, being due to irritation from particles or to biomechanical trauma, as perhaps by microfractures. Nevertheless, it is mostly the character of the inflammation that not infrequently makes it difficult to distinguish osteoarthritis from other varieties of arthritis. When most of the pathological changes in and near the joint are those of osteoarthritis but some secondary phenomenon, e.g., fracture of an osteophyte or secondary infection, is present, diagnosis of the concomitant but different entities may be difficult. On the other hand, when a different form of arthritis, e.g., traumatic or rheumatoid, evokes degenerative changes over time, one encounters the same dilemma.

Implications of Pathophysiological Data

Therefore the degenerative and reparative processes have pathophysiological features with diagnostic and surgical implications. One or another phase of the degeneration or the repair may predominate. Two examples illustrate the point.

Suppose a degenerative cyst at the hip or knee has become large. Radiologically, its presence may overshadow the changes in the articular surface to such an extent they obscure the arthritis. An acute onset of symptoms may have resulted from a pathological fracture through the wall of the cyst. The initiating condition might have been an osteochondritis dissecans of the femoral condyle that might pass unrecognized or might be considered an irrelevant finding. Removal of the cyst (and perhaps reconstruction with bone grafts) might be done with a diagnostic objective as well as a therapeutic one. However, degenerative cysts are indistinguishable histologically from a ganglionic of bone or from a ganglion of soft tissue.[60] It might then be the surgeon's opinion that a ganglion developed with other manifestations of degenerative joint disease or secondary changes (Fig. 8-10). The primary lesion, which should have been treated, would then be ignored.

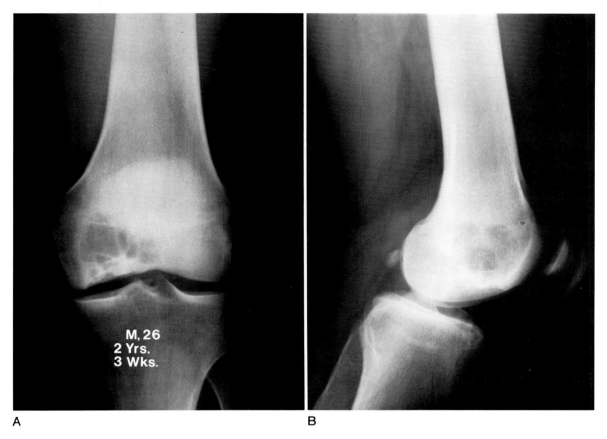

Fig. 8-10. Case 8-10. A 26-year-old man had had pain in the left knee for 2 years; it had become progressively worse and was acute for the past 3 weeks. It had been a dull, aching, intermittent pain until 3 weeks ago when it became sharp and piercing over the medial condyle of the femur. He noted crepitation at times. There was no recent or remote trauma. The medial aspect of the femoral condyle was tender. He had full range of motion. **(A&B)** Radiolucent lytic lesion of the medial femoral condyle of the left knee. Note the irregular subchondral cortex in the medial femoral condyle. *(Figure continues.)*

The second example is an osteophyte that, as mentioned above, has arisen at the fovea of the femoral head. Let us suppose that, except for this lesion, other changes in the hip attributable to degenerative joint disease are not severe (especially the changes in the cartilage), but the hip is painful and signs of impairment (especially subluxation) justify an operation. The removed marginal osteophyte shows a regenerated fibrocartilage on its surface. It and articular hyaline cartilage stain positively with safranin O, indicating that they contain normal mucopolysaccharides. Even the regenerated fibrocartilage of an osteophyte can undergo

the process of degenerative changes, and in this case it had an eburnated surface layer of bone under which there were remains of the original articular cartilage and of the regenerated osteophytic cartilage.

The reparative osteophyte that formed along the margins of the articular cartilage surfaces had surgical implications. It displaced the femoral head distally and, in concert with the osteophytes formed along the posteromedial aspect of the femoral head, also displaced the femoral head laterally and anteriorly. The surgical implication here is that removal of the foveal osteophytes and those on the

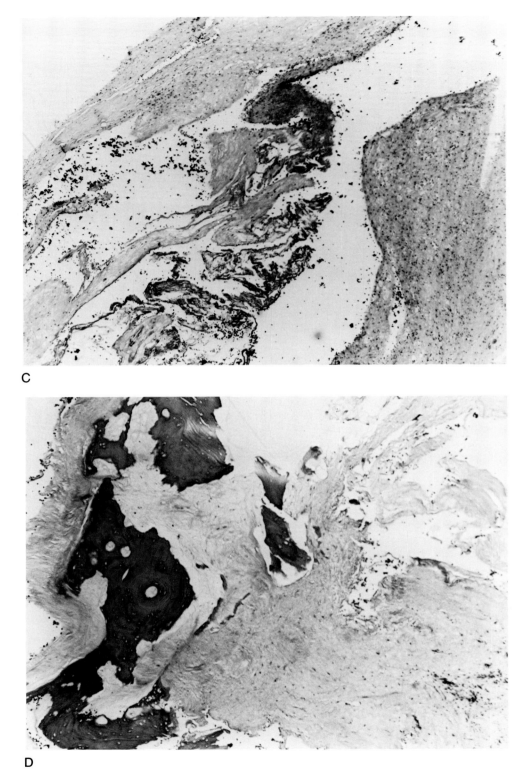

C

D

Fig. 8-10 *(Continued).* **(C)** Wall of the ganglion cyst (×20). It is similar to a degenerative cyst of bone. **(D)** The presence of repairing necrotic bone confirms the initial diagnosis of osteochondritis dissecans of the femoral condyle from which the secondary degenerative arthritis and cyst ensued. (×90)

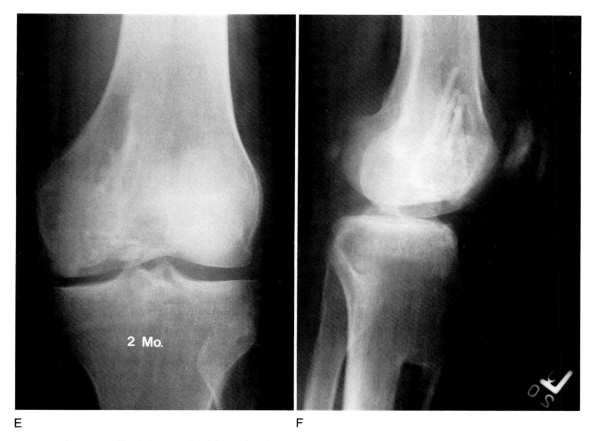

Fig. 8-10 *(Continued)*. **(E) AP** and **(F)** lateral radiographs 2 months after curettage and tibial bone graftings show healing of the cyst.

periphery of the femoral head might eliminate the main reason for subluxation of the joint. If the articular cartilage did not show an unacceptable degree of degeneration, it might be preferable to postpone a more radical procedure (i.e., replacement arthroplasty) and perhaps be content with removal of the osteophyte supplemented perhaps by an osteotomy. For this possibility to be entertained, the subluxation of the articular surface would have had to be of short duration. However, in the case under consideration the articular cartilage surface did undergo fibrillation, fragmentation, and eburnation. The marginal osteophytes had developed a reparative fibrocartilaginous surface. This repair process is the type to be expected when an osteotomy is performed to preserve joint function.

If that operation is to be done, the degenerative changes must not be severe and there must still be a reasonable range of motion in the affected joint. The idea is to preserve that function for a considerable period of time, i.e., at least 2 years. As with synovectomy for rheumatoid arthritis, the predictability of results is uncertain; yet it is advocated by some surgeons because it does extend the usefulness of the joint in a sufficient number of instances to make it a worthwhile treatment for the intermediate stages of degenerative joint disease.[4,5,16,32,47,49–51,54,59,66]

The rationale for osteotomy to treat osteoarthritis of the hip or the knee (see Fig. 8-21, below) is that it improves the hemodynamics in the bone substance and alters the direction of load transmission.[52] Some surgeons report good or excellent results when the hip is put in slight varus or valgus, with the benefit lasting 10 years or so. The results supposedly are better when the operation is performed early in the course of the arthritis, before there is marked restriction of motion and function.[50,54] The operation supposedly allows the remaining cartilage to regenerate a better articular surface.

It is this regenerative capacity that led to trials of arthroplasties with interposed materials. Metal cups between articular surfaces may still have a

place in therapy, particularly in the hip and especially for young patients with secondary degenerative joint disease.[34]

Case 8-11 A 29-year-old man had sustained a fracture dislocation of the right hip. He had reasonable function for 10 years but then developed severe secondary degenerative arthritis (Figs. 8-11A,B,C). Because of the pain and restricted function he underwent a cup arthroplasty. The range of motion preoperatively was only mildly restricted.

A successful cup arthroplasty depends on the

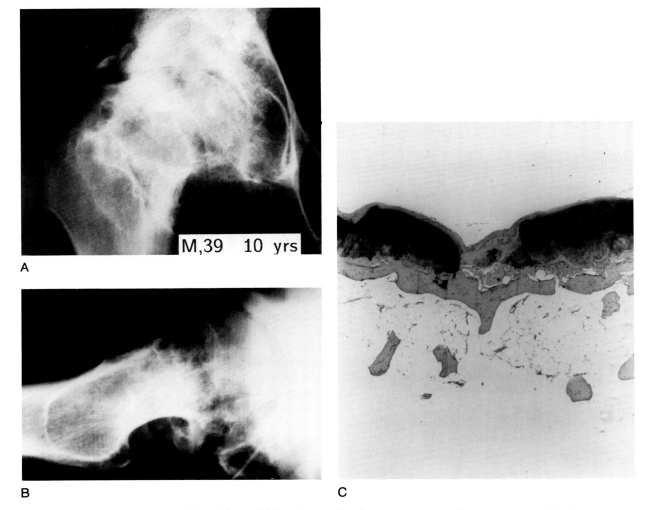

Fig. 8-11. Case 8-11. AP (**A**) and lateral (**B**) radiographs of posttraumatic arthritis 10 years after fracture dislocation of the right hip. (**C**) Photomicrograph of the irregular fibrocartilaginous surface of a medial osteophyte (×10).

formation of fibrocartilaginous surfaces to cover the denuded, and therefore bony, articular surfaces of the reshaped acetabulum and femoral head (Fig. 8-12). In case 8-11 several osteophytes were present and had to be completely removed, which meant that an inferior and more medial acetabular position had to be established for seating the acetabular cup. Inadequate excision or merely reaming the medial acetabular and central foveal osteophytes would have prevented this biomechanically desirable positioning for the cup. The time required for repair and regeneration of the articular cartilage surface with a functional fibrocartilage is a matter of many months, i.e., a minimum of 9 months and probably up to 2 years.

In case 8-11, treated during the 1940s, the options did not include total replacement arthroplasty. Cup arthroplasties generally have not been successful. In this case, one favorable factor was the patient's compliance with the rigorous regimen of postoperative treatment (non-weight-bearing for nearly a year and daily exercises). The success was achieved despite some unfavorable factors, i.e., the patient was heavy and active. As has been shown

for total hip arthroplasty (and incidentally for total knee arthroplasty as well) those two factors are adverse influences.

Total hip arthroplasty is now performed commonly, and much has been written concerning it. Controversy is evident on so many aspects of the subject that even the experts, despite confident pronouncements, disagree on the prerequisites for success. Cup arthroplasty, as a precursor to total hip replacement arthroplasty, evoked a lively controversy relative to several technical maneuvers, some of which also relate to total hip replacement arthroplasty (e.g., Is medialization of the hip desirable? What is the best position for the device?), but the cardinal pathophysiological principle of cup arthroplasty — promotion of a fibrocartilaginous surface — is not applicable when the articulating materials are metal and polymer. Controversy then is generated about which metal and which polymer is best; and for resolution of that controversy, only empirical evidence will be conclusive. For that evidence to be obtainable, many cases observed over more than a decade are needed, even though the study of the metals and polymers that might be

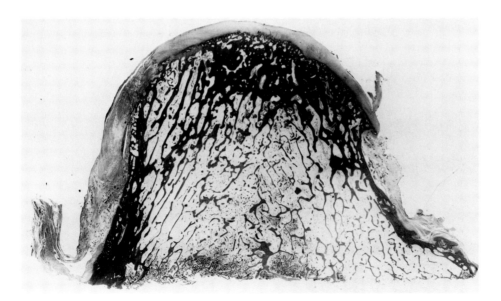

Fig. 8-12. Photomicrograph of a femoral head removed at autopsy 1.5 years after a cup arthroplasty had been performed for posttraumatic arthritis ($\times 3$). The articular surface is composed mostly of fibrocartilage. The cells along the surface are lined up along parallel bundles of collagen. Those cells near the subchondral cortex are shaped like cartilage cells in a homogeneous matrix. A synovial cell lining had formed about the cup. This kind of regeneration is the expected ideal.

appropriate for the application easily lends itself to laboratory techniques. This experimental evaluation has gone on for more than 30 years, so that much information is available relative to the materials and their properties (including tissue tolerance, as studied in animals); however, even with the limited aspects of the subject, the needed empirical data are not available. There are *no* reports of considerable numbers of cases for which there is follow-up of 10 years or more, for which the same materials were used, and for which there did not exist so many other variables that controlled observation was possible. These "other variables" therefore are at the heart of most of the controversy, and it is futile to attempt, by invocation of pathophysiological principles, to resolve the many controversial areas.

Empiricism, however, has revealed that certain technical matters jeopardize a total hip arthroplasty. Methylmethacrylate is a case in point. The development of total hip replacement depended in large part on firm, rapid fixation of the components of the prosthesis, and polymethylmethacrylate (PMMA) polymerized in situ was a crucial element for that fixation. Despite many advances in the technique of its use — inter alia, maneuvers to prevent bubbles and to prevent persistence of the monomer — there have been too many clinical failures attributable to the inadequacies of PMMA, especially in cases followed 5 years or more, for us to accept PMMA as a necessary part of total hip arthroplasty (ways are being devised to avoid its use) but nevertheless PMMA, based on empirical evidence primarily, remains essential for total hip arthroplasty in today's state of the art. Techniques that avoid its use can best regard as "under study" until at least a decade of observation yields enough evidence for proper judgment.

The foregoing discussion of materials merely illustrates some of the variables to be evaluated. There are many other variables — so many, in fact, as to preclude the mere listing of them much less any worthwhile discussion. We may mention, however, the numerous prosthetic designs and the various surgical approaches and technical maneuvers in insertion of each device. It is evident that one group of essential variables, i.e., the condition of the patient in regard to systemic factors, functional factors, and even the local pathological anatomy, must be accepted as impossible to control. Such

empirical evidence would have to be massive, if statistics can help the evaluation to some degree. The bioengineering evidence adduced for different devices merely supports decisions to conduct trial studies. Empirical evidence over the long term constitutes the only data on which valid judgments can be made. Pathophysiological principles usually play little or no part in that judgment.

One point in which pathological principles can play a part, however, is the following. Suppose the pathological changes in an arthritic joint lead to a marked deficiency in portions of the joint, such as the superior lateral aspect of the acetabulum and the femoral head. Suppose further that those portions of the femoral head and acetabulum have been worn away, and the surfaces have become eburnated. The surgical implication of treatment of that aspect of the pathological anatomy constitutes a dilemma: Should the prosthetic hip joint be devised so as to occupy a more nearly anatomical position, or should it be devised so it is more medial? The question may also arise as to whether to add a bone graft or additional methylmethacrylate to make up for the deficiency. Mention has been made that empirical failures of PMMA for long-term applications are not infrequent (see Fig. 10-3), but it also has been mentioned that there have been several advances in PMMA techniques. Pathophysiologically, it is preferable to avoid insertion of any foreign material if there is an alternative. Here the alternative is a bone graft. Despite decades of study, one still cannot be sure that a bone graft, applied to a site in which it will immediately be subject to loads, will retain its size and shape while being replaced by creeping substitution. The question of which type of bone graft (allograft or autograft) should be used also is still unanswered. Therefore pathophysiological principles cannot resolve the dilemma.

While we are on the subject of total hip arthroplasty, which is applicable to many cases of rheumatoid arthritis and nonspecific arthritis as well as to osteoarthritis, it should be mentioned that the surgeon should keep in mind the expected longevity of the prosthesis. If the patient is young, below age 20 for instance, and the patient's social and educational background is such that he or she is likely to go into work that demands a high level of physical activity, it may not be in his or her best interest to undergo an arthroplasty whose longevity may be about a decade. Many factors other than age and eventual choice of work would influence the choice of procedure, however, including, for example, involvement of other joints in the same extremity or in the contralateral one. Whereas osteoarthritis of the primary type is not a disease of the young, secondary osteoarthritis and nonspecific arthritis can commonly involve a single joint in young individuals. If total hip replacement is attempted and it has a limited period of success, whether in a young person or an elderly individual, salvage of the joint by revising the arthroplasty has a much poorer prognosis than did the original procedure. Often the alternative is an arthrodesis, in a young patient, or, in an older one, excision of the joint and formation of a pseudarthrosis. Neither of these salvage procedures introduces pathophysiological principles that are not obvious. It should be emphasized, however, that using arthrodesis as the original surgical maneuver in a young person may well be in the patient's best interest. After a decade or two the arthrodesed joint may be converted to an arthroplasty. This protocol would apply particularly to cases of tuberculosis or sepsis.

It has already been mentioned that on occasion subtrochanteric osteotomy for osteoarthritis of the hip would afford several years of good function perhaps prior to an arthroplasty. The same is true for osteoarthritis of the knee, when a tibial osteotomy is occasionally the operation indicated. Only rarely, if ever, is arthrodesis of the knee indicated as a first operation for osteoarthritis. It is primarily considered as a salvage procedure when another operation is unsuccessful, be it because of sepsis or other complication.

When the surgeon decides to do an osteotomy of the tibia, he or she should attempt not only to correct the alignment but also to utilize the more nearly normal compartment of the knee joint for maximal load bearing. The osteotomy should not just correct the angular deformity (usually varus) but also should restore the proper articulating biomechanics. It may be necessary to do a hemiarthroplasty, i.e., replace the medial tibial plateau and perhaps the medial femoral condyle as well. In any case, these procedures may defer the total joint arthroplasty, which in the knee is somewhat less predictably successful than in the hips.

The cases of osteoarthritis considered above were for the most part selected from the groups defined as primary (except case 8-11). It is important to differentiate that group from secondary cases, several of which have been considered in other chapters. The reason the differentiation is important is as follows. Every secondary case has had a primary lesion that contributed to the pathophysiology of the subsequent degenerative process. Many primary lesions can be culpable (e.g., sepsis, metabolic disease, aseptic necrosis). Although the histological sequences in the degeneration are similar—a final common pathway, if you will—the rapidity of the process depends to a major degree on the nature of the destruction caused by the primary process.

Posttraumatic Arthritis

One of the most frequent primary lesions that leads to secondary osteoarthritis is trauma,[23,38-40] and mostly for that reason posttraumatic arthritis is distinguished as a separate category. Another reason, perhaps, is the fact that in most of the cases of traumatic arthritis one can picture what the primary lesion was much more precisely than for nearly any other form of secondary osteoarthritis. Once the primary lesion is well in mind, its pathophysiological consequences can be understood.

An example of a posttraumatic (secondary) arthritis as the end-stage change of an intra-articular fracture of the head of the radius. Such a case was described in Chapter 5 (see Fig. 5-1). The pathological changes noted were those of synovitis and marked degeneration of the articular cartilage. There was resorption of the subchondral cortex by vascular buds breaking through into the hyaline cartilage. Those changes may also be seen with primary degenerative arthritis. The proliferation of the cells (but without elaboration of matrix) in the original articular cartilage is a reparative response characteristic of any degenerative arthritis. The synovial response in the case of posttraumatic arthritis was of an intensity compatible with that seen in primary degenerative arthritis. What appears to be important is that the marked alteration of joint congruity caused the extensive secondary degenerative arthritic changes that became the paramount cause of the disability.

The extensive alteration of joint congruity also was displayed by the patient in case 8-11. He had reasonably good function after 1 year of protected weight-bearing after the fracture dislocation of the hip, but he had never completely recovered full range of motion. During the year prior to his evaluation for increasing pain and stiffness of the hip (10 years after the traumatic episode), the patient had progressive loss of motion and function. His hip rating then was 55 (Iowa hip rating scale*), and radiographs of the hip showed extensive loss of articular cartilage space and large marginal osteophytes primarily on the femoral head (Figs. 8-11A,B). In addition, there was ossification of the medial soft tissue area of the capsule of the hip joint. The latter finding undoubtedly contributed to the restricted range of motion after the initial injury. The original fracture in this case involved the posterior lip of the acetabulum; and because a closed reduction was the treatment provided acutely, there is little doubt that the contour of the acetabulum's articular cartilage was not accurately restored. The ossification that developed in the capsule is evidence that, in addition, there was an extensive tear in the capsule. The stability of the hip and good function during the 9 posttraumatic years are evidence that the capsule healed. Therefore we can postulate no abnormal motion in the joint during those years; rather, there was gradual abrasive wear on the femoral head caused by the gap in the articular cartilage of the acetabulum and its sharp edges. The fibrillation on the femoral head, in turn, probably caused abnormal wear on the acetabular articular cartilage. The critical situation did not come about until the wear caused marked incongruity in the joint surfaces: Perhaps the wear, in spots, exposed the subchondral bone.

---

* Rating scales have been devised for the purpose of depicting quantitatively the status of the joint in order that longitudinal progression can be "precisely" delineated, including changes attributable to surgical procedures. Several systems exist for the hip, knee, etc. Points are assigned for such categories as range of motion, deformity, and radiographic changes. However, no one rating system for any one joint is in general use, and a comparison of systems relating to a single joint as applied to a series of patients shows disparities in the ratings so obtained. The main difficulty of quantitation rests in the delineation of categories that are entirely subjective (i.e., pain) or subjective in part (i.e., function). Another difficulty stems from the part that the joint often cannot be considered in isolation, particularly when there is multiarticular involvement or systemic disease.

This case therefore emphasizes the need for accurate reduction of intra-articular fractures; with the state-of-the-art open technique now generally practiced (i.e., open reduction and internal fixation) but not available at the time the patient was treated, the arthritis may well have been prevented. The case also reveals that a slight irregularity in the joint can be tolerated for years. At the time of the cup arthroplasty, no gap was grossly seen in the acetabular cartilage; i.e., the gap described above had filled with fibrocartilage. Therefore the wear in the femoral cartilage, at first attributed to the sharp edges of the fracture, later may either have been caused by the incongruity of the joint surface, the inferior quality of fibrocartilage (compared to articular cartilage), or both. Probably the articular surface of the femoral head was covered partly with fibrous tissue and partly with fibrocartilage, as noted histologically (Fig. 8-11C).

This situation was illustrated in the histological section from the femoral head of a similar case in which total replacement arthroplasty was done (Fig. 8-12). The thickness of the reparative tissue was less than one-third that of normal hyaline cartilage. The presence of areas of complete replacement of the articular surface by actively proliferation fibrous tissue and the evidence of active resorption of the subchondral cortex indicate that the surfaces were undergoing progressive reactive change.

In addition to the specimen of the radial head described earlier (see Fig. 5-1) and the present one, another specimen from a case of traumatic arthritis of the hip treated by a cup arthroplasty is shown in Figure 8-12.

Case 8-12 A 50-year-old man sustained intra-articular fractures of the metacarpophalangeal (MP) and proximal interphalangeal (PIP) joints. The fractures were reduced by open operation and fixed with Kirschner wires. In the MP joint the cartilage was found to be markedly comminuted, and the reduction was imperfect. After 3 weeks of this immobilization, the pins were removed. Motion was begun in the finger, but the finger remained stiff at the MP joint; after a few months it was amputated. The microscopic section showed the articular surface undergoing fibrosis with active granulation tissue resorbing cartilage where it had been involved in the intra-articular fracture (Fig. 8-13). In this specimen, in contrast to the others, a rather

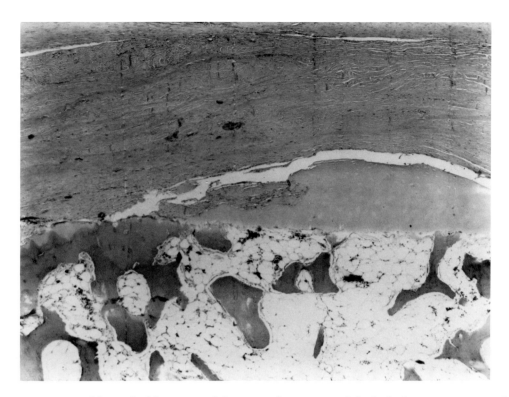

Fig. 8-13. A 50-year-old man had fractures of the MP and PIP joints of the little finger. An open reduction was performed to correct the comminuted articular surfaces of these joints. The pins were removed at 3 weeks, and joint motions were started. Persistent stiffness of the PIP and MP joints of the little finger was treated by amputation of the finger at the MP joint. This microscopic section of the articular surface of the PIP joint shows fibrosis, active granulation tissue, and resorption of the fracture site at 4 months (×40).

short period of time, 4 months, had elapsed during which the degenerative changes were proceeding. Those degenerative changes were severe, and the rapid deterioration may be ascribed mainly to the comminution of the fracture, which indicated a severe injury.

Arthritis Secondary to Nontraumatic Conditions

There are other examples of arthritis secondary to preexisting conditions in which emphasis must be placed on prevention when treating the condition, e.g., congenital dislocation or congenital dysplasia of the hip.[18,36,43,58,62,67] The emphasis here is on the fact that good treatment initially is the best prophylaxis against development of the arthritis.

Case 8-13 A 34-year-old woman first presented with pain in the left hip and then had an increasing limp over a period of 5 years. On presentation she had had congenital dislocations of the hips, for which allegedly a good result had been obtained with closed reduction and hip spica cast immobilization (Fig. 8-14A). She had a good range of motion of the hips, but both were tender at the extremes of all motions. The patient walked with a marked limp and with an abductor lurch on the left side; these signs were consistent with an instability indicative of a lateral or superior subluxation. A radiograph of the pelvis at age 39 showed that the right hip had a sloping acetabulum and a slightly narrowed articular cartilage space, but no other changes indicative of arthritis (Fig. 8-14B). In contrast, the left hip, which also showed acetabular dysplasia and narrowing of the articular cartilage, revealed displacement of the femoral head laterally.

The therapeutic problem presented by this patient was whether conservative or surgical treatment was most appropriate. Such patients should

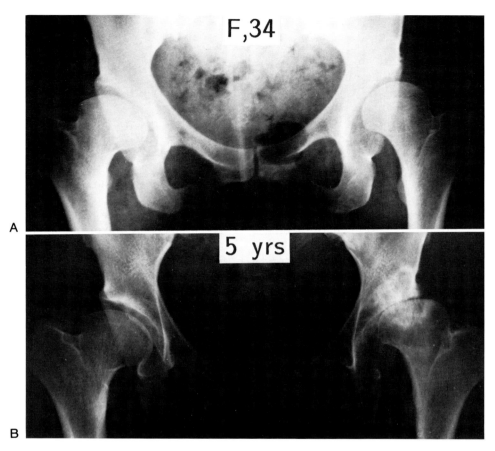

Fig. 8-14. (A) AP radiograph of the pelvis of a 34-year-old woman with congenital dislocation of the hips. Note the shallow acetabuli, thinning of the articular cartilage space, and the degenerative cyst of the superior acetabulum in the left hip. **(B)** Five years later the narrowing of the left hip is more marked. The degenerative cyst has enlarged, and more subluxation is present.

first try external supports, i.e., canes or crutches, to protect the symptomatic hip as well as to reduce activity. This treatment has one immediate objective, which can be interpreted as pathophysiological — reducing the irritation in the left hip. That irritation, evidenced by the restriction of motion and the pain, may be attributed to the subluxation that occurs at every step. If that subluxation causes exudation — thus a vicious cycle is begun — prevention of the progress of the subluxation might be beneficial. It should not be expected, however, that conservative treatment, even pursued over a period of months, would result in longstanding benefit.

The 5-year history of pain in the patient in case 8-13 would best be attributed, pathophysiologically, to an increasing degree of subluxation, which, in turn, would indicate increasing stretch of the hip capsule and perhaps resorption of the lateral part of the roof of the acetabulum. These two changes in the articulation cannot be reversed by conservative treatment. Another objective (of nonpathophysiological character) is establishment of a regimen of physical therapy. For the surgeon, ascertaining cooperation of the patient with the regimen is important because even though the surgeon expects to do a surgical procedure on the left hip in the near future and on the right in due course, the result will be better if the patient improves the abductor muscles by a regimen of reduced activity and appropriate exercises, no matter which surgical procedure is chosen.

Most orthopedists would probably consider the following surgical procedure appropriate. Subtrochanteric osteotomy of the femur might be done to centralize the femoral head in the acetabulum. It has the advantages of: (1) avoiding any intra-articular manipulations, including operative dislocation; (2) reducing the potential for operative complications; and (3) allowing use of an articulation that, despite the narrowed articular cartilage, might well be capable of years of good service. It has two distinct disadvantages: (1) It does not address all the pathological elements in the anatomy, notably the stretched capsule and the slope in the acetabular roof. It merely addresses a biomechanical deficiency, subluxation, (2) Even if it offers temporary benefit, it may be too transitory; and then, if total replacement is needed, the varus position of the upper end of the femur poses technical problems that may influence the operation adversely. Few pathophysiological principles that have not already been mentioned in the discussion of subtrochanteric osteotomy would be involved in the comparisons, and therefore readers are referred to the references for further details.

Another operation to be considered is correction of the acetabular insufficiency by an osteotomy of the ilium.[66] Several such operations have been advocated. Discussion of these techniques would require comparison of the advantages and disadvantages of each, not only with regard to the competing methods but also with regard to varus osteotomy; the comparisons would focus mostly on biomechanics (e.g., if medial displacement of the joint is advisable). The other option for treatment, of course, is a replacement arthroplasty. Because the patient in case 8-13 was relatively young and her arthritis not severe, one would try to preserve as much of the hip as possible for as long as possible; thus an osteotomy of one kind or another would be proper, recognizing that there would be no bridges burned by that approach. A total hip procedure could then be done should either conservative treatment be unsuccessful or the osteotomy not serve for a sufficient period of time. The rationale for a particular treatment in this case is discussed in greater detail in Chapter 10.

Other conditions, some of them discussed in Chapter 7 (see, for example, Fig. 7-37) — Legg-Perthes disease, slipped capital femoral epiphysis (see Fig. 5-11 & 5-17), sickle cell disease — produce extensive structural alterations and early degenerative arthritis during adult life. The treatment considerations were also discussed in Chapter 7.

Gout-Induced Arthritis

Several metabolic processes result in arthritic disease, i.e., crystal diseases such as gout and calcium pyrophosphate disease. These diseases are not difficult to identify when in full manifestation, but they may be difficult to diagnose during their early stages. At times they simulate other conditions. The first case is one of the crystal diseases. It was selected because of its unusual presentation, which made the diagnosis initially difficult.[17]

Case 8-14 A 29-year-old man complained of pain of 9 months' duration in the left knee that occurred only with weight-bearing. There were two episodes of locking of the knee, both times in extension. The locking did not last more than a few seconds, but for several weeks afterward he noted a fullness in the outer aspect of the knee and recently the fullness did not recede. He gave no history of trauma or symptoms of systemic disease. On examination there was mild tenderness at the left femoral condyle with a poorly defined fullness in the posteromedial aspect of the knee. The range of motion of the knee was full. The radiographs showed a lytic lesion of the posterior aspect of the lateral femoral condyle (Figs. 8-15A,B),[17] which was interpreted to be a benign process. Among the lesions considered were giant cell tumor, enchondroma, aneurysmal bone cyst, and degenerative cyst. Tomograms showed no communication of the "cyst" with the joint. The laboratory studies were normal except for a borderline serum uric acid level (10 mg/dl; normal 7.5 to 10.0 mg/dl).

An open biopsy was performed. This procedure was selected as the initial one in preference to arthroscopy of the knee for the following reasons. Although arthroscopy might reveal the reason for the fullness in the joint, it could not address the problem of diagnosis of the lytic osseous lesion. An open biopsy, on the other hand, would not only provide tissue samples from the cyst, it would also possibly allow definitive treatment, given the appropriate diagnosis. The tissue in the cyst proved to

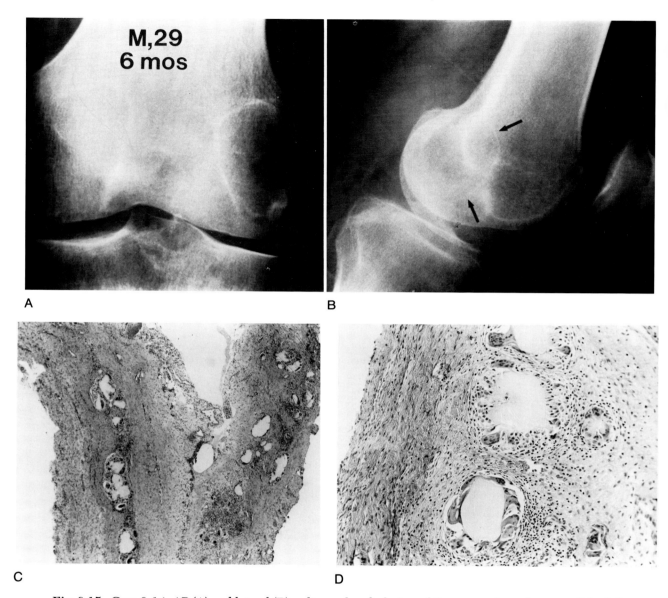

Fig. 8-15. Case 8-14. AP **(A)** and lateral **(B)** radiographs of a lesion of the posterolateral aspect of the left femoral condyle. (From Foucar et al.,[15] with permission.) **(C)** Photomicrograph of the wall of the cyst showing a urate deposit. **(D)** The gouty deposit is surrounded by the giant cells ($\times 63$). **(A&B** from Foucar et al.,[17] with permission.)

be connective tissue lining a cavity filled with yellow fluid. There were chalky-white crystalline granules attached to the lining membrane, which was peeled from the interior of the condyle. The cavity was packed with bone removed from the tibia. Histologically, the tissue consisted primarily of chronic inflammatory granulation tissue with a giant cell reaction (Figs. 8-15C,D) surrounding

crystalline material. Birefringent urate crystals were identified in the parts of the specimen fixed in alcohol, rather than in the other routine fixations.

On the second day postoperatively, the patient developed fever, acute pain, and redness and swelling of the left wrist, elbow, and ankle. Radiographs of the wrist revealed numerous radiolucent foci in the radius and carpus with reactive borders similar to those in the femur. The definitive diagnosis was reached 2 days postoperatively based on the demonstration of urate crystals in the specimen. It can be argued, mostly in retrospect, that arthroscopy, or even needle arthrocentesis, would have allowed a definitive diagnosis of gout; however, the lytic lesion still could not be so diagnosed definitively, given the possibility that it might be a separate, albeit benign, lesion. It also might be argued that the serum uric acid value should have been an indication for arthrocentesis. Had that procedure been done, the gouty exacerbation as a complication of the surgical procedure might have been prevented. However, that complication is one that should be recognized by orthopedic as well as other surgeons because it not uncommonly occurs in gouty patients who undergo any type of operation. Its pathophysiology is not understood, in contrast to the pathophysiology of gout itself, which has been extensively documented. It suffices here to point out that the giant cells in the tophus, as illustrated, often contain the urate crystals and often surround the aggregates of urate crystals. Those aggregates therefore simulate foreign bodies histologically; and one can postulate that the sharp borders of the crystals may well serve as irritants based on physical rather than chemical properties. The symptoms, signs, and postoperative exacerbations are classical for gout.

The lytic lesion in the femoral condyle healed, and the symptoms of gout were controlled with indomethacin. This case illustrates the principle that bony rather than articular manifestations of gout can be confused with other processes radiographically and clinically, particularly when the serum uric acid level is not markedly elevated, as is more commonly seen.

The more classical location and clinical and radiographic lesions of gout are shown in the next case.

Case 8-15 A 65-year-old man had a history of intermittent swelling and pain of 1 year's duration. The serum urate value was normal. There was a radiolucent lesion of the medial aspect of the distal end of the proximal phalanx of the great toe (Fig. 8-16). The radiographs were initially interpreted as diagnostic of degenerative joint disease with a plantar spur of the distal phalanx or endochondroma of the distal end of the proximal phalanx. Only when repeated serum urate assays were done

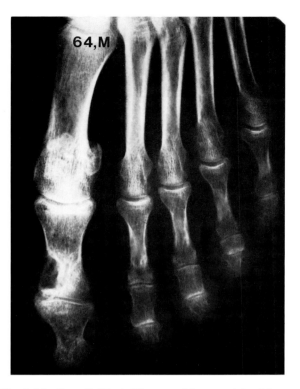

Fig. 8-16. Case 8-15. A 65-year-old man with a history of intermittent swelling and pain in his toe for a year displays a more classical location and clinical and radiographic form of gout. This radiograph shows a radiolucent lesion of the medial aspect of the distal end of the proximal phalanx of the great toe. It was first interpreted as degenerative joint disease with a plantar spur of the distal phalanx or endochondroma of the distal end of the proximal phalanx. A serum uric acid value was in the normal range initially. Only when repeated serum uric acid levels were seen to be elevated was the diagnosis changed to gout. The patient obtained good relief with allopurinol.

and a borderline elevation was demonstrated was the diagnosis of gout made. The patient obtained good relief with allopurinol. Gout continued to be suspected because of the characteristic location of the lesion and the absence of arthritic changes in other joints.

Chondrocalcinosis-Induced Arthritis
Another metabolic process affecting joints with symptoms simulating those of gout is *pseudogout* or *chondrocalcinosis*, now more popularly called calcium pyrophosphate dihydrate crystal disease (CPPD). When the condition presents in the acute

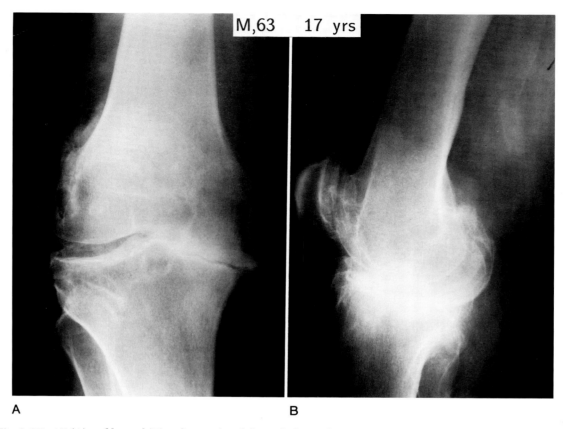

Fig. 8-17. AP (**A**) and lateral (**B**) radiographs of the right knee show extensive degenerative narrowing of the medial femoral condyle and the patellofemoral joint along with extensive marginal osteophytes. Increased densities are present in the meniscus and periarticular soft tissues around the lateral femoral condyle, the suprapatellar pouch, and the posterior capsule. *(Figure continues.)*

phase there often is an effusion into the joint that can cause transient difficulty with the diagnosis. Aspiration of the joint fluid makes it possible to identify the crystals, which requires that the fluid be examined under polarized light. The negatively birefringent urate crystals of both gout and CPPD are long, needle-like, or acicular, whereas those of calcium pyrophosphate are small, angular, or rhomboid-shaped and positively birefringent with a red compensatory filter. The more chronic form of CPPD does not differ greatly in clinical presentation from that of chronic degenerative arthritis where only one or two joints are affected, particularly the knees. The presence of an increased density in the meniscus and periarticular soft tissues often is there as an incidental finding indicative of CPPD.

Case 8-16 Such was the case in the radiographs (Figs. 8-17 A,B) of the knee of a 62-year-old man with a 17-year history of the knee initially locking, and later of its giving way accompanied by pain. He had had a meniscectomy at age 25 that had relieved the locking but not the pain and giving way. Examination showed a restricted range of motion and a varus deformity. At the time of a total knee arthroplasty, the synovial membrane and menisci were noted to feel gritty. Histologically, there was dark-staining crystal deposits dispersed throughout the synovial membrane (Figs. 8-17C,D). Otherwise, the histological findings were characteristic of degenerative arthritis.

Chondrocalcinosis is more common during the later decades of life. As many as 25 percent of cases present by the ninth decade of life with radiological

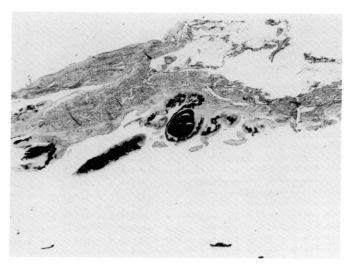
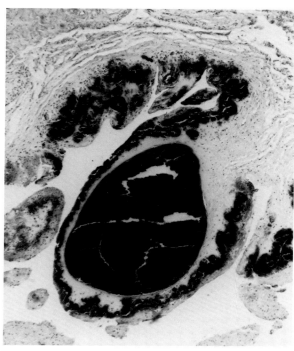

C   D

Fig. 8-17 *(Continued).* **(C&D)** Dark-staining crystal deposits of calcium pyrophosphate are dispersed throughout the synovial membrane. (**C** ×27; **D** ×63.)

findings. Treatment is symptomatic. The decision to perform total knee arthroplasty in the case illustrated was based on the functional impairment due to severe degenerative arthritis rather than the presence of the CPPD. The pathophysiology of the lesions, despite extensive study, is poorly understood.

Ochronosis-Induced Arthritis
One other "chemical" disease that affects joints, and that is the last example of metabolic arthritides to be mentioned, is ochronosis (alkaptonuria). Here a progressive and multiarticular arthropathy develops associated with an accumulation of homogentisic acid in the articular cartilage. The patients have an inherited deficiency of the enzyme homogentisic acid oxidase. The pigmented cartilage is brittle and fragments easily. The intervertebral discs in particular and the articular cartilage of major joints undergo changes similar to those of degenerative arthritis; however, there is a distinc-

tive brown to black pigmentation of the fibrocartilage of the ears, nose, and so on. This pigmentation is also seen in all hyaline cartilage shards within the hypertrophic synovial membrane of the joints whose articular surfaces have undergone the changes described for osteoarthritis.

Synovial Osteochondromatosis-Induced Arthritis, Pigmented Villonodular Synovitis
There are two kinds of lesions in joints that are evocative of degenerative changes by their nature. On occasion they present a diagnostic challenge, and often they are attended by a delay in diagnosis and treatment. The lesions in question are pigmented villonodular synovitis and synovial osteochondromatosis. One example of each follows.

Case 8-17 A 37-year-old woman complained of a sudden onset of pain and swelling in the left knee. She also was aware of a feeling of warmth in the distal part of the thigh just above the knee. The pain, at first acute, was followed by a mild aching

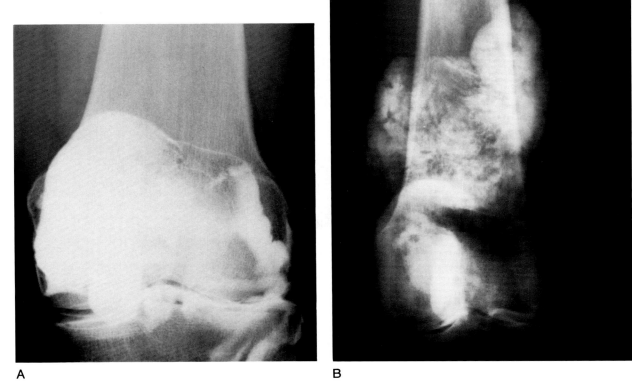

A   B

Fig. 8-18. Case 8-17. **(A)** AP arthrogram of the knee joint. **(B)** AP arthrogram of the suprapatellar pouch with extensive synovial proliferation. *(Figure continues.)*

whenever she walked. The family physician was consulted and aspirated a small amount of blood from the joint, but the swelling recurred. Two weeks after the aspiration she saw an orthopedic surgeon who again aspirated blood from the joint; but again swelling recurred and failed to resolve over the next month. She then underwent arthroscopy, which revealed no abnormality despite the presence of joint fluid that was serosanguineous. The knee continued to be achy, swollen, and warm; and occasionally she took anti-inflammatory medication, but it did not alleviate the symptoms. Radiographs of the knee at that time were normal, but there was a change in the location of the swelling, which instead of affecting the entire joint seemed to be predominantly in the suprapatellar area. The aching in the distal thigh did not diminish. She became aware of morning stiffness, but there was no

night pain or limitation of activity. The patient was otherwise well and without evidence of disease.

On examination the fullness that was present in the left suprapatellar area felt like spongy soft tissue, but there also was some fluid in the joint. An arthrogram revealed no abnormality in the articulating parts of the knee (Fig. 8-18A); when the contrast material was injected into the suprapatellar pouch, it revealed an outline of the spongy mass, which because of its nodular contour suggested pigmented villonodular synovitis (Fig. 8-18B). A partial synovectomy of the knee including most of the lining of the suprapatellar pouch was done. A large, dark brown pigmented ($10 \times 8 \times 2$ cm) mass, sharply delineated from adjacent normal synovial tissue, was removed. Histologically, the mass consisted of hypertrophic synovial membrane with villous proliferations (Fig. 8-18C). The villi had fi-

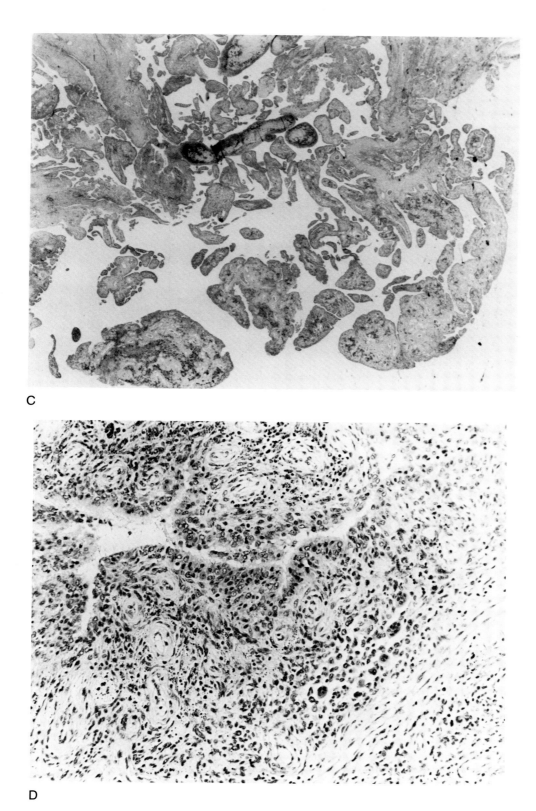

C

D

Fig. 8-18 *(Continued).* (**C**) Photomicrograph of the synovial membrane. Note the numerous villi (×25). (**D**) Photomicrograph showing compressed villi, histiocytes, foam cells, and reactive giant cells (×100). This picture is characteristic of pigmented villonodular synovitis.

brovascular centers with a large number of hemosiderophages within each villus (Fig. 8-18D). Other areas of the lesion showed sheets of histiocytes and foam cells, and there were foci of reactive giant cells.

Diagnosis in this case was delayed mostly because of failure to identify not only the nature of the process—recurrence of bleeding without trauma—but also the exact anatomical location of the lesion within the knee. The fact that the suprapatellar pouch rather than a structure in the knee joint itself was affected could not be determined by physical findings, as it could by means of routine radiography or an arthroscopic examination. Once the mass was excised, the joint returned to normal.

Despite that successful outcome, when the localized variety and in particular the generalized form of pigmented villonodular synovitis involves major joints, it does not respond to surgical treatment by return of the joint to a normal state. Secondary degenerative changes are common; usually with residual stiffness and loss of function. In some instances the process may be so extensive that it invades a bony surface adjacent to the joint. The extension of inflammatory tissue is similar to that described for rheumatoid arthritis when a cyst is formed that reaches into soft tissue some distance from the joint (Figs. 8-6B,C). It is to the patient's advantage that a diagnosis of pigmented villonodular synovitis is made early in the course of the disease, rather than late, so the destructive effects of the proliferation of this synovial process are minimized.

The pathophysiological implications of interest here do not concern those attending the nature of this lesion, as with other chronic inflammatory lesions in which there is no known etiological agent. Rather, they relate to therapy. The nature of the lesion need not be discussed because speculation has been controversial as to what it is. The role of histocytes in the lesion illustrates this controversy. They act as phagocytes of hemoglobin and red blood cell capsules. (But does lecithin from the capsule constitute the main component of the foam cell, and is the foam cell analogous to that seen with the lipidoses or perhaps in the lesion formerly known as giant cell tumor of the tendon sheath?) The therapeutic pathophysiological implication that is important is that the chronic inflammatory tissue, so far as is practical, should be removed. Because there is no evidence that an infectious agent is present, one need not worry about if the tissue is infectious, i.e., if antibiotics should be given prophylactically and if uninvolved tissue should be protected from exposure. In a generalized case, moreover, there should not be so meticulous an excision of involved tissue as to prejudice the function of the joint. Whether recurrence is thereby promoted is debatable, and the only way the debate can be settled is by empirical evidence, not yet available in suitable numbers of cases.

Case 8-18 The other process of unknown etiology that is an example of miscellaneous secondary osteoarthritides is illustrated by this case. A 26-year-old man had a history of pain and a grating sensation in the left hip joint of 4 years' duration. He was also aware of intermittent "popping." He gave no history of trauma. On examination there was tenderness in the left hip at the extremes of all ranges of motion and crepitation in the anterolateral aspect of the hip. The radiographs showed osteocartilaginous loose bodies in the area of the cotyloid notch (Fig. 8-19A). The articular cartilage space was of normal width, and there were osteophytes at the margin of the femoral head.

The osteocartilaginous loose bodies were removed from the hip, and in the process a dislocation was performed to allow complete exposure of the cotyloid notch. That area was particularly involved, with nodules of cartilage attached to the synovial membrane. A synovectomy was performed, and the loose bodies that were attached to the synovial membrane lining the ligamentum teres and elsewhere were removed. The cartilage of the femoral head appeared normal except for the margins, where there were small peripheral osteophytes. Histologically, the loose bodies within the synovial membrane were mostly cartilaginous, but some had osseous centers (Fig. 8-19B). The osteocartilaginous loose bodies, in this instance, were predominantly located in the fovea and cotyloid notch.

The usual effect on the articular cartilage surface in instances where there are intra-articular chondromas depends on their number, size, and in particular if they intervene between the articular surfaces to produce a mechanical injury to the cartilage. Owing to the pathway of nutrition of all

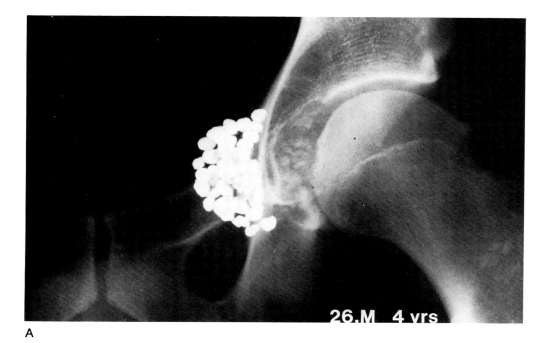

A

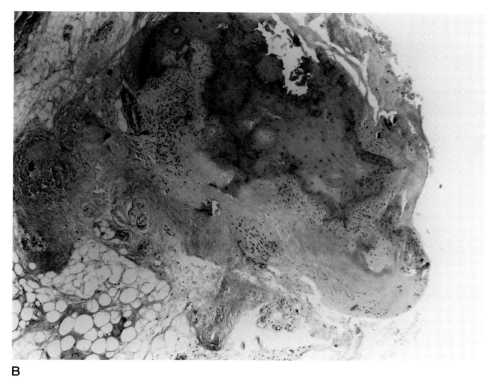

B

Fig. 8-19. Case 8-18. **(A)** Numerous areas of increased density surround the cotyloid notch. The photograph of the osteocartilaginous loose bodies is superimposed. **(B)** Photomicrograph of one of the nodules within the synovial membrane (×25).

intra-articular cartilage through the synovial fluid, the nodules that are detached not only remain alive but grow and often ossify. Large numbers of osteo-cartilaginous bodies may be the result, as they are the basis for the secondary arthritis. Because they tend to increase in size as well as number, early treatment (synovectomy) is indicated.

The pathophysiology of this lesion, as with pigmented villonodular synovitis and the other lesions that comprise the miscellaneous groups of osteoarthritides, is a matter of speculation and controversy, but one principle should be brought out. Undoubtably, there are cases in which there is trauma to a joint and release of cartilaginous particles. These particles remain alive and perhaps grow and become rounded. Early after the injury, they continue to have the characteristic orientation of the three zones of chondrocytes in articular cartilage and may even have a subchondral bony plate. After some months or years, however, those features disappear, and they may consist of just a cartilage nodule, with or without a bony center. At that point they are indistinguishable from the nodules of idiopathic synovial osteochondromatosis. One should not assume, however, that any given cartilage fragment from the articular surface will survive and grow in synovial fluid. If that were so, nearly all cases of osteoarthritis would be associated with loose bodies. That association is rare indeed, although the reason is not known.

SPECIAL CONSIDERATIONS — BY ANATOMICAL SITE

Throughout the book the emphasis on pathophysiology tends to focus on how an abnormal process affects tissues of the musculoskeletal system, whatever their location. In the present chapter, processes that affect joints are the focus; and although the illustrative cases depict a specific process (e.g., rheumatoid inflammation) in a specific joint, one may not infer that all joints are affected by the same process in the same way. For some processes, e.g., infection or tumor the inference may be valid, but for others, notably all types of arthritis except the septic type, the inference is not valid. It would be impossible to consider the various joints of the body separately, or even in groups, as they are affected by the various types of arthritis already discussed. There are entire books, as well as numerous articles devoted to single joints (hip, knee), and this part of the chapter does not attempt either to consider all the major joints or their principal idiosyncracies when they are affected by all or most of the types of arthritis. Instead, examples of single joints (knee, MP joint of the big toe[19,21,29]) or groups of joints (spine,[8–11,41,42,45,60,70] hand) illustrate a common type of arthritis in each of the four named parts.

Arthritis of the Knee

Evaluation of arthritis as it affects the knee deserves special consideration with respect to diagnosis as well as treatment. The knee lends itself to a variety of diagnostic investigational maneuvers more easily than do most other joints for two reasons. One is that it is superficially situated, and the other is that other joints are not so close that they obscure the findings. One of the most common lesions of the knee joint is osteoarthritis, which unless the patient is obese one can easily detect by physical examination, e.g., by the presence of fluid in the joint, or instability, or deformity, or if the articular surfaces are smooth or rough, and if there is weakness of the muscles moving the joint. With current radiographic techniques, including CT and arthrography, much can be found out about the bony structures and some of the nonosseous components, e.g., menisci, synovial membrane, and perhaps ligaments. Thus a diagnosis of osteoarthritis of the knee is usually simple and straightforward.

The current emphasis on arthroscopy for diagnosis has tended to deemphasize clinical diagnostic skills and the application of nonsurgical conservative treatment. All too frequently the diagnosis of osteoarthritis of the knee is evident from the history, physical findings, and radiographs. The surgeon should not be lured into performing arthroscopy on the specious grounds that it will provide information of value or, worse, that it will enable application of effective treatment to some aspect of the lesion. For example, if there if fibrillation of the cartilage, the surface can be smoothed off, a situation that is further discussed in Chapter 10. It is doubtful if that operation would be helpful, especially if weight-bearing surfaces are involved. A second example involves the menisci. A common cause for crepitation is an osteoarthritic knee with degeneration and a tear in the meniscus. The empirical evidence is convincing that meniscectomy for that lesion, as associated with osteoarthritis, will not be successful. In addition to those features of osteoarthritis in the knee, several others, e.g., deformity (mostly varus) may be surgically reparable, but each case must be carefully analyzed, with all pertinent factors in mind. One principle is that conservative measures should be an essential prerequisite for surgical treatment of the arthritic knee. Case 8-19 is a case in point.

Case 8-19 A 57-year-old moderately obese man developed pain in both knees over a period of several years. He had no history of antecedent trauma or relevant disease. His pain appeared only after long period of walking or standing and was relieved by nonsteroidal medication. He had a mild symmetrical varus deformity but no effusion. His range of flexion–extension was 130° on the right and 150° on the left. He felt mild crepitation when climbing stairs.

The radiographs showed a narrowed femoropatellar space and medial compartment space. The lateral compartment was normal. Degenerative subchondral cysts were present in both femoral condyles and in the tibia. A few small osteophytes were present (Fig. 8-20).

Because of the excellent range of motion in both knees and the lack of severe symptoms, and because the radiographs did not show marked articular damage, the patient was given a diet to lose weight, a cane to minimize weight-bearing on the right (the worse) knee, quadriceps and hamstring muscle strengthening exercises, and nonsteroidal anti-inflammatory medication. Although such

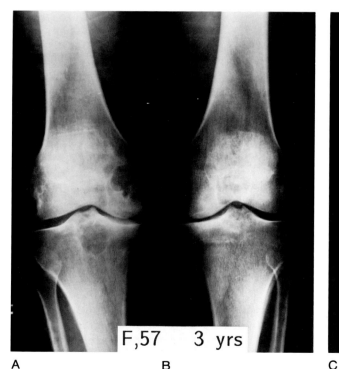
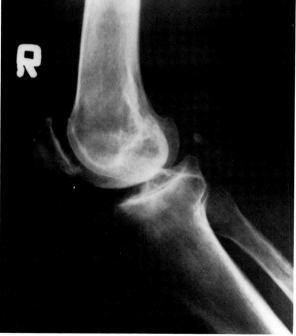

F,57   3 yrs

A   B   C

Fig. 8-20. Case 8-19. AP radiographs of the right (**A**) and left (**B**) knees. (**C**) Lateral radiograph of the right knee shows medial compartment cartilage space narrowing bilaterally. There are degenerative cysts of both femoral condyles.

measures were not expected to prevent progression of the degenerative process, it was hoped that they would improve his situation by minimizing symptoms. They would also prepare him for whatever surgical procedure was contemplated, if any. Osteotomy to realign the knee, hemiarthroplasty, or total knee replacement would be the principal choices.

This patient was not elderly, his degenerative arthritis involved mainly the medial or lateral compartment of the joint, and his range of motion was excellent; therefore he would be a good candidate for a high tibial osteotomy because the results of that procedure, as shown empirically, are predictably good. Although the mild varus deformity by itself would not be an indication for the procedure, the advantages of the procedure would include shifting the load of weight-bearing to the normal compartment of the joint. What the effects might be, including those on the patellofemoral joint, could not be shown because the conservative treatment was so effective that no operation (over a span of 5 years) was acceptable to the patient. His cysts disappeared within a year, and his pain decreased to the point where he needed a cane only occasionally. His range of motion did not change appreciably, nor did his varus deformity.

How successful a tibial osteotomy can be is illustrated by the next case.

Case 8-20 A 42-year-old male physical education teacher and coach complained of pain in the left knee with activity. He had had a torn medial meniscus that was excised at age 19. A second arthrotomy was done to remove the meniscal rim at age 27. He then had had only intermittent mild pain in the knee; but for the past 5 years, despite restricted activities and use of aspirin, the pain increased. On examination he had a 7° varus deformity of the knee, flexion from 0° to 110°, and crepitation through that range. The knee was stable. Radiographs showed a decreased medial articular cartilage space and a normal lateral joint cartilage space. However, there were several marginal osteophytes along the tibial, femoral, and patellar margins (Figs. 8-21A,B).

A tibial osteotomy was done, and the alignment was changed to 7° of valgus. There was marked relief of pain and improved function to the point where the patient now referees many basketball games in addition to teaching and coaching. He has been followed postoperatively for 3 years. The radiographs currently show no progression of the arthritis (Figs. 8-21C,D), and the medial joint cartilage space has not narrowed.

An increase in the cartilage space occurs rarely. When it does, as with subtrochanteric osteotomy for osteoarthritis of the hip, controversy arises as to how it can happen. It has been stated that the narrowing of the cartilage can be attributed to loss of cartilage matrix, mostly from abrasive wear on the surface (fibrillation and fissuring).[37,38,39] That surface, incapable of being restored to normal, would not be expected to elaborate new matrix, whether it be hyaline or fibrous. Nor would it be expected that the deeper cells in the cartilage would be stimulated to elaborate matrix production. The pathophysiology in these rare cases of thickening of cartilage remain an enigma, although two explanations have been suggested.[40] One is that in rare cases the narrowing is not mediated by the alterations just described so that wear and fibrillation have not occurred. Instead, possibly throughout the thickness of the articular cartilage, or perhaps in the zone where there is the most matrix surrounding chondrocytes, there has been resorption, possibly of water or of all the components of the matrix. It is postulated that this resorption is reversible in these rare cases. Another postulated explanation is that the thickening is an illusion, based on differences in the positioning of the knee for radiography. No histological evidence has been available to explain this rare phenomenon. With the osteotomy, preservation of the remaining cartilage is the most the surgeon can expect, although perhaps a halt in the growth of the osteophytes can be sought, as the architecture of the underlying subchondral cortex and cancellous bone is remodeled in response to the realigned muscular and weight-bearing stresses.[30]

One other operation might have been chosen for this patient: hemiarthroplasty. When only one compartment of the knee is compromised, usually more severely than in the present case, replacement of one-half of the joint, instead of replacing both compartments, may allow one to preserve the normal or minimally degenerated compartment. The end results of hemiarthroplasty are not nearly as predictable as the results of osteotomy; but when

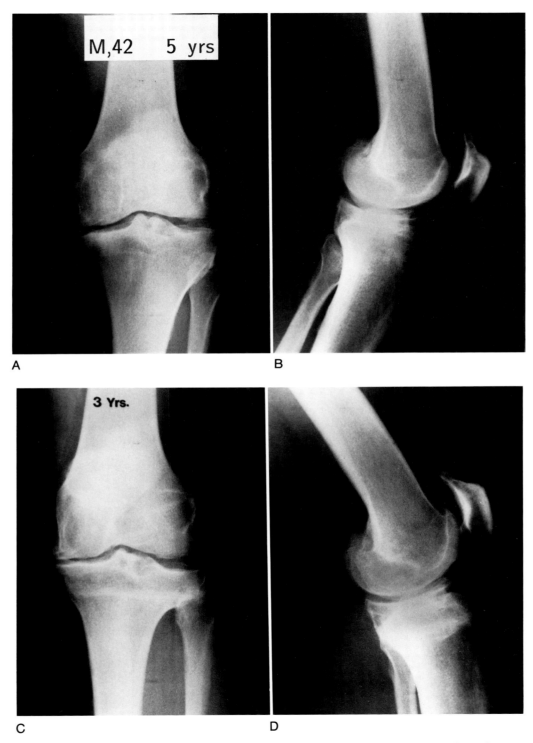

Fig. 8-21. Case 8-20. AP (**A**) and lateral (**B**) radiographs of the left knee show normal lateral joint space, small marginal osteophytes, decreased medial articular cartilage space, and a 4° varus deformity. No progression of the disease is seen in AP (**C**) and lateral (**D**) radiographs at 3 years.

successful, the success may be attributed to a more efficient correction of alignment. The need for a total knee replacement arthroplasty then may be deferred for years.

Patellofemoral Arthritis

Part of the pathological process in cases 8-19 and 8-20 was patellofemoral arthritis. No attention is paid to that lesion when an osteotomy or a hemiarthroplasty is done and justifiably so in view of the variable success recorded for both operations. It must be remembered that the patients selected for these two procedures are not those with severe osteoarthritis (total replacements usually are done for those patients). With that procedure the patellofemoral arthritis may deserve attention, but there still is controversy about what should be done: patellectomy, prosthetic replacement, and so on. It seems probable that the patellofemoral arthritis may be wrongfully accused as the culprit for causing pain in view of the fact that, in isolation, patellofemoral lesions do not cause serious impairment.[46]

This point is illustrated by the condition called *chondromalacia*. It raises the question of whether the alignment of the patella and knee is at fault. Usually chondromalacia occurs in patients who have more than the normal amount of valgus, a group that includes many young women or girls, especially those who are athletically active.[14] The articular cartilage of the patella becomes soft and fissured or fibrillated. When there is parapatellar pain and crepitation palpable at specific arcs of motion, depending on the area of patella that is involved, there is little doubt about the diagnosis. In most cases the pain is not so severe as to preclude some activity, and the patient's symptoms can be relieved by relatively simple measures, i.e., restriction of the extremes of activity and quadriceps strengthening exercises. The natural history of the process, however, includes some alleviation of the pain with time, particularly if the patient is a teenager and the physical activities become less rigorous. The degenerative changes in the cartilage may be expected to progress slowly and not to show repair. However, when it can be demonstrated that improper tracking of the patella in the patellofemoral groove is part of the problem, as revealed by standing radiographs of both knees or more sophisticated radiological or CT studies of the alignment of the patellofemoral joint, the surgeon may well consider how that alignment can be improved. This situation arises when, despite conservative therapy, the symptoms persist and the individual concerned is young and unwilling to forego athletics permanently. Surgical therapy then becomes a viable option, as illustrated in the following case.

Case 8-21 A 15-year-old girl had had pain in one knee for 2 years and femorotibial angle of 15° bilaterally. Arthrotomy of the knee showed marked degenerative changes of the articular surface of the patella, with loss of cartilage on its lateral face down to bare bone. Fibrillation of the remainder of the cartilage was evident. A patellectomy was performed. Because the angle the patellar tendon made with the tibia was so large, a release of the lateral retinaculum was done. The quadriceps and patellar tendon were realigned. In cases with less severe degenerative changes and less valgus, a realignment of the patellar ligament at its insertion with relocation of a block of tibial bone might be the procedure indicated if the patella then could be made to track more normally.

How extensive an operation is justified in the individual case is a difficult problem for the surgeon (be it a retinacular release arthroscopy, a Macquet procedure, or one of those mentioned above.) In principle, one should do the least extensive operation that can reliably relieve the symptoms. As noted earlier (see Ch. 6), repair of articular cartilage defects is impossible, if by "repair" one means complete restitution of the cartilage surface to normal. When a narrow hiatus, as by an experimental incision or a surgical incision, is devised in the cartilage, especially if it extends to the subchondral bone, it may be filled with fibrous repair tissue, which then is converted by metaplasia to fibrocartilage. The same phenomenon is evident when, as with a cup arthroplasty or similar procedure, cancellous bone is exposed and then subjected to cyclical motion. Metaplasia-to-cartilage transformation also occurs in cases of nonunion of fractures, where a pseudarthrosis develops (see Ch. 5). Arthroscopic treatment of chondromalacia by abrasion of eburnated bone and softened and fibrillated cartilage so that repair fibrocartilage will be formed may sound rational, but it is not likely to accomplish much more than does partial synovectomy with débridement of the arthritic joint in which osteophytes are removed along with loose bits of fissured or fibrillated cartilage with no attempt to "smooth off" the surface. That procedure has been shown to yield variable relief of pain of short duration. The arthroscopic release of the lateral bands for patellar chondromalacia has also been demonstrated to afford temporary relief at best, and the retinaculum then can be expected only to scar down and not to relieve the tracking abnormality.

The Macquet procedure mentioned above was designed to reduce the compression load on the patellofemoral joint. The tibial tubercle is osteotomized, and the block of bone so formed is elevated anteriorly from the tibia so as to shift the entire patella and quadriceps mechanism anteriorly. It too has not stood the test of time.

Arthritis of the MP Joint of the Great Toe

Another example of monarticular involvement, where the site of involvement introduces special pathophysiological principles, is arthritis of the metatarsal phalangeal (MP) joint of the great toe. This condition deserves mention because of the frequency of its occurrence.[29] Most commonly it seems to be caused by pressure from shoes, but sometimes the condition is hereditary. The arthritis most often accompanies a hallux valgus deformity; less commonly it occurs in the absence of valgus, i.e., as hallux rigidus. That there are so many surgical methods to treat the hallux valgus and the accompanying arthritis is evidence that no single method is without disadvantages. The importance of the associated hallux valgus deformity is a problem not often encountered with arthritis at other sites and arises because the individuals most often affected, women, insist on cosmetic considerations over and above functional considerations, both for the years during which the condition develops and postoperatively. The soft tissue enlargement about the joint in the form of a bunion complicates the problems. The following case is an

illustration of how several components of the composite lesion influence one another and how one method of surgical treatment was applied as it related to two or three components, but not all.

Case 8-22 A 57-year-old woman had a hallux valgus bilaterally, worse on the left. She did not have degenerative arthritis in parts other than the MP joint. A swelling along the medial border of the MP joint developed over the last few years and was getting worse. Shoe corrections (e.g., stretching of the leather over the involved joint, a pad, a metatarsal bar) were of only transitory benefit. There was a bunion over the first MP joint that was acutely inflamed. The hallux valgus was severe enough to cause slight medial deviation of the second toe. There was splaying of the fifth ray of the foot and a bunionette over the fifth metatarsal head that had appeared within the last year. Her foot had flattened out so that the transverse arch disappeared, and she began to experience metatarsalgia. Fitting a shoe became difficult because of the inability to get a shoe that was wide enough and that was comfortable.

The radiographs of the foot showed the soft tissue swellings over the first metatarsal head, the splaying of the first and fifth rays of the foot, and loss of the transverse arch. The hallux valgus was evident, and there was severe arthritis of the MP joint manifested by marginal osteophytes and narrowing of the joint cartilage space (Fig. 8-22A). The treatment chosen was the Keller procedure, supplemented by excision of the bursa with the underlying metatarsal prominence (Fig. 8-22B).

A major component (or the essence) of the Keller procedure is removal of the proximal part (one-half) of the proximal phalanx of the big toe. Adjuvant components may also be needed, however, e.g., removal of osteophytes or both sesamoid bones (if there is arthritis in their articulations with the metatarsal) or plastic repair of the medial connective tissue structures that have been made redundant because of the removal of the phalangeal bone. The pathophysiological rationale of the procedure, however extensive, is to convert a painful arthritic joint to a painless pseudarthrosis; it is accomplished by excising the inflamed synovial membrane. The mechanical rationale is to remove enough of the metatarsal head medially to relieve the pressure of that bone on the skin, pressure ex-

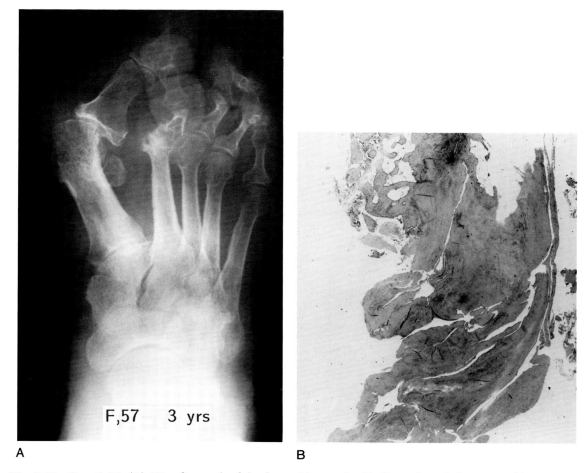

Fig. 8-22. Case 8-22. **(A)** AP radiograph of the foot with a marked hallux valgus deformity and bunion. **(B)** Photomicrograph of the bursa forming the bunion shows the clefts of the bursal tissue and the underlying bone of the osteotomy of the head of the metatarsal (×40).

erted because the maloriented metatarsal presses the skin against the medial border of the shoe. The procedure sacrifices much of the toe's function although potential for active flexion of the big toe remains; the function sacrificed is use of the toe flexors in take-off during gait. Much of that potential in women affected by the lesion had already been lost because of the habitual wearing of the culpable shoes (wedge-shaped or high heeled) that tend to make the take-off function of the hallux inoperative.

Other components of the lesion also were ignored by the Keller procedures: the bunionette,

splaying of the metatarsals, and loss of the transverse arch. Other procedures variably include attention to one or more of those components. Some, like the Mayo procedure, resemble the Keller method in that they fashion a pseudarthrosis but by removing the articular end of the metatarsal. Others try to retain the articulation if its alignment is not markedly disturbed, while correcting the alignment of the distal part of the metatarsal. The variability of the procedures described for this condition therefore is in some measure related to variations in the degree and composition of this multifactorial condition as well as the variation in the pathophysiological rationale of therapy. The patient in case 8-22 obtained relief of symptoms for at least 3 years.

The degree of arthritic pathological destruction of that joint is not as critical as the secondary mechanical effects on weight-bearing and shoeing. The advocates of resection arthroplasty and implant replacement cannot yet report predictable end results, although a number of prostheses are in use. Fusion in selected cases of posttraumatic arthritis relieves pain but may give problems with shoes because of the fixed angle of the fusion. Additional surgical considerations include osteotomies of the metatarsal (first or fifth) to achieve alignment for better shoeing or cosmesis, although usually neither is necessary for improving function or relieving pain. Coupled with the anatomical consideration in each patient is the associated disease (e.g., diabetes and its complications, rheumatoid arthritis, chronic alcoholic neuropathy), each of which would influence the selection of a particular treatment. With most of these complicating diseases, caution would dictate a conservative, not a surgical, approach to treatment. When a surgical procedure is needed, it usually should be a minimal one, simply to make shoe fitting simpler so the patient may continue to walk. A number of texts on surgical procedures of the foot and ankle are now available in addition to the standard ones on operative orthopedics.

Arthritis of the Spine

In contrast to the case just illustrated, where the arthritis under discussion involved mainly one joint, the metatarsophalangeal, and the secondary consequences of that lesion involved possibly all the structures of the forefoot, arthritis often involves several joints in concert. When it does, a somewhat similar pathophysiological principle in surgical therapy applies, i.e., that the totality of the involvement, not just that in a single articulation, must be kept in mind, even if one joint's involvement overshadows the others. It is illustrated by a case of degenerative arthritis of the spine, but the principle applies to any arthritis of the spine — rheumatoid, traumatic, metabolic.[2,31,45]

Degenerative arthritis of the spine can present in a variety of forms, some involving primarily the neck, others the back (usually the lower part of the back). Some involve several or many intervertebral levels, and some involve only one; but even when only one level is involved, at least four joints are directly affected: the syndesmosis (the two articulations of vertebral bone with intervertebral disc) and the two zygoapophyseal joints. It also should be emphasized that even when the histological changes are seen at only one level, functionally the other levels may be affected in that they may have to compensate for the loss of motion or the deformity at the involved level. In particular, because most of the muscles that move the vertebrae stretch over many levels, pain that is elicited by a structural or inflammatory change at one level usually causes spasm of muscles that affect entire regions of the spine. One obvious consequence is that when muscle spasm is a physical finding with little else to indicate a diagnosis, it is practically impossible to detect by physical examination the level or the joint that is affected.

As another illustration of how site of involvement influences pathophysiology, we have selected involvement of an intervertebral disc. Involvement of that structure is often associated with involvement of immediately adjacent structures (radiculopathy, spinal stenosis) (see Fig. 8-26, below), so the clinical spectrum is too wide to be considered. The illustration here was thus chosen merely to emphasize some morphological changes in the disc itself.

Intervertebral discs tend to undergo degeneration as a natural sequence of aging. The degeneration begins early in life, even before skeletal maturity, and progresses at varying rates in each individual. The writings of Schmorl,[61] Hirsch et al.,[25] Hirsch and Schajowicz,[24] and Coventry et al.[8-11] are particularly pertinent for describing the changes that may be called physiological, not pathological, as they occur with aging. However, the histological changes are indistinguishable from those that are called pathological changes; the distinction rests on gross patterns of change and their effects on adjacent structures.

Case 8-23 A 65-year-old man had no history of back pain. Photomicrographs show some loss of height of the disc, fissures within the disc substance

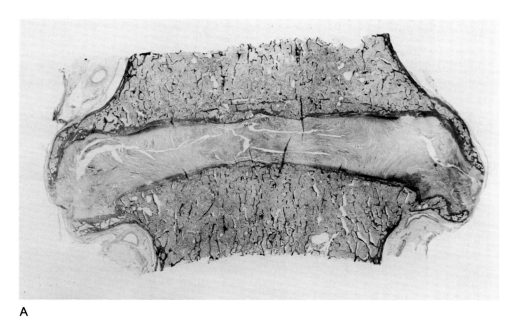

A

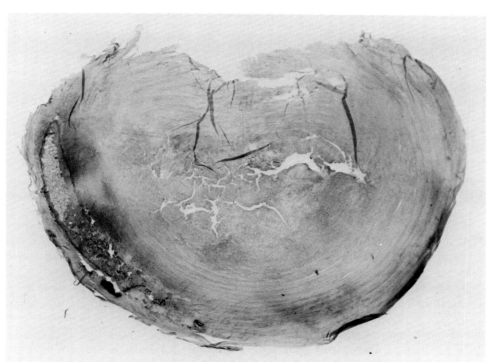

B

Fig. 8-23. Case 8-23. **(A)** Coronal section of the L4 intervertebral disc shows a loss of disc-height, fissures within the substance and ossification of the margins ($\times$4). **(B)** Horizontal section shows the annulus fibrous rings and the central fissures of the nucleus pulposus ($\times$4).

centrally and degeneration of that structure extending out to the margins where osteophytes extend from the vertebral bodies (Figs. 8-23A,B). These changes did not elicit either symptoms or signs, but one can readily postulate that in the natural course of events an incident of stress on such a disc can produce either a herniation of degenerated disc substance or accentuation of the loss of height. In either case, a series of events may ensue that cause pain.

Case 8-24 A 19-year-old football player developed acute low back pain during a particularly hard practice session. He became aware of a sharp, knife-like pain radiating from the right buttock into the posterior aspect of the thigh and down the lateral aspect of the leg. The outstanding physical findings were a positive straight-leg-raising test and a depressed ankle jerk. The clinical diagnosis of a herniated nucleus pulposus at the L4–L5 level was confirmed by CT and myelography (Fig. 8-24A,B), which showed that the herniated disc material compressed the dural sac. MRI in the sagittal plane also shows a filling defect in the spinal canal caused by fragment of herniated disc (Figs. 8-24C,D).

An operation was performed to remove the disc fragment that had herniated into the spinal canal, and it immediately relieved the pain. The surgical objective was based on the following pathophysiological concepts: (1) that continuing pressure from the fragment probably would make the neurological deficit permanent; and (2) possibly that deficit might be more extensive (i.e., sensory or motor loss) if the fragment elicited an inflammatory reaction. It would be expected that, with rest, the tear in the annulus fibrosus through which the disc fragment herniated would heal. It is probable that some of the more liquid substance from the center of the disc also had herniated but that material would be much more easily resorbed than would the fragment of fibrocartilage. Histologically, the fragment closely resembled the substance near the annulus fibrosis in Figure 8-23. The radiographs obtained postoperatively showed a reduction in disc height that was more than would be expected from loss of just the fragment removed, and that explained the suggestion (made above) that more than just the removed fragment had herniated.

The consequences of surgical removal of disc fragments is that surgical trauma is added to the effects of the rupture of the annulus fibrosis and the extrusion of disc fragments; moreover, the operation itself increases scar tissue at the site. The benefit of removing the fragment outweighs the disadvantages, however. Sometime later, perhaps years, the facet joints may develop secondary degenerative changes because of the altered stresses that follow the loss of disc height.

Examples of arthritis affecting the back have been provided in which morphological changes in the spine could be demonstrated and in which there were symptoms and signs (in addition to evidence of muscle spasm) that made surgical therapy appropriate. Preceding that therapy, radiological investigation (now ordinarily including CT and perhaps MRI) is performed to delineate the lesions in detail, as in case 8-25.

Case 8-25 (Fig. 8-25) A 63-year-old woman had complained of low back pain with intermittent leg pain bilaterally for 4 years. The leg pain was accompanied by paresthesias in both lower limbs below the knees when she walked one or two blocks. Both the pain and the paresthesias were relieved by rest. There was no associated weakness in the lower limbs. The patient did, however, have urinary stress incontinence with frequent urinary tract infection controlled by antibiotics. On examination the patient had 70° of flexion of the spine, 30° of lateral flexion, and negative straight-leg raising at 90° bilaterally. Motor power was normal, and ankle jerks were present but depressed bilaterally. Sensation and pulses were normal. Systematic evaluation indicated a mild weakness in bladder emptying and a small residual.

Such cases appear daily in one's ordinary practice — cases of back pain or cervical pain, with or without some radiological evidence of osteoarthritis, in which the lesions cannot be demonstrated. When the pain is intermittent or can be alleviated by conservative therapy, one may be at a loss to explain what lesion, if any, existed and how, pathophysiologically, our therapy could succeed. In such cases, it should be kept in mind that if one is dealing with an osteoarthritis or a traumatic arthritis, a component of those processes is inflammation.

Case 8-26 A 67-year-old man had had intermittent numbness and tingling of his left arm for 6

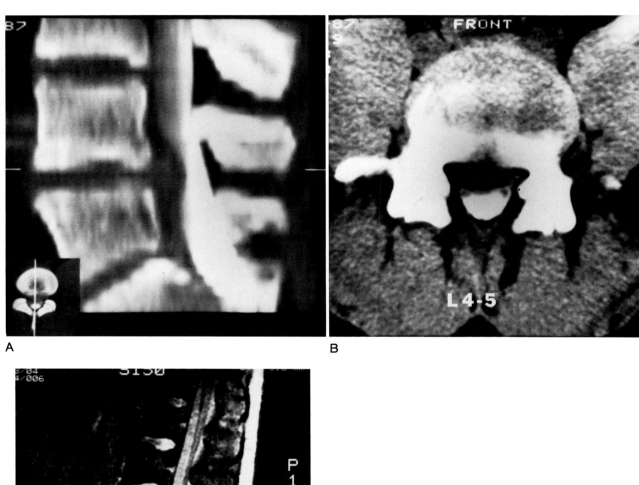

A

B

C

Fig. 8-24. Case 8-24. **(A)** Herniated disc material compressed the dural sac centrally and to the right **(B)** at L4–L5. **(C)** MRI in the sagittal plane reveals a defect of the disc at the L4–L5 level. *(Figure continues.)*

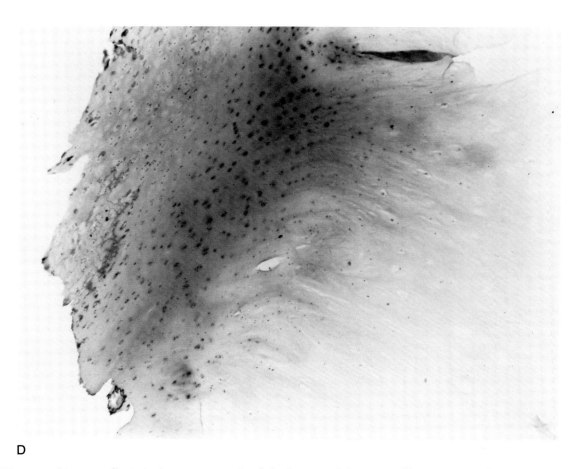

D

Fig. 8-24 *(Continued)*. **(D)** Photomicrograph of the herniated fragment, fibrocartilage of the annulus fibrosus, and the nucleus (×37).

months. On examination he had hypesthesia in the C5–C6 nerve root distribution. He had been unaware of a previous difficulty with his neck except for mild limitation in motion at the extremes.

In the narrow area of a facet joint in the spine, with an adjoining neural foramen (Fig. 8-26), only a small amount of edema fluid as part of the inflammation can exert sufficient pressure on the nerve root in the neural foramen (as in the synovial membrane and capsule of the facet joint) to be responsible for the pain. With conservative therapy that fluid may be resorbed within a few days or up to a week or two and might well explain the transience of the symptoms. The phenomenon can also be involved as a sequence adjacent to a herniated disc fragment. The obvious inference is that removal of

a herniated disc fragment is not mandatory, especially if a neurological deficit is not evident or is relatively minor and nonprogressive.[42,70]

Arthritis of the Hand

For the final illustration of how the site of involvement introduces important pathophysiological elements affecting surgical therapy, we have chosen a case of rheumatoid arthritis affecting the hand. A previous example of severe involvement in the hand (case 8-5) was included to illustrate how a sequence of operations is planned for step-by-step progress toward reducing the impairment and achieving a specific functional goal. The present

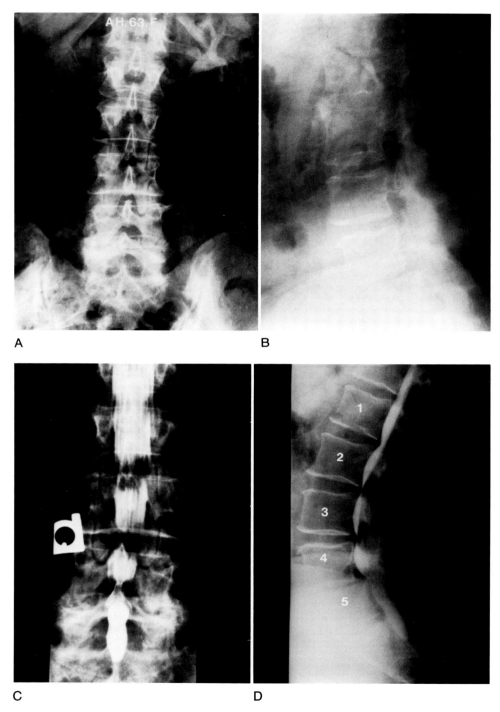

Fig. 8-25. **(A&B)** AP **(A)** and lateral **(B)** radiographs of the lumbosacral spine show degenerative disc and facet changes from L2 to S1. AP **(C)** and lateral **(D)** myelograms show multiple levels of indentation of the spinal canal consistent with a diagnosis of spinal stenosis. *(Figure continues.)*

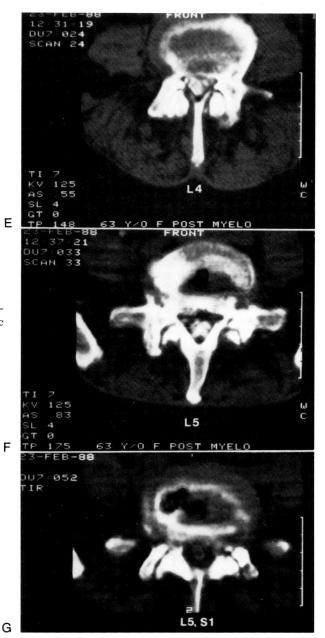

Fig. 8-25 *(Continued)*. (**E–G**) The anatomical configuration of the stenosis at L4–L5 and of the osteophytic facet joints at L5 are shown by these CT scans.

example, carpal tunnel syndrome, illustrates how the rheumatoid inflammatory process — here involving not only the joints but also nonarticular soft tissues — can introduce into the therapeutic regimen anatomical considerations peculiar to the site(s) of involvement.

Case 8-27 A 56-year-old patient had had rheumatoid arthritis for years, with major involvement of all four extremities. Nevertheless, she was doing fairly well as a housewife, although she noted that her normal activities (weaving, sewing) were being impeded by a progressive numbness in the right

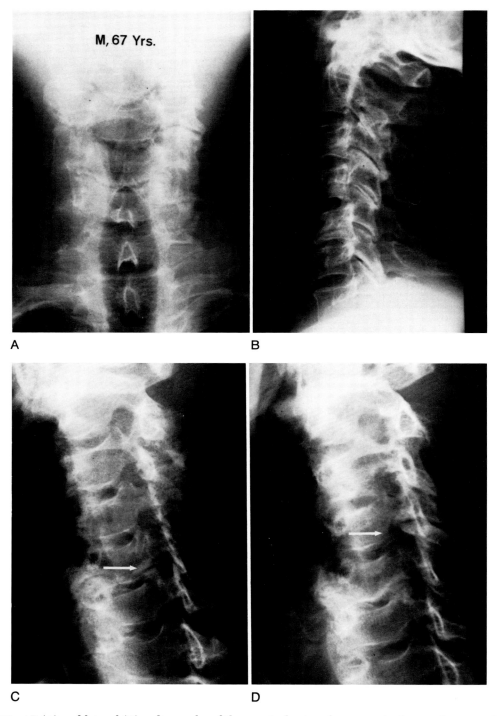

Fig. 8-26. AP (**A**) and lateral (**B**) radiographs of the cervical spine show marginal osteophytes at the facet joints. (**C&D**) Oblique views show encroachment of the neuroforamina of C5–C6 by the osteophytes (arrow). Treatment was symptomatic, with analgesics and a cervical collar.

hand and fingers. She had had years of known involvement of both hands with ulnar drift, but only during the last 2 months had the numbness become evident. Then, during the last week, she found that she was having trouble using the right thumb, which was the chief reason for consultation with an orthopedic surgeon, as suggested by her rheumatologist. There had been no recent exacerbation of the rheumatoid arthritis.

Examination of the right hand revealed all the classical signs of rheumatoid arthritis, affecting most of the interphalangeal joints and all of the MP joints. The wrist was swollen and showed a diminution in range of motion that had not changed significantly over the last few years. However, there was marked pain on passive as well as active flexion of the thumb, as well as hypesthesias in most of the hand and in the fingers. An electromyogram of the median nerve revealed findings of motor and sensory nerve involvement, and a carpal tunnel release was then done. As the tunnel was exposed, its synovial lining was seen to be thickened by chronic inflammation; in particular, the synovial sheath containing the flexor hallucis longus was more severely inflamed than was the synovial sheath of the other flexor tendons. Release of that sheath revealed that the layer covering the tendon was roughened and hypertrophied. A synovectomy of that tendon sheath was done; and other tendon sheaths, which were not so severely affected, were not débrided. The median nerve in the carpal canal was not directly involved in the inflammation.

Postoperatively, the thumb was able to flex without pain, and motion and use of the thumb and hand was encouraged as soon as possible. The numbness disappeared.

This case illustrates once more that when anatomical considerations include a restricted space that may be compromised, motion of tendons and passage of nerves through that space may be impeded. Arthritic swelling from adjacent joints, as well as actual inflammation with the space, may compromise the space.

In the case described, release of the carpal ligament and synovectomy were successful, but unfortunately the numbness recurred 2 years later. Although surgery was refused, the recurrence was attributed to reconstitution of the carpal ligament by scar and the continuing rheumatoid synovitis in the carpal tunnel.

This case also emphasizes the need for early motion of tendons that have been involved by an inflammatory process (or perhaps by a surgical procedure), the results of which might be expected to cause scarring and adhesions that ultimately would prevent the tendon from sliding within its sheath. Such motion must be started within days of the surgical procedure (here the removal of the synovial sheath) if motion is to be retained.

REFERENCES

1. Anderson CF, Ludowieg J, Harper HA: Engleman EP: The composition of the organic component of human articular cartilage: relationship to age and degenerative joint disease. J Bone Joint Surg [Am] 46:1176, 1964
2. Arnoldi CC, Brodsky AE, Cauchoix J, Crock HV, et al: Lumbar spinal stenosis and nerve root entrapment syndromes: definition and classification. CORR 115:4, 1976
3. Bennett GA, Waine H, Bauer W: Changes in the Knee Joint at Various Ages with Particular Reference to the Nature and Development of Degenerative Joint Disease. Commonwealth Fund, New York, 1942
4. Blount WP: Osteotomy in the treatment of osteoarthritis of the hip. J Bone Joint Surg [Am] 46:1297, 1964
5. Bombelli R: Osteoarthritis of the Hip Classification and Pathogenesis: The role of Osteotomy as a Consequent Therapy. 2nd Ed. Springer, Berlin, 1983
6. Brand RA: Joint lubrication, Ch. 10. In: The Scientific Basis of Orthopedics. Appleton-Century-Crofts, E Norwalk, CT, 1979
7. Brower TD: The growth and nutrition of articular cartilage. J Bone Joint Surg [Am] 49:1008, 1967
8. Coventry MB: Anatomy of the intervertebral disc. Clin Orthop 67:9, 1969
9. Coventry MB, Ghormley RK, Kernohan JW: The intervertebral disc: its microscopic anatomy and pathology. Part I. J Bone Joint Surg 27:105, 1945
10. Coventry MB, Ghormley RK, Kernohan JW: The intervertebral disc: its microscopic anatomy and pathology. Part II. Changes in the intervertebral disc with age. J Bone Joint Surg 27:233, 1945

11. Coventry MB, Ghormley RK, Kernohan JW: The intervertebral disc: its microscopic anatomy and pathology. Part III. Pathological changes in the intervertebral disc. J Bone Joint Surg 27:460, 1945

12. Curtiss Jr PH: Changes produced in the synovial membrane and synovial fluid by disease. J Bone Joint Surg [Am] 46:873, 1964

13. Curtiss Jr PH, Kincaid WE: Transitory demineralization of the hip in pregnancy. J Bone Joint Surg [Am] 41:1327, 1959

14. DeHaven KE, Dolan WA, Mayer PJ: Chondromalacia patellae in athletes. Am J Sports Med 7:5, 1979

15. Edwards CC, Chrisman OD: Articular cartilage. Ch. 9. In: The Scientific Basis of Orthopedics. Appleton-Century-Crofts, E Norwalk, CT, 1979

16. Ferguson AB: The pathological changes in degenerative arthritis of the hip and treatment by rotational osteotomy. J Bone Joint Surg [Am] 46:1337, 1964

17. Foucar E, Buckwalter JA, El-Khoury GY: Gout presenting as a femoral cyst. J Bone Joint Surg [Am] 66:294, 1984

18. Gibson DA: Congenital dislocation of the hip: a review of adults treated in childhood. Can J Surg 10:288, 1967

19. Gould N: Hallux rigidus, cheilotomy or implant? Foot Ankle 1:315, 1981

20. Greenwald AS, Haynes DW: Weight bearing areas in the human hip joint. J Bone Joint Surg [Br] 54:157, 1972

21. Guerra J, Resnick D: Arthritides affecting the foot: radiographic-pathologic correlation. Foot Ankle 2:325, 1982

22. Harrison MHM, Schajowicz F, Trueta J: Osteoarthritis of the hip: a study of the nature and evolution of the disease. J Bone Joint Surg [Br] 35:598, 1953

23. Hellman DB, Helms CA, Genant HK: Chronic repetitive trauma: a cause of atypical degenerative joint disease. Skeletal Radiol 10:236, 1983

24. Hirsch C, Schajowicz F: Studies in the lumbar annulus fibrosis. Acta Orthop Scand 22:184, 1952

25. Hirsch C, Paulson S, Sylven B, Snellman O: Characteristics of human nucleus pulposi during aging. Acta Orthop Scand 22:175, 1952

26. Hoaglund FT: Osteoarthritis: a general overview of the etiological factors, pathophysiology and physical findings in osteoarthritis. Orthop Clin North Am 2:3, 1971

27. Ishikawa H, Ohno O, Hirohata K: Long-term results of synovectomy in rheumatoid patients. J Bone Joint Surg [Am] 68:198, 1986

28. Johnson C: Kinetics of osteoarthritis. Lab Invest Armed Forces Inst Pathol 8:1223, 1959

29. Kelickian H: The hallux. p. 539. In: Jahss: Disorders of the Foot. Vol. I. WB Saunders, Philadelphia, 1982

30. Kettelkamp DB: Tibial osteotomy. p. 249. In McEverts C (ed): Surgery of the Musculoskeletal System. Vol. 3. Churchill Livingstone, New York, 1983

31. Kirkaldy-Willis WH, McIvor GWD: Lumbar spinal stenosis—editorial comment. Spine 115:2, 1976

32. Knodt H: Osteoarthritis of the hip joint: etiology and treatment by osteotomy. J Bone Joint Surg [Am] 46:1326, 1964

33. Larson CB: The wearing out of joints. J Am Geriatr Soc 10:558, 1962

34. Larson CB: "When" arthroplasty. In: Die Therapie der Koxarthrose. Georg Thieme Verlag, Stuttgart, 1969

35. Lothe K, Spycher MA, Ruttner JR: Focal lacunar resorption in the articular cartilage of femoral heads. J Bone Joint Surg [Br] 67:543, 1985

36. Malvitz T, Weinstein SW: Congenital hip dysplasia: review of 152 closed reductions with 31 year follow-up. To be published

37. Mankin, J: Biochemical and metabolic aspects of osteoarthritis. Orthop Clin North Am 2:19, 1971

38. Mankin HJ: The reaction of articular cartilage to injury and osteoarthritis, parts 1 and 2. N Engl J Med 291:1285, 1974

39. Mankin HJ: Current concepts, the response of articular cartilage to mechanical injury. J Bone Joint Surg [Am] 64:460, 1982

40. Mankin HJ, Lippiello LMS: Biochemical and metabolic abnormalities in articular cartilage from osteoarthritic human hips. J Bone Joint Surg [Am] 52:424, 1970

41. Martel W, Seeger JF, Wicks JD, Washburn RL: Traumatic lesions of the discovertebral junction in the lumbar spine. AJR 127:457, 1976

42. Massie WK: Chemonucleosis—editorial comment. Clin Orthop 67:2, 1959

43. Mardam-Beg TH, McEwen CD: Congenital dislocation of the hip after walking age. J Pediatr Orthop 2:478, 1982

44. McFarland JR, Sherman S: The synovial reactions of rheumatoid arthritis. Clin Orthop 36:10, 1964

45. McIvor GWD, Kirkaldy-Willis WH: Pathological and myelographic changes in major types of lumbar spinal stenosis. Clin Orthop 115:72, 1976

46. Merchant AC: Isolated patellofemoral arthritis. Contemp Orthop November:1015, 1981

47. Morscher W: Intertrochanteric osteotomy in osteoarthritis of the hip. p. 24. In: Proceedings of the 8th Open Scientific Meeting of the Hip Society, 1980

48. Nichols EH, Richardson FL: Arthritis deformans. J Med Res 2:149, 1909
49. Nissen KI: The arrest of primary osteoarthritis of the hip. J Bone Joint Surg [Br] 42:423, 1960
50. Nissen KI: The rationale of early osteotomy for idiopathic coxarthrosis (epichondro-osteoarthrosis of the hip). Clin Orthop 77:98, 1971
51. Olsson SE: Degenerative joint disease (osteoarthrosis): a review with special reference to the dog. J Small Anim Pract 12:333, 1971
52. Pauwels F: Biomechanics of the Normal and Diseased Hip. Springer, Berlin, 1976
53. Phillips CD, Keats TE: Development of post-traumatic cyst-like lesions in bone. Skeletal Radiol 15:631, 1986
53a. Ponseti IV, McClintock R: The pathology of slipping of the upper femoral epiphysis. J Bone Joint Surg [Am] 38:71, 1956
54. Poss R: The role of osteotomy in the treatment of osteoarthritis of the hip — current concepts review. J Bone Joint Surg [Am] 46:144, 1984
55. Radin EL, Paul IL, Tolkoff MJ: Subchondral bone changes in patients with early degenerative joint disease. Arthritis Rheum 13:400, 1970
56. Radin EL, Rose EM: Role of subchondral bone in the initiation and progression of cartilage damage. Clin Orthop 213:34, 1986
57. Ritchie JH, Fahrni WH: Age changes in lumbar intervertebral discs. Can J Surg 13:65, 1970
57a. Rodman GP, Schumacher HR (eds): Primer on Rheumatic Diseases, 8th ed. Arthritis Foundation, Atlanta, 1983
58. Salter RB, Kostuik J, Dallas S: Avascular necrosis of the femoral head as a complication of treatment for congenital dislocation of the hip in young children — a clinical and experimental investigation. Can J Surg, 12:44, Jan., 1969
59. Santore RF, Bombelli R: Long-term follow-up of the Bombelli experience with osteotomy for osteoarthritis: result at 11 years. p. 106. In: Proceedings of the 11th Open Scientific Meeting of the Hip Society. CV Mosby, St. Louis, 1983
60. Schajowicz F, Clavel Sainz M, Slullitel JA: Juxta articular bone cysts (intra-osseous ganglia). J Bone Joint Surg [Br] 61:107, 1979
61. Schmorl G, Junghanns H: The Human Spine in Health and Disease. 2nd American Ed. Grune & Stratton, New York, 1971, pp. 2–14, 158
62. Severin E: Congenital dislocation of the hip joint — late results of closed reduction and arthrographic studies of recent cases. Acta Orthop Scand [Suppl] 63:1, 1941
63. Sherman MS: The non-specificity of synovial reactions. Bull Hosp Joint Dis (NY) 12:110, 1951
64. Simmons DP, Chrisman OD: Salicylate inhibition of cartilage degradation. Arthritis Rheum 8:960, 1965
65. Smith WS, Badgley CE, Orwiz JB, Harper TW: Correlation of post reduction roentgenograms and thirty-one-year follow-up in congenital dislocations of the hip. J Bone Joint Surg [Am] 50:1081, 1968
66. Wedge JH, Salter RB: Innominate osteotomy: its role in the arrest of secondary degenerative arthritis of the hip in the adult. Clin Orthop 98:214, 1974
67. Weinstein SL: Natural history of congenital hip dislocation (CDH) and hip dysplasia. Clin Or RR 225:62, 1987
68. Wiberg G: Relation between congenital subluxation of the hip and arthritis deformans Acta Orthop Scand 10:351, 1939
69. Wiberg G: Studies on dysplastic acetabula and congenital subluxation of the hip joint with special reference to the complication of osteoarthritis. Acta Orthop Scand 58 (Suppl):1, 1939
70. Wiesel SW, Cuckler JM, Deluca F, Jones F, Zeide MS, Rothman RH: Acute low back pain: an objective analysis of conservation therapy. Spine 5:324, 1980

9

Musculoskeletal Tumors

When one suspects that the patient has a musculoskeletal tumor, the first problem is to prove that the lesion is indeed a tumor and then to identify it. Reference can be made to textbooks on the subject (see Ch. 11), but a differential diagnosis always is needed, and how to proceed with the evaluation and treatment is the focus of this chapter. The main emphasis again is on pathophysiology during the evaluation process. The goal is a diagnosis efficiently arrived at followed by application of the most efficacious treatment.

The first question is if the lesion under consideration is a tumor. If it is, whether the tumor is benign or malignant becomes the prime consideration. If malignant, the problem is whether the tumor is metastatic or primary. Only after these questions have been answered does the exact nature (specific diagnosis) of the tumor become important.

To illustrate the evaluation and treatment process we use examples not only of diagnostic problem cases but also of standard uncomplicated cases, both benign and malignant. In particular, we describe the approach used when, at the onset, one suspects that the tumor is a metastatic one. It is perhaps unfortunate that so much emphasis has been accorded primary malignancies of bone that, despite their relatively low incidence compared to either benign tumors or metastases, they have assumed so much importance in differential diagnosis.

There is no problem affecting the musculoskeletal system where the necessity for evaluation and correlation of the clinical, radiographic, and pathological aspects of the problem requires more skill than for the evaluation and treatment of musculoskeletal tumors. The orthopedic surgeon, after exercising that skill and arriving at a provisional diag-

nosis, must then decide what will be his or her role vis-à-vis the patient and the patient's family. At the very least, even during the evaluation procedures, the surgeon must advise the patient and family about what to expect from the process of evaluation and perhaps the treatment of the lesion. If the patient is to be referred for further evaluation and treatment, the specific reasons must be explained.

Suppose the physician decides that after the diagnostic tests a diagnosis can be reached that is not provisional and, further, that the patient can be treated definitively at his own institution, no matter what that diagnosis might be. The surgeon's role is then the standard one of the physician who is "in charge."

When the patient is being referred, that role changes, and the change depends on the reason for referral. The first reason for referral may be that the surgeon is not confident concerning his or her own expertise or that of colleagues in handling the case in question. Thus care in a medical center where a large number of patients with tumors are evaluated and treated is then advisable to minimize the risk of errors of evaluation (in particular, biopsy interpretation).

Another reason might be the need for special facilities, either diagnostic or therapeutic, not available locally. The important consideration of avoiding any delay in arriving at a diagnosis that might adversely affect the therapeutic decisions should be uppermost in the surgeon's mind, once a provisional diagnosis of tumor has been made. The physician who first encounters the patient and refers him or her to a center often needs to serve as the patient's "interpreter" concerning events preceding the evaluation and treatment process that is now being done elsewhere; moreover, in many in-

397

stances, the surgeon may also be involved with care of the patient once the definitive treatment is well under way.

It quickly becomes apparent why the foregoing remarks are needed, when it is considered on one hand, how infrequently individual surgeons treat patients with primary malignant tumors and, on the other, how frequently other patients who have metastatic or benign tumors come under the care of the same surgeons. Although statistics on cancer deaths in the United States indicate clearly that sarcomas in bone and soft tissue are relatively rare,[8,31] these data refer to primary malignant tumors only and do not include the much larger number of benign tumors and cancers metastatic to bone. The problems of diagnosis and evaluation in regard to treatment of these more frequent lesions ordinarily are similar to those of the primary malignant tumors, even though the treatment is not. Data on cancer deaths indicate that about 1,400 people in the United States die per year of bone sarcomas and 2,800 of soft tissue sarcomas. These figures represent less than 1 percent of all cancer deaths, but there are no statistics on what percentage of any of those groups of patients, who prior to their demise, have skeletal metastases that may require treatment. Undoubtedly, that percentage is high. The process of diagnosis by the patient's physician may at first be similar to that for any tumor; but once it becomes evident that there is a strong likelihood the tumor is malignant, and probably not metastatic, the patient may well be referred to another physician for further diagnostic tests.

No one institution or individual has a large experience in the evaluation and treatment of the sarcomas. Therefore one of the major problems in the treatment of musculoskeletal tumors is the lack of concentrations of patients who have similar lesions because it poses obstacles to the evaluation of any therapeutic regimen and to the development of surgical, radiological, and pharmacological therapy that will be more effective than the regimens used in the past. These obstacles are so formidable that the only way they can be circumvented is by collaborative studies using identical protocols, methods of assessment, and so on. It is equally important to note that at the collaborative centers the most modern and promising methods of diagnosis and treatment are applied. It therefore is preferable, when practical, for family practitioners and orthopedic surgeons who only see an occasional primary musculoskeletal neoplasm to refer such patients immediately, i.e., before a biopsy is done, to one of those centers. There it is routine for a team consisting of an orthopedic surgeon, a radiologist, a pathologist, a radiation therapist, a nuclear medicine physician, a medical oncologist, and an immunologist to take up the case.

Although this prescription of referral applies to most cases of sarcoma, it ordinarily does not apply to nearly all metastatic lesions or to most benign tumors. It may apply to some metastatic tumors where major problems in specific diagnosis are anticipated or where reconstructive surgery is part of the treatment. A major problem that has become evident in recent years is delays in treatment once the provisional diagnosis of malignant tumor is made. Multiple consultations regarding the histological slides may be sought, some of them by mail, especially if the local pathologists differ in their interpretations of the exact nature of the tumor. Most of these delays can be avoided if the surgeon with the clinical (but not biopsy) data at hand anticipates that there may be such a problem. In most instances, hospital laboratories that process only a few specimens from osseous lesions per year experience technical difficulties with these specimens; and when the surgeon is aware of that possibility, he or she can anticipate the problem. Referral prior to biopsy would then be best for the patient.

This type of practical problem is best discussed, briefly, as it is encountered when the patient is a child because primary bone tumors pose difficulties in diagnosis and treatment in children. It should be noted that one-third of all sarcomas occur in children under 15 years of age. In fact, primary tumors of the musculoskeletal system rank high on the list of causes of death in children (after leukemia and tumors of the central nervous system). When the surgeon has previously managed the preliminary diagnostic work-up in collaboration with the referring pediatrician and has referred the child to a center for definitive treatment, his or her role in the conduct of the case often is not finished.

There continue to be distressing problems that an orthopedic surgeon must face in fulfilling his or her appropriate and variable role. The orthopedist may have to rely heavily on the pediatrician for day-to-day prescription of analgesics and on an oncologist for supervision of chemotherapy. The orthopedist, rather than the pediatrician, may be called on to devise the support structure that is needed: if the child has had an amputation or a limb-sparing procedure, there is a need for social service personnel and possibly other paramedical specialists (e.g., a prosthetist familiar with the specific needs of the child). Sometimes the parents can be satisfied only by the team in a referral center. The child's disability may be dealt with by personnel accustomed to dealing only with adults, but the special needs of children (educational, psychosocial, and prosthetic — all influenced by growth) emphasize the advisability of referral of pediatric patients with tumors to an oncology center. There the team exists not only for the therapy but also for devising a local medical structure to carry on the aftercare, which may last many years.

Whatever the role of the orthopedic surgeon initially, with regard to an already anxious parent or patient who has entrusted him or her with any aspect of the responsibilities of diagnosis or care, the surgeon must keep in mind one primary duty to the patient, perhaps the epitome of the Hippocratic oath: *to do no harm.* Harm here may mean raising the level of anxiety of the patient or parents, e.g., overemphasizing the possibility of malignancy when it is actually remote. The overemphasis may be by implication alone or by pursuing an inordinately extensive testing regimen simply for the sake of a "complete" and thorough evaluation. The anxiety level may be unnecessarily heightened also by explicit emphasis by the surgeon during the discussion of possibilities in regard to "informed consent" to the treatment. It should be recognized that once the anxiety level is raised unduly, the surgeon may well be unable to convince the patient or parents thereafter that he or she is only fulfilling a principal duty — to assure them that all proper measures are being carried out with competence. This duty pertains when the surgeon is the primary physician (for triage) or the initial consultant who assumes the role of "captain of the ship"; the duty is assumed when the patient is referred to a center or when the surgeon provides a second opinion. The obligation always includes sensitive, tactful in-

teractions with the patient. The patient must be reassured that the problem is being addressed as well as possible. This precept can be violated in a number of ways, any one of which may prejudice either the result of treatment or, later, the patient's perception of how he was "handled" and the quality of the result. At one end of the spectrum of the evaluation process is an attitude that the "scientific" aspects of the tumor far outweigh the patient's needs. The other end of the spectrum is common during the triage segment of evaluation when the surgeon may discuss with the patient far too many details of possibilities in prospect that, as the evaluation proceeds, represent to the patient only psychological trauma. These areas are anxiety raisers that should be avoided.

CLASSIFICATION

Before discussing approaches to evaluation for establishing a diagnosis, a few words are appropriate about the classification of musculoskeletal tumors. It should be constantly kept in mind that a number of conditions simulate tumors (Table 9-1). A few of them have been illustrated in other chapters to clarify either some diagnostic or therapeutic aspect of the subject, e.g., stress fracture (see Ch. 3), ganglion cyst, and gout (see Ch. 8).

Considerable discussion has been devoted to schemes of classification of primary musculoskeletal tumors, but no one scheme has been universally accepted. One of the most recent that is commonly used is based on the histological typing of bone tumors. It was devised by the World Health Organization (WHO) and is available as two thin books, with beautiful and representative photomicrographs. One book covers the skeletal tumors[118] and the other the soft tissue sarcomas.[45,46] These classifications differ from others[150] only in minor ways, so that the others need not be considered here. We use a modified WHO classification for skeletal tumors (Table 9-2). Some controversy still exists over the grading of malignant tumors and the relative value of grading as associated with prognosis. The reader is referred to the publications of the American Joint Committee, the Union International Cancer Control (UICC), Spanier and Enne-

Table 9-1.   Conditions Simulating Tumors

Infections
   Syphilis tertiary: congenital, adult
   Pyogenic osteomyelitis
   Bone abscess
Developmental anomalies
   Anatomical variations of normal: cortical desmoid
   Metaphyseal (cortical) fibrous defect (nonosteo-
      genic fibroma)
   Osteogenic fibroma (Campanacci)
   Fibrous dysplasia
Circulatory disturbance in bone or aseptic necrosis:
   bone infarct
Metabolic disorders
   Gout
   Hyperparathyroidism: brown tumor
   Reticuloendotheliosis: all three forms of Histiocy-
      toses X
   Paget's disease
Injury and repair
   Stress fracture: osteoid osteoma, Ewing's sarcoma
   Avulsion fractures: especially ischium-cartilaginous
      tumor
   Heterotopic bone—soft tissue sarcoma: myositis os-
      sificans
   Aseptic necrosis, infarction, enchondroma, chon-
      drosarcoma
Miscellaneous
   Bone cyst
   Aneurysmal bone cyst
   Degenerative cyst: arthritis
   Ganglion cyst: injury and repair
   Paget's disease

Table 9-2.   Histological Typing of Primary Bone Tumors and Tumor-Like Lesions: WHO Classification (Modified)

I. Bone-forming tumors
   A. Benign
      1. Osteoma
      2. Osteoid osteoma
      3. Benign osteoblastoma
   B. Malignant
      1. Osteosarcoma
      2. Juxtacortical osteosarcoma
      3. Periosteal osteosarcoma
II. Cartilage-forming tumors
   A. Benign
      1. Chondroma
      2. Osteochondroma (osteocartilaginous exos-
         tosis)
      3. Chondroblastoma
      4. Chondromyxoid fibroma
   B. Malignant
      1. Chondrosarcoma
      2. Juxtacortical chondrosarcoma
      3. Mesenchymal chondrosarcoma
III. Fibrous or fibrohistiocytic tumors
   A. Benign
      1. Desmoplastic fibroma
   B. Intermediate or indeterminate
      1. Giant cell tumor
      2. Fibrous histiocytoma
   C. Malignant
      1. Fibrosarcoma
      2. Malignant fibrous histiocytoma
IV. Marrow tumors
      1. Ewing's sarcoma
      2. Reticulosarcoma of bone
      3. Lymphosarcoma of bone
      4. Myeloma
V. Vascular tumors
   A. Benign
      1. Hemangioma
      2. Lymphangioma
      3. Glomus tumor
   B. Intermediate or indeterminate
      1. Hemangiosarcoma
      2. Hemangiopericytoma
   C. Malignant
      1. Angiosarcoma
VI. Lipomatous tumors of bone
   A. Benign
      1. Lipoma
   B. Malignant
      1. Liposarcoma
VII. Other connective tissue tumors
      1. Malignant mesenchymoma
      2. Undifferentiated sarcoma

Continued

king,[2,39,42,43] and Suit et al.[142] for discussions of grading and staging.

   Much attention has been paid to surgical procedures for primary skeletal malignancies in the extremities, staging formulas, and protocols of treatment.[38] Each of these three topics requires considerable discussion, which can be found later in the chapter following a discussion of the diagnostic and therapeutic process. Staging formulas are important not only to the pathologist who is studying a series of cases in retrospect but also to the orthopedic surgeon who is treating patients. Each should know the end results of each treatment of the various malignant tumors according to each stage grouping. The Musculoskeletal Tumor Society has been actively involved in a variety of studies that range from the pitfalls of biopsy to collabora-

Table 9-2 *(continued)*

VIII. Neurogenic tumors
    1. Neurofibroma
    2. Neurilemoma (schwannoma)
  IX. Miscellaneous malignant tumors
    1. Adamantinoma
    2. Chordoma
   X. Tumors metastatic to bone

(Modified from Schajowicz et al.,[119] with permission.)

tive protocols for surgical treatment. These subjects are discussed later. The particulars of the evaluation procedures are reviewed first.

DIAGNOSTIC EVALUATION

When a patient is under consideration for a possible diagnosis of any skeletal tumor — be it primary, benign, malignant, or metastatic — ordinarily the possibility is first recognized because of radiographic findings. The patient's complaints only occasionally include an appreciation of the presence of a mass (perhaps mostly if the tumor is an osteochondroma). In contrast, the patient who has a tumor arising in soft tissue, whether it is benign or malignant, nearly always is aware that there is a mass. The clinical process of diagnosis therefore differs: When a mass is evident, the diagnostic thrust is toward as expeditious an ascertainment as possible as to what tissue constitutes the mass, whereas when the radiograph is the first order of business its interpretation is the focus of attention. Unlike the radiologist, who rarely sees the patient, the orthopedic surgeon usually knows the patient's complaints, physical findings, including age, sex, and so on before viewing the films. Such knowledge influences the approach to interpretation of any abnormal findings.

Conventional Radiography

There are several basic processes that one must be able to recognize during the radiographic evaluation of a lesion in bone. One is destruction (or lysis) of the normal pattern of bone by the lesion. The irregular erosive front, as evident when a cancellous pattern of trabeculae shows abrupt discontinuities or when a cortical density is irregularly rarefied or resorbed, is the radiographic picture of what histologically will be revealed as destruction. Its location, extent, and even to some degree its chronology become important elements in radiological interpretation.

A second process that must be recognized is the response of the bone, if any, to the lesion. The amount of new bone that is laid down, its location, and its pattern also must be factored into the diagnostic evaluation, and here too chronology plays an important role. It should be evident that these two "processes" represent pathophysiological abnormalities: in the first instance a concept of something eating away at the bone, and in the second instance an opposite concept — stimulation of the tissue to lay down more bone.

With respect to the chronology of lysis, it should be emphasized that much destruction of bone must have occurred before there is any visible evidence on conventional radiographs; therefore when cancellous bone in a localized site displays the characteristic signs, the lesion has been active for a considerable period of time. Because the two most common causes for pure lysis are acute infection and tumor, it should be emphasized that, in the absence of trauma, one is an acute process (i.e., days or weeks) whereas the other is not (probably months). The lytic process is recognized in the cancellous structure by a diminution in density and, more importantly, abrupt discontinuities in the trabecular structure. Those discontinuities often are best seen with the aid of a hand lens.

The chronology of the lytic process must not be inferred in isolation from the signs just described but should be deduced from the association of those radiological signs with any similar signs of bone production (to be described below) and, importantly, with clinical data (history of symptoms, physical signs).

When there is *pure* lysis of cortical bone at its internal or external surface, the only sign that allows one to judge if the lysis occurred acutely is the character of the eroded area. If it is smooth, rounded, and rather homogeneous in density, the lysis usually is chronic, as caused by pressure, rather than invasive, as caused by actively growing tissue. If, in contrast, it is rough, irregular, and variable in density, the lysis probably is acute. Rarely does one see lysis of cortical bone that is confined to the substance, not having affected one or both surfaces. Such a permeative appearance presupposes that a considerable volume of bone substance has been lost and that the lesion is long-standing. It also should be evident that features of the lesion other than these two "processes" must be evaluated in an orderly approach to a diagnosis.

When radiographic interpretation is considered in isolation, i.e., apart from the history, symptoms, and physical findings, the panorama of characteristics of bony lesions, in addition to lysis and deposition, are often used as a basis for characterizing a lesion. Those characteristics include longitudinal location in the bone (epiphyseal, metaphyseal, diaphyseal), transverse location (central, eccentric, peripheral), shape, and whether there are multiple lesions (generalized, disseminated, multifocal, paucifocal) or if it is an isolated lesion. Other characteristics are whether the lesion appears cystic or loculated, whether its content is homogeneously radiolucent or there are flocculent or other radiodensities, and if the lesion evokes a reaction (sclerosis) in the surrounding bone.

All of these elements are described in detail in texts on radiology,[106] and they receive detailed attention in texts on tumors of bone. However, given the long list of neoplasms (Table 9-2) and given the fact that nearly every tumor on the list is apt, to a variable degree, to include atypical instances, one should not be tempted to memorize the "typical" radiographic characteristics of even the more common lesions. As the experts expound on the characteristics in the case at hand, they nearly invariably call attention to one or more characteristics that may not be typical for the provisional diagnosis they favor. One often hears them say that "such and such" may on occasion also be seen in lesions B and C and rarely in lesion D, even though it is considered most typical (even pathognomonic) for lesion A. Rarely do they attempt precision, i.e., what percentage of lesion B, C, or D manifests the characteristic and if in x cases of lesion A the characteristic is always evident.

A word here may be appropriate as to the logical extrapolation of this item-by-item radiographic characterization. The clinician who is expected to have memorized all of the radiographic minutiae of even the most common lesions, or the expert who by a combination of memory and experience has, in his or her mind, a data bank, would have a diagnostic protocol that resembled a computer; the obvious fallacy in that extrapolation is that the data in the bank are not sufficient either in numbers of cases or "hardness" of observational records. For that reason, our emphasis in this chapter, as in the others, is that the problem-solving process should proceed with acquisition of bits of information — here represented by recognition of one or more radiological abnormalities (e.g., lysis) and concomitant realization of the implications, not in terms of a specific diagnosis but, rather, in terms of the pathophysiology.

The radiographic diagnosis always must be considered a provisional one because the necessary and sufficient elements of a definitive diagnosis for tumor cases lie in the histology. When considering the most likely diagnosis of the possible tumors or tumor-like lesions, further clinical, laboratory, or radiological studies may be indicated.

Laboratory Examinations

The clinical history, physical examination, and study of the conventional radiographs may suggest the need for some laboratory tests. They are most helpful for identifying certain metabolic diseases that may simulate bone tumors in radiographs. A complete blood count and urine examination is helpful in the general evaluation of the patient who may have a disseminated malignant disease, e.g., plasma cell myeloma, leukemia, lymphoma, or metastatic disease. Any one of these diseases may be suggested by the demonstration of significant anemia or an increased erythrocyte sedimentation rate (ESR). Other chemical or immunological tests may then be appropriate, e.g., for multiple myeloma (immunophoresis) or for metastatic carcinoma of the prostate (serum acid phosphatase). The serum alkaline phosphatase level is elevated in many conditions in which there is excessive osteoblastic activity, as in some cases of osteosarcoma, metastatic tumors, Paget's disease, and hyperparathyroidism. The serum calcium and phosphorus levels are of interest mainly for ruling out hyperparathyroidism in which the lesion can simulate a tumor (brown tumor) on the radiograph.

STAGING

To solve the problems of evaluation and treatment of a patient with a tumor from the point of view of the orthopedist, we begin with a case that illustrates the principles of staging.

Staging is a concept of classifying steps in the progress of a malignant tumor. However they are defined, the first step means that the tumor is localized, albeit infiltrating surrounding tissues, and the last step means that the tumor has metastasized. With sarcomas, in contrast to carcinomas, lymphatic metastases are uncommon. The concept admittedly may not apply to all types of tumor, but it can be applied to most; and it is a necessary tool for use in at least one important way: It allows patients to be grouped before treatment into meaningful categories so that a sizable number of patients with the specific lesion under study (i.e., the specific tumor at a specific stage) can be accorded prospectively a specific regimen of treatment, and an analogous group can be accorded another regimen. This protocol allows comparison of the results obtained by the two regimens. It also allows different types of tumor, in the same stage and treated with an identical regimen, to be compared in terms of response to the treatment.

Case 9-1   A 33-year-old man was seen because of pain in the left knee of 2 months' duration. He noted that the pain was more severe with weight-bearing to the point where he eventually had to resort to crutches to control the discomfort. On examination, he had an obvious but diffuse swelling of the thigh just above the knee. There was restricted range of motion of the knee during flexion and extension because of the discomfort. Tenderness was present along the medial and anterolateral aspects of the distal end of the femur.

The initial radiographs (Fig. 9-1A&B) showed an expanded radiolucent lesion of the lateral condyle, with the lateral cortex thinner anteriorly and laterally but no sign of lysis. The central part of the lesion included a zone of increased density, and there was a second radiolucent focus with a similar zone of increased density somewhat proximal to the main one in the lateral condyle. There was a suggestion of a subperiosteal area of increased density in the region of a minimal disruption in the cortex, suggesting a pathological fracture. A technetium bone scan for that area was positive (Fig. 9-1C). The initial radiographic interpretation was that the lesion was benign and cystic; an aneurysmal bone cyst, a giant cell tumor, and a chondromyxoid fibroma were considered the most likely diagnoses. Because of the uncertainty of the diagnosis and particularly because there were two foci of involvement in the femur, the patient was referred for further study and biopsy.

As the initial part of the staging, the physical findings revealed no sign of lesions in the lungs or lymph nodes, and pulmonary radiographs were negative. (Tomograms should have been obtained because there was some doubt as to whether the lesion was indeed benign.) The doubts about the above diagnoses stem from two observations on the conventional radiographs. The first was the fact that the lesion had two adjoining foci, and it was unclear whether the smaller, more proximal lesion was indeed separate or was an outgrowth of the larger one. The second was the presence in a lesion that was predominantly radiolucent, of densities of an irregularity and diffuse appearance that did not jibe with those associated with repair bone.

Computed tomography (CT) of the femur was done to ascertain the exact anatomical area of the tumor. It revealed, in addition, that there was a radiolucent, motheaten lesion extending around the popliteal vessels. This picture called into serious question the three alternatives of diagnosis just cited. The biopsy was performed from a lateral approach, as the cortex at its thinnest point was more easily penetrated and because that approach would not interfere with any subsequent operation that might be needed. There was a small amount of subperiosteal tumor that was identified grossly and a large mass of tumor inside the condyle. The tissue was grayish red and mushy with areas of what appeared to be necrotic tissue within. The histological (frozen section) diagnosis was that of a highly malignant fibrous histiocytoma (Fig. 9-1D). The patient was treated with a high thigh amputation. Three years after the amputation, there was no evidence of disease either locally or in the lung.

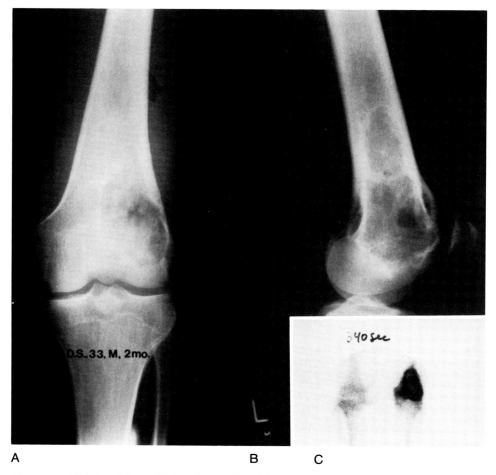

Fig. 9-1. Case 9-1. AP (**A**) and lateral (**B**) radiographs of the left femur with a radiolucent lesion in the distal anterolateral area. The cortex is thinned. Note a reactive zone of increased density along the medial aspect and a central, more proximal zone of lucency. (**C**) Positive technetium 99m bone scan. *(Figure continues.)*

This case illustrates the essential aspects of the procedures recommended for staging of bone tumors by the American Joint Commission on Cancer (AJCC).[2] The biopsy was planned and performed in relation to any possible surgical procedure that might be needed for definitive treatment. The options were either a wide (radical) resection or amputation. The final step in the staging process was accomplished after the amputation, and it consisted in applying the information obtained at operation to that obtained preoperatively. The fact that the tumor, as evident in the amputation specimen, had extended beyond the femoral cortex is a critical point. Whether it also infiltrated muscle could be determined only in the histological preparations. Whether it extended into the joint would be determined by dissection of the specimen removed during the definitive procedure.

SURGICAL CONSIDERATIONS

It is generally accepted that surgical procedures[38,42] targeted at removing tumors fall into four categories. *Intralesional resection* includes surgical entry into the tumor substance. In case 9-1 the biopsy might well have introduced tumor cells

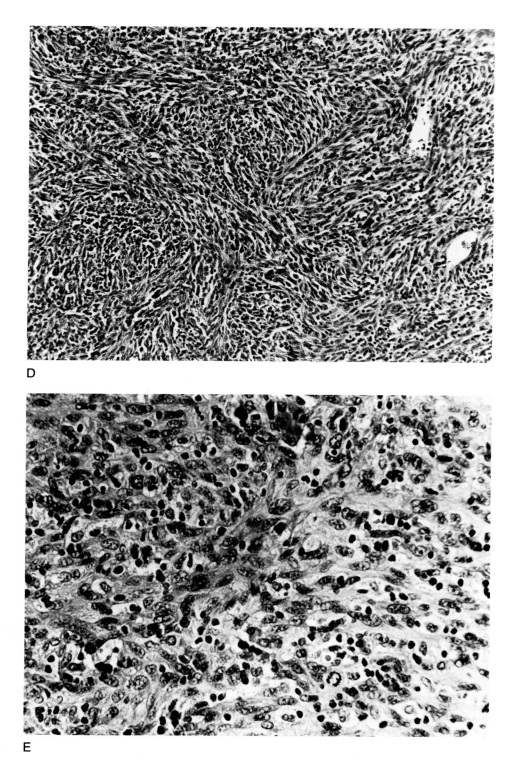

D

E

Fig. 9-1 *(Continued).* **(D)** Photomicrograph of the tissue shows the storiform pattern of a malignant fibrous histiocytoma (×100). **(E)** Hyperchromatic histiocytic and fibroblastic stromal cells (×250).

along the incision; and if that incision were used for the subsequent resection procedure, the resection would be called intralesional. Because the subsequent resection procedure (an amputation) was through an incision entirely proximal, the resection was defined as not intralesional. Two of the other three categories, defined as either *marginal resection* (i.e., through a margin of reactive, but not tumor, tissue) or *radical resection* (i.e., removing the entire involved bone and all the tissue compartments adjacent to the tumor), do not apply in this case. The definitive incision was made along the lateral aspect of the distal end of the thigh so that it could be extended if necessary for preparing proper flaps for an amputation. The same incision might be used for developing the anatomical planes for resection, once it is known that there is a clear tumor-free interval in the femur proximal and distal to the lesion. In this instance, because of the histological findings of a highly malignant grade IV fibrous histiocytoma and the difficulty of clearing the popliteal vessels and nerves, an amputation was chosen as the procedure of choice. The operation qualifies as the fourth staging category intermediate in degree between marginal and radical — *wide resection*, rather than radical resection — inasmuch as part of the femur and thigh muscles were retained. The CT scan of the lungs in a search for metastases to the lung as part of the selected procedures for staging as recommended by the AJCC[2] was obtained only after the biopsy proved there was a malignant tumor.

One of the surgical options that could be entertained, once the biopsy revealed a malignancy, might be a limb-sparing reconstruction after a wide resection.[17,20,35,41,87,111,112,131,151,153,156] Although many considerations are involved in establishing that option as viable (we consider the involvement of the popliteal vessels and nerves as absolute contraindications), it should be pointed out that so complicated a surgical regimen requires much preparation, special facilities, and techniques not available except in centers organized for the purpose. Even in such a center, a limb-sparing procedure rarely is done at the same time as the biopsy. Permanent sections to provide a definitive diagnosis are much more reliable than frozen sections. Moreover, it should be emphasized that if a limb-sparing option is contemplated by the referring physician the entire regimen of treatment, proba-

bly including the biopsy, had best be conducted at the referral center.

It is important for the surgeon who is not a part of that center to perform only those studies that add information either to lend support to a somewhat shaky provisional diagnosis or to allow staging of the tumor at the initial encounter. Additional studies may be performed, such as CT[12] or magnetic resonance imaging (MRI)[144] to determine the anatomical extent of the tumor or if there is some doubt about the most appropriate site for a biopsy if this physician plans to do the biopsy. In the case just presented, the need for CT and MRI before biopsy arose because the radiographic observations cast serious doubt that the tumor was benign. If the provisional diagnosis was strongly supported by typical radiographs, to the point that the surgeon might be confident of the diagnosis, CT and MRI would be unnecessary. In any case, the surgeon should always consider if additional diagnostic measures can raise the level of confidence. Tests should not be ordered routinely for the sake of accumulating diagnostic data or as a reflex, automatic routine. There is no justification for ordering tests to satisfy one's curiosity or for "complete" documentation when they are not necessary for the diagnosis or treatment. This rule applies especially when a test entails some risk, even though the risk may be minimal (but not negligible), e.g., radiation exposure of a CT scan. Risk is appreciable for invasive measures such as arteriography.[157] There are circumstances when knowledge of the arterial blood supply to a malignant primary or metastatic tumor is necessary for the ideal treatment of such a tumor. For procedures such as wide resections and elaborate, limb-sparing reconstructions, the blood supply to the area must be known.[152,153] One may have to plan the sites of ligation of some arteries, and those essential to the viability of the limb after the resection must be protected. In the case of a metastasis from a highly vascular tumor, such as a renal cell carcinoma, knowledge of the source of major arteries and veins to the lesion may be crucial to prevention of intraoperatively uncontrollable hemorrhage to the tumor. Possibly an interventionist angiographer might do selective thrombosis of those vessels preoperatively so that a definitive procedure such as intramedullary rod fixation or resection might then be done safely.[49,69]

In case 9-1 the biopsy was performed by the surgeon who planned and then performed the definitive surgical procedure. He was aware of the options available should the tumor prove to be malignant, and he began with the biopsy so the diagnosis would be firm. Thus no option was closed out. However, he also was aware that the institutional pathologist was an expert in tumors of bone. In this case, a consultation with the pathologist brought forth a recommendation against needle biopsy because the pathologist lacked confidence in his experience with that technique.[107,108]

In a study done under the auspices of the Musculoskeletal Tumor Society, the biopsy results from 340 cases randomly retrieved from tumors of bone and soft tissue were critically analyzed.[93] In 146 of the cases (slightly fewer than one-half) the biopsies were performed in the referring hospital, so that slightly more than one-half of the cases had had the biopsy done in the referral center. There were 82 cases (about one-fourth) in which an important difference existed between the biopsy diagnosis and the definitive diagnosis, as determined from studies of the resected specimen. In 56 of the 82 cases, the variances occurred in relation to the biopsies from the referring institutions. (In the other 26 the variances concerned mainly the type or grading of a malignancy, whereas in the 56 cases the variance often was between a benign and a malignant lesion.) In 60 patients (about one-sixth of the total) the changes in diagnosis based on review of the biopsy altered the plan of treatment of the patient. The biopsy procedure itself, as done in the referring institution, caused problems with the selection or performance of the definitive operation in 57 cases. In 15 patients the biopsy procedure done in the referring institution led to an unwarranted amputation, unwarranted either because, as assessed retrospectively, a more appropriate biopsy would have allowed a less radical operation or because complications of the biopsy compromised the extremity beyond salvage. In 28 cases the patient's course was affected adversely as a result of problems with the biopsy. It is for these reasons that we advocate that whenever possible the biopsy be performed by the surgeon who is to perform the definitive procedure; but in all cases there should be access to a radiologist, a pathologist, and perhaps an oncologist before, during, and after the surgery so as to ensure that the appropriate decisions are made. The decisions concerning the de-

tails of the biopsy should be thoroughly discussed beforehand, and the biopsy should be done only after the essential data are obtained. Although biopsy is technically a rather simple operation, it should not be relegated to an individual unaware of the pitfalls or the consequences of errors in judgment, even though he or she may be technically capable of doing the procedure well.[22,36,129] An example of how a biopsy can lead to difficulties in treatment is shown by the next case.

Case 9-2 A 33-year-old woman had had pain and swelling of the left buttock of 1 year's duration. The patient noted that the pain was becoming more severe, and the mass was increasing in size. There began to be tenderness in the buttock starting 4 months before she consulted her physician. The patient's fear of cancer delayed her going to the doctor.

On examination, a large mass was noted in the left buttock. A radiograph of the pelvis showed a lytic lesion of the posterior aspect of the ilium at the sacroiliac joint. A biopsy was done with the incision over the convexity of the mass, just lateral to the sacroiliac joint. The diagnosis was anaplastic undifferentiated sarcoma.

The patient was referred a week after the biopsy for definitive treatment. During that week increasing problems with the wound were evident, and at the time of referral the wound edges appeared edematous and the surrounding area erythematous (Fig. 9-2A). Several days elapsed before the microscopic slides become available to the referral center for review prior to planning the definitive treatment. During that time the sutures had to be removed because the tumor had enlarged to such a degree that it protruded through the biopsy incision (Fig. 9-2B).

This case illustrates several points, one of which is that the biopsy usually should be done by the surgeon who does the definitive surgical procedure. At the initial referring center, the desire to establish a histological diagnosis without thought to what the definitive diagnosis might be certainly reflects poor judgment. Second, the biopsy incision should have been placed in a location where either resection of the tumor or a hind-quarter amputation could be done. The posterior medial location of the incision precluded the development of flaps for an interilioabdominal amputation; furthermore, the tissue planes were so obscured by

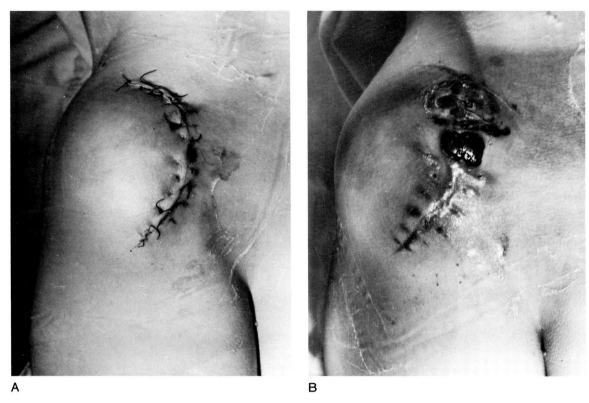

A   B

Fig. 9-2. Case 9-2. **(A)** Left buttock of a 33-year-old woman 7 days after biopsy of a mass arising from a fibrosarcoma of the left ilium at the sacroiliac joint. **(B)** Same patient 1 week later with tumor growing out of the biopsy wound. (From Cooper,[29] with permission.)

the surgical trauma that only a marginal excision or an intralesional excision were the options remaining to the surgeons at the referral center.

The biopsy procedure, simple as it was, may have been undertaken with little thought as to the alternative of needle biopsy, despite its disadvantage of possible (but not certain or even probable) difficulty in histological interpretation. Moreover, the surgeon who did the biopsy did not anticipate possible adverse local effects, which in the present instance included necrosis of tumor tissue, massive edema of the adjacent tissue, and intralesional hemorrhage. The cumulative result—massive swelling during the 2-week period between biopsy and referral—closed out the following therapeutic options: (1) Early application of radiation therapy might have been possible. If the tumor would be expected to be radiosensitive (as predictable

from its histology) or sensitive to chemotherapy, a preoperative course of radiotherapy, chemotherapy, or both might well have allowed, after an interval, a more conservative procedure than a hindquarter amputation. (2) The open biopsy, if performed in a less crucial site, might have permitted immediate amputation. Instead, the only operation that was in order was admittedly palliative. Therefore there was a disastrous chain of events attributable to what might be considered a simple routine procedure.

The lesion was rather superficial, at a location some distance from vital structures; thus one might justify the biopsy on the grounds that it was the most direct route to obtaining tissue for diagnosis. The chain of events mentioned includes several delays, as recorded. No doubt one important delay was due to the complications of the wound, but in this case, with a rapidly growing tumor mass and foreknowledge that the case would have to be referred, trouble should have been anticipated.

It should be emphasized that all of the diagnostic modalities used in this case and in case 9-1 yielded provisional diagnoses. The confidence level of each diagnosis varied, but none of the methods yielded a definitive diagnosis. It is the histological diagnosis that was definitive. As a necessary part of determining the extent (staging) of a primary malignant tumor, pulmonary CT or MRI is necessary to determine if metastasis has occurred. That situation influences the prognosis and the type of initial treatment of any tumor. It should be mentioned that, with MRI, what is revealed at present is water content, but in the near future MRI may well be able to

reveal the tissue content of other compounds or elements.[143-145] Additionally, MRI can demonstrate the presence of lesions so small they are impossible to detect in other ways. Cases are now on record of soft tissue tumors, e.g., a neuroma in an extremity, too small to be palpated, that have been revealed only by MRI. A number of examples are presented to illustrate how testing methods are used in specific cases.

Case 9-3 A 14-year-old boy had an osteosarcoma of the femoral diaphysis as provisionally diagnosed on radiographs (Fig. 9-3A&B). He was being considered for either amputation or disarticulation of the hip. One question — Are there metastases? — had to be answered in the negative if either of those procedures was to be appropriate. CT scan of the

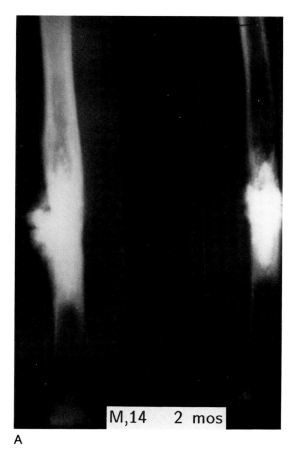

A

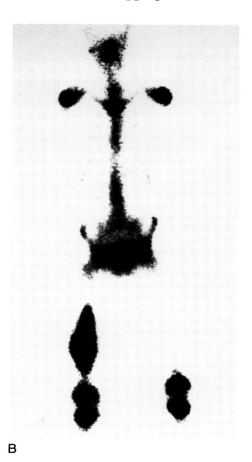

B

Fig. 9-3. Case 9-3. AP (**A**) and lateral (**B**) radiographs of the femur of a 14-year-old boy show a densely osteoblastic osteosarcoma of the mid-diaphysis. (**C**) Technetium 99m polyphosphate bone scan shows marked isotope uptake at the tumor and a tumor-free interval in the proximal third of the femur.

lungs revealed no pulmonary lesion. A technetium 99m polyphosphate scan revealed no other osteogenic lesion (Fig. 9-3C) and showed a tumor-free interval between the hip joint and the upper margin of the sarcoma.[73,84] Therefore a high thigh amputation with a removable, wide margin of normal tissue could be done and was. The patient has had no local recurrence during a 16-year follow-up. However, about 8 years after the amputation two small metastases to the periphery of the lung became evident and were removed by pulmonary wedge resection.[147] He is still alive with no evidence of disease 16 years after the initial diagnosis and amputation.

This case is noteworthy in that, first, so many years elapsed between removal of the primary tumor and the appearance of metastases (usually they appear within 2 years); second, the pulmonary tomogram initially failed to reveal the metastases; and third, routine yearly testing was carried out for so long postoperatively.

This case also raises a series of important pathophysiological questions: Were the two metastases present in the lungs at the time of the amputation? If so, were they so small as to be undetectable by tomography? If so, why would they remain undetectable for 2 years, only to suddenly grow? These questions and others concerning the process of malignant transformation of cells belong to the oncologists, who are in a field that is somewhat peripheral to the focus of orthopedic surgery. Oncology requires so many references to technology in a variety of disciplines, especially when chemotherapy is at issue, that in this chapter there is only passing mention of special items, as illustrated in the next case.

Case 9-4   A 13-year-old boy had an osteosarcoma of the distal end of the femur identified radiographically 3 weeks after a football injury that had caused effusion in the knee. He had developed pain and limp on that side, and the radiographs obtained by the family doctor showed a lesion (Fig. 9-4A&B) characterized by a mottled increase in density of the metaphysis reaching to the epiphyseal plate. The lateral cortex was lysed in a permeative fashion, and there was a zone of reactive periosteal new bone in the metaphyseal diaphyseal area ("Codman triangle"). An indistinct soft tissue swelling was evident posterolaterally.

The patient was referred for further evaluation with a provisional diagnosis of osteosarcoma that was confirmed by biopsy. One question that arose in the further work-up was the extent of infiltration of soft tissue by the tumor. In addition to chemotherapy, there was consideration of either a limb salvage procedure or an amputation. One surgical consideration, similar to that discussed in case 9-1, i.e., if the tumor involved the popliteal vessels, was resolved here by MRI (in case 9-1 a CT scan served the purpose). The MRI showed a tumor with enhanced T_2 value delineation (Fig. 9-4D&E) that infiltrated the popliteal structures. That finding prevented the limb salvage option, so a high mid-thigh amputation was performed. This mode of imaging is generally superior to CT for defining the soft tissue extent of the tumor.[144,151] Follow-up after 3 years showed no evidence of disease.

Consideration of chemotherapy (not entertained in case 9-2 because of refusal by the patient's parents) had to be pursued in view of the dramatic rise in survival rate of patients with osteosarcoma since the advent of chemotherapy (a rise from approximately 10 percent to approximately 50 percent).[55,80] A decision had to be made as to which drugs to use as well as the regimen (doses, chronology, monitoring). Several regimens have been advocated, each with a theoretical and different pathophysiological rationale. No one regimen has achieved general acceptance, and results with the various regimens now being tried clinically have not settled the question of which is best. As matters now stand, each center has agreed to participate in a collaborative study supervised nationally in the United States and to some extent in other countries. The chemotherapeutic regimen to be used on our particular patient depended not on pathophysiological principles applicable to that case (e.g., tissue culture tests of sensitivity of the cells to particular drugs or tests of analogous import) but, rather, to the assigned protocol, for the center in question.

Case 9-5   A 47-year-old patient had a chondrosarcoma that arose in one of multiple osteocartilaginous exostoses of which the patient had been aware for years (they were palpable masses)(Fig. 9-5A). The tumor arose from the inner aspect of the wing of the ilium (Fig. 9-5D), had recently become symptomatic, and had grown to a large size. A bar-

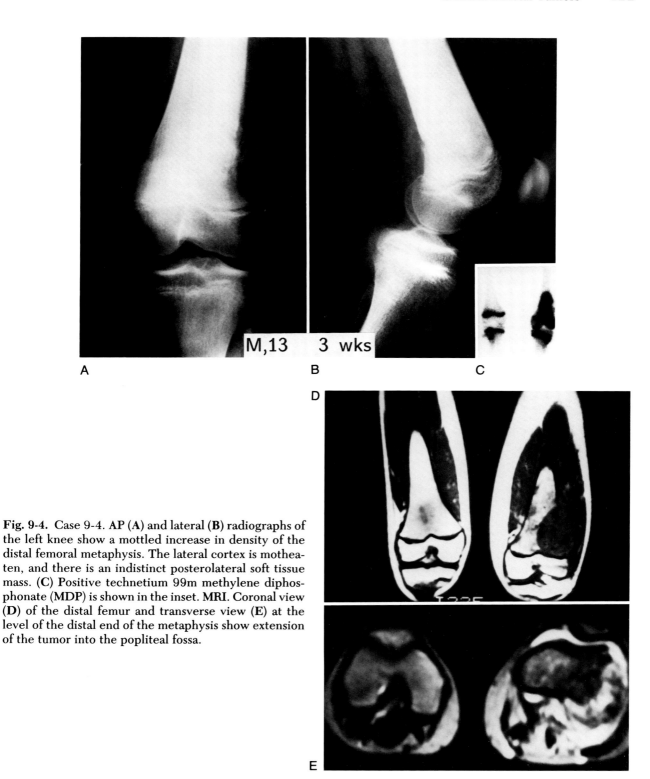

Fig. 9-4. Case 9-4. AP (**A**) and lateral (**B**) radiographs of the left knee show a mottled increase in density of the distal femoral metaphysis. The lateral cortex is motheaten, and there is an indistinct posterolateral soft tissue mass. (**C**) Positive technetium 99m methylene diphosphonate (MDP) is shown in the inset. **MRI.** Coronal view (**D**) of the distal femur and transverse view (**E**) at the level of the distal end of the metaphysis show extension of the tumor into the popliteal fossa.

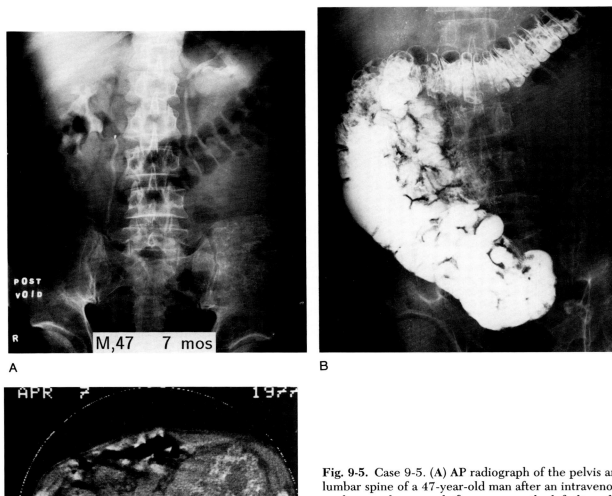

A

B

C

Fig. 9-5. Case 9-5. **(A)** AP radiograph of the pelvis and lumbar spine of a 47-year-old man after an intravenous pyelogram shows a calcific mass over the left ilium distorting the ureter and renal pelvis. **(B)** Barium study of the bowel shows the displacement by the tumor. **(C)** CT scan at the level of the sacroiliac joint displays the calcific mass arising from an exostosis of the ilium at the sacroiliac joint. *(Figure continues.)*

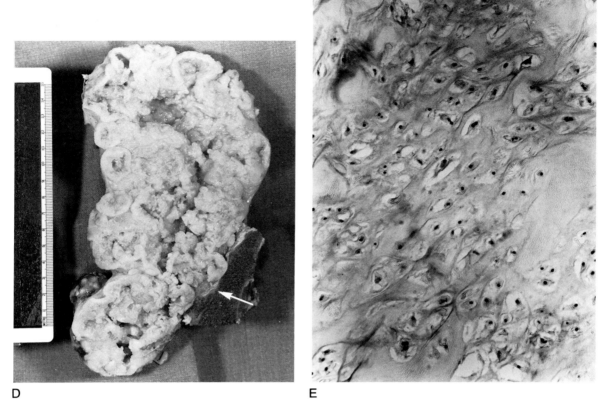

Fig. 9-5 *(Continued).* (**D**) Gross split specimen of the resected chondrosarcoma shows the tumor arising from the ilium (arrow). (**E**) Characteristic appearance of a low grade chondrosarcoma with numerous double-nucleated cells (×180). (**A–E,** From El Khoury and Bonfiglio,[34a] with permission.)

ium enema study (Fig. 9-5B) was useful for outlining the location and extent of the tumor, as was a CT study (Fig. 9-5C). It could not be determined whether the increase in size was recent or dated back several years. In any case, it was decided that a "marginal resection" could be undertaken. It was understood at the outset that cure of this type of tumor in this location by any surgical procedure would be unlikely. The tumor extended from the inner aspect of the pelvis to the diaphragm. The resection had to include the proximal half of the ilium, a small portion of the sacroiliac joint, and the fibrous tissue capsule that had formed between the tumor and the retroperitoneal space (Fig. 9-5D). A local recurrence became evident 2 years later, and a second marginal resection was done. The patient is still alive 10 years after the last surgical procedure.

This case illustrates one principle that must be understood if therapy for malignant tumors is to be conducted appropriately. It is the fact that the biology and natural history of different kinds of tumor differ greatly. Those differences are reflected in the differences in their response to and their indications for specific therapeutic regimens. In this case (a secondary chondrosarcoma,[109,125] i.e., one secondary to a primary osteochondroma) the surgeon was aware of the special character of the disease, multiple osteochondromatosis.[121] If the case history indicated familial involvement, i.e., if other family members had secondary chondrosarcomas (they did not), or if there was unequivocal evidence of recent enlargement of the mass of tumor, the surgeon would be compelled by that evidence to do as radical a resection as was practical. In this case, lacking that evidence, the procedure was a "marginal" resection, which as has already been defined means that the line of section passed through reactive tissue, not tumor tissue. It was the location of the tumor that precluded a wider resection. The concept of wide resection, which includes removal of muscle compartments, is mainly applicable to tumors in the extremities; therefore with an iliac tumor, that delineation cannot be made. Yet it should be understood that, for the purposes of systematic therapeutic studies, the compartment concept, despite its shortcomings, serves a good purpose.[38]

Before proceeding to other examples of the treatment of bone tumors, further discussion is appropriate at this point on the systems of staging malignant musculoskeletal tumors. The system devised by the AJCC[2] has been adopted by the International Union on Cancer Control (IUCC) and is similar to that for soft tissue sarcoma.[117] It has not proved as practical for the surgeon as the staging system described by Enneking et al.,[42,43] which was adopted by the Musculoskeletal Tumor Society for their preliminary studies.[39] With the latter system, which applies to tumors arising in soft tissues as well as those arising in bone, an essential feature of the staging is the determination whether the tumor is contained in one "compartment" or has violated the compartmental limits. The compartments are defined conceptually; e.g., a soft tissue tumor may be confined to one of the three muscular compartments of the leg, and a bone tumor may be entirely within the cortical limits of the bone. In either case, removal of the entire compartment would constitute a radical resection. In the AJCC system no reference is made to compartments, mainly because the data on the cases with which that system was devised did not allow characterization of the more than 2,000 cases with respect to compartments.[30] Most musculoskeletal tumors of high grade malignancy fall into stage II according to the system of Enneking et al.; i.e., they have violated their compartment of origin. It should be pointed out, however, that as in cases 9-1 and 9-3, where each tumor arose in the bone and extended into the popliteal fossa, the anatomical concept of compart-

ments, nicely delineated in other locations, is not strictly applicable. In those two cases there may be questions as to exactly what constitute the compartments and which structures are involved, e.g., perhaps the joint. The concept of violation of a compartment here was not nearly so important to the therapy as the demonstration of arterial compromise.

With either staging system, once metastases are present (whether to regional nodes, bone, or lungs), the tumor is classified as stage III and the outcome is generally predictably poor, although there are exceptions. Some studies now under way suggest that the size and location of the tumor (superficial versus deep) may be important factors for the prognosis, but these two properties, although amenable to quantitation, are difficult to incorporate into any system of staging.

Surgical treatment remains an essential element for any regimen of treatment of all musculoskeletal tumors; but before the specific regimen is decided on, there should always be a correlation of clinical, radiographic, gross, and microscopical findings. This correlation, everyone agrees, requires consultation between the surgeon (as head of the team) and, at a minimum, the radiologist and pathologist. The radiation therapist and chemotherapist become part of the team whenever the question is raised about irradiation or chemotherapy.

It was recommended in the introductory part of this chapter that most *primary* malignant tumors be referred to medical centers for treatment. This recommendation implies that in most hospitals orthopedic surgeons have available consultants in the specialties just named, and if a case of a primary malignant tumor of bone appears there is an ad hoc team that can pursue the diagnostic process but that it ordinarily does not attempt treatment. Of course, it may not always be possible (for practical reasons) to have the patient referred appropriately, so that each orthopedic surgeon then must recognize the therapeutic options. Consultation with an expert at the nearest medical center is probably in order. At such centers there is much concern about the pathophysiology of many of the tumors listed in Table 9-2, particularly those that lead to frequent failure of treatment, however radical.

Although some tumors are notoriously fulminating whereas others are slow-growing, the biological behavior of any specific tumor (i.e., its growth) does not always follow the "characteristic" pattern for the tumor under study.[90,104,152] Some undergo gradual enlargement in all directions except when they encounter anatomical obstacles. The obstacle may be cartilage, as when a conventional osteosarcoma in a metaphysis abuts against the epiphyseal plate or the periosteum. When it breaks through the cortex and periosteum, it may be the fascia that demarcates a muscle compartment. Efforts have been made to grade histologically several specific types of malignant tumor and then to compare the grades as manifested in groups of cases. It has proved impossible, however, to predict what influences there may be that cause any single tumor to be contained in the fascial planes or in well defined compartments. If each tumor could be so characterized, there would be higher rates of cure than are presently being reported.

Tumors spread not only by infiltration but also by invasion of blood vessels, large and small. When that occurs tumor cells can escape into the circulation to seed at other sites. As is well known, not all of those seedlings grow to become visible metastases. Many, if not most, of the tumor emboli do not find fertile ground in which to grow. Tumor cells have been recovered from the blood in a high percentage of cases of osteosarcoma. They arise from the original site of the tumors either spontaneously or after palpation or biopsy.[52] Despite intensive studies (including genetic and immunological ones) of this problem (rarely involving musculoskeletal tumors,[48,70] however) the pathophysiology of metastasis, infiltrative growth, and indeed unrestrained growth of any cancer cell remain unsolved mysteries. As these factors concern primary malignant tumors of the musculoskeletal system in particular because of their diversity, it may not be assumed that one tumor necessarily has in common with others any particular mechanism that is responsible for any one of the three processes just mentioned. However, in the absence of a pathophysiological schema, certain empirical observations must be kept in mind.

The more quickly a tumor grows and the larger its extent when it is first recognized, the greater are its potentials for invasion, recurrence, and metastases. Yet this generalization has many exceptions,

not just a few. One cannot come to the logical conclusion that a tumor that is large and destructive when first seen means that a wide resection or an amputation must be done, even after consideration of the specific tumor diagnosis and the "typical" biological behavior of that particular tumor.

The surgical procedure of choice is one tailormade to all the elements of the situation. First, it must minimize the possibility of local recurrence.[112] When there is a local recurrence of a tumor of either bone or soft tissue, the prognosis for patient survival is diminished, but this element in the situation does not mean that the surgical procedure should always be so radical as to overshadow the third element, which is to provide the patient with as good a functional result as the situation permits. The factors over which a surgeon has no control include the tendency of the particular tumor to vascular invasion and spread and the immune defense of the body to those tumor cells that have escaped the local site. The surgeon's choice of operation depends strongly on the histological examination of the biopsy specimen. If there is no vascular invasion and the tumor cells are recognized as being likely to be sensitive to chemotherapy, a wide resection may be the best operation.[17,20,35,41,87,111,131,151,153,156]

To conclude the general considerations that apply to the surgical aspect of tumors, i.e., how one chooses a resection technique, three cases are described, all of giant cell tumors that were not unequivocally benign.[20,21,62,78,125,155] Cases of unequivocally benign tumors are discussed later because those lesions rarely if ever require radical procedures. Even if part of a benign tumor is not removed through necessity or inadvertently, the consequences are rarely serious, and the local residual lesion usually can be removed secondarily when it becomes evident.

Case 9-6 The radiographs of the knee of a 41-year-old man showed a characteristic giant cell tumor of the proximal end of the tibia (Fig. 9-6A&B). The tumor had extended to and expanded the cortex on the lateral side of the proximal part of the tibia, and extended up to the subchondral layer of bone. The provisional (radiographic) diagnosis of this rather common tumor (characteristic in location and pattern but larger than usual, although characteristically showing

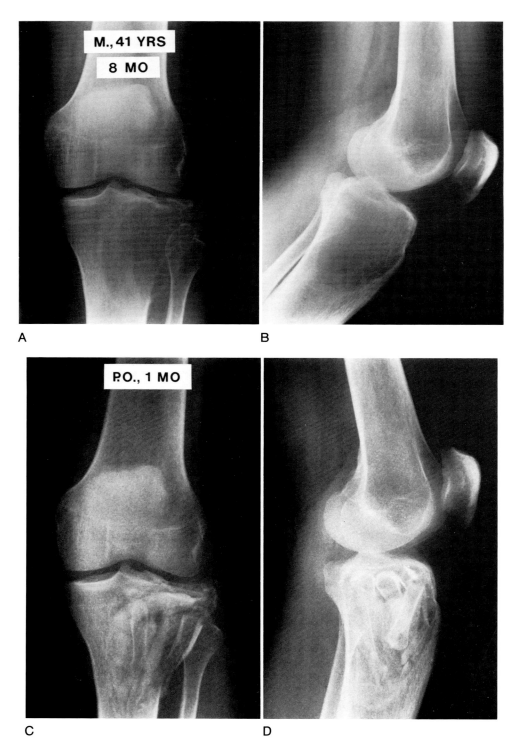

Fig. 9-6. Case 9-6. **AP (A)** and lateral **(B)** radiographs of the left knee of a 41-year-old man with a giant cell tumor of the lateral aspect of the proximal tibia. The lateral cortex has been eroded, and the outer half of the subchondral cortex of the lateral plateau is radiolucent. **AP (C)** and lateral **(D)** radiographs 1 month after curettage and insertion of an iliac crest bone graft. *(Figure continues.)*

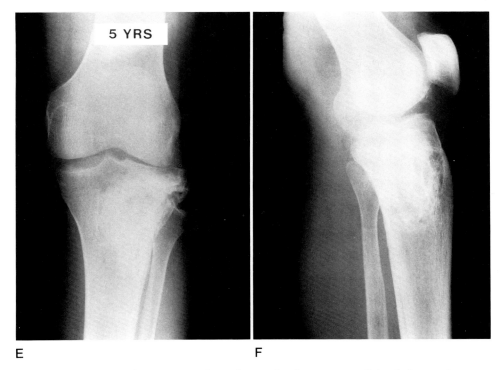

E   F

Fig. 9-6 *(Continued)*. **(E&F)** At 5 years the radiographs show repair of the defect and no recurrence.

only lysis) was made despite the unusual size; that diagnosis was made so confidently that the plan of treatment called for no preliminary biopsy. The surgical option chosen included frozen section histology to be followed immediately by definitive surgical resection. The procedure of choice, then, was one in which the knee joint would not be compromised. The plan could be followed, however, only if the histology was not that of fulminant malignancy.

That being the case, the lesion was first curetted as a biopsy through a wide window in the anterolateral aspect of the tibia through which all portions of the tumor could be visualized. After the curettage was completed, initially with hand tools (chisel, curette) and then with a power burr, a zone of normal bone was removed posteriorly, medially, and distally, including all of the subchondral bone down to the cartilage. When processed, the frozen section revealed typical histological findings of a giant cell tumor with no evidence of extreme anaplasia that might influence the surgeon to proceed

to a more radical resection. The surgical procedure that was done falls into the category of an intralesional resection. This resection procedure was chosen despite the surgeon's recognition that there is a high percentage of local recurrence following curettage of giant cell tumors.[21,62,78,103,155] The defect was then reconstructed with the use of the window in the lateral wall that was large enough to accommodate large pieces of the iliac crest, which were used to support the subchondral cartilage and fill the bony defect. Pieces of iliac crest were also used as struts to support the articular cartilage (Fig. 9-6C&D). After 5 years this patient had no evidence of recurrence or metastasis. The knee had been well reconstituted by the autogenous iliac bone grafts and functioned normally (Fig. 9-6E&F).

The main factor that impelled the surgeon to use what might be considered a resection short of the ideal was his judgment that the evidence concerning the propensity of giant cell tumors to recur following curettage is fairly weak. It is based on

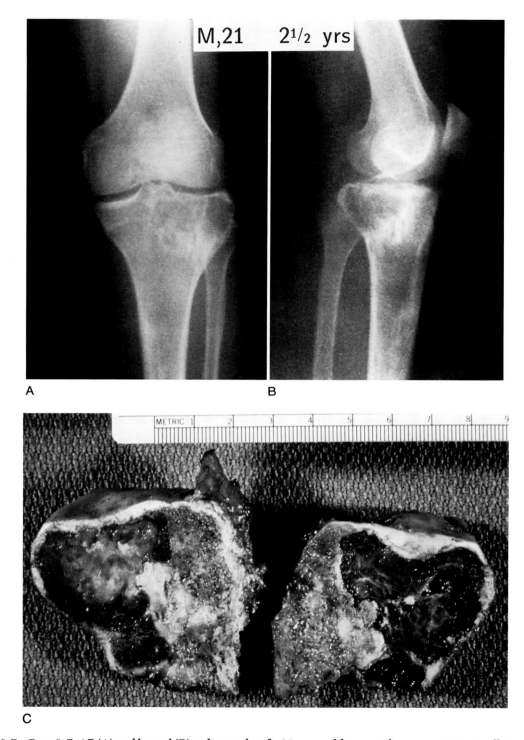

Fig. 9-7. Case 9-7. AP (**A**) and lateral (**B**) radiographs of a 21-year-old man with recurrent giant cell tumor of the posterolateral aspect of the proximal tibia 2½ years after curettage and bone grafting. (**C**) Gross specimen. *(Figure continues.)*

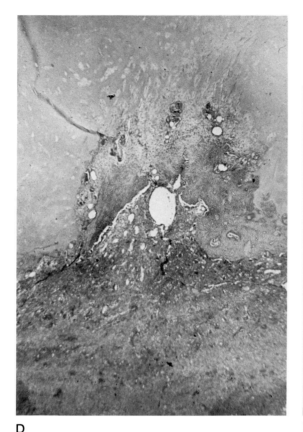

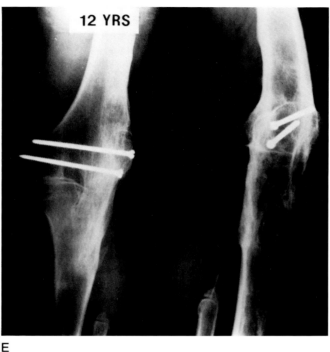

D   E

Fig. 9-7 *(Continued)*. **(D)** Photomicrograph of the tissue shows a giant cell tumor replacing the subchondral cortex and invading the articular cartilage (×40). AP **(E)** and lateral **(F)** radiographs of the knee 12 years after resection and fusion.

statistics derived from collections of cases in which the curettage depended on the experience of many surgeons, so in some cases the curettage was not as thorough as it should be. Second, the surgeon knew that, even were there to be a local recurrence, experience with such a complication (when radiotherapy has not been given) has not shown that the recurrent tumor is more anaplastic than the primary. If there were a recurrence, the salvage procedure would not necessarily be a difficult or radical one. Third, the surgeon did not think that the resection that might be considered ideal, i.e., block removal of the upper end of the tibia, would allow any reconstruction other than a total prosthetic replacement of the entire knee joint, and that procedure would not only be difficult, given the exten-

sive tibial defect, but also would not promise as good function as the reconstruction chosen. Finally, the surgeon was aware of the unusual nature of giant cell tumors in regard to metastasis; i.e., even when that complication becomes evident, the pulmonary lesion is often a single nodule, which often is easily resectable and usually not one that threatens the life of the patient.

Case 9-7 A 21-year-old male farmer presented with a recurrence of a giant cell tumor. He had had curettage for that lesion in the proximal end of the tibia and presented 2.5 years afterward with aching in the knee of 2 months' duration. The radiographs showed a radiolucent lesion in the posterolateral aspect of the proximal part of the tibia, the distal margin of which was radiopaque. The sclerosis that was present probably represented repair from previously inserted bone grafts plus some residual grafted bone (Fig. 9-7A&B). This situation represented a local recurrence without other complications, and a block resection of the tumor was planned. Because of the youth of the patient and his occupation, a knee fusion was the procedure chosen for reconstruction. The proximal end of the tibia was excised, and a portion of the femur was turned down to fill the interval of resected proximal tibia. The proximal end of the fibula was excised and inserted in the defect created by turning down the lateral condyle of the femur. The femur was fixed by screws into the medial femoral condyle and into the medial portion of the tibia. Radiographs showed solid fusion at 12 years after the marginal resection and reconstruction, and no metastases or additional local recurrence had occurred (Fig. 9-7E&F).

A photograph of the gross specimen shows the recurrent giant cell tumor in the proximal aspect of the lateral tibial plateau. The tumor encroached on the articular cartilage of the plateau (Fig. 9-7C). The histological features of the recurrence were those of a classical giant cell tumor without anaplasia.

One reason for recurrence of a giant cell tumor that is abutting the subchondral cortex is invasion of the subchondral bony layer. The invading tumor cells may easily be missed on curettage. There may even be perforation of the articular cartilage (Fig. 9-7D). This encroachment on subchondral bone and cartilage is one reason for inadequate curettage. When an effort is made to completely remove the subchondral cortex with a high speed burr, as was done in case 9-6, and when the cartilage has not been invaded (or perforated), this technique has a good chance of success.

Case 9-8 A 28-year-old woman presented with an essentially painless but palpable mass in the right arm of 8 months' duration. The radiographs showed a bony tumor adjacent to the humerus but not arising from it. There was some erosion of the cortex. The tumor represented what was essentially an extraosseous mass. The medullary canal of the humerus appeared clear (Fig. 9-8A&B). Because this patient was treated before the era of computed tomography (CT), it could not be unequivocally ascertained preoperatively that the

medullary cavity had not been invaded by tumor. The provisional diagnosis was parosteal osteosarcoma, which was confirmed by open biopsy. A wide surgical excision was performed.

The surgical plan was to remove the tumor along with a zone of what appeared to be normal tissue about 2 cm thick; thus the excision would be wide of the tumor on all sides, as might be judged by radiography preoperatively and by palpation intraoperatively. That thickness was achieved proximally and circumferentially but not distally; the distal margin of the resection was only about 1 cm. To have excised more of the humerus would have meant compromising the elbow joint, which would have caused difficulty in controlling the distal fragment of the humerus with the method of fixation that was chosen. The gross specimen included the biopsy wound along with a cuff of muscle and bone on either side of the tumor, as well as a segment of the radial nerve (Fig. 9-8C). A photomicrograph of the transected entire specimen shows that there was indeed medullary extension of this low grade parosteal osteosarcoma. Histologically, the photomicrograph displayed active fibrogenesis and active osteoblasts forming bone in the fibrous tissue.

Reconstruction was accomplished by inserting an intramedullary rod and a large autogenous tibial graft between the proximal and distal portions of the humerus. The graft was held in place with sutures, aided by the remaining muscle envelope. At 1 year the defect in the humerus had been sufficiently repaired to allow removal of all external support. Tendon transfers were done for the wrist drop and loss of finger extensors that were caused by resecting the radial nerve. Two years after the resection, the intramedullary rod was replaced with a shorter one to allow unrestricted motion of the shoulder.

At a 17-year follow-up visit the bony reconstruction appeared intact, and the patient had excellent function of the limb. The radiographs showed complete replacement of the bone graft about the internal fixation device (Fig. 9-8D&E). There was no local recurrence and no metastasis.

This case highlights one of the difficulties with the definition of what constitutes a wide resection. A wide resection ordinarily means that approximately 5 cm of normal tissue between the periphery of the tumor and the line of resection has been

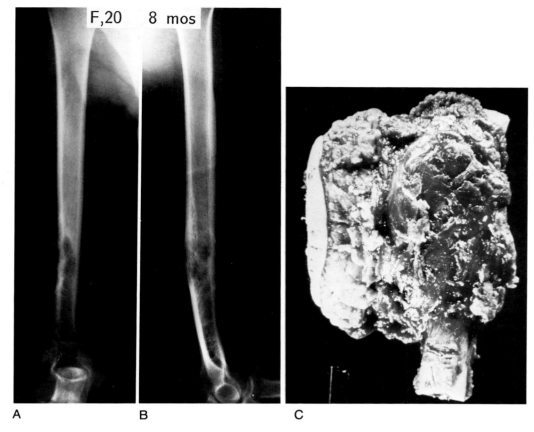

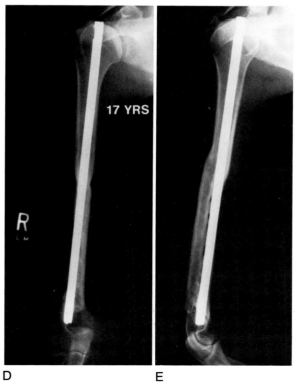

Fig. 9-8. Case 9-8. AP (**A**) and lateral (**B**) radiographs of the right humerus of a 20-year-old woman with a parosteal osteosarcoma which was symptomatic for 8 months. (**C**) Resected tumor includes the biopsy wound, radial nerve, and 10 cm of bone. AP (**D**) and lateral (**E**) radiographs of the reconstructed humerus (tibial bone graft and intramedullary rod) 17 years after resection.

removed. One cannot always be sure how wide the interval is, even when the specimen is examined grossly after it is removed; therefore until the specimen is examined histologically by the pathologist, the exact width of the margin is indeterminate. This fact suggests that perhaps there should be two designations in the surgical staging system as definitions of resection: the clinical definition and the pathological definition. The first is a provisional, planning designation made during the preoperative and intraoperative phases of treatment. The second is the definitive designation and should be the only one used for analytical definitive studies.

In the case under discussion, although the margins of normal tissue planned for resection fell short of the definition of a "wide resection," it was appreciated that the tumor, a parosteal osteosarcoma, is not one that rapidly and insidiously infiltrates the adjacent tissue.[7,29,31,34,60,65,66,81,99] That one consideration, which depended on a confident interpretation of the radiographs and a fortiori on the histological preparations, justified the less radical procedure. Fortunately, the brachial artery was far enough from the tumor that vascular compromise could be avoided. For practical reasons, the fact that normal tissue intervened between the line of resection and the marginal reactive tissue at the edges of the tumor justifies classifying the resection as "wide" rather than "marginal." Had there been reactive tissue (not tumor) in the line of resection, the margin of resection would have conformed to what has been ineptly called *marginal*. No example of a marginal resection is illustrated here for the following reasons: When such a margin has been obtained, it represents a surgical failure to achieve a wider margin, either because the surgeon could not determine the tumor's boundary with accuracy or because anatomical factors (presence of vital structures) prevented. No series of cases of "marginal" resections in substantial numbers for individual tumors have been collected for study. When they do appear in a study of large size, they nearly always constitute a heterogeneous group, for the reasons given, and must be categorized apart from cases of intralesional or wide resection. Therefore the designation serves merely to purify those two groups and eliminates overlapping. To minimize the incidence of local recurrence of a tumor, the best the surgeon can do is to delineate as accurately as possible the anatomical extent and to resect a margin of normal tissue, adequate in thickness, around it. That procedure is the best way to prevent tumor spread along the usual pathways, i.e., along tissue planes and through blood vessels and lymphatics. Even if a wide resection is accomplished, but especially with less extensive resections, the surgeon during dissection should never expose tumor tissue and should refrain from handling or forcibly retracting tumor tissue, which might free a few cells for embolization[52] or local spread of tumor. For these reasons also, if inadvertently or perhaps without recognizing that the tumor was exposed, the surgeon should avoid any unnecessary exposure and opening of fascial planes. These techniques are the best ways to avoid potential surgical seeding of tumor cells in vessels and lymphatics. The dissection should be sharp and minimally traumatic, with careful hemostasis.

Unfortunately, the surgeon has no other guide to identifying tumor except its gross appearance. The tissues nearby or at a varying distance from the major mass, and the tumor tissue itself, may be altered from their pristine appearance by fibrosis, necrosis, edema, or hemorrhage, so the surgeon's guides and landmarks for dissection may be indistinct. The uppermost prohibition during the surgical process must be exposure of tumor tissue (if it is malignant). If no tumor has been exposed during the resection, the surgeon has done his or her best to prevent local recurrence and metastasis.

The other factors that determine the location and growth of a recurrence of the tumor, either local or abscopal, reflects the biological behavior of the specific tumor. It is known, empirically, that tumors with high grade anaplasia more commonly seed in new locations than do tumors of low grade anaplasia. An example of that phenomenon is shown in the next case. The case also illustrates the most extensive (i.e., radical) procedure of resection—one that includes the entire compartment containing the tumor.

Case 9-9   A 23-year-old man was in good health until 6 months prior to presentation, when he bumped his knee. Within a few days there was pain and local ecchymosis that had barely disappeared when 2 weeks later he bumped it again. Thereafter he noticed a growing, painful mass below the knee, and he was unable to bend the knee fully. His complaints at the time of initial examination therefore were a painful swelling on the medial aspect of the left leg below the knee and restriction of motion of the knee. The radiographs revealed an increase in density on the medial and posterior aspects of the proximal part of the tibia adjacent to a soft tissue swelling (Fig. 9-9A&B). After the appropriate diagnostic studies were done (including pulmonary CT) and it was ascertained that there was no evidence of metastasis, an open biopsy of the tumor was performed. A high grade osteosarcoma was diagnosed (Fig. 9-9C). The periosteum had been lifted from the cortex by tumor, and there was considerable invasion of the medullary canal and soft tissues. A mid-thigh amputation was performed.

A cross section of the split specimen shows the extent of the soft tissue mass (Fig. 9-9D), which had invaded the muscles of the posterior compartment of the calf. A photomicrograph from the periphery of the tumor demonstrates a large artery in which there is a tumor thrombus. No tumor bone within the thrombus or in the immediate subperiosteal margin of the tumor was evident (Fig. 9-9E).

Finding a major vessel containing a tumor thrombus usually portends a grave prognosis, and the patient developed metastases in the lungs within 3 months of the amputation. He died within 6 months after presentation.

There may be invasion of tumor cells into venous channels (Fig. 9-10) as well as into the artery. It is this microvascular invasion that is invoked as the explanation for how metastasis develops; but the mere presence of circulating tumor cells, which ultimately form the metastatic foci, does not completely explain the spread of some tumors and not of others.[52] As an example of the enigmas in this matter, consider these facts: Many carcinomas spread by lymphatics to lymph nodes and then beyond, whereas osteosarcomas rarely do so. They tend to metastasize mainly to lung and to other bones, presumably via the veins. Pathologists have made valiant efforts to define grades of anaplasia in an objective, quantitative fashion.[30,47,102,126] They have used, inter alia, counts of cells showing mitoses in defined volumes of tumor tissue, chemical indicators of excessive nuclear activity,[91,92] and delineation of the ability of sarcoma cells to produce an intercellular matrix (be it in a nearly normal or a bizarre pattern) for this purpose. All these methods

have been shown to correlate roughly, but not precisely, with the outcomes of well delineated regimens of treatment, but they are most helpful for the evaluation of chemotherapeutic agents.[55,80]

In case 9-9, the demonstration of tumorous bone in the intramedullary part of the tumor (probably the older part of the lesion) but not in the subperiosteal or soft tissue mass invites speculation that there was an anaplastic progression in the tumor over time. If true, it supports the generally accepted concept that the earlier the treatment is instituted the better. The three, somewhat obvious reasons for this concept are that at an early stage the lesion is small, and its rate of growth and potential for metastasis are not fully developed. In the present case one cannot date the onset of tumor formation because, as is so often the case, the two injuries, incurred 6 months before the patient's presentation, may merely have called attention to the progression of the lesion, which earlier was not detected (no radiographs were obtained).

A correlation also has been demonstrated, as mentioned, between the size of a tumor at presentation and the prognosis. It is presumed that a large tumor allows a large number of cells to be released into the circulation (cell dose).

The cell dose may be a factor in whether a metastasis takes root. Many believe that there are immunological factors that are responsible for the destruction of circulating cells.[70] They speculate that the competence of the hypothetically immune substances as well as their amounts may well be such that they can be overwhelmed by a large cell dose. That idea is the rationale for such therapeutic maneuvers as debulking of large tumors as a first stage in definitive chemotherapy or administration of radiation. Chemotherapy then is part of the treatment protocol in cases such as the one just described. Before chemotherapy was available the only treatment of a metastasis was irradiation or surgery, the latter being appropriate in only a small percentage of cases where there were few and localized metastases, e.g., wedge resection of one or two pulmonary metastases (Fig. 9-11C&D). That such a regimen is on occasion successful is shown by the next case.

Case 9-10 A 20-year-old man had an osteosarcoma of the distal part of the left femur treated by a high thigh amputation (Fig. 9-11A&B). He devel-

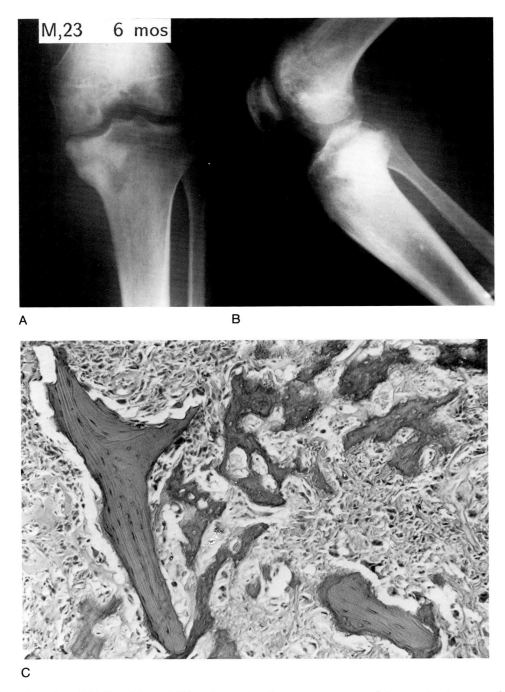

Fig. 9-9. Case 9-9. **AP (A)** and lateral **(B)** radiographs of an osteosarcoma of the proximal aspect of the left tibia show increased tumor density medially and posteriorly. An above-knee amputation was done. **(C)** Photomicrograph demonstrates the tumor bone in a high grade malignant stroma replacing the marrow (×100). *(Figure continues.)*

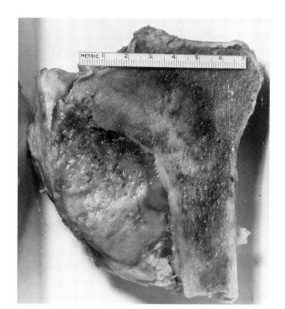

Fig. 9-9 *(Continued)*. (**D**) Coronal section of the specimen shows extension of the tumor. (**E**) Photomicrograph of tumor thrombi in vessels at the popliteal periphery of the tumor (×8).

D

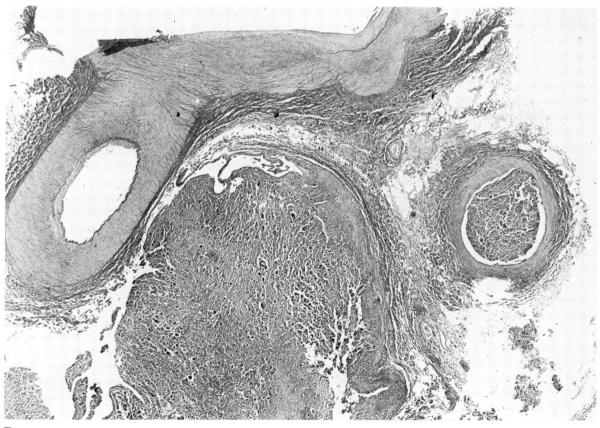

E

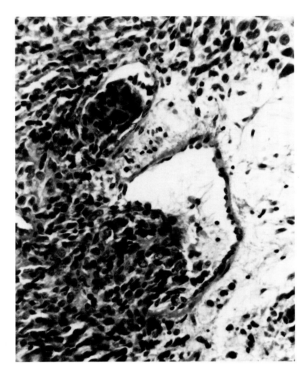

Fig. 9-10. Photomicrograph of an intramedullary osteosarcoma of the femur in an 11-year-old boy shows tumor invasion of a venous channel (×250).

oped a metastatic lesion in the lower lobe of the left lung 2 years after the amputation. The primary lesion was shown by radiography to be a destructive process with posterior invasion of the soft tissue (Fig. 9-11A&B). The radiograph of the lung 2 years later showed an area of increased density that was a metastasis in the left lower lobe (Fig. 9-11C). A wedge resection of the left lower lobe containing the metastasis was performed; 12 years after that procedure and 14 years after the amputation the chest radiograph showed no evidence of disease (Fig. 9-11D).

We have given a few examples of the evaluation and treatment of primary musculoskeletal tumors and have described the staging of the various types of primary malignant tumor. The definitions of sur-

gical treatment have been delineated. The next section amplifies some of the points made as they apply to categories of tumors and discusses some of the problems of evaluation and treatment. To discuss any further the use of adjunctive therapy (i.e., chemotherapy or radiotherapy) for controlling micrometastases or the local lesion is beyond the scope of this book. However, these modes of therapy are mentioned in the specific examples.

SPECIAL CONSIDERATIONS BY TUMOR TYPE

Benign Tumors

Benign tumors (which for classification purposes arbitrarily include lesions that probably represent some nonneoplastic harmartomatous malformations and some reactive lesions)[15] are listed (Table 9-2) in the classification by cell type. Thus under bone-forming tumors there are three lesions that produce osteoid or bone,[19,25,74,89,96] but it is questionable if osteoid osteomas[123,124] or osteomas are really neoplasms. The most common of all bone "tumors," the osteochondroma,[15,125] or exostosis, despite its bone-forming character has been listed under cartilage-forming lesions to call attention to its probable origin as an anomaly of growth of those cells. Many believe that osteoid osteoma and osteomas are reactive changes to as yet unidentified infectious agents. The chondroblastoma[28,67,76,154] is a nearly pure collection of chondroblasts, whereas the chondromyxoid fibroma,[77] as the name implies, has a variable mixture of cells. That variability is responsible for the confusion in the older nomenclature about lesions such as myxomas. Benign fibrous tissues other than giant cell tumors are rare in bone, except for the so-called nonosteogenic fibroma, which may indeed be a variant of the metaphyseal fibrous defect, now generally considered a nonneoplastic developmental anomaly. That lesion has been tabulated (Table 9-1) under conditions simulating tumors. The giant cell tumor is classified

Fig. 9-11. Case 9-10. AP (**A**) and lateral (**B**) radiographs of the right femur shows a lytic osteosarcoma with posterior extension into soft tissue (arrows). (**C**) PA radiograph of the chest shows a metastasis in the lower lobe of the left lung 2 years after a high-thigh amputation. (**D**) There is no evidence of recurrence in a PA radiograph of the chest 12 years after wedge resection of the lung and 14 years after amputation.

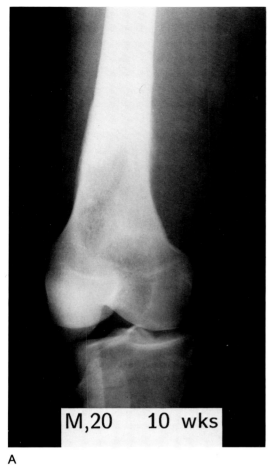

A

M,20   10 wks

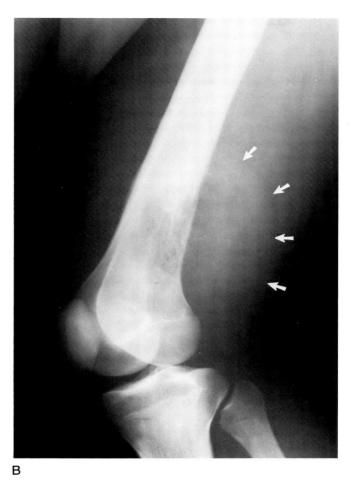

B

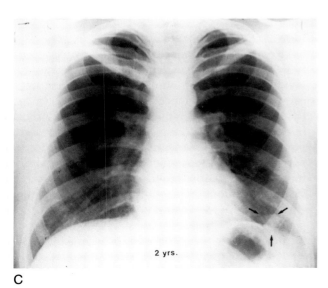

C

2 yrs.

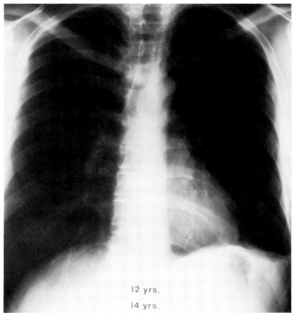

D

12 yrs.

14 yrs.

as a fibrous-tissue-forming tumor even though it has, at best, only small amounts of collagen. Its stem cell, here listed as presumably a collagen producer, is best regarded as a mesenchymal cell capable of differentiating (in groups) as an osteoclast, an osteoblast, or a fibroblast.

When considering benign lesions of bone, the spectrum of biological behavior from innocuous to aggressive must be kept in mind, the latter being evident in such lesions as osteoblastoma, chondromyxoid fibroma, and giant cell tumor. Sometimes osteocartilaginous exostoses can be considered premalignant tumors,[121] in particular solitary enchondromas in specific locations[59] or multiple enchondromas of long bones in hereditary manifestation.

As a group, benign lesions of bone infrequently pose problems in diagnosis of treatment. It is worth repeating, however, that an accurate diagnosis requires a correlation of all of the features of the lesion, especially the chronological and radiological features, in order to avoid errors of interpretation that may lead to either overtreatment or undertreatment.

As a rule, benign lesions produce much less pain than do malignant lesions. As discussed in Chapter 1, there rarely is the distinctive pain pattern exemplified in *osteoid osteoma,* i.e., a deep, mild to moderate bone pain present at night that is sufficiently severe to awake the patient but that can be relieved by aspirin. Osteoblastomas, chondroblastomas, and chondromyxoid fibromas, produce pain of an intermittent nature without a nocturnal predilection. A hemangioma, when symptomatic, produces a dull, aching pain at the site of involvement. In the spine, when it presses on nerve roots it may produce radiating pain or neurological deficits. Giant cell tumor only occasionally presents with a local swelling in addition to the dull, aching pain and restriction of motion of the adjacent joint. Swelling uncommonly accompanies the benign tumors unless the lesion has been known to be there for years. A slow and perceptible increase of size of the mass may then be its only outstanding symptomatic characteristic. A history of recent rapid increase in size or a sudden change in the character of the pain suggests a pathological fracture or a malignant transformation. The *location* of the lesion may be a clue to the diagnosis. Thus a lesion in the epiphysis of a long bone in a youngster before closure of the

epiphyseal plate should bring to mind a chondroblastoma rather than other lesions.[15,67,76,154] After skeletal maturity has been reached, such a lesion would bring to mind a giant cell tumor instead.[62,155] Osteoblastomas have a predilection for the spine but may be found in any bone of the appendicular skeleton.[96] The same is true for osteoid osteomas. The radiographic findings of any of these lesions may not be diagnostic (as they often are with osteochondromas and endochondromas), but the radiolucent lesions include chondroblastoma, chondromyxoid fibroma, enchondroma, and giant cell tumor, although other possibilities, including eosinophilic granuloma and a localized indolent infection, must also be entertained.

The radiological aspects of *osteoid osteoma* present so distinctive a pattern (i.e., diffusely increased density around a small radiodense fleck surrounded by a slightly decreased density) that it may be diagnostic if accompanied by the typical symptom complex. The diagnosis is particularly easy when the lesion is located in proximity to the cortex but in cancellous bone. However, when the lesion is adjacent to joints, it may be difficult to detect radiologically, and the symptoms may relate mainly to the reactive synovitis[123] (Fig. 9-12A). Neurological symptoms may be present as a result of nerve irritation from a lesion in bone near it, and then the soft tissues adjacent to the nerve show chronic inflammation (Fig. 9-12B). In such cases special diagnostic tests may be pursued. A bone scan,[63,84] ordinary tomography, CT scan[12] (Fig. 9-13), and angiography[58] have been of help in localizing and identifying such a lesion.

The next case illustrates the difficulty of identifying a lesion arising in a small bone of the wrist that produces symptoms evocative of a median nerve carpal tunnel syndrome.

Case 9-11 A 19-year-old man presented with pain in the wrist and paresthesias along the course of the median nerve in the right hand. These symptoms had been progressive for a year. The physical findings were exquisite tenderness in the wrist over the distal carpal bones and at the base of the third metacarpal. His radiographs showed a radiolucent lesion at the corner of the capitate bone (Fig. 9-12A). Radiographs of the hand and wrist made early in the course of the process were read as normal. There was a small area of increased density within the radiolucency.

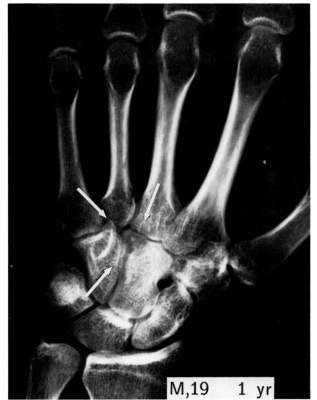

A

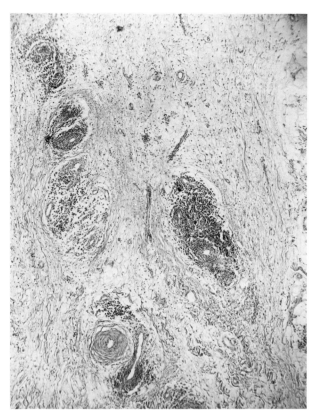

B

Fig. 9-12. Case 9-11. (A) AP radiograph of the wrist and hand of a 19-year-old man with wrist pain and median nerve paresthesias of 1 year's duration. The capitate bone shows a small area of increased density surrounded by a radiolucent area (arrows). The lesion was excised. (B) Photomicrograph of the adjacent soft tissues dorsally demonstrates an intense perivascular inflammatory reaction. This finding occurs with osteoid osteoma near joints (×100). (C) Photomicrograph of the curetted lesion shows the new bone and osteoid in a vascular stroma (×250).

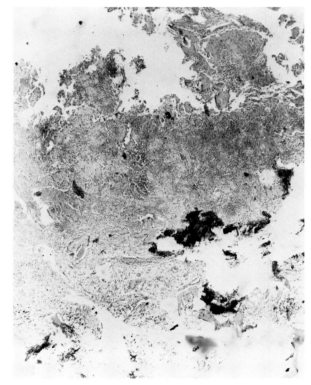

C

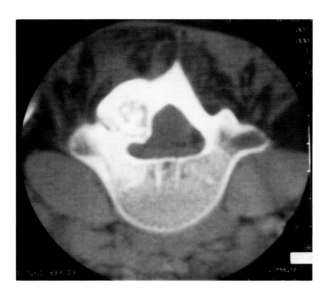

Fig. 9-13. CT scan of the L4 level shows an osteoid osteoma in the lamina near the facet joint (see case 2-2, Fig. 2-1).

In addition to the tenderness mentioned above, the median nerve at the carpal tunnel was tender, and there was an area of hypesthesia along the thenar eminence and the index finger. The ordinary radiographs in this case were so typical of osteoid osteoma and the localization of the lesion so definite that other imaging modalities (CT, MRI, angiography) were not used. They might generate pretty pictures, true, but they could not alter the surgical plan, which was to remove the involved part of the capitate bone. Grossly, at operation the carpal capsule over the capitate was edematous and swollen, but there were no gross abnormalities in the segment of capitate that was excised. Histologically, the lesion shows osteoid and new bone in that excised segment. The interpretation was osteoid osteoma, somewhat atypical in that the usual pattern, evident in lesions excised en bloc, was not found (Fig. 9-12B&C). A histological section of the capsular tissue showed intense perivascular inflammatory infiltrate. The patient's symptoms cleared after the surgery.

Because of the small size of osteoid osteomas and their tendency to be located in "problem locations" (in posterior spinal elements or near joints or the lesser trochanter) their localization and treatment often require the special diagnostic strategies already mentioned.[1,58,63] We have shown in Figure 1-1 how a radioactive isotope bone scan can help localize a lesion involving the junction of the lamina and facet joint of a vertebrae. In that case, a localized additional definition was needed before excision could be undertaken; therefore a CT scan was performed, and it revealed the precise location of the lesion anatomically. In the case just reviewed, where the lesion was in the capitate, it should be emphasized that there were no gross abnormalities the surgeon could recognize on the exposed bone, so that in essence the excision was blind: He had to rely entirely on the diagnostic tests to plan the removal of the lesion; furthermore, it would be well for him to have been aware that a piecemeal resection of fragments would militate against a confident diagnosis from the pathologist. The lesion's character stems largely from the overall relations of the three zonal elements (nidus, pericenter, and periphery), and only a block removal allows these relations to be recognized. A number of techniques in addition to those mentioned have been developed to make it possible to identify the lesion at surgery.[1,58,63] One of those techniques is use of an intraoperative radiosensitive probe that is activated by a radioactive isotope (of short half-life) given to the patient at an appropriate time prior to surgery.[63] The isotope becomes concentrated in the lesion. In the patient with a spinal lesion, excision of the lesion required removal of the lamina and pedicle, which left a potentially unstable spinal segment, necessitating fusion of the adjacent vertebrae (L4 with L5).

An *osteoblastoma* may vary in size from small, 3 to 4 cm in diameter (Fig. 2-1F&G) to extremely large (Fig. 9-14).[96] Even after doing the special studies mentioned, there may be delay in diagnosis, particularly when the lesion involves only cancellous bone near a joint or in the trunk. Although delay probably would stem from elaborate testing (e.g., to rule in or out any of several primary sites of tumors on the chance that the bony lesion is a metastasis), such delay per se would not do the patient substantial harm. When such uncertainty prevails and the expense of testing or prolonged delay must be avoided, the most efficient course of evaluation is to proceed, early, with a biopsy.

There are no abnormal blood chemical values in

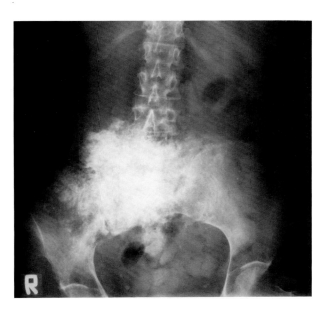

Fig. 9-14. AP radiograph of the lumbosacral spine and pelvis of a 45-year-old woman 2 years after biopsy and 7 years after the onset of pain. Note the large osteoblastoma over the sacrum, right ilium, and fifth lumbar vertebra. (From Marsh et al.,[96] with permission.)

association with benign tumors so there would be no need for special tests. The histological examination is the essential requirement (necessary and sufficient) for a definite diagnosis.

An *osteocartilaginous exostosis* (as mentioned above) is considered to be an aberration of bone development. The lesion is usually treated as a benign tumor, and when it has to be removed the reason for doing so may vary. It may encroach on a vessel[26] or nerve, or it may interfere with the motion of a joint or of overlying muscular or fascial structures. It may be associated with a deformity that requires correction (osteotomy) and may be removed as part of that procedure. It may be injured (fracture), and questions may then arise as to whether the symptoms stem from the fracture or its repair, or if there has been a malignant transformation.[121] We have already discussed in this chapter an example of a chondrosarcoma arising from an *osteocartilaginous exostosis* of the ilium in an adult with multiple hereditary osteocartilaginous exostoses (Fig. 9-5).

In most cases removal of the anomalous tissue poses no surgical problems; care must be taken to remove all the cartilaginous cap (plus the overlying bursa, if there is one), otherwise there is a substantial risk of local recurrence. Sometimes in unusual locations, a part that is dispensable is best removed. For instance, if the lesion arises from the proximal end of the fibula, as in the next example, a resection of the fibular head along with the exostosis may be necessary. Careful dissection of the peroneal nerve is then mandatory, as the sequelae of injury to this nerve may be more troublesome than the exostosis.

Case 9-12 A 13-year-old girl had multiple hereditary osteocartilaginous exostoses. One large lesion arose (Fig. 9-15A) from the proximal end of the right fibula and caused pain and intermittent numbness in the lateral aspect of the right calf and leg. The symptoms had been evident for 9 months. Although several members of the family also had the condition, none had had a malignancy arise from one of the lesions. A radiograph and histological section of the split specimen demonstrated the main features of the lesion (Fig. 9-15B&C). There was a partial but increased sensory deficit in the peroneal nerve distribution resulting from the dissection. The irritated nerve had to be freed from the neck of the fibula during the resection. It took more than a year for complete recovery from the sensory deficit. A microsection of the complete specimen showed the broad base of the exostosis which had, in its stalk, a medullary cavity continuous with that of the fibula (Fig. 9-15C). This finding is unusual.

There are reasons for removal of an exostosis other than those mentioned. Instances of soft tissue irritation include a *painful bursa* produced by motion of the soft tissues over the exostosis that may cause intermittent swelling and be reported as fluctuation in the size of the mass. A *false aneurysm* rarely may develop is an artery (particularly the popliteal)[26] abuts the lesion because of constant friction over the exostosis.

Although the pathogenesis of any osteochondroma is unknown, special attention has been paid to the hereditary multiple manifestation, which is uncommon but not rare.[134] Inheritance is by an autosomal dominant gene of variable expressivity. Fewer than 1 percent of patients with a *solitary* exostosis develop a chondrosarcoma during adult life, whereas about 10 percent of patients with multiple exostoses develop a chondrosarcoma in

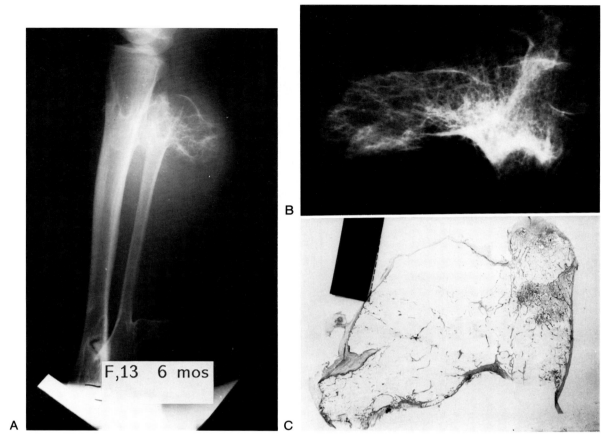

Fig. 9-15. Case 9-12. **(A)** Lateral radiograph of the tibia and fibula shows an osteocartilaginous exostosis in a 13-year-old girl with hereditary multiple osteocartilaginous exostoses. The large proximal fibular exostosis was painful when it was bumped. Radiograph of the specimen **(B)** and a microscopic section of the whole specimen (×1) **(C)** show the cartilage cap and fatty marrow and its origin from the fibula.

one of the lesions some time during their lives. The clinical clue that is most significant in this and other cartilaginous lesions, whether solitary or multiple, is that any sudden growth or distinct change in symptoms or radiological character unaccounted for by friction or specific injury is highly suspicious for a malignant transformation.

Some benign tumors (and some malignant ones) cause difficulty with clinical interpretation of symptoms because of their location. For instance, the mechanical effect of the tumor on the adjacent tissues, e.g., the joint, may delude the physician into attributing the pain or dysfunction to a disease of the synovial membrane or other soft tissue in-

volved. Some of the most egregious errors are so generated, even when radiographs (usually in retrospect) reveal a pararticular tumor. At the knee, for instance, when the lesion has been missed on the radiograph, arthroscopy may be undertaken, and then when it proves negative a course of irrelevant therapy may be pursued that only delays institution of the appropriate treatment. We have discussed this problem twice in Chapter 8 once relative to the nonspecific synovitis caused by an osteoid osteoma adjacent to the hip where the synovitis simulated arthritis and subsequently in the case of a chondroblastoma (see Fig. 8-2).

One aspect of benign tumors that deserves pass-

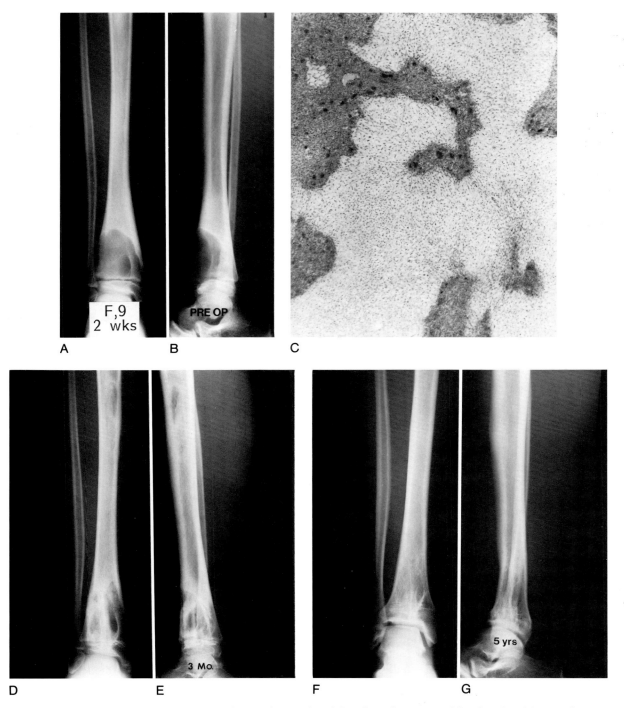

Fig. 9-16. Case 9-13. **AP (A)** and lateral **(B)** radiographs of the tibia of a 9-year-old girl with ankle pain for 2 weeks shows a radiolucent lesion of the distal metaphysis crossing the physis into the epiphysis. **(C)** Photomicrograph shows chondromyxoid fibroma with hemorrhagic spaces of an aneurysmal bone cyst ($\times 40$). **AP (D)** and lateral **(E)** radiographs 3 months after curettage and bone grafting. **(F&G)** Radiographs at 5 years show no recurrence.

ing mention is the association of some of them with aneurysmal bone cysts.[6,24,27,32,96,98,118] It has become increasingly evident that there are certain benign tumors that are associated rarely with an aberration of the vascularity of the lesion. When it happens, large and small vascular spaces with an inconspicuous endothelial lining devoid of muscular or fibrous support become engorged, so that the lesion becomes cyst-like and expands to complicate and distort the usual appearance of the original lesion. We mentioned one such case in Chapter 2 (see Figs. 1-2F&G). There a small osteoblastoma of the pedicle of L4 was involved. Osteoblastoma may be associated with aneurysmal bone cysts in as many as 20 percent of cases. When the aneurysmal features of the lesion predominate, the histology of the original tumor may be so obscured as to prevent the pathologist from recognizing the lesion. This situation may occur particularly in the spine.[96] It has surgical implications beyond the problem of bleeding, as discussed earlier (see Ch. 2). How to cope with the sometimes large defect created by the "cyst" is one such problem.

There is one other aspect of benign tumors that needs to be mentioned. When the lesion occurs in a child and is within or near an epiphysis and its growth plate, growth may be inhibited or distorted.[24]

Case 9-13 A 9-year-old girl had a lytic lesion of the distal tibial metaphysis extending across the epiphyseal plate into the epiphysis (Fig. 9-16A&B). Biopsy and curettage of the lesion (a chondromyxoid fibroma) revealed an associated aneurysmal bone cyst (Fig. 9-16C). Premature closure of the distal tibial epiphysis resulted (Fig. 9-16D&E). The limb length discrepancy at 5 years was small because of the relatively small contribution of that epiphyseal plate to the overall limb growth (Fig. 9-16F&G), and there was no deformity of the ankle despite the asymmetrical position of the lesion.

Case 9-14 A 14-year-old girl complained of pain in the shoulder. She had limited motion of the shoulder, and a radiograph revealed a lytic lesion occupying the entire epiphysis of the head of the humerus (Fig. 9-17A). The extent of the involvement of the epiphyseal plate is not clearly delineated, but the lesion was considered clinically to be either a chondroblastoma or an enchondroma. A

CT scan was performed that showed a more extensive lytic process than was evident on the radiographs (Fig. 9-17B). A biopsy revealed a chondroblastoma with an associated aneurysmal bone cyst, and curettage was performed. In this instance the effect of the lesion on the growth plate (and its treatment) would be expected to be minimal because the patient was close to skeletal maturity when her epiphyseal plate was damaged.

Malignant Primary Tumors

Several attempts have been made to evolve systems to quantitatively assess the aggressiveness of both benign and malignant tumors.[47,91,92,97,102,104,117,126] Radiographic[90] as well as histological criteria ordinarily are defined in these systems, in addition to the other elements that go into the staging (as described above). Unfortunately, these measures have not clearly delineated those tumors that will not be at all aggressive from those that behave in an aggressive manner or from those that are not only aggressive but also have a propensity, great or small, to metastasize. The difficulty of determining the prognosis of so many tumors brings up a concept that stems from the empirical observations accumulated on the biological behavior of tumors in general and musculoskeletal tumors in particular. The concept is that there is a spectrum of biological aggressiveness that is different for each of four cell lines — osteoblastic cells, cartilaginous cells, fibrous cells, and marrow cells,[115,116] the latter including reticulum cells[146] and stem cells but not the hematopoietic precursor cells. The degree of aggressiveness is from benign to the most malignant. Examples of the latter in the osteoblastic cell line were shown earlier in this chapter (Figs. 9-8, 9-9, 9-10, and 9-14). A few additional examples serve to illustrate this concept in more detail and reveal how it may affect treatment.

With the osteoblastic tumor line, lesions such as osteoid osteoma rarely recur. There the tumor is localized and usually can be excised in toto. However, if it is curetted and a residue remains, it can again manifest. This rule also applies to the osteoblastoma, which, however, rarely becomes aggressive. It may grow to so large a size as to simulate an

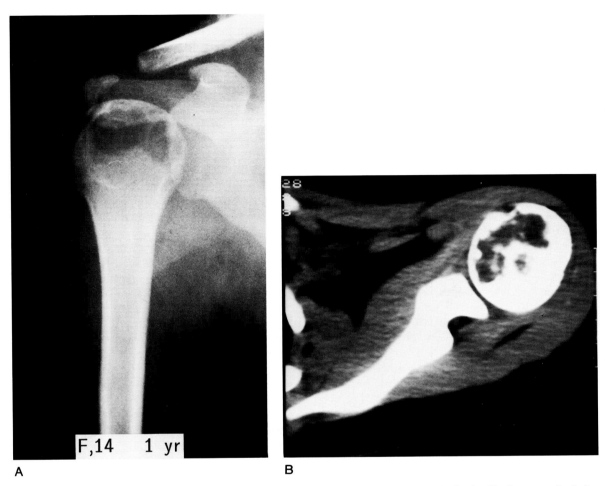

A   B

Fig. 9-17. Case 9-14. (A) AP radiograph of the left humerus of a 14-year-old girl who had had pain in the left shoulder for 1 year shows a lytic lesion of the head of the humerus. It was diagnosed as a chondroblastoma. (B) CT scan shows a larger lucent area than was evident on the radiograph. Histologically, a chondroblastoma with aneurysmal bone cyst features was found.

osteosarcoma and still remain benign.[79,96,100] The osteoblastic tumor pictured in Figure 9-14 appeared to be aggressive histologically, and it grew to a large size but did not metastasize. A more aggressive osteoblastic tumor, i.e., one of intermediate grade of malignancy, is the parosteal osteosarcoma, as was shown in Figure 9-8. Its histological grade was similar to that of the femoral tumor in the 14-year-old boy discussed above (Fig. 9-3), but the boy developed metastases. (The metastases were amenable to resection; i.e., wedge resection of a lobe of the lung was successful.) Parosteal osteosarcomas in general are known to have a good prognosis—better than 50 percent survival—with surgery alone (without chemotherapy). The tumor cells, even within a single tumor, vary in grade, from cells that produce a bone matrix of a mature type to those not so well differentiated. Occasional parosteal osteosarcomas do have some cells that exhibit a high degree of pleomorphism, abnormal mitoses, and bizarre hyperchromatism (all features of high grade tumors).

However, parosteal osteosarcomas are not seen in profusion even in oncology centers, so that no valid correlation between the anaplastic degree of a tumor and the prognosis with any type of treatment has been possible to date.

Osteoblastic tumors of higher degrees of anaplasia — the various osteosarcomas — have already been discussed. They were represented by the rather typical conventional case (case 9-4), a case that also was rather typical except for the appearance of metastases after a latent interval of years (case 9-3), a case of a highly undifferentiated type (case 9-9), and even a case (case 9-2) where the cells were so anaplastic that no bone was produced in the tumor, thereby making classification of it as an osteosarcoma inappropriate because one of the criteria for that designation is production of tumor bone.

Consideration of these cases and of the various other subgroups of osteosarcoma (i.e., the parosteal, sometimes called juxtacortical, osteosarcoma and the highly undifferentiated periosteal osteosarcoma) has led to many studies, the objective of which was to correlate prognosis with whatever features of the tumors and the patients could be documented with precision, e.g., location of tumor, age of patient, size of tumor, compartmentalization. As applied to osteoblastic malignant tumors, no correlation has been established as having so high a correlation coefficient that it is worthy of emphasis.[33] Thus central densely osteoblastic tumors *seem* to have a better prognosis than central lesions that are more osteolytic in their appearance, but here compartmentalization also has to be factored in, as do other features. Obviously, the pathologist is the one most concerned with histological grading, i.e., quantitation of anaplasia. Some of the pathologist's concerns have already been mentioned, e.g., number of abnormal mitoses, number of cells per unit volume of tissue. These concerns apply not only to osteoblastic tumors but to all malignant tumors. There have been many attempts to assess anaplasia by chemical rather than morphological techniques,[91,92] but the obstacles to all of the methods are formidable, not least among them the almost unsolvable problem of grouping sufficient numbers of patients who meet narrow criteria of selection and then subjecting them to identical treatment. Such treatment must then proceed for a year or two, during which interval other treatments will have been developed and may be proposed. If the latter are instituted, assessment of the original treatment may be impossible.

The cartilaginous tumors display a benign to aggressive spectrum of behavior more clearly than do any of the other tumor cell lines.[102] It is said that with cartilage tumors, in particular, one cannot depend on the histological appearance of the cartilage cells to predict the behavior of the tumor. Instead, one must depend on a combination of the clinical course, radiographic appearance, and histological features to make a prognosis. Three examples are cited.

Case 9-15 An asymptomatic lytic lesion was noted incidentally in the proximal end of the humerus when radiographs were obtained because of a minor injury to the shoulder of a 38-year-old man. The radiographs showed a stippled calcification irregularly distributed in a radiolucent, well demarcated area within the bone (Fig. 9-18A). Despite the typical radiological features, because there was some concern about possible fracture the lesion was removed by curettement. The specimen showed typical hyaline cartilage (Fig. 9-18B). This histological appearance is typical of an enchondroma.

Case 9-16 A 29-year-old man had had an aching intermittent pain in the upper part of the thigh of several year's duration. There was local tenderness but no functional impairment. Radiographs showed a lytic lesion of the proximal third of the femur with slight expansion of a thickened cortex (Fig. 9-19A&B). The biopsy showed a cartilaginous lesion with some double-nucleated cartilage cells but no unequivocal evidence of malignancy (Fig. 9-19C). This picture was interpreted either as a chondroma or a low grade chondrosarcoma. The latter possibility was entertained because the patient had symptoms and there was, radiologically, an expansion of the cortex as evidence of growth of the tumor. Therefore a wide resection was undertaken, and reconstruction was done with tibial bone grafts and an intramedullary rod. The long-term follow-up at 25 years was satisfactory except for slight limb shortening compensated for by a shoe lift (Fig. 9-19D&E).

Case 9-17 A 22-year-old woman had a history of

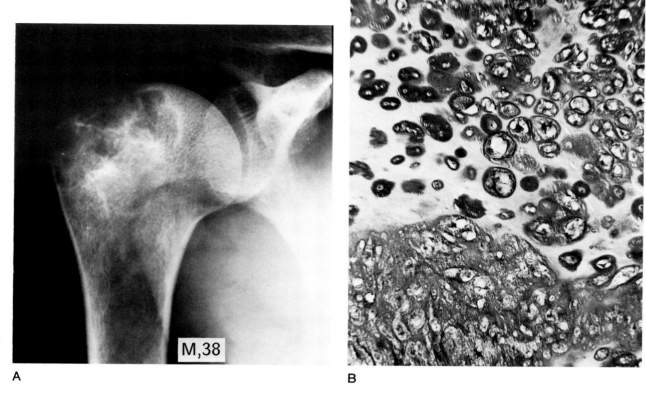

A   B

Fig. 9-18. Case 9-15. (A) AP radiograph of the right shoulder of a 38-year-old man shows a radiolucent irregular lesion that contains calcification. Note the reactive border of increased density, suggesting an endochondroma. (B) Photomicrograph of the lesion shows that it is composed of cartilage cells in a hyaline matrix with calcification in the matrix and about the cells. Occasional binucleated cartilage cells are present. The diagnosis was enchondroma.

pain and swelling of the upper thigh of 10 weeks' duration. The pain had been of increasing severity, enough to interfere with sleep. The patient also had been losing some weight recently. Radiographs of the femur showed a destructive lesion of the proximal half of the femur with a large extra-cortical mass. There was ossification within the subperiosteal component of the tumor, best seen on the radiograph of the specimen (Fig. 9-20A). The diagnosis of a malignant tumor was clear enough, and the prebiopsy question was whether it was an osteosarcoma or a chondrosarcoma. The biopsy showed rapidly infiltrating tumor cells characteristic of a chondrosarcoma, but there also were many undifferentiated (mesenchymal?) cells.

The ossification was occurring within the hyaline cartilage of the tumor (Fig. 9-20B). The histological evidence of severe anaplasia included a large number of cells with double or triple nuclei, and some of the abnormal cells were in foci of more than 20 per high-power field. The patient had a hip disarticulation, but died of her tumor 27 months later. In the amputation specimen it was evident that the tumor had invaded the femoral vein (Fig. 9-20C). The latter behavior is not unusual for chondrosarcoma. Venous extension of a thrombus from the tumor to the lungs through the heart has been reported.[110]

The spectrum from enchondroma to frank chondrosarcoma depends on cellular morphology to a

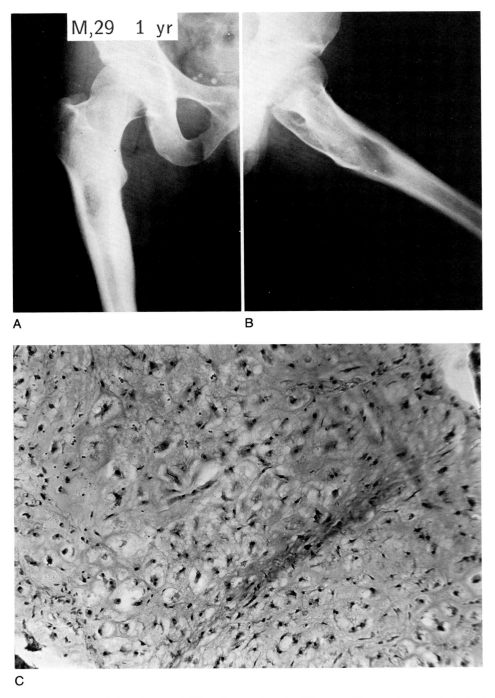

Fig. 9-19. Case 9-16. AP (**A**) and lateral (**B**) radiographs of a 29-year-old man shows a lytic lesion of the proximal femur with cortical thickening and a stippled calcification, noted best in the lateral view. The patient had had aching pain in the upper thigh for at last 1 year. (**C**) Photomicrograph demonstrates scattered binucleated and pleomorphic cartilage cells throughout a hyaline cartilage matrix of a low grade chondrosarcoma (×250). *(Figure continues.)*

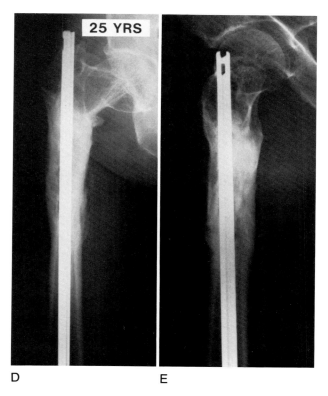

D   E

Fig. 9-19 *(Continued).* AP **(D)** and lateral **(E)** radiographs 25 years after resection and recontruction with autogenous bone grafts and intramedullary rod fixation show that the defect has healed and there is no recurrence.

lesser degree than does, for example, the spectrum in osteoblastic and fibrous tumor groups. Thus there were clinical features in case 9-17 in addition to the histological features that suggested a fulminating malignancy. The story of rapid growth of a preexisting cartilaginous lesion is similar to that in case 9-5, the patient with multiple exostoses and a chondrosarcoma arising from one of them in the ilium (Fig. 9-5). Enchondromas arising in small tubular bones, particularly those of the hands and feet, are with rare exception benign.[59,125] Only rarely does the patient recognize a sudden onset of pain in those (usually multiple) lesions, unless there has been specific trauma, and rarely do these lesions show an unusual spurt of growth. They may be treated simply by curettage and packing with bone should there be a fracture through the lesion.

The prognosis for enchondromas and for most low grade chondrosarcomas is excellent, whereas the prognosis for high grade chondrosarcomas resembles that for osteosarcoma. Radiation treatment is ineffectual, as all of the cartilage tumors are radioresistant.

The increasing attention being paid by pathologists to the grading of osteosarcomas and chondrosarcomas has had not only the objective of better defining the aggressiveness of the tumor (as part of the staging) but also of determining the probable response of a given tumor to adjuvant chemotherapy. This therapy, given prior to the surgical procedure, may allow the surgeon to attempt to salvage the limb[87,131,151] rather than do a radical amputation. When there is a high degree of cell necrosis after a short period of chemotherapy, as determined by sequential biopsies, the surgeon might perform a limb salvage procedure, whereas a poorly responsive tumor might indicate the need for amputation or palliative resection.[53,80] In either

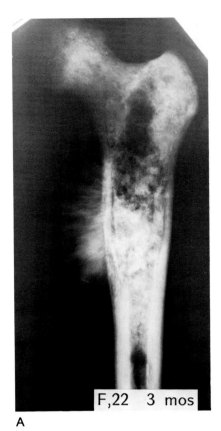

A

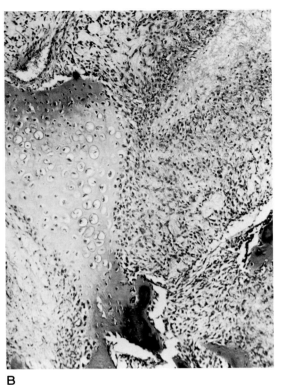

B

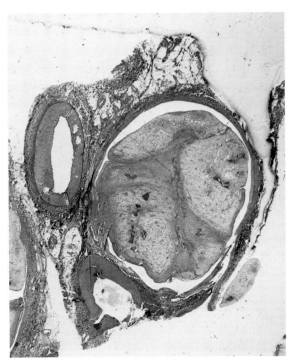

C

Fig. 9-20. Case 9-17. (**A**) AP radiograph of a highly malignant chondrosarcoma of the proximal femur shows a calcified tumor that has expanded into the cortex and extended into the soft tissue, producing a "sunburst" ossification. (**B**) Photomicrograph shows large, bizarre chondrocytes in a myxomatous and hyaline cartilage matrix. Enchondral ossification is also present (×105). (**C**) Tumor has invaded the femoral vein (×10).

case the operation would be followed by continuation of the chemotherapy regimen. Primary malignant tumors of bone that two decades ago would have been treated by amputation or disarticulation[14,16,53,54,66,88,148] are now being treated by limb-sparing techniques: Varying protocols of adjuvant chemotherapy are used followed by resection, followed by reconstruction of the resected area with either an internal prosthesis, allografts, or autografts.[9,17,20,35,41,61,68,82,83,156]

This approach to the treatment of sarcoma means that the degree of responsiveness of the tumor cells to the chemotherapy must be assessed at the time of diagnostic biopsy and within a few weeks after the chemotherapy regimen has been initiated. Such techniques are under study at present, and some of the problems of comparing them have been previously discussed. One additional problem is that there appears to be an increase in the number of short-term survivors of highly malignant musculoskeletal tumors (compared to historical controls) no matter which technique of therapy is used.[130,135,149] As was indicated earlier, the rarity of primary malignant tumors of bone means that no one institution can accumulate sufficient numbers of patients to classify them into meaningful groups so as to evaluate the effectiveness of a particular treatment protocol.

Malignant tumors that have been categorized as arising from a mesenchymal cell line include some giant cell tumors of bone, fibrosarcomas, and malignant fibrus histiocytoma. Although it is true that mesenchymal cells also serve as precursors to osteoblasts and chondroblasts, as well as some other cells of mesodermal origin, the mixtures of cells in the lesions of the group under discussion may call attention to the variation in the cells' potential for differentiation along lines other than chondrogenesis or osteogenesis.[97,102,117] We presented examples of malignant fibrous histiocytoma in Figure 9-1 and of giant cell tumor in Figures 9-6 and 9-7. When a giant cell tumor develops aggressive characteristics, as those cases demonstrated, it is difficult to determine whether the tumor is benign or behaving like a fibrosarcoma or a malignant fibrous histiocytoma.[21,78,122,136] It may share certain features of either or both of those tumors. An uncommon fibrous tumor designated desmoplastic fibroma has been reported at the lowest end of the

spectrum of malignancy.[3] This tumor has a propensity for local recurrence but does not metastasize. Histologically, it resembles its soft tissue counterpart, aggressive fibromatosis of the soft tissues,[71] or the desmoplastic fibroma of the abdominal wall.

The reclassification of many tumors previously considered fibrosarcomas or reticulum cell sarcomas into the more modern grouping known as malignant fibrous histiocytoma has the virtue of calling attention to the diversity of cell morphology seen in the members of the grouping. However, the various members can have a prognosis that is relatively good or decidedly poor, and the morphology of the tumor cells is not well correlated with the prognosis. In addition, this "mesenchymal" group of tumors may well contain foci not only of malignant fibrous cells, histiocytes, and so on but also chondroblasts or osteoblasts, although there may be only sparse production of the characteristic intercellular matrix.[101] Nevertheless, the processes of differentiation, dedifferentiation, or both in this set of tumors, from the pathophysiological point of view, are crucial to understanding how malignancy develops; unfortunately, the evidence on such matters is nearly all empirical as well as morphological, and the few experimental approaches that have been attempted produced little but interesting speculation.

When discussing the first three categories of tumors in Table 9-2 (of the ten listed), aspects of both diagnosis and treatment are described that depend on the biological behavior of each specific tumor and on the pathophysiology of tumors, benign and malignant. It is not convenient now to discuss the other seven categories. The reader can find each tumor type covered in any one of the recommended texts. The emphasis should be on the influence of diagnostic variables on treatment.

In cases 9-1 and 9-4 involvement of popliteal structures was demonstrated with preoperative imaging studies, so the decision to perform an amputation rather than limb salvage was clear. The preservation of function must never take priority over local control of the tumor. The surgeon may not have any choice but to take the risk of local recurrence should the patient or the family refuse to consent to an amputation or disarticulation when either of those procedures offers the best chance at local control of the tumor. In either case (resection or amputation), adjunctive chemotherapy (as noted) would be in order.

Metastatic Tumors in Bone

A metastasis or multiple metastases in bone may be discovered after the primary tumor has made its presence known (most of the time), but not infrequently the metastasis may cause the presenting symptoms.[18,57,80,127,132,138] In that case, pain may be caused by an outright fracture. For a description of such cases the reader should review Chapter 5 (see Figs. 5-45 through 5-48).

Tumors metastatic to bone comprise most of the tumors affecting bone. For this reason and because patients with all types of cancer are living longer, the orthopedic surgeon is increasingly involved in treating those patients. Tumors metastatic to bone may not cause an overt pathological fracture, however, but may cause symptoms by destroying bone trabeculae; in such cases the microfractures are not visible radiologically, i.e., there is pure lysis.[56] That situation arises frequently when the patient is known to have, or have had, a malignancy (breast, prostate, kidney). It also arises when there is no reason to suspect that the patient has a cancer, e.g., hidden primary carcinoma (or sarcoma). In the latter situation, once the radiographs have revealed a skeletal lesion whose differential diagnosis includes a malignant tumor, possible metastatic, a search ordinarily is instituted for a primary tumor. Whether the primary is identified as a result of the search, or if the search is unsuccessful but a biopsy of the lesion identifies the metastasis, treatment of that lesion then becomes the problem. Because many of the lesions in question affect the spine, needle biopsy plays an essential role in diagnosis.[107,108] This section of the chapter deals, in particular, with orthopedic treatment of metastases to the skeleton.[4,18,57,120,127,128,138]

It is important to differentiate metastatic tumors not only from primary tumors of bone but also from an inflammatory process or one of various metabolic diseases. It has been estimated that for every six cases where the primary tumor is known to be present, the initial manifestation of a cancer is its metastasis.[75]

Case 9-18 A 66-year-old woman had complained of aching pain in the right thigh intermittently for 6 years. On examination she had tenderness in the upper thigh but normal range of motion of the hip and knee. Radiographs of the right femur showed a purely lytic lesion of the proximal femoral diaphysis with thinning of the femoral cortex surrounding the lesion (Fig. 9-21A&B). The important findings on laboratory work-up included no Bence Jones protein in the urine and negative plasmaphoresis and immunophoresis for plasma cell myeloma. A bone scan revealed no other bony lesions except that in the femur.

Because the patient was thought to have an impending fracture, the operated area was strengthened by inserting an intramedullary Zickel nail after a curettage biopsy of the lesion was done at the time of reaming the femoral canal. The histological diagnosis by frozen and permanent sections of the lesions, as well as the touch preparation, was plasma cell myeloma.

During insertion of the device, the thin shell of femoral cortex fractured (as was anticipated). At 6 weeks the fracture was healing (Fig. 9-21C). Now, at 11 years, the medial cortex is intact and thicker but the lesion has not completely healed despite treatment of the disease with radiation therapy and chemotherapeutic agents (Fig. 9-21D). Nevertheless, the patient is able to bear weight comfortably with use of a cane.

This case has been presented here, in the subsection on metastatic tumors, despite the fact that it is really an example of category IV in Table 9-2. The case is unusual in that myelomas are not commonly encountered as solitary lesions. The surgical treatment (curettage and so on) was predicated on the anticipation that multiple lesions were to be expected; prior to treatment, it was expected that the disseminated character of the disease would manifest in positive immunological tests. Therefore in some respects myeloma can be regarded as a systemic condition, even though a solitary lesion, as in this case, may precede the typical manifestations. Although such a lesion may require treatment, as in this case, it should not be subjected to the same radical treatment as a primary malignancy for prophylaxis against local recurrence or metastasis. Surgery under those circumstances becomes an adjunctive treatment to oncological management of the disease.

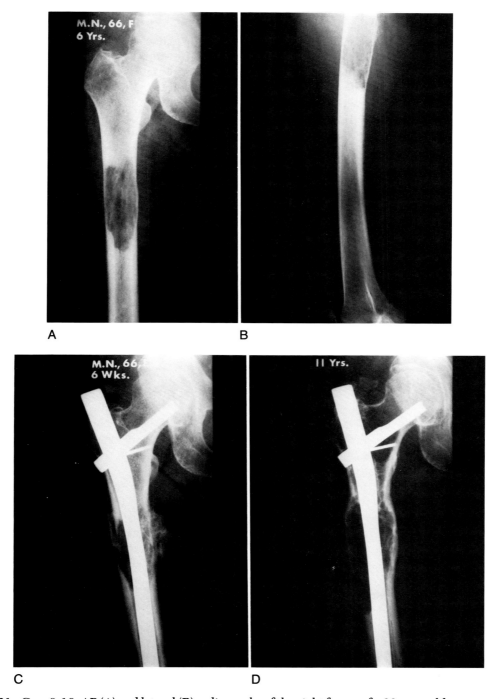

Fig. 9-21. Case 9-18. AP (**A**) and lateral (**B**) radiographs of the right femur of a 66-year-old woman who had had pain in the right thigh for 6 months. Six months earlier she had been treated for an adenocarcinoma of the endometrium and has had no evidence of that disease since. The lytic lesion (thought to be a metastasis) was treated by biopsy and insertion of a Zickel nail. Plasma cell myeloma was diagnosed. (**C&D**) AP radiographs at 6 weeks and 11 years show repair of the medial cortex but persistence of the myelomatous focus while the patient underwent chemotherapy for the tumor and irradiation to the femur.

Once the diagnosis of a marrow tumor — myeloma, lymphoma and its variants (reticulum cell sarcoma) — is made, the tumor is treated by medical oncologists with chemotherapy, irradiation, or both.[115] Exceptions occur when only a solitary focus of these tumors is present.[114,146] An impending fracture of such a lesion in a long bone treated by internal fixation with an intramedullary rod can prevent (or control) the fracture (Fig. 9-21). Adjunctive radiotherapy and chemotherapy relieve pain and may prevent progression of the tumor at the site. There is no evidence that reaming of the medullary canal or insertion of an intramedullary device without reaming spreads the tumor cells to form a new focus distal to the primary one.

When it is suspected that a lesion might be a cancer metastatic to bone, one should follow the AJCC protocol for evaluation, as mentioned earlier in this chapter. The protocol consists in a detailed family history regarding malignancy as well as a personal history. The physical examination and radiographic examination must be thorough and would include films of the sites identified by the history and physical examination as being possibly involved. As a practical matter, a biopsy might well be done early in the course of the evaluation once routine radiographs reveal a lesion, so the histological findings would give direction to studies that might identify the hitherto unknown primary lesion. For example, a carcinoma of the thyroid (case 9-19; Fig. 9-22) or kidney (case 9-20; Fig. 9-23) can easily be recognized by histological evidence, as can other visceral tumors on occasion. The biopsy might also identify some lesion other than metastatic cancer simulating the disease radiographically (infection perhaps). This identification would obviate a misdirected extensive and expensive diagnostic test sequence including perhaps an intravenous pyelogram or a barium enema.

A search for the primary site should not be done pro forma but, rather, as a part of the evaluation of the extent of the disease, thereby allowing the best

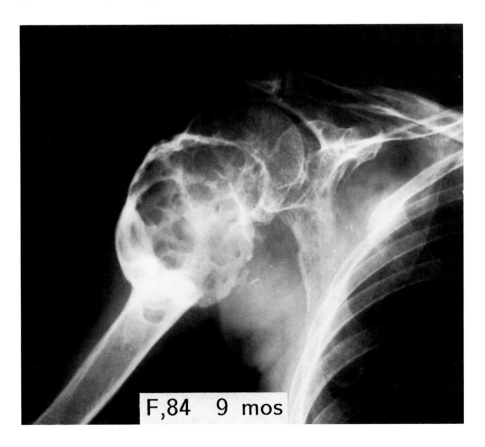

Fig. 9-22. Case 9-19. AP radiograph of the right shoulder of an 84-year-old woman with a large lytic, soap bubble metastasis from a carcinoma of the thyroid gland. Uptake of ^{131}I in the metastasis and thyroid gland made the isotope the principal means of treating the tumor. The biopsy identified the primary tumor with reasonable certainty in this case.

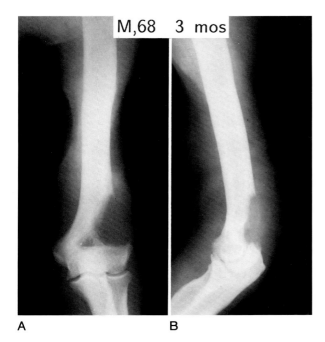

A   B

Fig. 9-23. Case 9-20. AP (**A**) and lateral (**B**) radiographs of the left humerus and elbow show a lytic lesion of the lateral area of the distal humerus. The mass pulsated. Biopsy confirmed the diagnosis of a renal cell carcinoma metastasis.

regimen of treatment to be followed. It should be remembered that in one-sixth of cases in which skeletal metastases are diagnosed the primary site is never identified despite an extensive search.[75,132] Treatment of the primary tumor, when it *is* identified, is based on the present local and systemic effects of the primary tumor as well as any anticipated effects, rather than on the effects of treatment for a given metastasis.

Case 9-21 A 39-year-old man complained that he had had pain in the leg just below the knee for 6 months. There was tenderness and swelling localized to the tibia below the tubercle, and radiographs (Fig. 9-24) showed an osteolytic lesion of the proximal part of the tibia that expanded the cortex. Routine laboratory tests were negative. A needle biopsy prior to any further testing showed an epidermoid carcinoma, probably from the lung; the involvement of the lung was then revealed by tracheal washings. The tibia was treated by irradiation only (for palliation).[4,120]

If the site identified as tumorous is less accessible for biopsy than the tibia, a radioisotope scan might be a good way to identify a second, more readily accessible site.[84] The surgeon should have in mind two objectives: (1) establish a definitive diagnosis by obtaining a tissue sample; and (2) if needed, apply appropriate surgical treatment to the skeletal lesion. If the first objective can be gained by a needle biopsy without further compromising the structural integrity of the bone, that procedure alone might be done so that later the second objective can be achieved more effectively, i.e., better information about exactly what type of tumor is under consideration and exactly what operation is best. In case 9-21, there was no need for elaborate tests (scans, MRI, CT) and no need for reconstructive surgical measures prior to performing the biopsy. Only when one would have planned a resection would a CT scan or MRI have been needed.

The orthopedic surgeon is increasingly involved in the care of patients with metastatic disease in two ways. One is to assist the oncologist by obtaining tissue. That examination then enables the pathologist to predict the sensitivity of the cancer to hormonal treatment or chemotherapy. The other is to determine the nature of the tumor and its grading. Whatever orthopedic treatment is needed for the musculoskeletal metastasis is then the orthopedist's responsibility.

Treatment

Many if not most sites of metastatic disease in the skeleton do not result in, or threaten to result in, a pathological fracture.[14b] Only when there is a fracture of importance (or a threat of the same) is surgical treatment indicated.[18,127,128,138] The surgeon must use a method of treatment appropriate to the situation. Surgery would not be indicated, for instance, for a metastasis from an adenocarcinoma of the thyroid. That lesion takes up radioactive iodine[130] and thus may well respond to treatment with that isotope (Fig. 9-22A).

Fractures of importance include those of vertebrae, which threaten neurological integrity, or those causing so much pain as to reduce the patient to virtually complete immobility. Additionally, the prognosis concerning duration of life must justify whatever procedure is to be done; i.e., the empirical evidence for (1) the type of tumor involved, (2)

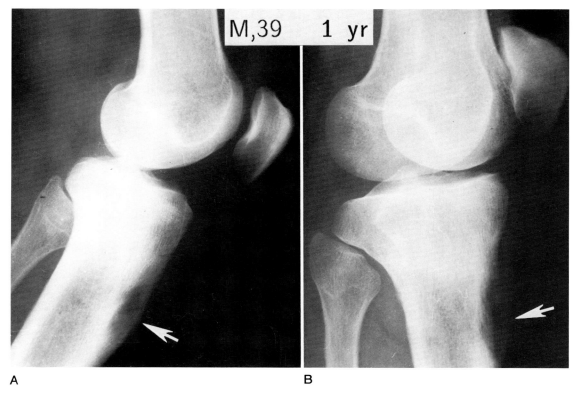

Fig. 9-24. AP (**A**) and lateral (**B**) radiographs of the left knee of a 39-year-old man who had had pain in the anterior aspect of the knee for 1 year. Biopsy of the lytic area of the anterior cortex showed an epidermoid carcinoma metastatic from the lung.

the extent of involvement, and (3) the general condition of the patient must not be a contraindication. Unfortunately, this judgment rests primarily on the opinions of the physicians involved, and they have little or no help either from published material on the specific subject or general knowledge of pathophysiology. As indicated in the discussion of malignancies, there are so many controversies concerning the nature of anaplasia, metastasis, and other basic aspects of neoplasia that the application of principles — which are far from clear or in general acceptance — is impossible.

Of equal importance to the involvement of vertebrae, although far less common, are involvements of the femur and tibia. These structures also constitute sites of "important" pathological fractures or impending fractures. In vertebral cases, one option is excision of the tumor-bearing bone by resection or curettage and reconstruction with

bone grafts, polymethylmethacrylate (**PMMA**) and posterior fusion, or both. These alternatives apply to the cervical spine[3a] whereas anterior interbody fusion combined with fixation rods contoured posteriorly may be appropriate for lesions in the thoracic or lumbar spine. These techniques should provide stabilization and relief of pain, and they prevent immobilization of the patient.

A patient who has a pathological fracture of the humerus, femur, or tibia, or who is at high risk for developing that complication, also is a candidate for prophylactic internal fixation to meet not only those objectives just mentioned but also, at the very least, to ease nursing care (Fig. 9-25). Internal fixation with any of several intramedullary devices (Küntscher rods, Zickle nails, Ender rods) possibly with wire mesh (Fig. 9-26) at the site of the fracture or structural weakness, with or without the incorporation of threaded pins and PMMA, may serve to

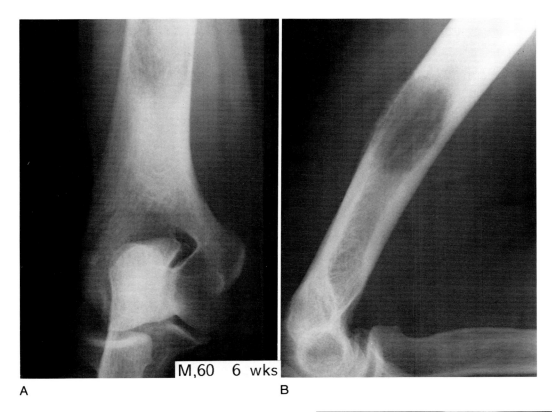

A   M,60   6 wks   B

Fig. 9-25. AP (**A**) and lateral (**B**) radiographs of the right humerus of a 60-year-old man with an osteolytic squamous cell carcinoma of the lung. The metastasis at the junction of the middle and distal thirds of the humerus had been symptomatic for 6 weeks. (**C**) The deposit was biopsied, curetted, and filled with polymethacrylate, and the site was stabilized with dual plates.

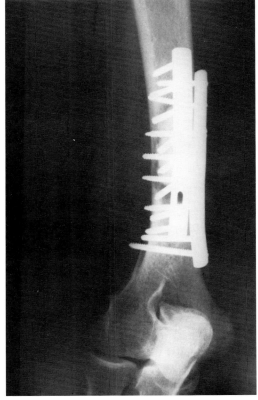

C

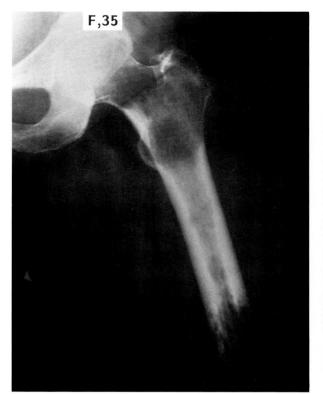

A

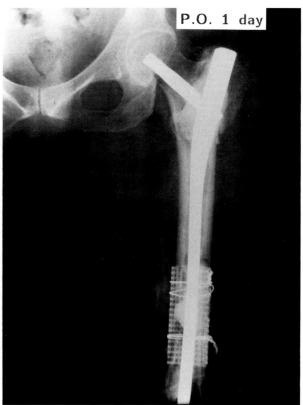

B

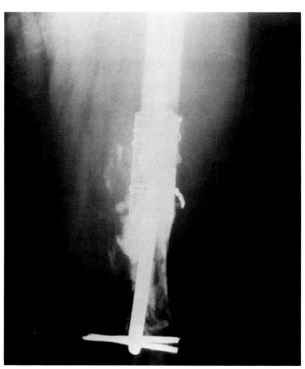

C

Fig. 9-26. (A) AP radiograph of the left femur of a 35-year-old woman with carcinoma of the breast shows lytic metastases in the intertrochanteric and mid-diaphysis of the femur. A third focus was present in the distal third of the femur. (B) For ease of nursing care and to honor a wish by the patient and her family to be at home during her terminal illness, each focus was curetted and filled with PMMA; the femur was then stabilized by internal fixation with a Zickel nail and wire mesh about the mid-femur focus. (C) Threaded pins were placed at the distal focus.

return the extremity to useful function.[14a] It should be emphasized that these techniques challenge the surgeon's ingenuity in devising a sturdy reconstruction and are not such that they can be well portrayed in atlases of operations. There are articles on specific operations for specific sites of involvement, but the surgeon should bear in mind that the reconstruction, unlike reconstructions for resected primary tumors or for conditions such as arthritis, cannot depend even in part on the patient's reparative potential. The reconstruction should be usable immediately after the patient recovers from the operation; i.e., it should be well carpentered, albeit for the short rather than the long term. Curettage of the tumor for the purpose of removing tissue that may impair the structural integrity of the reconstruction may be of value, but it should not be so vigorous as to represent an attempt at complete removal of tumor. All of the affected sites may then be subjected to adjunctive radiation therapy to suppress, if possible, further local spread of the tumor.[4,18,120]

Soft Tissue Tumors

As with the discussion of tumors in bone, we concentrate here on the orthopedic aspects of tumors of the soft tissues rather than the pathological or oncological aspects.[44,94,95,137,139–141] Soft tissue tumors are different from bone tumors in terms of evaluation and treatment. Sarcomas of the soft tissues lend themselves to a discussion of principles as a group, rather than as subgroups delineated by their origin from a specific stem cell. We do not cover each tumor, and specific characteristics can be readily reviewed in other texts.[46,139]

The patient who presents with a mass in the soft tissue should make the physician think of three categories of lesion: a nonneoplastic process (Table 9-3), a benign neoplasm, or a malignant soft tissue lesion (Table 9-4). Most masses that are encountered are nonmalignant; it has been estimated that only 1 percent of such masses are malignant tumors.

The orthopedist sees only a small fraction of the soft tissue masses, as most are treated by general surgeons. Nevertheless, a sizable number are referred, if not for primary treatment, then for rea-

Table 9-3. Nonneoplastic Soft Tissue Lesions Simulating Tumors

Injury and repair
    Chronic Hematoma acute injury
    Contusion
    Myositis ossificans
    Pseudosarcomatous tumor
Infection
    Abscess, pyogenic, tuberculous, fungal
Foreign body [metal, wood, plastic (silicone)]
Fibromatosis
    Sternocleidomastoid tumor of infancy
    Palmar, plantar
Degenerative disease
    Bursitis with or without calcification
    Ganglion cyst
Rheumatoid cyst
Gout

sons such as recurrence, the need for reconstruction, or treatment of functional disability.

All the steps outlined earlier for diagnosis in regard to bone tumors including biopsy are applicable here. A careful history and physical examination, of course, come first.

The history relating to a soft tissue mass often includes an injury to the soft tissues. It may have occurred long before the presentation and may be forgotten by the patient until the physician persists in the questioning on that subject. We discussed several such lesions in Chapter 6 (Figs. 6-9, 6-10, 6-11). One case proved to be a chronic hematoma, another myositis ossificans, and a third a sternocleidomastoid tumor.

The physical examination is equally important. It differs from the examination described for a malignant bone tumor in that the latter rarely presents as a mass (it usually is first revealed by radiographs). When a bone tumor does include a mass in its manifestations, it is of little consequence to record the various properties of the mass, whereas with the soft tissue sarcoma those characteristics may be of paramount importance. In fact, the size of the mass may be the most crucial of its features with regard to staging. Also important are the location of the mass (superficial or deep, proximal or distal), the relation of the mass to the surrounding tissues (skin, muscle, or bone) as determined by palpation,

Table 9-4. International Histological Classifications of Tumors No. 3: Soft Tissue Tumors

I. Tumors and tumor-like lesions of fibrous tissue
  A. Fibromas
    1. Fibroma durum
    2. Fibroma molle (fibrolipoma)
    3. Dermatofibroma (histiocytoma, sclerosing hemangioma)
    4. Elastofibroma (dorsi)
  B. Fibromatosis
    1. Cicatricial fibromatosis
    2. Keloid
    3. Nodular fasciitis (pseudosarcomatous fibromatosis)
    4. Irradiation fibromatosis
    5. Penile fibromatosis (Peyronie's disease)
    6. Fibromatosis colli
    7. Palmar fibromatosis
    8. Juvenile aponeurotic fibroma (calcifying fibroma)
    9. Plantar fibromatosis
    10. Nasopharyngeal fibroma (juvenile angiofibroma)
    11. Abdominal fibromatosis (abdominal desmoid)
    12. Fibromatosis or aggressive fibromatois (extra-abdominal desmoid)
    13. Congenital generalized fibromatosis
  C. Dermatofibrosarcoma protuberans
  D. Fibrosarcoma
II. Tumors and tumor-like lesions of adipose tissue
  A. Benign
    1. Lipoma (including fibrolipoma, angiolipoma, etc.)
    2. Intramuscular lipoma (infiltrating lipoma)
    3. Hibernoma
    4. Angiomyolipoma (of renal origin)
    5. Myelolipoma
    6. Lipoblastomatosis (fetal lipoma)
    7. Diffuse lipomatosis
  B. Malignant
    1. Liposarcoma
      a. Predominantly well differentiated
      b. Predominantly myxoid (embryonal)
      c. Predominantly round cell
      d. Predominantly pleomorphic (poorly differentiated)
      e. Mixed type (combining features of a, b, c, or d)
III. Tumors of muscle tissue
  A. Smooth muscle
    1. Benign
      a. Leiomyoma
      b. Angiomyoma (vascular leiomyoma)
      c. Epithelioid leiomyoma (bizarre leiomyoma, leiomyoblastoma)

    2. Malignant
      a. Leiomyosarcoma
  B. Striated muscle
    1. Benign
      a. Rhabdomyoma
    2. Malignant
      a. Rhabdomyosarcoma
        (1) Predominantly embroyonal
        (2) Predominantly alveolar
        (3) Predominantly pleomorphic
        (4) Mixed (combining the features of (1), (2), or (3)
IV. Tumors and tumor-like lesions of blood vessels
  A. Benign
    1. Hemangioma
      a. Benign hemangioendothelioma
      b. Capillary hemangioma (juvenile hemangioma)
      c. Cavernous hemangioma
      d. Venous hemangioma
      e. Racemose (cirsoid) hemangioma (arterial, venous, arteriovenous)
    2. Intramuscular hemangioma (capillary, cavernous, or arteriovenous)
    3. Systemic hemangiomatosis
    4. Hemangiomatosis with or without congenital arteriovenous fistula
    5. Benign hemangiopericytoma
    6. Glomus tumor (glomangioma)
    7. Angiomyoma (vascular leiomyoma)
    8. "Hemangioma" or granulation-tissue type (granuloma pyogenicum)
  B. Malignant
    1. Malignant hemangioendothelioma (angiosarcoma)
    2. Malignant hemangiopericytoma
V. Tumors and tumor-like lesions of lymph vessels
  A. Benign
    1. Lymphangioma
      a. Capillary
      b. Cavernous
      c. Cystic (hygroma)
    2. Lymphangiomyoma
    3. Systemic lymphangiomatosis
  B. Malignant
    1. Malignant lymphangioendothelioma (lymphangiosarcoma)
VI. Tumors of synovial tissues
  A. Malignant
    1. Synovial sarcoma (malignant synovioma)
      a. Predominantly biphasic (spindle cell and epithelioid patterns)
      b. Predominantly monophasic (spindle cell or epithelioid pattern)
  B. Benign
    1. Benign synovioma

Continued

Table 9-4 *(continued)*

VII. Tumors of mesothelial tissue
    A. Benign mesothelioma
        1. Predominantly epithelioid
        2. Predominantly fibrous (spindle cell)
        3. Biphasic
    B. Malignant mesothelioma
        1. Predominantly epithelioid
        2. Predominantly fibrous (spindle cell)
        3. Biphasic
VIII. Tumors and tumor-like lesions of peripheral nerves
    A. Benign
        1. Traumatic neuroma (amputation neuroma)
        2. Neurofibroma
        3. Neurilemoma (schwannoma)
        4. Neurofibromatosis (von Recklinghausen's disease)
    B. Malignant
        1. Malignant schwannoma (neurogenic sarcoma, neurofibrosarcoma)
        2. Peripheral tumors of primitive neuroectoderm
IX. Tumors of sympathetic ganglia
    A. Benign
        1. Ganglioneuroma
    B. Malignant
        1. Neuroblastoma (sympathicoblastoma, symphathicogonioma)
        2. Ganglioneuroblastoma
X. Tumors of paraganglionic structures
    A. Peochromocytoma
        1. Benign
        2. Malignant
    B. Chemodectoma (nonchromaffin paraganglioma)
        1. Benign
        2. Malignant
    C. Paraganglioma, unclassified
XI. Tumors and tumor-like lesions of pluripotential mesenchyme
    A. Benign
        1. Mesenchymoma
    B. Malignant
        1. Malignant mesenchymoma
XII. Tumors of vestigial embryonic structures
    A. Benign
        1. Chordoma
    B. Malignant
        1. Malignant chordoma
XIII. Tumors of possible extragonadal germ cell origin
    A. Benign
        1. Teratoma (dermoid cyst)
    B. Malignant
        1. Teratocarcinoma

        2. Embryonal carcinoma
        3. Choriocarcinoma
XIV. Tumors of disputed or uncertain histogenesis
    A. Benign
        1. Granular cell tumor (granular cell "myoblastoma")
        2. Chondroma of soft parts
        3. Osteoma of soft parts
        4. Nasal glioma (ganglioglioma)
        5. Pacinian tumor
        6. Adenomatoid tumor of genital tract
        7. Myxoma
        8. Melanotic progonoma (retinal anlage tumor, melanotic neuroectodermal tumor of infancy)
        9. Fibrous hamartoma of infancy
    B. Malignant
        1. Alveolar soft-part sarcoma (malignant organoid granular cell "myoblastoma")
        2. Malignant granular cell tumor [malignant (monorganoid) granular cell "myoblastoma"]
        3. Chondrosarcoma of soft parts
        4. Osteosarcoma of soft parts
        5. Malignant giant cell tumor of soft parts
        6. Malignant fibroxanthoma (malignant histiocytoma)
        7. Kaposi's sarcoma
        8. Clear-cell sarcoma of tendons and aponeuroses
XV. Non-neoplastic or questionably neoplastic lesions of soft tissues — of interest because of their resemblance to true neoplasm
    A. Xanthoma group
        1. Fibroxanthoma (fibrous histiocytoma)
        2. Xanthoma
        3. Juvenile xanthogranuloma (nevoxanthoendothelioma)
        4. Retroperitoneal xanthogranuloma (Oberling)
        5. Nodular tenosynovitis (giant cell tumor of tendon sheath) and pigmented villonodular synovitis
    B. Ganglion
    C. Localized myxedema
    D. Myositis ossificans
    E. Proliferative myositis
XVI. Soft tissue tumor, unclassified

(Modified from Enzinger et al.,[46] with permission.)

and its physical properties (softness, nodularity, heterogeneity). Finally, it may be of the essence to find that the mass is pulsatile, which may have to be determined using a stethoscope. Examination of an extremity that is the site of a soft tissue mass always should include an assessment of any nerve deficit or circulatory deficit. Such deficits are rarely caused by tumors of bone, possibly with the exception of osteochondromas.

Radiographs of the involved part are called for routinely to reveal differences in density of the soft tissues and to show if there is distortion of the normal anatomical structures at the site. The lower density of fat compared to that of muscle should be recognized; and if fat is present, as revealed on films taken with an exposure designed to bring out the low density, the affected area may well be delineated anatomically and may be diagnosable by such a film even before other tests (especially CT and MRI) are done. Demonstration of calcifications or ossification within the mass is helpful to distinguish injury and repair reactions from neoplasm. Only a few neoplasms show calcifications (i.e., synovial sarcoma[13] or fibrosarcoma) — and infrequently at that. An abutting periosteal response or actual invasion of the bone by an aggressive sarcoma on rare occasion is evident on the radiograph. Other imaging methods would then be indicated: bone scans,[40,50,71,72,83] ultrasound,[85] CT scans,[12] MRI,[143] angiography.[157] Only when the mass has been shown to abut against bone are tests such as scintigraphy necessary. Technetium bone scintigraphy demonstrates only that the proximity of the soft tissue sarcoma to bone has evoked a reaction. Gallium scintigraphy may be highly specific for demonstrating the presence of a soft tissue sarcoma.[83] Both procedures are recommended for initial *clinical* staging of the tumors.[2,44,45,46,117,142] The other methods (CT, MRI) may be of value for revealing the tumor's anatomy; ultrasound or angiography can also be used in selected cases.

Ultrasound studies sometimes distinguish a malignant from a benign tumor.[85] A CT scan may show the outline of a lipoma with reasonable certainty. MRI of a patient with sarcoma shows a high signal intensity with a T_1-weighted image, but chronic hematomas, a hemangioma, a well differentiated liposarcoma, or a hemorrhagic popliteal cyst produce the same image. In these cases pulsing may help delineate the extent of the mass.[143]

Although imaging tests are useful, none can with certainty determine whether the lesion is a tumor or other lesion or whether it is benign or malignant. That determination, as with bone tumors, must be made on the basis of the histological evidence, so a biopsy is always in order.

The biopsy of any soft tissue mass deserves special comment because there is a major difference between the biopsy done for bone tumors and that done for soft tissue tumors. The latter lesions often are easily accessible, particularly when superficial. Most of the principles applied are the same, except for the following. Malignant tumors of bone, in contrast to benign tumors, rarely are amenable to excisional biopsy, whereas soft tissue masses frequently can be removed in their entirety. If the soft tissue mass is obviously a benign tumor as evaluated preoperatively, and if intraoperatively its presentation includes a capsule, the surgeon usually proceeds correctly to "shell" it out. When the preoperative evidence is not so unequivocal, the surgeon still is tempted to expose the mass and, once that is done, to attempt to shell it out. Exposure of the mass then introduces a heightened risk of recurrence of the tumor should it prove to be malignant. If the tumor is relatively small and not associated with vital structures (nerves, arteries) — and therefore amenable to removal en bloc with a margin of normal tissue — excisional biopsy may be possible. If it can be done, subsequent staging of the lesion, according to the surgical procedure, allows one to avoid the inferior "intralesional" designation of the operation performed. The operation would then be either a marginal or a wide excision, depending on the rim of nontumorous tissue that is removed. The temptation (to be resisted) to "shell out" the tumor as an excisional biopsy is a procedure to be strongly discouraged if there is the slightest doubt about the malignant status of the lesion. If the lesion is small, excisional biopsy should include a margin of at least 2 cm of normal tissue, which minimizes the risk of local recurrence should the tumor prove to be malignant. There is strong evidence that local recurrence of soft tissue sarcomas greatly increases the potential for metastasis.[37,38,44,94]

When an intralesional or marginal excision of a mass has been done, and the lesion is diagnosed as a sarcoma, the surgeon faces a dilemma. Should there be a wider excision of the site, should radiation therapy be applied, or should both be done? None of the three options is completely satisfactory because the surgical exercise probably has disseminated tumor cells along the tissue planes of the compartment(s) containing the tumor, and dissemination of tumor cells into the circulation by the manipulation of the tumor may also have occurred. If radiation is prescribed, should it be a high dose targeted at the entire surgical field? Should the lungs be irradiated on the grounds of prophylaxis against tumor cells released into the circulation? Would any one of the three options be more applicable if the tumor is low grade than if the tumor is of high grade? Probably the best choice would be a secondary, wider excision of the tumor if it is a low grade lesion and the excision was intralesional or marginal. That choice also might be worthwhile if the tumor was of high grade and the excision was intralesional. Local irradiation would possibly be best if the lesion is high grade and the excision was either marginal or wide.[140,141]

Incisional biopsy of larger or deeper tumor masses is the procedure of choice, particularly if it appears on imaging studies that the mass is not resectable. The tumor may then be shrunk by either irradiation or selective embolization of its arterial supply, thereby rendering it resectable.

As with bone tumors, placement of the biopsy incision is an important consideration, especially as it affects the potential option of a limb-sparing procedure. Soft tissue sarcomas in the limbs tend to occupy either one or two compartments. Excision of the tumor-bearing muscle compartment(s) often is readily accomplished, and then the limb can be preserved. When the bone is involved, this potential to spare the limb is greatly reduced. An amputation then should be done that includes the bone and all of the muscles surrounding the tumor.

The staging of soft tissue tumors differs somewhat from that of bone.[2,43,44,117,142] Stage 3 (i.e., involvement of lymph nodes) is included in the scheme for soft tissue tumors, whereas it rarely applies to bone tumors. Approximately 8 percent of soft tissue sarcomas spread to lymph nodes, so a lymphangiogram is indicated when regional lymph nodes are enlarged or demonstrably involved. At times a lymph node dissection is part of the tumor surgery.

The treatment of choice of any resectable soft tissue sarcoma is radical excision. Conservative surgery has a place in protocols that combine radiation therapy either pre- or postoperatively, or

both, with less radical excisional procedures.[142] The outcome of treatment of low grade tumors is usually excellent, but tumors such as malignant histiocytic fibromas may recur or progress to a more malignant form. Moreover, some benign tumors such as myxoid lipomas, pleomorphic lipomas, and angiolipomas have a propensity for local recurrence or recrudescence. It is well known that a neurofibroma as part of neurofibromatosis may become a neurogenic sarcoma.

The prognosis of soft tissue sarcoma varies with the type of tumor and grade of malignancy. In terms of long-term survival, the latter appears to be a more significant factor than the size or the location of the tumor.

REFERENCES

1. Ayala AG, Murray JA, Erling MA, Raymond AK: Osteoid-osteoma: intraoperative tetracycline-fluorescence demonstration of the nidus. J Bone Joint Surg [Am] 68:747, 1986
2. Beahrs O, Myers MH (eds): Musculoskeletal sites. p. 107. Soft tissues. p. 111. In: Manual for Staging of Cancer. 2nd Ed. JB Lippincott, Philadelphia, 1983
3. Bertoni F: Desmoplastic fibroma of bone. J Bone Joint Surg [Br] 66:265, 1984
3a. Bilos ZJ, Hui PWT: Dorsal dislocation of lunate with carpal collapse. J Bone Joint Surg [Am] 63:1484, 1981
4. Blake DD: Radiation treatment of metastatic bone disease. Clin Orthop 73:89, 1970
5. Bloen JL, Mulder JD: Chondroblastoma: a clinical and radiological study of 104 cases. Skeletal Radiol 14:1, 1985
6. Bonakdarpour A, Levy WM, Aegerter E: Primary and secondary aneurysmal bone cyst: a radiologic study of 75 cases. Radiology 126:75, 1978
7. Bonfiglio M: Malignant Tumors Primary in Bone (Osteosarcoma, Fibrosarcoma, Malignant Giant Cell Tumor). Sixth National Cancer Conference Proceedings. JB Lippincott, Philadelphia, 1971
8. Bonfiglio M: On musculoskeletal tumors. J Iowa Med Soc January:20, 1973 (editorial)
9. Bonfiglio M, Jeter WS: Immunologic responses to bone. Clin Orthop 87:19, 1972
10. Brennhovd IO: The treatment of soft tissue sarcomas — a plea for a more urgent and aggressive approach. Acta Chir Scand 131:438, 1966

11. Brown KLB, Cruess RL: Bone cartilage transplantation in orthopaedic surgery. J Bone Joint Surg [Am] 64A:270, 1982

12. Brown KT, Kattapuram SV, Rosenthal DI: Computed tomography analysis of bone tumors: patterns of cortical destruction and soft tissue extension. Skeletal Radiol 15:448, 1986

13. Buck P, Mickelson MR, Bonfiglio M: Synovial sarcoma. Clin Orthop 156:211, 1981

14. Cade S: Osteogenic sarcoma: a study based on 131 patients. J R Coll Surg Edinb 1:79, 1955

14a. Calandruccio RA, Anderson III WE: Post-fracture avascular necrosis of the femoral head: correlation of experimental and clinical studies. Clin Orthop 152:49, 1980

14b. Campbell CJ: Aseptic necrosis of the hip as complication of disease not associated with trauma. In: Proceedings of the Conference on Aseptic Necrosis of the Femoral Head, 1964, p. 109

15. Campbell CJ: Benign Tumors of Bone. Fifth National Cancer Conference Proceedings. JB Lippincott, Philadelphia, 1965, pp. 345–358

16. Campbell CJ: Indications and Principles of Amputation for Bone Sarcoma. Sixth National Cancer Conference. JB Lippincott, Philadelphia, 1968

17. Campbell CJ: Massive resection and autogenous bone grafting: its place in the management of primary bone tumors. Kanto J Orthop 6:577, 1975

18. Campbell CJ: Orthopedic aspects of management in metastatic disease. In Horton J, Hill GJ (eds): Clinical Oncology. WB Saunders, Philadelphia, 1974

19. Campbell CJ: Osteoblastoma and osteoid osteoma. p. 177. In Evarts CM (ed): Surgery of the Musculoskeletal System. Vol. 4. 1983, Churchill Livingstone, New York, 1983

20. Campbell CJ, Akbarnia BA: Giant cell tumor of the radius treated by massive resection and tibial bone graft. J Bone Joint Surg [Am] 57:982, 1975

21. Campbell CJ, Bonfiglio M: Aggressiveness and malignancy in giant cell tumors of bone. Proc Symp Colston Res Soc 24:15, 1973

22. Campbell CJ, Cohen J, Enneking WF: New therapies for osteogenic sarcoma. J Bone Joint Surg [Am] 57:143, 1975 (editorial)

23. Capanna R, Bertoni F, Bettelli G, Picci P, et al: Dedifferentiated chondrosarcoma. J Bone Joint Surg [Am] 70:60, 1988

24. Capanna R, Springfield DS, Springfield DS, Biagini R, Ruggieri P, Giunti A: Juxtaepiphyseal aneurysmal bone cyst. Skeletal Radiol 13:21, 1985

25. Capanna R, Van Horn JR, Ayala A, Picci R, Bettelli G: Osteoid osteoma and osteoblastoma of the talus. Skeletal Radiol 15:360, 1986

26. Clark PM, Keokarn T: Popliteal aneurysm complicating benign osteocartilaginous exostosis. J Bone Joint Surg [Am] 47:1386, 1965

27. Clough JR, Price CHG: Aneurysmal bone cyst: pathogenesis and long-term results of treatment. Clin Orthop 97:52, 1973

28. Codman EA: Epiphyseal chondromatous tumors of the upper end of the humerus. Surg Gynecol Obstet 52:543, 1931

29. Cooper RR: Primary malignant tumors of bone. p. 527. In: Cancer Management. JB Lippincott, Philadelphia, 1968

30. Copeland MD, Robbins GF, Meyers MH: Development of a clinical staging system for primary malignant tumors of bone. p. 35. In: Management of Primary Bone and Soft Tissue Tumors. Year Book Medical Publishers, Chicago, 1976

31. Copeland MM: Primary malignant tumors of bone: evaluation of current diagnosis and treatment. Cancer 20:738, 1967

32. Dahlin DC: Aneurysmal bone cyst and other nonneoplastic conditions. Skeletal Radiol 8:243, 1982

33. Dahlin DC: Problems in the interpretation of results of treatment for osteosarcoma. Mayo Clin Proc 54:612, 1979 (editorial)

34. Dahlin DC, Coventry MD: Osteogenic sarcoma: a study of 600 cases. J Bone Joint Surg [Am] 49:101, 1967

34a. El Khoury GY, Bonfiglio M: Case report 60: Chondrosarcoma occurring in a patient with multiple herditary exostoses. Skeletal Radiol 3:49, 1978

35. D'Aubigne RM, Meary R, Thornine JM: La Resection dans le traitment des tumeurs des os. Rev Chir Orthop 52:303, 1966

36. Enneking WF: Issue of the biopsy. J Bone Joint Surg [Am] 64:119, 1982 (editorial)

37. Enneking WF: Local resection of malignant lesions of the hip and pelvis. J Bone Joint Surg [Am] 48:991, 1966

38. Enneking WF: Musculoskeletal Tumor Surgery. Churchill Livingstone, New York, 1983, p. 31

39. Enneking WF: Staging of musculoskeletal neoplasms. Skeletal Radiol 13:183, 1985

40. Enneking WF, Chiew FS, Springfield DS, et al: The role of radionucleide bone scanning in determining the resectability of soft tissue sarcomas. J Bone Joint Surg [Am] 63:249, 1981

41. Enneking WF, Eady JL, Burchardt H: Autogenous cortical bone grafts in the reconstruction of segmental skeletal defects. J Bone Joint Surg [Am] 62:1039, 1980

42. Enneking WF, Spanier SS, Goodman MA: A system for surgical staging of musculoskeletal sarcoma. Clin Orthop 153:106, 1980

43. Enneking WF, Spanier SS, Goodman MA: The surgical staging of musculoskeletal sarcoma. J Bone Joint Surg [Am] 62:1027, 1980

44. Enneking WF, Spanier SS, Malawer MD: The effect of anatomic setting on the results of surgical procedures for soft parts sarcoma of the thigh. Cancer 47:1005, 1981

45. Enzinger FM: Recent developments in the classification of soft-tissue sarcomas. In: Management of Primary Bone and Soft-Tissue Tumors. Year Book Medical Publishers, Chicago, 1977, p. 219

46. Enzinger FM, Lattes R, Torloni H: Histological Typing of Soft Tissue Tumors. International Classification of Tumors No. 3. World Health Organization, Geneva, 1969

47. Evans JL, Ayala AB, Romsdehl MM: Prognostic factors in chondrosarcoma of bone: a clinicopathologic analysis with emphasis on histologic grading. Cancer 40:818, 1977

48. Farrandes PA, Perkins A, Sully L, et al: Localization of human osteosarcoma by antitumor, monoclonal antibody. J Bone Joint Surg [Br] 65:638, 1983

49. Feldman F, Casarella WJ, Dick HM, Hollander BA: Selective intraarterial embolization of bone tumors. Am J Radiol 123:130, 1975

50. Finn HA, Simon MA, Martin WB, Darakjian H: Scintigraphy with gallium-67 citrate in staging of soft-tissue sarcoma of the extremity. J Bone Joint Surg [Am] 69:886, 1987

51. Fitzgerald Jr RH, Berquist TH: Magnetic resonance imaging. J Bone Joint Surg [Am] 68:799, 1986 (editorial)

52. Foss OP, Brennhovd IO, Messett OT, Erskind J, Liverud K: Invasion of tumor cells into the blood stream caused by palpation or biopsy of the tumor. Surgery 59:691, 1966

53. Francis KC: Massive preoperative irradiation in the treatment of osteogenic sarcoma. Prog Clin Cancer 1:774, 1965

54. Francis KC: The role of amputation in the treatment of metastatic bone cancer. Clin Orthop 73:61, 1970

55. Frei III E, Jaffe N, Gero M, Skipper H, Watts H: Adjuvant chemotherapy of osteogenic sarcoma, progress and perspective. J Natl Cancer Inst 60:3, 1978 (guest editorial)

56. Galasko CS: Mechanisms of lytic and blastic metastatic disease of bone. Clin Orthop 169:20, 1982

57. Galasko CSB: Skeletal Metastases. Butterworth, London, 1986

58. Ghelman B, Thompson FM, Arnold WD: Intraoperative localization of an osteoid osteoma. J Bone Joint Surg [Am] 63:826, 1981

59. Gilmore Jr WS, Kilgore W, Smith H: Central cartilage tumors of bone. Clin Orthop 26:81, 1963

60. Goidanich IF: I Tumori Primitive dell Osso. Soc. per Azioni, Poligrafica II Resto del Carlino, Bologna, 1957

61. Goldberg VM, Howell A, Shaffer JW, et al: Bone grafting: role of histocompatibility in transplantation. J Orthop Res 3:389, 1985

62. Goldenberg RR, Campbell CJ, Bonfiglio M: Giant cell tumor of bone: an analysis of 218 cases. J Bone Joint Surg [Am] 42:619, 1970

63. Harcke HT, Conway JJ, Tachdjan MD, Dias LS, Nobel HB, et al: Scintigraphic localization of bone lesions during surgery. Skeletal Radiol 13:211, 1985

64. Harrington KD, Sim FH, Enis JE, et al: Methylmethacrylate as an adjunct in the internal fixation of pathological fractures. J Bone Joint Surg [Am] 58:1047, 1976

65. Hatcher CH: The diagnosis of bone sarcoma. Rocky Mountain Med Journal, November 1948

66. Hatcher CH: Treatment of Bone Sarcoma. Rocky Mt Med J November 1948

67. Hatcher H, Campbell C: Benign chondroblastoma of bone. Bull Hosp Joint Dis 12:411, 1951

68. Heiple KG, Chase SW, Herndon CH: A comparative study of the healing process following different types of bone transplantation. J Bone Joint Surg 45:1593, 1963

69. Hemmingway AP, Allison DJ: Complications of embolization: analysis of 410 procedures. Radiology 166:669, 1988

70. Holmes EC, Eilber FR, Morton DL: Immunotherapy of malignancy in humans. JAMA 232:1052, 1975

71. Hudson TM, Bertoni F, Enneking WF: Scintigraphy of aggressive fibromatosis. Skeletal Radiol 13:26, 1986

72. Hudson TM, Schakel M 2nd, Springfield DS, Spanier SS, Enneking WF: The comparative value of bone scintigraphy and computed tomography in determining bone involvement by soft-tissue sarcomas. J Bone Joint Surg [Am] 66:1400, 1984

73. Hudson TM, Schliber M, Springfield DS, et al: Radiologic imaging of osteosarcoma: role in planning surgical treatment. Skeletal Radiol 10:137, 1982

74. Jaffe HL: A benign osteoblastic tumor composed of osteoid and atypical bone. Arch Surg 31:709, 1935

75. Jaffe HL: Tumors and Tumorous Conditions of the Bones and Joints. Lea & Febiger, Philadelphia, 1958, pp. 164–166

76. Jaffe HL, Lichtenstein L: Benign chondroblastoma of bone. Am J Pathol 18:989, 1942

77. Jaffe HL, Lichtenstein L: Chondromyxoid fibroma

of bone: distinctive benign tumor likely to be mistaken especially for chondrosarcoma. Arch Pathol 45:541, 1948

78. Jaffe HL, Lichtenstein L, Portis RB: Giant tumor of bone: its pathologic appearance, grading, supposed variants and treatment. Arch Pathol 30:993, 1940

79. Jaffe HL, Mayer L: An osteoblastic osteoid tissue forming tumor. Arch Surg 24:550, 1932

80. Jaffe N, Traggis D, Cassady JR, et al: Multidisciplinary treatment of macrometastatic osteogenic sarcoma. Br Med J 2:1039, 1976

81. Johnson RJ, Bonfiglio M, Cooper RR: Osteosarcoma. Clin Orthop 78:314, 1971

82. Kettlekamp DB, Alexander AH, Dolan J: A comparison of metacarpal replacement experimental arthroplasty. J Bone Joint Surg [Am] 50:1564, 1968

83. Kirchner PT, Simon MA: Clinical value of bone and galluim scintigraphy for soft tissue sarcomas of the extremities. J Bone Joint Surg [Am] 66:319, 1984

84. Kirchner PT, Simon MA: Radioisotope evaluation of skeletal disease. J Bone Joint Surg [Am] 63:673, 1981

85. Lange TA, Austin CW, Seibert JJ, et al: Ultrasound imaging as a screening study for malignant soft-tissue tumors. J Bone Joint Surg [Am] 69:100, 1987

86. Lateur L, Baert AL: Localization and diagnosis of osteoid osteoma of the carpal area by angiography. Skeletal Radiol 2:75, 1977

87. Lawrence Jr W: Limb Sparing Treatment of Adult Soft Tissue Sarcomas and Osteosarcomas. Consensus Development Conference on Limb Sparing Treatment of Adult Soft Tissue Sarcomas and Osteosarcomas. Vol. 5, No. 6. National Institutes of Health, Bethesda, 1984

88. Lee ES, MacKenzie DH: Osteosarcoma: a study of the value of preoperative megavoltage radiotherapy. Br J Surg 51:252, 1964

89. Lichtenstein L: Benign osteoblastoma. Cancer 9:1044, 1956

90. Lodwick GS, Wilson AJ, Farrel C, et al: Determining growth rates of focal lesions of bone from radiographs. Radiology 134:577, 1980

91. Mankin HJ, Cantley RP, Lippiello L, Schiller AL, et al: The biology of human chondrosarcoma. I. Description of the series, grading and biochemical analysis. J Bone Joint Surg [Am] 62:160, 1980

92. Mankin HJ, Cantley RP, Schiller AL, Lippiello L: The biology of human chondrosarcoma. II. Variations in chemical composition among types and subtypes of benign and malignant cartilage tumors. J Bone Joint Surg [Am] 62:176, 1980

93. Mankin HJ, Lange T, Spanier S: The hazard of biopsy in patients with malignant primary and soft tissue tumors. J Bone Joint Surg [Am] 64:1121, 1982

94. Markhede G, Angerwall L, Stener B: A multivariate analysis of the prognosis after surgical treatment of malignant soft tissue tumors. Cancer 49:1721, 1982

95. Markhede G, Stener B: Function after removal of various hip and thigh muscles for extirpation of tumors. Acta Orthop Scand 52:373, 1981

96. Marsh BW, Bonfiglio M, Brady LP, Enneking WF: Benign osteoblastoma; range of manifestations. J Bone Joint Surg [Am] 57:1, 1975

97. McCarthy EE, Dorfman HD: Chondrosarcoma of bone with dedifferentation: a study of eighteen cases. Hum Pathol 13:36, 1982

98. McCarthy SM, Ogden JA: Epiphyseal extension of an aneurysmal bone cyst. J Pediatr Orthop 2:171, 1982

99. McKenna RJ, et al: Sarcomata of the osteogenic series. J Bone Joint Surg [Am] 48:1, 1966

100. Merryweather R, Middlemiss JH, Sanerkin NG: Malignant transformation of osteoblastoma. J Bone Joint Surg [Br] 62:381, 1980

101. Mindell ER, Shah NK, Webster JH: Postradiation sarcoma of bone and soft tissues: symposium on tumors of the musculoskeletal system. Orthop Clin North Am 8:821, 1977

102. Mirra JM, Gold R, Downs J, Eckardt JJ: A new histologic approach to the differentiation of enchondroma and chondrosarcoma of the bones. Clin Orthop 201:214, 1985

103. Mnaymneh WA, Dudley HR, Mnaymneh LG: Giant cell tumor of bone. J Bone Joint Surg [Am] 46:63, 1964

104. Morton DL: Tumor doubling time. Ann Surg 178:360, 1973

105. Murphy WA, Strecker EB, Schoenecker PL: Transcatheter embolization therapy of an ischial aneurysmal bone cyst. J Bone Joint Surg [Br] 64:166, 1982

106. Murray RO, Jacobson HC: The Radiology of Skeletal Disorders. Churchill Livingstone, Edinburgh, 1971

107. Ottolenghi CE: Diagnosis of orthopaedic lesions by aspiration biopsy of the cervical spine. J Bone Joint Surg [Am] 37:443, 1965

108. Ottolenghi CE, Schajowicz F, DeSchant FA: Aspiration biopsy of the cervical spine. J Bone Joint Surg [Am] 46:715, 1964

109. Phemister DB: Cancer of the bone and joint. JAMA 136:545, 1948

110. Phemister DB: Chondrosarcoma of bone. Surg Gynecol Obstet 50:216, 1930

111. Phemister DB: Conservative surgery in the treatment of bone tumors. Surg Gynecol Obstet 70:355, 1940

112. Phemister DB: Local resection of malignant tumors of bone. Arch Surg 63:715, 1951 (editorial)

113. Phemister DB: Rapid repair of defect of femur by massive bone grafts after resection for tumors. Surg Gynecol Obstet 81:120, 1945

114. Pritchard DJ: Indications for surgical treatment of localized Ewing's sarcoma of bone. Clin Orthop 153:39, 1980

115. Pritchard DJ: Small round cell tumors. p. 247. In Evarts (ed): Surgery of the Musculoskeletal System. Vol. 4. Churchill Livingstone, New York, 1983

116. Russell WO, Cohen J, Enzinger FM, et al: A clinical and pathological staging system for soft tissue sarcomas. Cancer 40:1562, 1977

117. Sanerkin NG, Woods CG: Fibrosarcomata and malignant fibrous histiocytoma arising in relation to enchondromata. J Bone Joint Surg [Br] 61:366, 1979

118. Schajowicz F: Aneurysmal bone cyst (multilocular hematic bone cyst). p. 424. In: Tumors and Tumor-Like Lesions of Bone. Springer-Verlag, New York, 1981

119. Schajowicz F, Ackerman LV, Sissons HA: Histological Typing of Bone Tumours. International Histological Classification of Tumours No. 6. WHO, Geneva, 1972

120. Schocker JD, Brady LW: Radiation therapy for bone metastasis. Clin Orthop 169:38, 1982

121. Schwartz HS, Zimmerman NB, Simon MA, et al: The malignant potential of enchondromatosis. J Bone Joint Surg [Am] 69:269, 1987

122. Sherman M: Giant cell tumor of bone. In: Tumors of Bone and Soft Tissue (Eighth Annual Clinical Conference on Cancer, University of Texas, 1963). Year Book Medical Publishers, Chicago, 1965

123. Sherman M: Osteoid osteoma associated with changes in adjacent joint. J Bone Joint Surg 29:483, 1947

124. Sherman M: Osteoid osteoma — review of literature and 30 case reports. J Bone Joint Surg [Am] 29:483, 1947

125. Sherman MS: Cartilaginous Tumors of Bone. AAOS Instructional Course Lectures. Vol. 12, 1955, p. 233

126. Sherman MS: Histogenesis of bone tumors. p. 15. In: Tumors of Bone and Soft Tissue. Year Book Medical Publishers, Chicago, 1965

127. Sherry HS, Levy RN, Siffert RS: Metastatic disease of bone in orthopaedic surgery. Clin Orthop 169:44, 1982

128. Sim FH, Pritchard DJ: Metastatic disease in the upper extremity. Clin Orthop 169:83, 1982

129. Simon MA: Biopsy of musculoskeletal tumors, current concepts review. J Bone Joint Surg [Am] 64:1253, 1982

130. Simon MA: Causes of increased survival of patients with osteosarcoma: current controversies. J Bone Joint Surg [Am] 66:306, 1984

131. Simon MA: Limb salvage for osteosarcoma. J Bone Joint Surg [Am] 70:307, 1988

132. Simon MA, Kavluk MB: Skeletal metastases of unknown origin. Clin Orthop 166:96, 1982

133. Slowick FA, Campbell CJ, Kettelkamp DB: Aneurysmal bone cysts: an analysis of 13 cases. J Bone Joint Surg [Am] 50:1142, 1968

134. Solomon L: Hereditary multiple exostosis. J Bone Joint Surg [Br] 45:292, 1963

135. Souhami RL, Craft AW: Annotation: progress in management of malignant bone tumors. J Bone Joint Surg [Br] 70:345, 1988

136. Spanier SS, Enneking WF, Enriquez P: Primary malignant fibrous histiocytoma of bone. Cancer 36:2084, 1975

137. Stener B, Stener J: Malignant tumors of the soft tissues of the thigh. Acta Chir Scand 115:457, 1958

138. Stoll BA, Parbhoo S: Bone Metastasis Monitoring and Treatment. Raven Press, New York, 1983

139. Stout AP, Lattes R: Tumors of the Soft Tissues. Armed Forces Institute of Pathology, Washington, DC, 1966

140. Suit HD, Russell WO, Mankin R: Management of patients with sarcoma of the soft tissue in an extremity. Cancer 31:1247, 1973

141. Suit HD, Russell WO, Martin RG: Sarcoma of soft tissue: clinical and histopathologic parameters and response to treatment. Cancer 35:1478, 1975

142. Suit HG, Mankin HJ, Schiller AL, et al: Staging systems for sarcoma of soft tissue and sarcoma of bone. In: Cancer Treatment Symposia, Vol. 3, 1985, p. 29

143. Sundaram M, McGuire MH, Herbold DR, et al: High signal intensity soft tissue masses on T_1 weighted pulsing sequences. Skeletal Radiol 16:30, 1987

144. Sundaram M, McGuire MH, Herbold DR: Magnetic resonance imaging of osteosarcoma. Skeletal Radiol 16:23, 1987

145. Sundaram M, McGuire MH, Herbold DR, et al: Magnetic resonance imaging in planning limb sal-

vage surgery for primary malignant tumors of bone. J Bone Joint Surg [Am] 68:809, 1986

146. Sweet DL, Mass DP, Simon MA, Shapiro CM: Histiocytic lymphoma (reticulum cell sarcoma) of bone: current strategy for orthopaedic surgeons). J Bone Joint Surg [Am] 63:79, 1981

147. Sweetnam DR, Ross K: Surgical treatment of pulmonary metastases from primary tumors of bone. J Bone Joint Surg [Br] 49:74, 1967

148. Sweetnam R, Knoweldon J, Seddon H: Bone sarcoma: treatment by irradiation, amputation or a combination of the two. Br Med J 2:363, 1971

149. Taylor WF, Ivins JC, Dahlin DC, et al: Trends and variability in survival from osteosarcoma. Mayo Clin Proc 53:695, 1978

150. The Netherlands Committee on Bone Tumors: Radiologic Atlas of Bone Tumors. Vols. 1 and 2. Williams & Wilkins, Baltimore, 1966 (Vol. 1) and 1973 (Vol. 2)

151. Uyttendaele D, DeSchryver A, Claessens H, et al: Limb conservation in primary bone tumors by resection, extracorporeal irradiation, and re-implantation. J Bone Joint Surg [Br] 70:348, 1988

152. VanRijssel TG: Progression in bone tumors. Proc Symp Colston Res Soc 24:88, 1973

153. Weiland AJ: Vascularized free bone transplants. J Bone Joint Surg [Am] 63:166, 1981

154. Welsh RA, Meyer AT: A histogenetic study of chondroblastoma. Cancer 17:578, 1964

155. Williams RR, Dahlin DC, Ghormley PK: Giant cell tumor of bone. Cancer 7:764, 1954

156. Wilson PD, Lance EM: Surgical reconstruction of the skeleton following segmental resection for bone tumors. J Bone Joint Surg [Am] 47:1629, 1965

157. Yaghmi I, Zia A, Shariat S, Afshari R: Value of arteriography in diagnosis of benign and malignant bone lesions. Cancer 27:1134, 1971

10

Surgical Process

Many surgeons view their operating skills as the supreme expression of the art of medicine. Too often the mechanics of the performance, the development of new apparatus, and extension of the application of operating to more and more situations takes so major a part in their thinking that the pathophysiology of the tissue on which they operate, normal or lesional, is virtually ignored. The price, all too often, is a failed operation. When that occurs, the surgeon may well seek extenuating circumstances, e.g., the serious condition of the patient. Only rarely is the possibility considered that one or more facets of the surgical process put too-heavy reliance on the tissues' potential for repair. In other words, there was too little knowledge of pathophysiology.

All surgery involves, to some extent, injury to normal tissue and as a result all of the fundamental sequences that were described in the chapters on inflammation and injury: on the one hand, necrosis, hemorrhage, exudation, thrombosis, and the cellular changes of inflammation; on the other hand, cleanup of the individual part and healing by scar. Added to these processes may be reactions to a variety of foreign materials—sutures, hardware, even prostheses. Because the operated tissues' cumulative reactions during the immediate postoperative period constitute a summation of several influences, no one of which can be isolated from the others as it affects the end result, it usually is impossible to detect the real villain in the play when it ends in tragedy. Nevertheless, the cast of characters can be portrayed individually as they play out their parts in the surgical process, and important inferences may be drawn from their characteristics.

NECROSIS

No surgical procedure can be done without killing some cells. Even the sharpest scalpel leaves a thin layer of dead cells on either side of it as it cuts through tissue, and usually a cautery knife leaves a zone of necrosis that is wider, unless the scalpel blade is so dull as to lacerate rather than cut. It follows therefore that the more extensive the dissection, the more the necrosis. Special criticism falls on the surgeon who in orderly, even obsessive routine lays extensive tissue planes wide open on the pretext of achieving good exposure of the operative site or for ensuring the safety of nerves and vessels. Whether done by sharp or blunt dissection, necrosis of most of the tissue so devascularized is inevitable, all to satisfy the surgeon's desire to display the anatomy. The opposite extreme is to make as small an incision as possible. The pretext here is to minimize the scar or to lay open as small an expanse of any tissue plane as possible. However, this action also may lead to necrosis, this time because such forceful retraction is necessary that a massive thickness of tissue underneath the retractors can well undergo pressure necrosis (Fig. 10-1). When the surgeon plans an operation (see below) and when it is carried out, necrosis should be kept to a minimum. The amount of necrosis, whether by scalpel, retraction, osteotome, or even just pro-

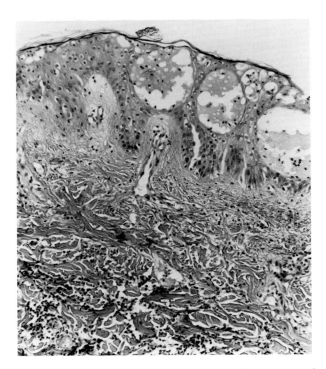

Fig. 10-1. Microskin crush at 7 days. Note the necrosis of the epidermis and the inflammatory exudate in the dermis.

stages, resorption of extravasated blood may be rapid. Because of diapedesis the red blood cells return intact to the circulation; but after a few days in the tissues, these cells become part of a hematoma and are lysed by enzymatic degradation of their walls. The precepts the surgeon follows to minimize hemorrhage are well known: ligation of vessels prior to cutting them, coagulation of bleeding points, and prophylactic use of a tourniquet when indicated.

Postoperatively, minimizing the trauma that might disrupt fragile vessels and initiate recurrence or even cyclic hemorrhage is good practice. Also well known are the measures taken to minimize accumulation of hematoma: minimizing "deadspace" when operations require removal of large amounts of tissue or repositioning large volumes of muscle or other tissue; striving for complete hemostasis before closure of the operative sites; drainage by continuous suction if necessary when deadspace exists that may have been unavoidable; suction applied to structures (e.g., cut surfaces of cancellous bone) from which seepage of blood is to be expected and surgical hemostasis is therefore impossible; and finally, postoperative pressure dressings.

longed exposure to drying, can make the difference between success and failure.

HEMORRHAGE

Much of what has just been described as relating to necrosis pertains to hemorrhage. If there is a copious volume of hematoma remaining in the operative site when the operation is finished, some necrosis not only of hematoma but of adjacent tissue inevitably results. The time it takes for absorption of the hematoma, depending inter alia on its anatomical distribution and the blood flow through the part, may be a week or two, but in many cases resorption may not be complete even after a few months.

Chronicity in the resorptive process is always productive of scarring, and the resulting process, as it concerns hematoma in its latest stages, is identical to that relating to necrotic tissue. In the acute

EXUDATION

Exudation was referred to in the description of inflammation (see Ch. 2) but requires more elaborate consideration regarding the two roles it plays in the surgical process. One role is as a diffuse accumulation of fluid in tissues or as the main component of the fluid emitted from the operative wound when it weeps. The second role of exudation we call "extrinsic" to reflect the idea that there is or may be an avenue for egress or tracking of the fluid and that when the fluid collects, as in a deadspace, it is pocketed as a unit, demarcated from the tissues. The fluid, serum, can clot or remain syrupy or viscous; and when it dries on the skin or the epithelialized healing wound, it forms the well known scab under which epithelium must creep as the wound heals. The first effect of an exudate in the surgical process is to swell the tissue, separating whatever cells and extracellular materials composed the involved tissues.

With extrinsic exudation, obviously the volume exuded depends largely on the cumulative surgical trauma inflicted on the several tissues directly handled in the operation. All of them weep exudate into the wound, and the amount may well conform to the formula intensity × area. The intensity refers to the severity of the trauma, i.e., the spectrum from a clean incision and delicacy of manipulation to any more vigorous measures (rough wiping, strong retraction) that lead to a thick zone of necrosis. Because the necrotic tissue, in which the capillaries, venules, and lymphatics presumably are thrombosed, does not form exudate, it is the immediately adjacent tissue that does so. However, the very presence of the necrosis allows that tissue to exude fluid for a protracted period. Hence the severity of the trauma directly affects the amount of exudate per unit area. That unit refers to the surface area of all tissues (be they bone, fascia, ligaments, fat) that have been exposed during the operation.

An ideal surgical procedure minimizes not only the severity of the trauma but also the area exposed. Inevitably, some exudate forms, but many of the measures mentioned above that minimize the accumulation of hematoma also tend to have the same effect on exudate. Two of them may not, however. One is the process of achieving hemostasis prior to closure of the wound. When a coagulating device is used to excess, or when the wound is allowed to dry out while meticulous (and perhaps delicate) attention is being paid to minute bleeding points, the result is more exudate, even though there is less hematoma. Another procedure that may limit hemorrhage but increase exudation is too-prolonged tourniquet application.

The second effect of exudation, that which occurs into tissues and for which drainage is not feasible, also follows the formula of intensity × area, but here the area factor is more properly a volume factor; i.e., the tissue affected is not merely the viable surface of the operative wound but tissue to a depth exceeding the dimensions of the necrotic surface layer. Often the depth is several millimeters. This exudate-laden tissue is invaded by inflammatory cells during the early postoperative hours and days; needless to say, the wider the zone affected and the more severe the inflammation, the longer it takes for the edges of the wound in its depths to heal.

One additional factor in this "intrinsic" exudation must be borne in mind, and that is systemic influences. The predilection of malnourished patients to postoperative complications has attracted some attention, and it deserves mention not only because, for elective procedures, prophylaxis is obviously mandatory but also because even for nonelective (or urgent or emergency) surgery diagnosis and treatment of the concomitant deficiencies with perioperative and postoperative attention to the condition are beneficial. The subject pertains to the discussion of exudation because the principal culprit generating the complication is hypoproteinemia, which plays a crucial role in the regulation of interstitial fluid formation and resorption. Hypoproteinemia deserves emphasis here because of its pathophysiology and because during the care of all surgical patients, particularly those who have to be hospitalized for months (e.g., patients with multiple injuries or multiple reconstructive operations) as well as those whose malnutrition is not directly related to their orthopedic problem the monitoring of blood proteins is essential.

The outstanding local consequence of intrinsic exudation as it affects the repair process in soft tissues is retardation of healing. The exudate must be resorbed before the fibroblasts can lay their collagen fibers across discontinuities in the tissue. Another consequence is that intrinsic exudate serves as an obstacle to resorption of extrinsic exudate, if it exists, just as necrotic tissue acts as an obstacle. A third consequence is that the exudate serves as a bed in which fibroblasts develop and accumulate, so that when intrinsic exudate persists more than a few days scarring is more profuse than would have been the case if the involved tissue had not accumulated the exudate. A good example of this phenomenon is a chronic ulcer that often develops in patients with varicose veins. Its border is swollen and progressively scarred, so that often healing does not occur even if the venous stasis is alleviated.

From the therapeutic point of view, intrinsic exudation is not easily targeted by a pharmacological approach. It is best alleviated by mechanical means, i.e., anything that tends to press the fluid back into circulation. The usual modalities are pressure dressings and elevation of the part. Elevation causes gravity to work to counter the venous (or capillary) pressure. As has been mentioned (see Ch. 2), intrinsic exudation in bone presents the additional hazard of depriving the surrounding marrow tissue (because the walls of cancellous spaces are rigid) of the small communications between them; necrosis is the result.

Extrinsic exudation in mild or moderate amount is an inevitable consequence of any operation. Any incision creates a discontinuity of tissues, and inevitably it is occupied by exudate (and some hematoma as well). The surgeon who minimizes the volume of the discontinuity gives the patient optimal conditions for healing. It is done by suturing across the discontinuity, opposing layers of tissue that are to be reconstituted mechanically. However, such suturing is not without its hazards, so that attention exclusively paid to minimizing deadspace may not be entirely beneficial—perhaps quite the opposite. Sutures placed under great tension cause necrosis of all the tissues they strangulate; in addition, they add foreign material that in itself may inflame the tissue. The surgical art, in this situation, consists in avoiding as far as possible the negative influences and using, also as far as possible, the positive ones. When the tissues at the depths of the wound cannot be apposed without suturing the tissue under great tensile force, the surgeon should know just how far to stretch the tissues and the minimum number of sutures that will minimize the deadspace. To promote removal of the extrinsic exudate (and hematoma) in that cavity the surgeon should know how to use drains and suction.

To conclude the consideration of exudation, two examples can briefly illustrate the two ends of the spectrum of the surgical process. One is the linear crust that forms on the incised wound within minutes of suturing. As the exudate dries and as the thin layer of necrotic tissue (plus necrotic hematoma and clotted serum) stimulate the adjacent viable tissue to initiate the process of resorption (as described in Chapter 2), the viable tissue is protected by the shell of dry exudate. Under that shell, at its periphery, the epithelial cells multiply and edge under the scab. When the crust does not change much from day to day, except to become somewhat harder, darker and contracted, it serves a positive function—protection of the wound, which underneath is elaborating the scar (which will heal the depths of the wound), and the epithelial edges (which will seal it over). If the crust shows any tendency to become soupy, however, even in focal areas (e.g., at a suture), or when the wound edges on either side of the crust become swollen or inflamed, those changes signify that exudation is continuing. The scab, even though it was protective at first, may now be serving as a culture medium for bacteria. Removal of the crust then serves not only to minimize the volume of culture medium but also to allow drainage of the newly formed fluid exudate. Removal of sutures around an area where pus has formed (microabscesses) serves the same purpose. Proper handling of such an infected incision may involve removal of crust and exudate at least daily.

The other end of the spectrum is illustrated by a dehisced wound whose edges are swollen with intrinsic exudate. In the depths of such a wound there may be a considerable volume of clotted exudate, degenerating hematoma, and necrotic tissue. Perhaps in most instances such a situation could have been prevented by all of the measures mentioned. When it does occur, however, the pathophysiological basis for treatment certainly includes removal of dead tissue (as much as can be identified grossly) along with all collected hematoma and exudate, followed by progressive mechanical diminution of the deadspace. Measures should then be taken to relieve the intrinsic exudation and, finally, to encourage healthy coverage of the exposed tissue either by granulation stimulated by local pressure or by epithelium produced either at the edges or by skin graft.

INFECTION

During the surgical process, from its inception through the operative maneuvers, and then comprising all postoperative measures, one must envisage not only the inflammation that inevitably is part of the repair process but also that which occurs in more acute and extensive form when there is infection. Infection therefore should always be a preoperative consideration (i.e., prophylaxis) as well as a possible intraoperative and postoperative phenomenon. The following three situations deserve separate attention.

Preoperatively, when a patient is about to undergo an elective procedure he or she should be monitored for an infection anywhere, not just on the skin at the site of the incision or in the structure to be operated on. That infection should be cured before the operation if possible. Not only should an appropriate antibiotic be used for therapy, it also should be continued prophylactically intraoperatively and for a reasonable period of time thereafter. Pathophysiologically, this regimen is justified by the possibility that all the organisms in an infected focus may not be killed. Although the focus may seem quiescent, it may release organisms into the bloodstream under the stress of the operation, and these organisms may lodge in the operative site. The above sequence has repeatedly been implicated in late secondary infection after many operations, particularly total joint arthroplasty.

Perioperatively and intraoperatively, in addition to the usual strict asepsis, a number of adjuvant optional routines have been advocated. Although its actual prevalence is not high (as assessed in percentages), sepsis leads to the occasional catastrophe. Whether the result is prolonged morbidity but no decrease in the benefit of the operation or a variable decrease in the patient's activity level (perhaps even death), a vigorous attempt at prophylaxis becomes justified. The attempt may consist in prophylactic administration of one or another antibiotic drug given a day or two preoperatively, intraoperatively, and for some time (1 day to 1 week) postoperatively. The obvious pathophysiological rationale is to kill any bacteria that may have wandered into the wound via the air or blood. In medical centers where large numbers of operations are done, the intraoperative hazard may be diminished by any of several devices to minimize the number of bacteria that possibly could enter the operative site: laminar airflow, shielding the patient from the bacteria derived from operative personnel, and so on.

PLANNING THE OPERATION

The surgical process, as implied above, must be viewed as a continuum from operation to final follow-up. However, so much of what happens intra-operatively depends on prior planning by the surgeon that it is convenient to discuss at this point the process of planning. Let us assume that the diagnosis (be it fracture, tumor, infection) has been made. Let us assume further that the anatomical details or other relevant information has been investigated to the extent needed. As an example, there are some fractures for which the surgeon needs no further information than that provided by routine radiographs because from them the surgeon decides that the maneuver needed is a closed reduction and a plaster cast. On the other hand, there are many fractures whose details are not clearly appreciated from routine radiographs. As required, computed tomography (CT) or other modalities of diagnosis might be indicated. However, assuming that adequate diagnostic information is at hand, the obvious goal of the operation for a fracture would ordinarily be reduction and fixation of the fracture fragments.

Using the example just cited, where closed reduction would be adequate treatment, we can examine the facets of surgical treatment, including, for example, the risks of anesthesia. The essential pathophysiology for a closed procedure would not differ from that for an open reduction (without internal fixation).

The pathophysiology of the reactions of the injured tissues and of the repair process, as they affect the planning of treatment, takes priority over all other considerations if *ideal* treatment is contemplated. However, one must define what the word "ideal" means in the particular context. For any definition to be generally accepted, a number of competing concepts must be assigned their relative values and then all of them weighed in the balance. For example, with a closed fracture of the tibia, the concepts involved may be minimal risk of nonunion, earliest inception of weight-bearing and functional activities of daily living, and reasonable availability of facilities and competent personnel. The relations between each of these concepts and pathophysiology are variable. It is the surgeon's responsibility to recognize in the individual case the relative importance of each variable. They cannot be regarded as isolated elements because no one variable exists in isolation.

How the variables interact may be illustrated in the example just posed, by considering whether immediate weight-bearing (2 to 3 days post injury), perhaps in a skin-tight plaster cast, would most closely approach what would be called ideal treatment. The arguments in favor might be minimal morbidity, minimal (ordinarily zero) surgical risk, immediate compression of fracture fragments, and minimal gap between fracture fragments (if the reduction is a good one). All of these factors weigh heavily in the balance, but there are also important variables on the negative side. One is the fact that risks other than the surgical risk are introduced: Skin-tight plaster casts introduce the risks of pressure sores and circulatory deprivation. Another is the need for superb expertise in cast application, a technique that has been in decline over the last few years. The final influence is the cooperation of the patient.

Unfortunately, as treatment for fractures becomes more and more impersonal because patients become less rooted in particular localities, the surgeon may become less willing or less able to establish the close follow-up required for treatment, as with tight casts. Such reluctance may also be seen in the context of unknown "socioeconomic" influences (e.g., alcoholism, unfavorable home environment). The surgeon, juggling so many unknowns, may therefore opt for what is deemed definitive treatment, e.g., compression internal fixation. He or she chooses and accepts certain surgical risks so as to avoid others. Under those circumstances pathophysiology may, perhaps deservedly, take a back seat (note the comments on internal fixation and fracture repair in Chapter 3).

It is obviously impossible to consider every surgical procedure individually in terms of the surgical process, as planned and put into action. For fractures there are several textbooks (see Ch. 11) that describe the various operations for the numerous categories of fractures as they occur in each bone. Similar compendia of operations for orthopedic conditions other than fractures are also available; but in them, regretfully, we find usually inadequate consideration of indications and contraindications for particular procedures that might be relevant to pathophysiology.

In each of the illustrative cases that were introduced in Chapters 2 through 9 of this book, emphasis was laid on pathophysiology as an essential component of decision-making at every stage of the treatment. Nowhere is it more important than in the planning stage. Here pathophysiology enters as it should be perceived in prospect, i.e., as a probability, based on all the available data in the individual case. Those data include, as mentioned in Chapter 1, historical information, the signs and symptoms of physical findings at the time planning options are formulated in broad outline, laboratory data that have been accumulated to support diagnostic possibilities and treatment options, and so on. As new facts enter the data matrix, each has the potential of altering the probabilities of the pathophysiological perception. When the alteration is minor, it may change the pathophysiological conceptualization only to a minor degree, e.g., prolongation of the estimated duration of one of the repair processes. Sometimes there is no essential change in the planned treatment based on such an enlarged estimate. Alternatively, the alteration may be so major (e.g., appearance of signs of infection after an elective procedure or the prospect of immobilizing a major joint for several months) that the entire plan of treatment must be changed.

This principle has been discussed in the chapters on trauma, arthritis, and tumors and also as it relates to follow-up evaluation systems. In Chapter 8 we discussed planning a sequence of procedures for patients with rheumatoid arthritis affecting many joints and planning a hip operation with considerations of a prosthesis using either polymethylmethacrylate cement or a porous metal coating without cement. These examples are just a few of those previously considered that reveal how important a role pathophysiological considerations play when planning elective procedures.

Planning surgical therapy therefore should never be the mindless application of a routine chosen from a compendium of routines, as a cook chooses a recipe from a cookbook. Planning is a continuum; and at every point in time pathophysiological processes are at work, preoperatively as well as intraoperatively and postoperatively. The therapeutic modality at any moment should be designed to potentiate the positive aspects of the process—to veer it toward normal physiology and morphology while avoiding, so far as possible, the risk of worsening the condition.

BIOMECHANICS
AND BIOMATERIALS

The musculoskeletal system is the machine whose function is essential to the motion of the body as whole or of its parts. Study of that system has therefore been of interest not only to orthopedic surgeons but also to others whose primary discipline may be in mechanical engineering or material science. Our emphasis in this book is on pathophysiology; but because any machine may have a defect of a mechanical nature, it invites study of that defect from the point of view of engineers. There have been many studies of biomechanics and biomaterials pertinent to orthopedic surgery. When the defect in the musculoskeletal system is in the material from which the machine is made, it may invite study by researchers in several disciplines. For example, if a joint is defective, lubrication may be the focus of study, as may the composition of the articulating surfaces, their design, or the loading parameters, both static and dynamic.

It has become apparent that the immense fund of knowledge in these areas, which for convenience can be called biomechanics and biomaterials, has attracted the attention of firms whose interest in the practical applications of the knowledge may be subordinate to their interest in profit, even though they allege to have as their primary purpose the betterment of orthopedic treatment. Consider the interest of a surgeon who devises a technique for treatment of a condition and then applies it, regardless of proper indications, and tries to popularize it in ways that thinly disguise self-interest.

Biomechanics originally was concerned, during the presurgical era, with restoration of the normal alignment of fracture fragments or betterment of the alignment of joint, e.g., by bracing. It now has become applicable, by surgical procedures, to an ever-enlarging field of application. Special tools and devices are so strongly advocated that the surgeon may well be misled to use the tools and devices for the alleged biomechanical advantages they provide with little attention to pathophysiology.

As one example of this phenomenon, consider scoliosis. The diagnosis is usually first made when a deformity becomes apparent and hardly ever when the condition is causing pain or, worse, has decreased the patient's respiratory reserve to a low level. When either of these symptoms becomes noteworthy, usually the patient has had the curvature of the spine for many years; furthermore, the curve has become severe. Because the curvature most often starts (for reasons unknown) during childhood or adolescence and then, almost without exception, is asymptomatic, recognition of the condition, first by postural abnormalities and then radiographically, ordinarily initiates a train of treatment. It may consist in exercises, braces, or muscle stimulation. Each may be pursued for months or years, during which time the physician can ascertain the rate of progression of the curve. He or she may judge whether the degree of curvature ultimately will be great enough to justify prophylactic surgical correction and may decide on a surgical procedure before the curve is severe. "Severe" in this usage may mean that the simpler operation that is planned cannot straighten the curve to the satisfaction of the surgeon and perhaps that a more radical (therefore more risky) procedure may be "needed." The emphasis in delineating the indications therefore are biomechanical, and little attention is paid to the fact that little information is available about the correlation between the ultimate symptoms and the degree of curvature, i.e., the natural history of scoliosis of defined severity over several decades. It has been well demonstrated that *severe* curves (for this purpose they may be defined as 60° or more) do tend to cause pain when a patient becomes middle-aged, and very severe curves (e.g., over 90°) are often associated with cardiorespiratory impairment (also during middle age). However, extrapolation of this information to scoliosis curves that are substantially less severe is questionable, and little substantiation of this extrapolation has been forthcoming.

In this situation the pathophysiological basis for the symptoms can be firmly assayed by well known respiratory tests. Whether biomechanical malalignment is or is not related to pain in patients with scoliosis is difficult to prove. Yet at present this biomechanical argument not only convinces many surgeons to perform prophylactic straightening operations but often leads them to choose methods and devices with considerable risks. For them, the fact that most curves of 30° or less never become symptomatic has little importance compared to the satisfaction of getting the degree of curvature to a minimum.

It is apparent that when the emphasis is on biomechanics to the exclusion of all else, the situation described tends to channel research into more and more sophisticated aspects of scoliosis. The orthopedic surgeon in charge of planning and carrying out treatment may well be unable to thread his or her way through the research data that frequently ignore clinical data, which may be of the essence (location of curves, flexibility, rate of progression). Instead, the surgeon is exposed to static representations of computerized models, calculations of forces, and many other tools of modern physicists. The physicists or engineers attracted by the human application of their disciplines have studied whatever conditions are considered appropriate by their orthopedic colleagues. Although the information derived from studies of such topics as scoliosis may further the understanding, it has not yet affected therapy to any substantial degree.

However, the orthopedic topic that has undoubtedly attracted most attention biomechanically is total joint replacement, and in that case the information that has been and is being derived often is of immediate practical value. It should be pointed out that rarely is a biomechanical study in the field of total joint replacement integrated *prospectively* with pathophysiological considerations. Those considerations would include tissue reactions to the materials and their wear products, tissue reactions to anticipated loads, or altered dynamics. More often than not the biomechanical considerations lead to experimental trials, often done on human subjects, with inadequate prefatory use of animals to establish the nature of some of the unknown risks. Happily, this situation is changing for the better—witness the extensive experiments done on porous surface implants.

Total joint replacement as a subject for biomechanical investigation may reflect concern in regard to all aspects of the design of the device, but pathophysiological concerns are necessarily focused on the interactions of the device and the tissues against which it rests. This same focus pertains to the use of any material implanted in the body to serve a mechanical function. The material may be as complex as a massive allograft used in limb salvage tumor surgery or one as simple as a suture. In principle, any material, whether fabricated by a chemical or metallurgical process or derived from natural sources (which may include autografts as well as allografts or heterografts), when inserted in the tissues evokes some reaction in those tissues. This reaction in soft tissue can range from acute inflammation, even suppuration, to formation of a thin membrane. In bone the same spectrum of reaction exists (Fig. 10-2).

The studies on and development of biomaterials have progressed along many lines over the last century, during which time these materials have come into everyday use for the routines of surgery. The initial concern was mainly whether a suture was absorbable (catgut) or would be encased in scar (silk, cotton, steel). This concern depended largely on the frequent occurrence of infection, often associated with foreign material in a wound. Before antibiotics became available, this issue was critical. Two other issues now are the main concerns regarding implants in pathophysiology. They are, first, that the implant function properly over the period of time expected and, second, that the severity of the tissue reaction fall short of rejection. Whether the rejection phenomenon is an acute one or one that simmers over months or years, the interaction between tissue and the material(s) of the device is crucial. The act of implantation of any device whatsoever is one that, at a minimum, exposes a plane of tissue whose surface undergoes necrosis. At the least, this necrosis involves only the exposed cells; and for the implant to be "accepted," i.e., for the tissues to tolerate it, they must react by resorbing the necrotic cells (and associated matrix if the tissue is fibrous, cartilaginous, or bony). This reaction is analogous to that following a clean incision, so that the end result in soft tissue is a minimal scar.

Bone, cancellous or cortical, as has been described in Chapter 3, also develops a surface necrosis when it is traumatized. In bone, instead of scalpel incisions, the trauma is provided by a drill, saw, or osteotome. The surface that becomes necrotic is that exposed by the tool used; but the thickness of the layer of necrotic tissue, even under optimal circumstances, far exceeds that described

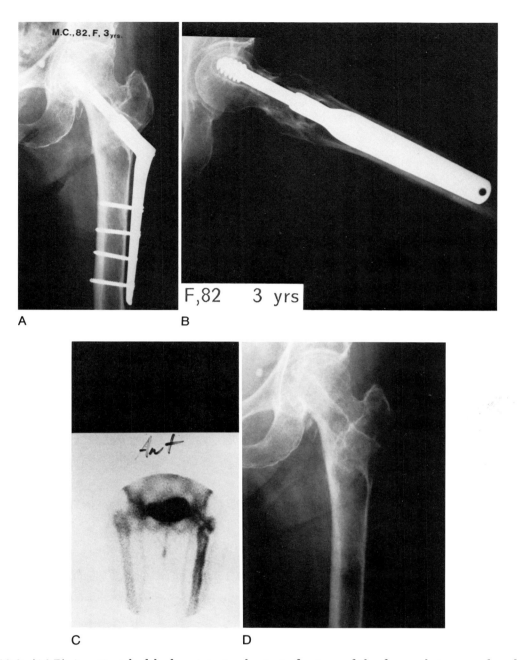

Fig. 10-2. (A&B) A patient had had an intertrochanteric fracture of the femur that was reduced and immobilized by a screw and side plate and screws. The metal of the plate and screws was steel that conformed to modern specifications. **(C&D)** An abscess developed after the fixation approach had been in situ for 3 years and the fracture had healed. Culture of the abscess yielded no bacteria. Drainage of the pus and removal of the hardware cured the abscess. One severe area of corrosion at a screw–plate junction was evident on the removed hardware. *(Figure continues.)*

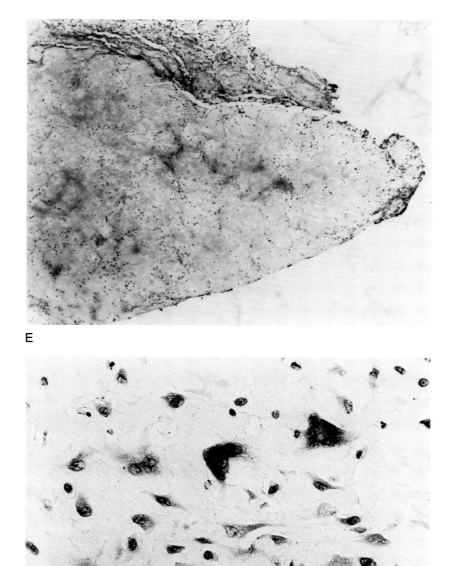

E

F

Fig. 10-2 *(Continued)*. **(E)** Granulation tissue from the wall of an abscess that was formed adjacent to a metallic fixation device (×40). **(F)** In addition to the usual inflammatory elements, rust particles are evident both extracellularly and in macrophages (×250).

for soft tissue. Nevertheless, that necrotic zone undergoes resorption; but whether a permanent thin membrane or a thicker scarred membrane develops is contingent on the character of the opposed implant and mechanical factors (e.g., cyclic motion, overloading) (Fig. 10-3).

However, in bone, to a degree more obvious than in soft tissue, the two main factors in the equation that depicts the reaction of the tissues to an implant are the chemical character of the surface of the material and the mechanical character of its motion and loading. Neither of these factors remains constant or can be studied separately.

Only one hypothetical example of the thousands of possible clinical situations in which an implant is used serves to depict the complexities of the interactions. Suppose a small long bone, e.g., a metatarsal, has suffered an oblique uncomminuted fracture that has been reduced by the orthopedic surgeon under direct vision, with one lag screw used to fix the fragments. Suppose further that the carpentry is superb, as is the surgeon's understanding of tissue reactions to surgical maneuvers. He or she has predrilled the fragments so that the self-tapping screw engages the bony substance with the precise firmness of fixation needed to supplement the fixation provided by the opposed oblique surfaces of the fracture; the drill hole was made with minimum production of bone dust (subsequently washed away from the soft tissue), and the drilling was done slowly and with saline irrigation to avoid heat necrosis. Concluding the supposed operative maneuvers, the lag screw has been inserted, cutting out just the right (and minimal) amount of cortical bone to ensure firm apposition of the threads to bony substance.

It is a temptation from the mechanical standpoint to view the bone–screw construct as if the broken item were analogous to situations and constructs of materials familiar to all — a broken wood beam, for instance. One then can devise corrections in engineering formulas for the disparate physical properties (elasticity, tensile strength) of bone versus wood, or steel, or even masonry. One can also devise methods to allow comparison of the essentially tubular bone vis-à-vis a metal or wooden pipe. One can then emerge triumphant with data, calculations, and analyses — impeccable from the point of view of the mechanical engineer — that elucidate

the many parameters and questions that apply. (How large should be the diameter of the screw? How deep its threads?)

What is missing from such a mechanical study are the pathophysiological verities, the changes that occur in the living tissues that over periods of days or weeks invalidate the mechanical parameters. In the hypothetical example above, the screw threads tightly engage cortical bone, and the bone substance immediately apposed to the metal is necrotic and does not change its properties over short periods of time. Adjacent to the necrosis, however, the cortical bone will become hyperemic and, over a period of a week or two some of its substance will be resorbed. Depending then on such factors as micromotion (with the cyclic stresses that occur, even in bones that are not bearing weight or are protected by devices such as casts) the micromotion becomes amplified, and that in itself may accelerate the resorption. The vicious cycle so initiated is impeded after 2 weeks or so by the formation of periosteal bone and the other reparative reactions in the soft tissues that restrict the micromotion. These reparative processes, when sufficient to restrict the micromotion to such a degree as to break the vicious cycle, allow the fracture to unite. The surgeon's treatment is then deemed successful.

It should be emphasized, however, that several factors, in addition to the mechanically "superb" construct, were essential to the success. They may be summarized under the phrase concerning the surgeon's "superb . . . understanding of tissue reactions to surgical maneuvers"; some have been mentioned (e.g., avoiding heat necrosis of bone during drilling), but others have not, e.g., protecting the viability of the periosteum. This single element in this situation might be the critical one regarding success or failure. If little periosteum remained, viable periosteal callus might well be delayed for so long a time that the vicious cycle of bone resorption and increased micromotion might not be impeded during the crucial time (the 2- to 5-week postoperative interval) when the stimulus to periosteal bone formation is maximal.

In the hypothetical case just described, one may justifiably dismiss tissue reactions to the metal of the screw as inconsequential. During the last few decades, the metals used for screws and other fas-

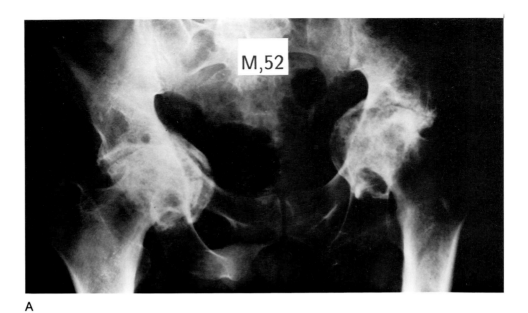

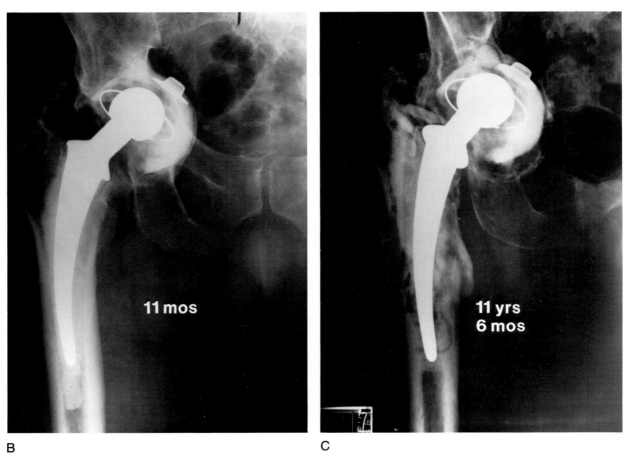

Fig. 10-3. (A) AP radiograph of the pelvis of a 52-year-old man with protrusio acetabuli and symptomatic degenerative joint disease. (B) AP radiograph of the right hip with a Charnley total hip replacement with PMMA. (C) AP radiograph of a loose total hip replacement 11.5 years later. (*Figure continues.*)

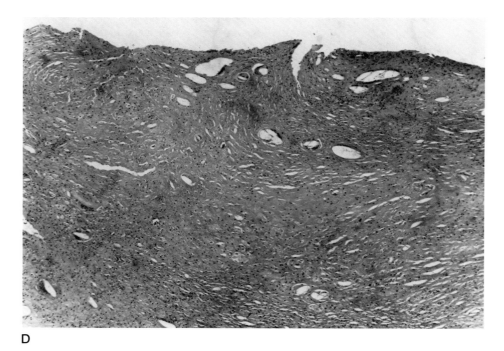

D

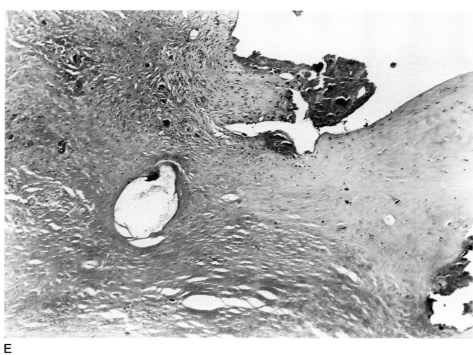

E

Fig. 10-3 *(Continued)*. **(D)** Photomicrograph of a fibrous tissue membrane removed at the time of revision of a loose total hip arthroplasty of the right hip shows embedded shards of PMMA engulfed by foreign body giant cells (×40). **(E)** Many histiocytes are in the tissue (×100).

tener devices have been improved to such a degree (in regard to their propensity to irritate tissues) that inordinate reactivity is rare. The possibility should not be dismissed, however, for several reasons.

1. Although the metal of a device may have met the generally accepted specifications prior to fabrication of the device, improper fabrication methods can alter the metal's composition, perhaps not in the main body of the device but, importantly, in spots on the surface. A burr left on the thread of the screw might be so altered as to be reactive, as can an area called a "stress-raiser." Such an area therefore is vulnerable to failure on both chemical and mechanical grounds. Obviously, these possibilities make it important for the orthopedic surgeon to make sure the devices are of optimal quality.

2. Metals used initially for fasteners that were expected to fulfill a mechanical function for relatively short periods (weeks or perhaps a few months at most) are now able to fulfill their mechanical function for many months or even many years. A slow chemical reaction on the metal's surface (and *no* metal can be shown to be completely devoid of reaction to tissue fluids) may over the weeks or months (and even years) yield negligible volumes of products (corrosion), and those products also may well be negligible in regard to reactivity with the tissue. Yet over longer periods, neither the volume nor the reactivity may be negligible. As devices are used for fractures, this danger may not be consequential: Should such a device (e.g., an intramedullary nail) prove to be irritative, it can be removed, the fracture having healed long before the irritation became evident. When the metal is part of a device that is expected to function mechanically over years, as for total joint arthroplasty, the possibility of chemical irritation must be reduced to a minimum. Not only must the metal used to fabricate the device be carefully chosen, but, as already mentioned, the fabrication maneuvers must also be such as to minimize any increase in the metal's low propensity to reaction.

As an example of how the chemical and mechanical factors interact, consider the use, now of immediate interest, of the so-called porous-surfaced prosthesis. The mechanical purpose for such surfacing is to allow ingrowth of bony substance. One method of devising the surface is by coating the device, in a desired area, with small balls of the metal that are welded by pressure to one another and to the core of the component of the prosthesis. Whether the welds chemically are not sufficiently reactive to cause trouble has not yet been proved. In some cases, at least a few balls of the metal have separated (indicating that micromotion has occurred). The resolution of this question requires years of observation of large numbers of cases.

3. The devising of metal fasteners that are more and more complex introduces situations that predispose the device to adverse reactions. Two such situations fall under the headings of *crevice corrosion* and *corrosion wear*. In the first, crevices are introduced (as when a screw attaches a plate to a bone). Minute crevices are sites of predilection for corrosion even in the best of metals. When such a crevice also is subjected to cyclic micromotion, as also occurs with a screw – plate construct, the reaction is potentiated (Fig. 10-2).

Corrosion wear is a term usually applied to the deteriorative process as it pertains to gross motion rather than micromotion. The original total joint prostheses had metal-to-metal articulations, and the wear particles produced by them soon caused the devices to fail. Relatively large volumes of wear product were produced from pure abrasion. Some corrosion also was evident that was attributable to the heightened reactions of the surface as it was being abraded. Lastly, the wear particles were shown to be more reactive than the parent metal.

Although prostheses at present are rarely if ever designed to have metal articulating with metal, some crevice corrosion and some corrosion wear occur when a metal surface articulates with any surface, including the polyethylene now in general use. It should be mentioned that some wear of the polyethylene occurs as well, and that some other chemical changes in that polymer (and other polymers that have been tried out) can be expected during the years they are to be used.

Case 10-1 A 25-year-old man had had a silicone prosthesis inserted 6 years before for a fracture of the carpal lunate followed by aseptic necrosis. During those 6 years he gradually developed an arthritis of the wrist, attributable to a foreign body reaction to silicone particles (Fig. 10-4).

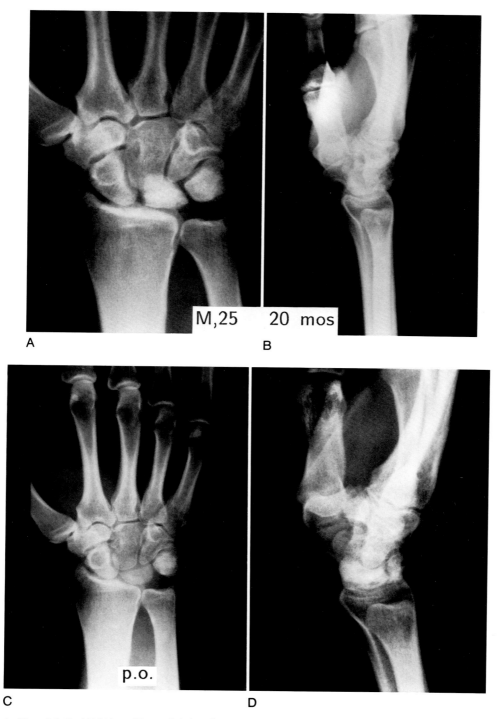

Fig. 10-4. Case 10-1. AP (**A**) and lateral (**B**) radiographs of the left wrist of a 25-year-old man who had had pain in the wrist for 20 months show aseptic necrosis of the carpal lunate with collapse. AP (**C**) and lateral (**D**) radiographs of the wrist after insertion of a silicone prosthesis. *(Figure continues.)*

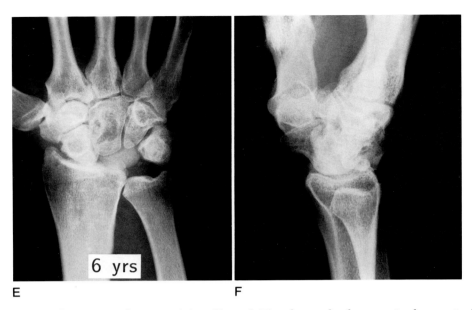

E   F

Fig. 10-4 *(Continued).* Six years later, AP (**E**) and lateral (**F**) radiographs show cystic changes in the scaphoid, capitate, and triquetrum secondary to silicone synovitis.

The surgical procedures used in orthopedic cases can be classified into several types, and often more than one type is involved in specific cases. Examples of such procedures are osteotomies for alignment; replacement of a joint, ligament, or bone; rearrangement of tendons or ligaments. They often involve biomaterials, as has been discussed.

Another type of procedure, now to be considered, is concerned with the abnormal growth of a bone (or several bones). A simple example is the group of operations designed to achieve equality of the lengths of the lower extremity. Obviously, disparity of leg lengths of important degree (perhaps 2 cm or more) is undesirable; and when it may be predicted with certainty that a child whose growth center or centers in one extremity have been damaged at an early age will have that kind of impairment when he achieves skeletal maturity, the goal of surgical treatment is to minimize the disparity.

In this type of situation, growth is an essential consideration. The surgeon must have in mind several variables, any one of which, if ignored, will render the treatment program, including the operation, less effective than it should have been. Many of those variables are concerned with quantitative predictions of linear growth; and the surgeon must be aware of uncertainties that characterize nearly any prediction. Only a few are mentioned here.

One is heredity, and perhaps race. Children of tall parents tend to be tall, but even in the same family exceptions are common so that predictions of height, and length of bones at maturity are somewhat uncertain. A second variable is time-related, possibly under hormonal control. The growth curve of a child, not only with regard to total height but also with regard to the length of a long bone, is not a steady, straight curve; rather, there are a series of growth spurts separated by periods of relative latency. Some children reach skeletal maturity at a much earlier age than others, and a prediction based on average figures is often wrong to an important degree. A third factor is nutrition, as illustrated by the fact that over the last several decades, in countries where measurements have been made (and they always have been made in affluent areas), there has been a notable increase in the average height of the population, which in the main has been attributed to better nutrition.

The type of damage that has occurred to one or more growth centers is a key factor. When a single epiphyseal center has been damaged to the extent that it can no longer contribute any growth in length to the bone involved, it may not be difficult to calculate the approximate number of centimeters of growth that will be lost in the involved extremity. The data required for the calculation are the number of centimeters per year of growth that will be contributed by the contralateral epiphysis, the age and sex of the child, and the projected age when skeletal maturity will be reached. Tables exist for these data, and once the surgeon has enough observations of the patient, e.g., over a year or two, so as to verify that (1) no growth in length is contributed by the damaged epiphysis, (2) the contralateral epiphysis is contributing x centimeters per year, and (3) skeletal maturity is not going to be either delayed or accelerated (as revealed by determinations of skeletal age from radiographs of the wrist) appropriate plans can be made. From the calculation, one can determine the amount of growth retardation that is to be incurred in the contralateral extremity for the child to have extremities of equal length at maturity. One can also factor in other considerations that affect the type of procedure that would be optimal, e.g., selection of the epiphysis that should have an epiphysiodesis and at what age. The surgeon should be able to predict, for example, if the epiphysiodesis will cause the knees to be too asymmetrical in position and if the patient will be shortened excessively.

When an epiphysiodesis is so damaged as to lose *all* potential for contributing to the length of the bone, whether the lesion is traumatic, infectious, congenital, or neurological (e.g., after poliomyelitis or other muscle-wasting diseases), one's options for treatment include the low risk epiphysiodesis. However, when contraindications exist, the higher-risk operation of lengthening the affected bone may be appropriate; or in cases of extreme discrepancy, both operations may be appropriate.

However, in most cases the epiphysis that is affected is not so greatly damaged as to lose all potential for growth. When the damage is asymmetrical, the growth will be asymmetrical, so there will be progressive deformity as well as retardation, and in such cases prevention of deformity may outweigh the achievement of equal length of the extremities. This situation is commonly seen when a fracture occurs in a child and the involved epiphy-

sis is traumatized primarily on one side. Even when good reduction of the fragments is obtained or when there is little or no displacement, but the damage has been severe, the pathophysiology of the repair process may be such as to compromise growth. When scar tissue forms at the site of the fracture just peripheral to the epiphysis and in the gap between fracture fragments, it constitutes an important impediment to the growth of the injured side of the epiphysis. The uninjured side grows, however, either normally or with only slight retardation, and a progressive deformity is the result. Obviously, one cannot wait for months or years to accumulate longitudinal data on growth because in the interval the scar would become denser and more restrictive. Prophylactically, soon after the injury the growth of the affected side of the epiphysis, if any potential of growth remains, must be allowed to proceed if possible. It may be done by preventing scar from developing in the spot where it can inhibit growth, i.e., where it will bond the bony epiphysis to the diaphysis. Langenskiold devised an operation wherein an autogenous fat graft is inserted at the appropriate spot; others have used different biomaterials for the same purpose.

Although there are many pediatric orthopedic conditions for which the factor of growth plays an important or even primary role in the rationale of treatment (e.g., clubfoot, scoliosis), the above discussion on the importance of the pathophysiology of skeletal growth must suffice. It must be emphasized, however, that any treatment of pediatric orthopedic lesions may involve possible complications caused by a disturbance in growth. Even when epiphyses are not involved, any inflammatory condition adjacent to an epiphysis, e.g., rheumatoid arthritis, can either accelerate the growth of that epiphysis (by enhancing its blood flow) or retard it (by forming scar).

Finally, there is one more category of surgical procedures for which the rationale of the surgical process differs from those already discussed. The difference is that in this category one aims at a functional goal for extremities that have a neuromuscular impairment. This category is biomechanical in a sense different from the one considered earlier in which one corrects the alignment of a deformed bone or joint, replaces a load-bearing structure, and so on. Here the impairment may be loss of strength in particular muscles or loss of control, as through spasticity or paralysis. This category includes many procedures performed to correct for imbalances of musculature (e.g., adductor myotomy in cerebral palsy) or for loss of certain muscular functions, (e.g., footdrop in a stroke victim or a series of tendon transfers in leprous patients whose hands have been seriously impaired by neuropathy). Tendon transfers to balance muscular forces around a joint, remove a deforming force, or provide an active motor to replace one that has been lost are examples of this set of procedures.

Because of the diversity of the conditions under consideration, no attempt is made in this chapter to illustrate or discuss further the physiology and pathophysiology of such intricate functional activities as ordinary gait, professional athletics, or other aspects of manual and other coordination, e.g., grasp or pinch. Suffice it to say that any abnormality in the neuromuscular category requires of the surgeon a reasonable appreciation of much research involving a good deal of electronic technology (e.g., studies on electromyography, nerve conduction time) and empirical clinical trials of soft tissue surgery before a decision on reasonable surgical treatment can be made.

Nevertheless, once the relevant information is assembled and the plan of the operation established, the cardinal principles of the healing process must be kept in mind. In contrast to the healing of bone, as described in Chapters 3 through 5, most of the procedures involving neuromuscular deficits and many associated with joints, in particular disabilities that now are considered the domain of sports medicine, involve the soft tissue healing process. Whether the surgeon is transferring the attachment of a tendon to a new site of insertion or rerouting a ligamentous structure with a bony attachment to restore some stability to an unstable joint, the pathophysiological objective is to have a firm scar form to anchor the transferred insertional end of connective tissue. For that to occur within a reasonable time frame, and with the knowledge that the evolution of fibrous tissue to mature sufficiently to carry the load under consideration certainly will take weeks if not months depending on the dimensions of the tissue and the load, the surgeon must not violate principles already empha-

sized: avoiding necrosis, maintaining vascularity, and so on. A small zone of necrosis in just the spot where a transferred element is designed to insert may make it impossible for a scar to join the donor tissue to the recipient site. The surgeon should envisage that critical process in the same light as he or she does a split-thickness skin graft, which under the surgeon's direct observation can be observed to "take" when the graft bed is healthy and, in contrast, can be observed to slough when any amount of hemorrhage, exudate, or necrosis intervenes between graft and bed.

Furthermore, the surgeon must have in mind pathological processes that may be at work, e.g., degeneration in the tissues undergoing surgery. Those processes may not always be obvious to the naked eye, especially in the early stages. The surgeon should be aware of sites of predilection for degeneration (e.g., intervertebral discs, menisci, shoulder cuffs) because degenerated tissues do not heal well, and an operation that depends on normal healing by scar may fail if degenerated tissues are expected to repair normally.

This chapter would be seriously deficient if no mention were made of major changes that have occurred recently and are occurring repeatedly in the tools used for operating. The introduction of some of those tools has served in a major way to emphasize technical niceties, often with a parallel deemphasis on pathophysiology. One example of this phenomenon is the development of motorized equipment that allows markedly improved precision when shaping bone. The demonstration by Japanese surgeons of ways to amplify the volume of the spinal canal in patients with spinal stenosis by forming a hinged trapdoor posteriorly, the hinge being formed by bending the vertebral laminae posteriorly, exemplifies the point. It is further illustrated by the huge armamentarium of jigs, templates, and countless accessory devices that comprise systems for inserting individual models of arthroplasty prostheses. In these examples and in several others that relate mostly to treatment of fractures, there usually is an adequate pathophysiological rationale for the procedure in question. Widening a stenotic spinal canal, replacing a joint that has been destroyed, or reducing a fracture and immobilizing the fragments are indisputably sound objectives of surgical therapy; and the use of better tools to do the job more effectively cannot be criticized. However, expertise in their use requires that the surgeon be educated in the technique. Therein lies the rub. If that education is to "pay off," the technique cannot be used sparingly; it must be applied often. The result is that indications for its use become broader and broader, often at the expense of pathophysiological principles. Each technique is advertised not only in the media (and that includes books, oral presentations at conventions, and "courses") but also in articles written by advocates who presumably have developed their skills to levels rarely to be reached by the rank and file. In those articles it is unusual to find the necessary caveats and documentation of the errors that are inevitably part of the "learning curve."

Perhaps the phenomenal rise in popularity of arthroscopy will serve to illustrate how pathophysiological principles must be accorded their essential role in therapy, especially when technical advances allow a surgeon to develop new therapeutic maneuvers. An arthroscopic technique for suturing a torn meniscus, now being tried out, is an appropriate case in point. It is well known that articular cartilage does not have the potential for healing by scar. Given a tear that involves only the body or inner edge of the meniscus, suture of such a tear presupposes that the sutures will not only restore the architecture to a functional level but will also maintain that architecture. The surgeon should be aware that over months and years of use sutures used in that way are not likely to hold. Only empirical observations can answer the question of whether they will hold for a substantial (and worthwhile) period of time. Lacking such a body of observations, a conservative surgeon would better excise the part of the meniscus that is torn. Another appropriate case in point is the applicability of power tools to smooth off a roughened, degenerated articular cartilage. Although empirical observations on the results of that technical maneuver will be the ultimate test, the pathophysiological implications of the maneuver do not bode well for its success. It is granted that it is well to remove the fronds of cartilage that are degenerated and perhaps necrotic, which roughen the surface and that over time slough into the joint. To assert that removing those fronds by a scalpel does not smooth the articular surface enough to have it function well may be a valid argument against such a procedure, but to assert that removing them with a power tool yields such a surface ignores two important pathophysiological concepts. One is that a surface composed of mostly necrotic tissue elicits an inflammatory reaction in the adjoining viable tissue, and the power-abraded but smooth surface achieved by the surgeon is, for the most part, a necrotic expanse. The second is that even if the surface is smooth it does not conform to the surface of the opposite member of the joint, and therefore it cannot function well.

CONCLUSION

Attention has been called to the many factors that enter into the surgical process. Those attracting most attention at present—the new biomaterials and the new tools in particular—should not be applied without strict attention to the older, but proved principles of pathophysiology.

REFERENCES

There are no references for this chapter because no specific details can be singled out for the many areas discussed that are worthy of emphasis by citation. The fields of tissue reaction to injury, systemic reaction to injury, biomechanics, biomaterials, total joint replacement, allografts, and reconstructive surgery—to mention just a few of the subjects in the chapter—are discussed in hundreds of articles per year in the orthopedic literature. The reader must seek out articles pertaining to his or her specific interest and is directed to the more prestigious journals for the same. Some of those journals have periodically issued accumulated indices covering several years that facilitate the retrieval of information.

11

Critical Bibliography

A critical bibliography is included here as a separate chapter because the mere listing of books and articles at the end of chapters often fails to meet the needs of the reader. Even when the text of an article or book cites a reference to a specific book with or without the page number, a limited purpose usually is served, i.e., documentation of a detail. The reader then has no guide to further reading, except in regard to that specific detail. Moreover, a voluminous bibliography usually includes so many articles that references to the most valuable books on specific subjects tend to be buried among the citations, and one is not sure whether the book cited is good for further reading on the topic at hand or it is mentioned merely to document a specific detail. General experience with bibliographic material that ranges in volume from practically zero in some articles and books to pages and pages in others has brought home to the authors the fact that a bibliography that is of practical use is rare indeed.

This bibliography is not designed to document details. It does have many other purposes, however, one of which is to emphasize that in the many books available on orthopedic surgery pathophysiology is not considered as the permeating essence of a general text, as it is in this book. When pathophysiology is an important element in a text listed in the general bibliography here it is emphasized with three or two stars. Undoubtedly many books with lower ratings are good books, but they do not emphasize pathophysiology. It was not our purpose to rate the books on other criteria.

With these reflections in mind, we thought it would be a service to the reader to provide a chapter about the current relevant orthopedic books.

We first include here reviews of a few books we think well of from the viewpoint of pathophysiology, discussed according to the chapter to which they pertain; journal articles are relegated to the ends of the individual chapters. We have drawn the boundaries around our reviews as closely as we could in order to avoid a proliferation of titles about subjects only peripheral to this book.

We went about the task by assembling from the indices of the *Journal of Bone and Joint Surgery (JBJS)* the titles of all the English-language orthopedic publications we could retrieve that were published during the decade prior to the writing of this book. More than 600 titles form the pool. We examined the catalogues of most of the publishers of books on orthopedics, noting citations of books in the articles listed in the bibliography to each chapter and in several books we are using for reference. We included in the pool only those books that were reviewed in *JBJS* during the decade referred to above and a few older books with which we were familiar.

We decided for reasons that should be obvious to omit rating many monographs, many collections of reviews, the bound volumes that record proceedings of meetings or symposia, and so on. However, they are listed in the General Bibliography, which cites the year, volume, and page where a review appeared in the *JBJS*.

The format of this chapter therefore is as follows: First is an explanation of the General Bibliography. Second, we discuss some well known general texts that are commonly used as references to the entire field. Third to be considered are those texts that serve as supplemental reading relative to some of the chapters in this book. The fourth section is the General Bibliography, and the fifth is a list of orthopedic journals and books available as serial publications. Finally there is a Selected Bibliography by special subject.

EXPLANATION OF GENERAL BIBLIOGRAPHY

The list of books in the General Bibliography is so formidable it would take years to read them all, even if it were necessary to do that. The authors of the present book have read for review, or use as references, a relatively small number on the list, selected for a variety of reasons. We did not think that we could make a useful selection of books to shorten the General Bibliography for the various purposes readers might have, so we decided that the judgments of the editors of the *Journal of Bone and Joint Surgery* should be followed. They decided which books should be reviewed. We elected not to include the other books submitted to them by publishers. They are listed by title only in the book review sections of the *Journal*. We have also omitted the older listing of any book which during the decade underwent republication as a more recent edition. It was obvious during the tabulation of books and study of reviews that the newer editions of a popular book often contained only minor revisions despite the publisher's assertions that the text was expanded and new material introduced. In contrast, many of the books listed indeed are obsolete, particularly those involving rapidly advancing technology, e.g., books on magnetic resonance imaging or arthroscopy. For practical purposes we chose to include such books in the listing; they are not rated. We do not imply thereby that they are not recommended but, rather, that they do not amplify pathophysiologic principles. The decision as to whether they are obsolete must be left to the reader.

We have rated some books in the Selected Bibliography using asterisks. This rating system measures the coverage of pathophysiology in the book. It is not a measure of value of the book in other respects. Thus an atlas of radiographs may be superb for its purpose (ribbon-matching) but the book is not rated, as would be compendia of surgical approaches, operations, and, as mentioned, symposia. Ratings for the books we have not read or with which we are not particularly familiar are based on the *Journals'* reviews, all of which we have studied. All readers recognize that reviewers vary extensively in how well they summarize a book's contents and what they find fault with or choose to praise. So on that shaky ground, our rating system may well be far from precise and for that possible weakness we take whatever blame is due.

GENERAL BOOKS ON ORTHOPEDIC SURGERY

Campbells Operative Orthopaedics, now in its seventh edition, occupies so strong a position in the libraries of orthopedic surgeons, hospitals, and orthopedic departments that it deserves first place in a discussion of general books on orthopedic surgery. Notwithstanding its special utility as a first rate guide to how all the essential and popular operations are done — and therefore its serviceability as a "night before" reference to an operation — it also provides short reviews of most orthopedic conditions. Yet the question arises as to whether it should be supplemented by other books for either of the purposes just mentioned. One recent competitor, Evarts' *Surgery of the Musculoskeletal System*, has the advantage of conveying the views of a select group of coauthors. It contrasts with Campbell's book, which relies almost exclusively on the practice as carried out in a single center (Memphis, Tennessee). One weakness of the Evarts work is that, in its present edition (the first), the several omissions and idiosyncracies noted in reviews have not been addressed, as is probable in the next edition (available soon). The Evarts and Campbell books are weakest in their portrayal of indications and contraindications for the various operations; the bulk of each of those books emphasized the "how to do it" and paid little attention to what can be done, short of operation, when there are contraindications.

Both books are targeted at orthopedic surgeons — those in practice and in training stages — although the readers of our volume may well be satisfied in their quest for specific information by consulting either book or both. The multiple volumes of each, needless to say, are not meant for sequential reading or study.

Turek's book, *Orthopaedics: Principles and Their Application*, which tries to cover the field of orthopedic operations as well as to summarize the basic sciences that relate to those operations and the conditions they serve, does not succeed nearly as well as the Campbell and Evarts books in the first regard. As to the second, the personal and often idiosyncratic views of the single author do not recommend the text to students interested in pursuing the basic sciences in orthopedics. Those subjects had better be studied in separate texts.

If the reader requires a general text in orthopedic surgery that does not emphasize the operations, Duthie and Bentley's revision of *Mercer's Orthopaedic Surgery* can meet most purposes. It can serve as a primary source for medical students or beginning trainees in orthopedic surgery, but it is too large for a read-through and contains too much material for anyone who wants a quick overview of this subject. Each chapter can serve as a good take-off for the individual interested in a specific topic in a chapter; for most students, however, the prerequisite of a medical school education may make the material too advanced for easy use.

There are a number of shorter books designed for review purposes or for general depiction of the conditions amenable to orthopedic treatment. Each has its virtues, and the following may be mentioned: Shand's text (as edited by Raney and Brashear) as well as those by Apley, Aston Adams, and Gartland. These texts are narrowly restricted regarding the depth of their materials and for that reason qualify somewhat as general texts. However, it is questionable if one who is interested in more than a "feel" for what orthopedic surgery is all about would want to own, or have available, any of these books. One can imagine a beginning nursing or medical student, or an emergency technician, reading any one of them to glean general information.

It is evident from study of the General Bibliography that authors have attempted in many ways to focus on some conceptual delineation of the diverse body of medical knowledge that is now thought of as the orthopedic domain. Authors have chosen such topics as age (e.g., the book on adult orthopedics by Cruess or the several books on pediatric orthopedics by Tachdjian, Sharrard, Rang,

et al.), a regional subject, or a technical approach (including a radiographic focus). The reader can ascertain the reviewers' opinions on the items culled and then examine those books that seem to have promise regarding his or her purposes.

INTERPRETIVE SKILLS (CHAPTER 1)

Chapter 1 is aimed primarily at orthopedic trainees and practitioners — mostly surgeons at all levels of expertise — and therefore it presupposes that the reader has completed medical school and has had some hospital training. Such an audience may well have available for reference the textbooks that each has accumulated during medical school. However infrequently reference is made to these volumes, it is probably done to refresh the memory or to verify details, not for further study. Other readers, particular those who have not gone through the courses ordinarily constituting medical school, may find the chapter somewhat frustrating. Conceivably, it may provide them with an idea of some thought processes that are elicited by a physician's recognition of a detail of observation and the inferences drawn from that detail.

Because the structural basis of this book is its emphasis on pathophysiology, one might well presume that physiology and pathology textbooks would provide all kinds of readers with the necessary background to this chapter. That these texts help is true, but only in small part. Unfortunately, experience has shown that those textbooks do not lend themselves to extending the reader's grasp of the subject contained in Chapter 1. General textbooks on pathology treat the musculoskeletal system from the point of view of the pathologist-author (whose principal duty is diagnosis of a lesion from a histologic preparation). Texts on physiology are written by physiologists, whose goal is the understanding of process, not necessarily a targeting of the process to clinical ends. Neither viewpoint is of much value to a clinician who is interested in sharpening interpretive skills. Certainly such texts do not constitute good material for studying a clinical approach in depth.

Hence a back-up bibliography for Chapter 1 requires a list of books that is extensive. More importantly than in any other chapter in the book, specific textbooks on each of the subjects that contributes to the material of the chapter cannot be cited. Any standard textbook on anatomy, can serve adequately, as can a single textbook on physical diagnosis. The medical student or practitioner has had courses in the "basic sciences," and thus most readers here are familiar with pathology or physiology books and may even have them in his or her own library. Other readers can consult the textbook list of any medical library.

That there is a need for special books for "polishing one's interpretive skills" in orthopedic surgery has been made evident in some publications (those of DeBrunner McRae, D'Ambrosia, Post, and Hoppenfeld), each of which has provided physical diagnostic routines limited to the musculoskeletal system. How one examines that system is usually not taught well in medical school courses. Each of the five texts noted adequately demonstrates how to elicit abnormal physical signs and record them. Necessarily, these texts cannot go into the minute detail pertaining to a single part of the motor system, as does Ritter and Gosling on the knee, for example. Monographs directed at single parts (hand, foot, spine) usually contain large chapters devoted to the examination of the part under study, often supplemented by anatomic data.

"Interpretive skills" includes much more than elicitation of physical findings, however, as important, even essential, as physical findings are to the diagnosis and treatment. It might be thought, then, that specific books on diagnosis are appropriate reference materials for the chapter. One expects to find in those books material on history taking as well as symptoms and signs. Consideration of laboratory aids to diagnosis also would be expected, even though one or more special books on laboratory examinations appear on any medical student's required reading list. Those books on diagnosis, however, are mostly structured on a framework of diagnoses *that have already been made,* no matter how specific or general, provisional or final, those diagnoses are. Even when they are especially devised for radiologic observations (e.g., Ferguson, Eideken and Hodes, Murray and Jacobsen), they presuppose that when the reader is using the book for reference he or she already has an idea of the diagnosis of the case in question. Of course, the same comment applies to textbooks on pathology, arthrography, arthroscopy, angiography, computed tomography, and diagnostic modalities.

As this book was being written, it became evident that, once the subject of interpretive skills was dealt with, the material given related to all the substantive subjects that followed. Unfortunately, those subjects did not appear in any logical order.

For that reason, this critical bibliography, from this point on, considers books that pertain to the subsequent chapters, in order. The reader may well choose to read the relevant parts of this bibliographic critique just before, during, or after studying each chapter.

INFECTION AND INFLAMMATION (CHAPTER 2)

The classic features of infection and inflammation are well described in the standard textbooks on pathology, not one of which pays particular attention to the musculoskeletal system as especially affected. One book (Burris) is totally devoted to a single type of orthopedic infection (posttraumatic) but is not particularly concerned with the process in general. Others are narrowly focused on infections of specific regions (e.g., hand — Carter, Connolly; hip — Eftekhar), but there is no one book that treats infections and inflammations as they affect the musculoskeletal system. As is evident when Chapter 2 is examined, the modern emphasis is on treatment of infections by antibiotic drugs, with the newer experimental approaches involving alteration (by drugs) of the inflammatory sequence; these two fields are changing so rapidly, however, that specifics had best be sought in journals rather than in books. Several textbooks on the pathology of the nontumorous affections of the musculoskeletal system address chapters to inflammation and infection. Perhaps the one most oriented to the needs of the clinician is that by Enneking. Another, that of Woods, is useful for the paramedical reader and for all those who have not taken standard courses in pathology. For residents and practitioners, however, it is inadequate. For lack of an adequate reference, those readers are directed to the texts of Lichtenstein and Jaffe, neither of which do much more than portray the material that a pathologist must process in the course of hospital service. Aegerter and Kirkpatrick, attempting to correlate those portrayals with radiographic and longitudinal study of the progress of infection and inflammation, are much more successful in portraying that group of diseases (and others too), and their text is highly recommended.

Still another book attempts to portray the pathology of inflammation (Sissons, Murray, and Kemp), and selected case histories are recounted and illustrated by radiographs and microphotographs. The portrayal of the morphologic patterns is static, however, and the book omits any attempt at the ebb and flow of physiologic processes that is the essence of the content of Chapter 2 of this book.

There are several books targeted at infections in special settings (Eftekhar — after joint replacement; Epps — as complications of operations; Carter — as they occur in the hand), and all of these books can be used if the special setting is the focus of interest rather than the nature of the infection per se. Only one book (Hughes and Fitzgerald) treats that process, but with greater emphasis on antibiotic therapy than on pathophysiology. Uhthoff has compiled a large series of essays on the subject by many authors, most of the essays addressing a subject as restricted as the use of gentamicin in the cement of joint replacements as prophylaxis against infection. (Here too it is all very well if the focus is the setting, but first the process must be understood.)

INJURY AND REPAIR: FRACTURES (CHAPTERS 3 – 5)

There is little doubt that one source of information cannot suffice for exposition of the subject of injury and repair of bone and soft tissue. The subject is too broad and too important to be encompassed in one place. The reader may want to use one general text on fractures for ready reference and others for specific details or specific methods of treatment.

At least one textbook on fractures should grace the bookshelf of most readers of this book. Our choice, which is designed mostly for reference about problems encountered daily in the emergency room, is Rockwood and Green's°° *Fractures*

in Adults (Vols. 1 and 2) and Wilkins and King's *Fractures in Children* (Vol. 3). These volumes are not for the medical student and certainly not for interested paramedical personnel, e.g., nurse practitioners, orthopedic nurses, or physical therapists. In addition to providing a ready reference about most fractures, this work meets the needs of orthopedic surgeons and other readers who want to study some specific fracture in particular in that it serves as a springboard to the periodical literature. For medical students and others in training, the chapter in Rockwood and Green's work on basic processes in the healing of fractures, tendons, and ligaments during the initial stage is recommended. After that the first four chapters become essential reading for anyone — including, for example, emergency technicians — involved in the evaluation and treatment of fractures. It includes a chapter by Harkess on principles that is filled with pearls of wisdom concerning the closed treatment of fractures by plaster immobilization or traction. Harkess provided practical suggestions as to methods and complications from those two most commonly used methods. The chapter by Gregory on open fractures also rates high praise.

For its emphasis on principles of treatment and thoughtful concern with prognosis and functional results, Blount's *Fractures in Children* is essential reading for everyone before reading any other basic text on fractures (perhaps with the exception of the book by Rockwood and Green). Blount's approach to fracture treatment, sound and conservative, is based on many decades of personal experience. The reader must go to other texts (Wilkins, Sharrard, King, Rang, Ogden) to obtain information on pediatric specifics, e.g., classification of epiphyseal fracture separations or the modern treatment of slipped femoral capital epiphysis. On the other hand, Blount's book serves well as an introduction to the subject of fractures in children even for medical students, physical therapists, and interested laymen.

Concerning fractures in adults, the text originally by Watson-Jones, *Fractures and Injuries* (5th edition, edited by J. N. Wilson), also serves as a good reference, but it is not quite as good as that of Rockwood and Green. It may be consulted before undertaking treatment of a specific problem fracture, and it provides a generally more conservative approach than do Rockwood and Green for treatment of musculoskeletal injuries. It has excellent line drawings of fractures and, in particular, of the blood supply to bone: It emphasizes the effect of adequate blood supply on the healing of fractures.

Another standard text useful primarily for reference in an emergency facility is the one based on experience at the Massachusetts General Hospital Fracture Clinic by Cave, Burke, and Boyd: *Fractures and Other Injuries*. A balanced approach between nonsurgical and surgical treatment of fractures and emphasis on end-result evaluation make it an excellent reference book. The chapters on shoulder injuries and metal implants are particularly well worth reading.

We would recommend that there should be at least three books specifically on fractures in an emergency facility: Rockwood and Green, Blount, and Cave et al. (plus any others favored by the consultant staff). Practitioners who maintain personal libraries would do well to supplement the books that represent their special interests with these three books if for no other reason than occasional reference.

Charnley's *Closed Treatment of Common Fractures* has three virtues that recommend it particularly to medical students and paramedical personnel: It is short, eminently readable, and straightforward in its advocacy of conservative treatment. Charnley's portrayal of the aim of treatment as elimination of all adverse influences on healing is not only sound but helpful because it provides the student with a better perception of the relation between basic science and clinical practice. Unfortunately, as for nearly all cases in which closed manipulation of a fracture is advocated as treatment, surgical experience cannot be learned from words or pictures but requires "hands on" manipulation. A similar comment is appropriate in regard to plaster casts.

The book by Sarmiento and Latta, *Closed Functional Treatment of Fractures*, is not to be overlooked even though its main focus is on cast bracing as a method of fracture treatment. The authors have described the method in considerable, well illustrated detail, giving the reader the benefit of their extensive experience. For each type of fracture the reader can get a good idea of the effectiveness of the method and the contraindications to its use.

In contrast to the books describing the conservative, nonoperative end of the spectrum, the *Fracture Manual of Internal Fixation* by Mueller et al. describes the details of a single, highly publicized system of internal fixation. The book is well illustrated and is useful for anyone performing internal fixation by the method being advocated. It has one important disadvantage, however. It advocates one "principle" above all others: that open fixation of a fracture nearly always provides the means for accurate reduction and secure fixation of the fracture fragments. The word "principle" is placed within quotation marks because these authors strongly imply in their book and in all their writings that it is desirable if not imperative to achieve anatomic reduction and secure fixation — if possible. We discuss that subject at length in Chapter 4, but here we must emphasize that this advocacy is not a principle to be adopted universally. Advocacy of one brand of instrumentation also smacks of some measure of self-interest. Mueller et al. used new words to define biologic events that are well known, and their book is recommended only to experienced orthopedic surgeons. It contains perhaps the clearest portrayal of one good internal fixation method, and such readers can recognize that, although the book is doctrinaire, much can be learned, mostly on a technical level, for specific situations.

Emergency room texts should include those that deal with *Emergency Care and Transportation of the Sick and Injured,* developed by the Committee on Injuries of the American Academy of Orthopaedic Surgeons (Charles Rockwood, editor). Written in clear language with extensive use of line drawings, it is especially written for the emergency medical technician but can serve as a quick review for others caring for the acutely injured person, along with the other consensus book, *Early Care of the Injured Patient,* noted below. Once the general texts on the care of the traumatized patient are considered, each emergency room can add those specialty texts most often used by the practicing specialist.

A word should be said about a textbook on the general care of the traumatized patient. One book, *Care of the Trauma Patient* (2nd ed., edited by Shires), is worthy of consideration. There are excellent chapters by Paradies and Gregory. The book is based largely on the experience at one hospital and provides a good review of the general principles of treatment for systemic problems such as shock, cardiovascular complications, and burns. For fractures associated with injuries involving the head or abdominal viscera or those of the chest or pelvis, this book is a useful guide to the principles and specifics of treatment as well as diagnosis. The book is especially valuable for students, interns, residents, and "emergency room" physicians, i.e., those who may be involved in the care of the patients who present immediately after an accident. It provides good information on the administration of fluids and treatment of cardiovascular and respiratory injuries, genitourinary disturbances, and such complications as pancreatitis and stress ulcers.

Another book on the subject, but not designed for use in an emergency facility, consists of a useful, up-to-date series of short chapters on several (18) topics dealing with systemic problems: *Trauma, Sepsis and Shock* by Clowes. The basic science background for the three general subjects in the title is found in this book, which is perhaps better organized than most texts in terms of being an introduction to the scientific context of specific topics, e.g., anticoagulation therapy and action of antibiotics.

Other books of this kind are not to be overlooked especially when amassing a personal library of some breadth. *Management of Trauma* (3rd ed., edited by Zuidema) is especially recommended for its chapter on initial evaluation and resuscitation of the injured patient. *Management of Trauma, Pitfalls and Practice* by Walt and Wilson emphasizes the axioms of good treatment and the pitfalls one should avoid. It is based largely on emergency room experience (at the Detroit Receiving Hospital).

A book (manual) that is particularly useful for students, paramedical individuals, nurses, and residents is *Early Care of the Injured Patient* (edited by Walt). Written by the Committee on Trauma of the American College of Surgeons, it contains as good and concise a summary of the evaluation and treatment of fractures and dislocations as any general text on orthopedic surgery. The description is accompanied by excellent line drawings. Because a consensus of the committee was required, the controversial aspects of fracture treatment were reduced to a minimum.

In passing, we mention *Shands Handbook of Or-thopedic Surgery* by Brashear and Raney as a good book for students and for review. The chapter on musculoskeletal injuries is a reasonable introduction to the beginning medical student or paramedical student or practitioner. Also worth attention as an introduction to the subject are the three chapters devoted to injuries in the book by Salter, *Textbook of Disorders and Injuries of the Musculoskeletal System*. More than a passing glance is recommended for such individuals to Apley's *System of Orthopedics and Fractures*. His five chapters on musculoskeletal injuries provide a good introduction and summary of fracture evaluation and treatment, including complications. He makes excellent use of composite radiographs and presents the information in concise outline form, discussing each area. The beginning medical student and paramedical person will find the chapter on orthopedics by Cooper in *Synopsis of Surgery* (edited by Liechty and Soper) worthy of attention as an introduction to trauma of the musculoskeletal system.

The chapter "Principles and Management of Fractures and Dislocations" in Gartland's *Fundamentals of Orthopedics* is much too brief and too simple to be of value to anyone other than the very beginning student.

SOFT TISSUE INJURY AND WOUND REPAIR (CHAPTER 6)

No consideration of injury and repair would be complete without a discussion of wound repair and injuries to soft tissues. The texts available in this area are few indeed. There are two worthy of our consideration. One, *Fundamentals of Wound Management* by Hunt and Dunphy, is the more current and more worth having. An outgrowth of a series of monographs on various aspects of the subject, it has 16 contributors in addition to the 12 members of the editorial advisory board. The book is well organized. There are chapters on normal repair and on the broader aspects of wound healing based on the concept of the dependence of repair on tissue perfusion, oxygenation, and nutrition, all of which a good blood supply provides. The chapter "Disorders of Repair and Their Management" is especially useful because of the emphasis it places on the negative effect on repair following massive injury as a result of greater catabolic responses, when there is reduced oxygenation of injured tissue. There is a good summary with practical advice concerning the care of wounded tissue, much of which is summarized in standard surgical and fracture texts but not discussed in adequate detail. The chapter on the repair of selected tissues provides a good summary of tendon repair; that on bone healing is not covered as well as in other texts.

The second book, *Wound Repair,* by Peacock and VanWinkle (WB Saunders, 1970, 2nd ed.), is out of date, although it is particularly valuable for its descriptions of the cellular response to injury and the cellular phases of wound repair. These subjects are exposited in considerable detail in regard to experimental studies and clinical observations. In addition, it covers as well as any text the repair of tendons and the restoration of function. The book needs updating to reflect major advances in technique and instrumentation, e.g., the operating microscope and microvascular surgery.

Another book that deserves mention as a useful reference is *The Biologic Basis of Wound Healing* by Mencker. This book, with 20 contributors, has detailed various aspects of hemostasis, platelets, blood coagulation, and acute inflammation and its chemical mediators. The descriptions of acute inflammation and its chemical mediators and hypersensitivity reactions are more detailed than is needed by clinicians and all but special students. The description of antibody structure and function and the relevance to wound healing is not clearly stated other than to discuss briefly the altered immune response in burn patients. However, the value of antibiotic treatment and skin grafting to reduce infection in burn patients is emphasized. The description of the effect of hormones and stress, nutrition, and protein synthesis on wound healing is well covered, as are the structure, chemistry, and function of collagen. The book serves as a good general overview of wound healing; unfortunately, there is not enough concentration on soft tissue injuries and bone to recommend it as a book to own.

Also deserving of mention is the chapter by Glynn, *"Tissue Repair and Regeneration,"* in Volume 3 of the *Handbook of Inflammation,* a five-volume series with multiple contributors that contains a detailed consideration of the fibroblast, collagen, proteoglycans, and regeneration in the healing of bone, cartilage, and connective tissue. It covers in particular the regulation of wound healing by autocoids, substances that form locally to regulate metabolic processes. (Histamine, bradykinin, and serotonin are examples of autocoids.) After one reads one of the other less intensive chapters in texts on wound healing, Glynn's chapter is a logical extension of details on subjects of basic importance, but it is too complicated for the nonspecialist.

Sports Medicine

Despite the explosion of interest and emphasis on injuries incurred during sports and exercise in all parts of the world and its pervading involvement of all age groups and both sexes, it is truly surprising that so few general texts have been written on the subject. The best known and still the most useful is *The Treatment of Injuries to Athletes* by O'Donohue. Its descriptions of common and unusual problems are simple and unpretentious.

Several other texts probably are worthy of inclusion in the library of anyone specializing in sports medicine, particularly the physician who plans to be a team physician. *The Injured Athlete* by Kulund and Ervin has considerable text devoted to the problems of the ordinary avocational or competitive athlete. The principles of training, diet, and fitness are well covered, but the major part of the book is devoted to injuries. A small volume, *Injuries in Sports* (color atlas, 1980, by Williams), focuses on mechanisms and recommendations for treatment of injuries.

Every orthopedist involved in the care of athletes should know and value the book by Smillie, *Injuries of the Knee Joint.* It records the experience of a physician who has been concerned with the treatment of meniscal and ligamentous injuries of the knee for four decades. Although ultramodern subjects such as arthroscopy and reconstruction of ligaments are not the forte of the book and controversial views are presented as fact, e.g., the pathogenesis of osteochondritis dissecans, they do not detract from the value of the book, which lies principally in chapters on diagnosis, history taking, and office practice.

ASEPTIC NECROSIS OF BONE (CHAPTER 7)

Of the two most recent books published on aseptic necrosis of bone in adults, the recommended text is that by Davidson. It presents the essential information on the clinical, pathologic, and radiologic observations and their correlations. The chapter by Catto on pathology, in particular, deserves a preliminary reading as it serves to highlight what follows. The essentials of the clinical and radiographic observations in aseptic necrosis as it develops after trauma or in dysbaric osteonecrosis are lucid and detailed. Davidson's own exposition of decompression sickness—its manifestations, prevalence, distribution, and classification—serves as a monograph on that subject. Pertinent advice is offered on the best technique for obtaining quality radiographs that are crucial to the detection of necrosis.

A second text or, rather, monograph on the subject is by Ficat and Arlet, edited and adapted by Hungerford. These authors present, in particular, newer methods for studying bone circulation in patients suspected of necrosis of the femoral head and a classification based on pressure measurements as well as radiographic and histologic observations. They suggest a plan of treatment related to the classification, and in particular they advocate core decompression as early treatment. Other reading suggested on the subject includes Chapters 19 through 22 in Jaffe's book, *Metabolic and Degenerative Inflammatory Diseases of Bones and Joints.*

Because there are so few books on coxa plana, a monograph by Catterall, *Legg-Calve-Perthes Disease,* should be read by anyone who treats even a few cases of that entity. This monograph makes an effort to correlate much of what has been written on the subject with some original observations on specimens; it attempts a classification, still somewhat controversial, that divides lesions into stages that bear on prognosis as well as treatment.

ARTHRITIS (CHAPTER 8)

The texts on arthritis fall into three major groups, textbooks on the medical aspects of rheumatic diseases, those concerned with surgical treatment, and those with a special focus, e.g. juvenile polyarthritis or by anatomic location, e.g., spine, hand, foot, knee, or hip.

The Primer on the Rheumatic Diseases is a well organized basic text essential to anyone's library. It contains succinct descriptions of essential information concerning each major type of rheumatic disease. Because it is based on a consensus of rheumatologists, it can serve as an up-to-date summary of information—but not of matters still in controversy. For that reason it is of particular value to medical students, residents, and all physicians and surgeons as a quick reference on the subject. It should be a starting point for study and reference, although one often needs more extensive discussion. The appendices in *The Primer* on accepted criteria for the diagnosis and classification of the many types of rheumatic disease are of particular value. This book therefore is essential reading for anyone beginning a study of the diagnosis and treatment of the arthritic patient. It should be read before using one of the reference texts or special focus books discussed below.

Among the general textbooks there are two that stand out. One is *The Textbook of Rheumatology* (edited by Kelly, Harris, Ruddy, and Sledge, published in one or two volumes by WB Saunders, 1981). In addition to the four editors, there are many authors who wrote separate chapters. The text is designed to serve mainly as a reference. A similarly multiauthored and equally satisfactory reference textbook for one's library is *Arthritis and Allied Conditions* (9th ed., 1979, edited by McCarty; formerly edited by Hollander and before that by Comroe). It has long served as the standard text in rheumatology, whereas that of Kelly et al. is more recent; each has relatively well known authors in their respective areas. Each chapter is focused so that reference to pathophysiology of each disease entity and its clinical and therapeutic aspects can be readily reviewed.

Our choice as to which group of well known authorities we prefer in these two textbooks of generally equal depth and coverage falls to McCarty, but there are four chapters (see below) that are better in the text of Kelly et al. The many tables constitute useful summaries of information for the reader. We advocate starting with the chapter entitled "The Scientific Basis of Rheumatoid Arthritis and Differential Diagnosis" and then "Bone Formation and Resorption" (by Sledge) and "Biomechanics of Joints" (by Simon) before proceeding to other, more specific subjects. The chapters on synovial fluid analysis and radiology are particularly good, as are "Correction of Arthritic Deformities of the Upper and Lower Limbs" (Flatt and Sledge), the general exposition of "Osteoarthritis" (Sokoloff and Howell), and "Pathogenesis and Treatment of Crystal Induced Inflammation and Pseudogout."

There are a few exceptional chapters in the text by Kelly et al. Each provides more detailed coverage of a specific topic. One chapter we found particularly useful and practical with excellent diagrams is "Aspiration and Injection of Joints and Soft Tissues." Part of a section on diagnostic tests, it is particularly valuable for any physician planning to undertake any regimen of diagnostic procedures.

A second section, that on the clinical pharmacology of the antirheumatic drugs, newly written (1981) for McCarty's current edition, is more modern than Kelly's analogous section (1979) but will probably change dramatically by the time the next edition appears what with the frequent introduction of new antiarthritic drugs. As experience on the short- and long-term usefulness of a drug accumulates, it can be seen that many drugs have short lives. As this book is written, a nonsteroidal drug for arthritis that had shown early promise of success and wide usage was reported fatal to some patients and has therefore been withdrawn from the market. Although both of the texts under discussion have chapters on those aspects of the disease that relate to surgical treatment, the relevant text is designed mainly to acquaint nonsurgical readers with the armamentarium of surgeons but is not detailed enough for those who are studying or performing the surgical procedures themselves.

The chapter in Kelly's text that is most valuable for the orthopedic surgeon is "The Examination of Joints." It discusses in clear detail functional evaluation and diagnostic tests. This subject is particularly difficult because each major joint poses not only the preoperative problem of quantitative impairment (pain, range of motion, deformity, function) in isolation but also as it affects the rest of the extremity and the patient as a whole. Then too, the effectiveness of any operation must be portrayed as

it affects the preoperative quantitations; for example, how much will fusion of a severely affected wrist allow a patient who has to use crutches to extend his sphere of activity? Among the ten chapters on reconstructive surgery there is one exceptional one, on synovectomy, that deserves particular attention because that subject is seldom covered in one place in such depth and clarity with respect to the indications and contraindications for the operation on each joint affected.

Both textbooks have excellent chapters on the analysis of synovial fluid, and one should be read by anyone who performs diagnostic or therapeutic arthrocentesis.

In Kelly's book the chapter on medical orthopedics provides a useful description of common minor problems encountered by rheumatologists in office practice or emergency rooms. This chapter would be of value for the medical student and emergency room physician.

Because of its special focus on juvenile rheumatoid arthritis, *Rheumatoid Disorders in Childhood* by Ansel (Butterworth, 1980) serves as the best text for anyone especially interested in pediatric orthopedics. Similarly, *The Care of The Arthritic Hand,* by Flatt (CV Mosby, 4th ed., 1983), is particularly valuable for the principles regarding the care of rheumatoid diseases as they affect the hand, and the same can be said for the book by Freeman, *Arthritis of the Knee: Clinical Features and Surgical Management* (Springer-Verlag, 1981).

Two other primarily medical (rather than surgical) books that deserve mention are Coperman's *Textbook of Rheumatic Diseases* edited by Scott, (5th ed., 1978, Churchill Livingstone), and *Rheumatic Diseases—Diagnosis and Management* by Katz (JB Lippincott, 1977).

TUMORS AND TUMOR-LIKE LESIONS (CHAPTER 9)

A few textbooks concerning tumors are recommended. Some are described at some length below, and about a dozen other books are considered as well. Of the standard textbooks, the first is the classic text by Jaffe, *Tumors and Tumorous Conditions of the Bones and Joints* (Lea & Febiger, 1958). Although this book is comparatively old, and at the present writing undergoing revision by Sissons, it is the first choice for systematic descriptions of the gross, radiologic, and histologic fractures of each tumor.

The fascicle (really an atlas) *Tumors of Bone and Cartilage,* by Spjut, Dorfman, Fechner, and Ackerman, is not generally available from bookstores. Its value lies largely in its profuse illustrations of histology, although it is also valuable for its radiographs. This low-cost book may be purchased by writing to the Armed Forces Institute of Pathology (Bethesda, Maryland).

The best of recent texts (reviewed below) is *Tumors and Tumor-like Lesions of Bone and Joints* by Schajowicz. Dahlin's text, *Bone Tumors — General Aspects and Data on 6221 Cases* (Charles C Thomas, 1981; reviewed below) is also a valuable reference because it is derived from a huge personal experience at the Mayo Clinic.

There is a relatively large number of recent textbooks on bone tumors, and they present one with the dilemma of which to choose for a library, for a review, or for special purposes. In addition to the three books that are recommended above, which serve most purposes, several others have special features that deserve mention. General texts that are somewhat less complete than that of Schajowicz, are those by Mirra and Huvos; they have the advantage of being based in large part on an extensive American experience mainly with malignant tumors from one institution (the same one) to which patients with malignancies are frequently referred. Huvos's book contains more historical data than do any of the others. Mirra's book is somewhat doctrinaire in regard to therapy of certain tumors but is readable and is a well organized text; it is suitable for review of the subject and has an excellent bibliography. Also readable and about as satisfactory as any for review (as before an examination) is the text of Lichtenstein, *Bone Tumors,* (CV Mosby, 1977).

Of special importance is the book *Histologic Typing of Bone Tumors* by Schajowicz, Ackerman, and Sissons, a publication of The World Health Organization. This small volume consists mainly of photomicrographs collated by a committee of experts to establish standards that meet with general agreement as to histologic diagnosis and nomenclature.

It serves to supplement the photomicrographs in the *Atlas* of Spjut et al. Another book that is devoted only to cytologic diagnosis is that of Sanerkin and Jeffree, *Cytology of Bone Tumors.*

A text mostly devoted to radiologic illustrations is a collection from The Netherlands, *Radiologic Atlas of Bone Tumors.* It is written by a large group of clinicians who had available to them all, or nearly all, the cases in that small, well organized country, and it contains a wide selection of radiographs on nearly all the major types of neoplasm. It is best used for recognition of those classic lesions, but also, like ribbon matching, it has so many illustrations of each tumor that one can use it to find the best fit for an atypical lesion in each accepted diagnostic category.

Certain books are available on special topics relating to osseous neoplasms. One is a report of recent research: Price and Ross's *Bone — Certain Aspects of Neoplasia.* Another is that of Marcove, *The Surgery of Tumors of Bone and Cartilage,* concerning his own surgical approaches to therapy. Still another is Jaffe's *Bone Tumors in Childhood.* These books are of interest only to one pursuing special studies, however.

Tumors of soft tissues are seldom singled out for textbook exposition, although if one wishes to be permissive in defining what one calls a soft tissue tumor or even a soft tissue tumor of the extremity, the incidence of such lesions would be much larger than that of tumors of bone. Under present patterns of medical care, most tumors of bone are considered the province of orthopedic surgeons, whereas many of the soft tissue tumors, even if those of the skin are excluded, are treated by general surgeons, particularly those benign neoplasms that undergo simple excision, with no reconstructive operation being indicated afterward. Not only are such tumors plentiful (e.g., lipomas), they also are of many types because of the several types of soft tissue represented in the extremities. Were this book to restrict its purview only to the musculoskeletal system, soft tissue tumors arising from nerves, vessels, etc. but not from muscle or fascia might be considered irrelevant; but in practice many of those tumors come to be treated by orthopedic surgeons, particularly the large ones and those that interfere with the function of an extremity.

There is not much reason to praise Hajdu's text on *Tumors of the Soft Tissue* more than that of Enzinger and Weiss, *Soft Tissue Tumors*. Both books can serve as references, but neither, because of the low incidence of the lesions encountered in orthopedic practice, belongs in any but reference libraries or in the library of someone especially interested in tumors. It is doubtful that these books will be consulted, except when one actually encounters one of the tumors. Perhaps it is unfortunate that the subject of tumors is being so compartmentalized that there is no one textbook that covers all the neoplasms of interest in orthopedic practice.

Of special interest are the two texts by Enneking (see General Bibliography). The one on surgical treatment of bone tumors reflects his personal experience with bone and soft tissue tumors at the University of Florida. This text is particularly useful for its emphasis on the natural history, staging, and clinical aspects as they relate to initial treatment and surgical technique. The other book, which discusses tumors in only one-third of its 500 pages, constitutes an excellent, well illustrated summary of not only tumors but the entire orthopedic domain viewed from the standpoint of a clinician well versed in pathology. It is targeted at medical students and orthopedic surgeons in training and is not of much service to others.

THE SURGICAL PROCESS (CHAPTER 10)

As was remarked in the section in the chapter regarding interpretative skills, a large variety of texts pertain to the subject of surgical process, and one's medical school texts on anatomy and surgery, in particular, relate to much that is in Chapter 10 of this book. We prefer, as a basic exposé of the pathophysiology of ordinary surgical procedures involving soft tissues, the recent text by Sabiston, the title of which—*Textbook of Surgery: The Biological Basis of Surgical Practice*—indicates an emphasis on pathophysiology not common in most other analogous texts. However, further reading of that text is inappropriate for surgeons in training or practice, although it is appropriate for other orthopedic personnel.

With regard to the planning of operations, the principles emphasized in the chapter involve not only the processes that accompany each step in the surgery, from preoperative preparations through the continuum from incision to rehabilitation, but also the tools, the materials, and the mechanics. Consider first the incision. Several texts are available describing surgical approaches to all parts of the musculoskeletal system. Inasmuch as most of those approaches are pictured in Campbell and Evarts, the argument for separate books, e.g., the classic books by Henry (*Extensile Exposure Applied to Limb Surgery*, Williams & Wilkins, 1945) or newer texts (Adams, Nicola, or Hoppenfeld) might be mainly convenience. Further reading on the other intraoperative topics is governed by the particular topic under scrutiny, and the titles in the General Bibliography may serve as a guide to any of the multitude of possible topics. The field of biomechanical engineering is advancing so rapidly the texts can merely indicate to the reader the fundamental disciplines involved and the methods in use in those disciplines as they can be applied to the particular constructs or material under consideration. The data on specific constructs or materials must be sought out in periodicals.

PERIODICALS

Let us turn now from the consideration of books relevant to individual chapters in the present book to the relevant periodicals. A list of orthopedic journals follows the General Bibliography. Under the heading of serial publications in orthopedics and traumatology the *Medical and Health Care Books and Serials in Print 1988* lists 136 titles (in all languages). The list herein represents our selection from that list, based on our familiarity with the publications. To our knowledge, none of the periodicals omitted here meets all our criteria: written in English, composed mainly of original articles, subjected to peer review, easily available. We omitted all directories, newsletters, almanacs, product news, collections of excerpts, institutional journals, and proceedings of meetings. From this list, one can select a group of publications that would be eminently serviceable to the office of a large or small group of orthopedic surgeons or similar facility. To have the entire list on file would be appropriate only for a medical library serving an entire region. Most orthopedic departmental libraries would be well enough served with only *Clinical Orthopedics and Related Research, JBJS* (American), and *JBJS* (British) supplemented by any others that cover the domains of special interest of the individuals concerned. For instance, for a department with major interests in sports medicine, in addition to the classic texts of O'Donoghue and Smillie the library might include several books on that subject chosen from the General Bibliography. The appropriate journal(s) would depend on the special interests of the department. In contrast, an orthopedic department associated with a medical school would have to include books and periodicals servicing the needs of all the personnel attached to the department, even those (e.g., medical students, nursing students) whose attachment is temporary, and others (e.g., emergency technicians, orthopedic nurses) whose needs have a narrow focus, somewhat apart from the needs of the surgeons and house officers.

GENERAL BIBLIOGRAPHY*,†

° Abramson DI, Miller DS: *Vascular Problems in Musculoskeletal Disorders of the Limbs,* Springer-Verlag (**1981;64B:651**)

° Ackroyd CE, O'Connor BT, de Bruyn PF: *The Severely Injured Limb,* Churchill Livingstone (Edinburgh) (**1983;66A:638; 66B:622**)

Adams JC: *Outline of Fractures,* Churchill Livingstone (Edinburgh) (**1983;66B:155**)

Adams JC: *Outline of Orthopaedics,* 9th ed., Churchill Livingstone (Edinburgh) (**1981;63B:649**)

Adams JC: *Standard Orthopaedic Operations: A Guide for the Junior Surgeon,* 3rd ed., Churchill Livingstone (Edinburgh) (**1985;68B:169**)

° Aitken M: *Osteoporosis in Clinical Practice,* Wright (**1984; 68B:171**)

°° Albright JA, Brand RA (eds): *The Scientific Basis of Orthopaedics,* Appleton-Century-Crofts (**1979;61A:958; 63B:311**)

Alexander RM: *Animal Mechanics,* 2nd ed., Blackwell Scientific Publishers (**1983;66B:467**)

American Academy of Orthopaedic Surgeons. *Athletic Training and Sports Medicine,* CV Mosby (**1984;67A:669**)

American Academy of Orthopaedic Surgeons: *Atlas of Limb Prosthetics,* CV Mosby (**1981;63A:1038; 64B:266**)

American Academy of Orthopaedic Surgeons: *Instructional Course Lectures,* Vol. 26, CV Mosby (**1977;61B:132**). Vol. 29, CV Mosby (**1980;64B:148**). Vol. 30, CV Mosby (**1981;65B:528**). Vol. 32, CV Mosby (**1983;66B:619**). Vol. 31, CV Mosby (**1982;66B:153**)

American Academy of Orthopaedic Surgeons: *Orthopaedic Knowledge Update I: Home Study Syllabus,* CV Mosby (**1984;66A:814**)

American Academy of Orthopaedic Surgeons: *Symposium on the Athlete's Knee,* CV Mosby (**1980;63A:174, 63B:648**)

American Academy of Orthopaedic Surgeons: *Symposium on the Foot and Ankle,* CV Mosby (**1983;65A:1036**)

American Academy of Orthopaedic Surgeons: *Symposium on the Foot and Leg in Running Sports,* CV Mosby (**1980;66B:154**)

American Academy of Orthopaedic Surgeons: *Symposium on Heritable Disorders of Connective Tissue,* 3rd ed., CV Mosby (**1982;66B:156**)

American Academy of Orthopaedic Surgeons: *Symposium on the Lumbar Spine,* CV Mosby (**1981;64B:650**)

American Academy of Orthopaedic Surgeons: *Symposium on Microsurgery,* CV Mosby (**1979;62A:318**)

American Academy of Orthopaedic Surgeons: *Symposium on Reconstructive Surgery of the Knee,* CV Mosby (**1978; 61B:390**)

American Academy of Orthopaedic Surgeons: *Symposium on Total Joint Replacement of the Upper Extremity,* CV Mosby (**1982;65B:683**)

American Academy of Orthopaedic Surgeons: *Symposium on Trauma to the Leg and Its Sequelae,* CV Mosby (**1981;64B:650**)

° American Society for Surgery of the Hand: *The Hand: Examination and Diagnosis,* Churchill Livingstone (Edinburgh) (**1983;66B:468**)

Anderson JR: *Atlas of Skeletal Muscle Pathology* (**1985;68B:344**)

°° *Apley's System of Orthopaedics and Fractures,* 5th ed., Butterworth (Publishers) (**1977;60B:299**), 6th ed., Butterworth (Publishers) (**1982;64B:649**)

---

* Note that the authors or editors, the book title and publisher are given. For further information about the book, consult the *Journal of Bone and Joint Surgery* issue in which the book was reviewed. The year of book publication, volume, and page of the *JBJS* issue are given in boldface in parentheses at the end of each reference.

† See page 506.

Arden GP, Ansel BM (eds): *Surgical Management of Juvenile Chronic Polyarthritis,* Grune & Stratton (1978;61A:957; 62B:413)

Ariyan S: *The Hand Book,* 2nd ed., Williams & Wilkins (1980;66B:623)

° Arlet J, Ficat RP, Hungerford DS: *Bone Circulation,* Williams & Wilkins (1984;68B:170)

Arndt RD, Horns JW, Gold RH: *Clinical Arthrography,* 2nd ed., Williams & Wilkins (1985;67A:1310)

Aston's Short Textbook of Orthopaedics and Traumatology, 3rd ed., Hodder and Stoughton (1983;66B:464)

Austin RT: *Robert Chessher of Hinkley 1750–1831: First English Orthopaedist,* Leicestershire Libraries and Information Services (1981;65B:108)

° Avioli LV, Krane SM (eds): *Metabolic Bone Disease,* Academic Press (1977/1978;61A:638)

Back Pain Association: *Low Back Pain and Industrial and Social Disablement,* Backpain Association (1983;66B:793)

Backhouse KM, Harrison SH, Hutchings RT: *Color Atlas of Rheumatoid Hand Surgery,* Yearbook Medical Publishers (1981;65A:285; 64B:391)

Banna M: *Clinical Radiology of the Spine and Spinal Cord,* Aspen Publishers (1985;68A:1309)

Barron JN, Saad MN (eds): *Operative Plastic and Reconstructive Surgery, Vol. 3: The Hand,* Churchill Livingstone (Edinburgh) (1980;63B:482)

Barry H: *Orthopaedics in Australia,* Williams & Wilkins (1983;67B:519)

Basmajian JV: *Muscles Alive: Their Function Revealed by Electromyography,* 4th ed., Williams & Wilkins (1978;61A:478)

Basmajian JV (ed): *Therapeutic Exercises,* student edition, Williams & Wilkins (1980;62A:1229)

Bateman JE: *The Shoulder and Neck,* 2nd ed., WB Saunders (1978;61B:525)

Bateman JE, Trott AW (eds): *The Foot and Ankle,* Thieme (1980;63A:174)

Bayley I, Kessell L (eds): *Shoulder Surgery,* Springer-Verlag (1982;65B:107)

Beasley RW: *Hand Injuries,* WB Saunders (1981;64A:638; 64B:391)

Bedbrook GM (ed): *Lifetime Care of the Paraplegic Patient,* Churchill Livingstone (Edinburgh) (1985;67A:1150)

Bedbrook Sir GM (ed): *Lifetime Care of the Paraplegic Patient,* Churchill Livingstone (Edinburgh) (1985;68B:166)

Beighton P: *Inherited Disorders of the Skeleton,* Springer-Verlag (1978;61B:389)

° Beighton P, Cremin BJ: *Sclerosing Bone Dysplasias,* Springer-Verlag (1980;63A:509)

Beighton P, Beighton G: *The Man Behind the Syndrome,* Churchill Livingstone (Edinburgh) (1986;69B:516)

Beighton P, Grahame R, Bird H: *Hypermobility of Joints,* Springer-Verlag (1983;65A:1213; 66B:310)

Bell Sir C: *The Hand: Its Mechanism and Vital Endowments as Evincing Design,* Pilgrims Press [1833 (facsimile edition, 1979); 62B:139]

Benini A: *Ischias Ohne Bandscheibenvortall die Stenose des Lumbalen Wirbelkanals,* Hans Huber Publishers (1986;69A:478)

Benjamin A, Helal B: *Surgical Repair and Reconstruction in Rheumatoid Disease,* Macmillan Press (1980;63B:306)

Bernau A, Berquist TH: *Orthopaedic Positioning in Diagnostic Radiology,* Appleton-Century-Crofts (1983;66A:477)

Bernbeck R, Simos A: *Neuro-orthopedic Screening in Infancy,* Urban and Schwarzenberg (1978;60A:1159)

° Berquist TH (ed): *Imaging of Orthopedic Trauma and Surgery,* Urban and Schwarzenberg (1985;68A:478)

Berquist TH: *Diagnostic Imaging of the Acutely Injured Patient,* WB Saunders (1985;68A:957)

Berquist TH (ed): *Magnetic Resonance of the Musculoskeletal System,* Raven Press (1986;69B:859)

Birch R, Brooks D (eds): *Rob & Smith's Operative Surgery: The Hand,* 4th ed., Springer-Verlag (1984;67B:686)

Black J, Dumbleton JH (eds): *Clinical Biomechanics,* Churchill Livingstone (New York) (1981;64B:266)

Blauth W, Schneider-Sickert FR: *Congenital Deformities of the Hand,* Springer-Verlag (1981;64A:637; 64B:391)

Blauvelt CT, Nelson FRT: *Manual of Orthopaedic Terminology,* CV Mosby (1977;61B:132; 62A:318). 2nd ed. (1981;63A:1358)

Bleck EE: *Orthopaedic Management of Cerebral Palsy,* WB Saunders (1979;63B:145)

° Blockey NJ: *Congenital Dislocation of the Hip,* Glasgow University Press (1985;68B:860)

Blount WP, Moe JH: *The Milwaukee Brace,* 2nd ed., Williams & Wilkins (1980;63A:510; 64B:267)

° Bogumill GP, Schwamm HA: *Orthopaedic Pathology: A Synopsis with Clinical and Radiographic Correlation,* Springer-Verlag (1984;67B:513)

Bowerman JW: *Radiology and Injury in Sport,* Appleton-Century-Crofts (1977;60A:141)

Boijsen E, Ekelund L (eds): *Computed Tomography in Orthopedic Radiology,* Thieme (1983;66B:312)

Bonola A, Caroli A, Celli C: *La Mano,* Piein Editorial (1981;65B:107)

Bora FW Jr (ed): *The Pediatric Upper Extremity*, Springer-Verlag (1986;68A:1133)

Boswick JA (ed): *Current Concepts in Hand Surgery*, Lea & Febiger (1983;66B:623)

Boswick JA Jr (ed): *Complications in Hand Surgery*, WB Saunders (1986;68A:797; 69B:514)

Bourdillon JF: *Spinal Manipulation*, Appleton-Century-Crofts (1982;65B:232)

Bowers WH (ed): *Interphalangeal Joints, Vol. 1: The Hand and Upper Limb*, Churchill Livingstone (Edinburgh) (1987;69A:1309)

Bradford DS, Hensinger RM (eds): *The Paediatric Spine*, Charles C Thomas (1985;68B:516)

°° Brand PW: *Clinical Mechanics of the Hand*, CV Mosby (1985;68B:514)

Braune W, Fischer O: *On the Centre of Gravity of the Human Body: As Related to the Equipment of the German Infantry Soldier*, Springer-Verlag (1985;67B:852)

Brighton CT, et al (eds): *Electrical Properties of Bone and Cartilage*, Grune & Stratton (1979;62A:494; 62B:539)

° Brooke MH: *A Clinician's View of Neuromuscular Diseases*, Williams & Wilkins (1977;60A:141)

Brooker AF Jr, Cooney WP III, Chao EY: *Principles of External Fixation*, Williams & Wilkins (1983;66A:317; 67B:171)

Brooker AF Jr, Schmeisser G: *Orthopaedic Traction Manual*, Williams & Wilkins (1980;63B:147)

Brown JE, Nordby EJ, Smith L (eds): *Chemonucleolysis*, CB Slack (1985;67A:1454)

Brown MD: *Intradiscal Therapy: Chymopapain or Collagenase*, Yearbook Medical Publishers (1983;65A:1214; 66B:310)

° Browne PSH: *Basic Facts in Orthopaedics*, 2nd ed., Blackwell Scientific Publishers (1985;68B:344)

° Brunelli G (ed): *Ischemia and Reimplantation*, Liviana Editrice (1981;64B:652)

Brunner CF, Weber BG: *Special Techniques in Internal Fixation*, Springer-Verlag (1982;64A:797, 1401 — (correspondence)

Bucholz RW, Lippert FG III, Wenger DR, Ezaki, M: *Orthopaedic Decision Making*, CV Mosby (1984;67B:344)

Buck-Gramcko D, et al: *Hand Trauma: A Practical Guide*, Charles C Thomas (1986;68A:1310)

Bulcke JA, Baert KU: *Clinical and Radiological Aspects of Myopathies: CT Scanning, EMG, Radioisotopes*, Springer-Verlag (1982;66B:312)

° Bullough PG, Vigorita VJ: *Atlas of Orthopaedic Pathology with Clinical and Radiologic Correlations*, Butterworth (Publishers) (1984;66A:812; 67B:165)

Bunch WH, et al (eds): *Atlas of Orthotics*, 2nd ed., CV Mosby (1985;68B:515)

Burnett W (ed): *Clinical Science for Surgeons*, Butterworth (Publishers) (1981;64B:389)

Burri C, Claes L (eds): *Alloplastic Ligament Replacement*, Hans Huber Publishers (1983;66B:467)

Cahuzac M, Claverie P, Nichil J: *L'Enfant Infirme Moteur d'Origine Cérébrale*, Masson Press (1977;60A:1158)

Calenoff L (ed): *Radiology of Spinal Cord Injury*, CV Mosby (1981;64A:477; 64B:513)

Camins MB, O'Leary PF (eds): *The Lumbar Spine*, Raven Press (1986;69A:797)

°° *Campbell's Operative Orthopaedics*, 6th ed., CV Mosby (1980;62A:1392; 63B:481)

Carter PR: *Common Hand Injuries and Infections: A Practical Approach to Early Treatment*, WB Saunders (1983;66A:478; 66B:622)

Caruso G, Ludin HP (eds): *Electromyography in the Diagnosis and Management of Peripheral Nerve Impulses*, Hans Huber Publishers (1983;67B:171)

Catterall A: *Legg-Calvé-Perthes' Disease*, Churchill Livingstone (Edinburgh) (1982;65A:877; 65B:525)

Cauthen JC (ed): *Lumbar Spine Surgery: Indications, Techniques, Failures and Alternatives*, Williams & Wilkins (1983;65A:1036; 66B:310)

Cervical Spine Research Society Editorial Subcommittee (eds): *The Cervical Spine*, JB Lippincott (1983;65A:1037; 66B:624)

Chapchal G (ed): *Injuries of the Ligaments and Their Repair: Hand–Knee–Foot*, Charles C Thomas (1977;60A:277)

Chapchal G (ed): *Pseudarthroses and Their Treatment*, Charles C Thomas (1979;61A:1263; 62B:287)

° Charnley Sir J: *Low Friction Arthroplasty of the Hip*, Springer-Verlag (1979;62A:156; 62B:137)

Chase RA: *Atlas of Hand Surgery*, Vol. 2, WB Saunders (1984;66A:1150; 67B:170)

Chen Zhong-wei, Yang Dong-yeu, Chang Di-sheng: *Microsurgery*, Springer-Verlag (1982;66B:153)

Chung SMK: *Handbook of Pediatric Orthopaedics*, Van Nostrand Reinhold (1986;69A:318)

° Clark JMP: *Tether, Contracture and Deformity*, William Heinemann (1976;60B:147)

° *Clinics in Rheumatic Diseases, Vo. 4, No. 2: Surgical Management of Rheumatoid Arthritis*, WB Saunders (1978;61B:391) Vol. 6, No. 1: Low Back Pain (1980;63B:148)

° Cochran GVB: *A Primer of Orthopaedic Biomechanics*, Churchill Livingstone (New York) (1982;65B:682)

Coleman SS: *Complex Foot Deformities*, Lea & Febiger (1983;66B:154)

Conolly WB: *Atlas of Hand Conditions*, Yearbook Medical Publishers (1980;63A:1198)

Conolly WB, Kilgore ES Jr: *Hand Injuries and Infections*, Edward Arnold Publishers (1979;62B:139)

° Connor JM: *Soft Tissue Ossification*, Springer-Verlag (1983;66A:637; 66B:621)

°° Copeman's Textbook of the Rheumatic Diseases, 5th ed., Churchill Livingstone (Edinburgh) (1978;60B:591)

Cowen NJ (ed): *Practical Hand Surgery*, Yearbook Medical Publishers (1980;64B:514)

Cremin BJ, Beighton P: *Bone Dysplasias of Infancy*, Springer-Verlag (1978;62B:137)

°° Crenshaw AH (ed): *Campbell's Operative Orthopaedics*, 7th ed., CV Mosby (1987;69A:1310)

Crock HV: *Practice of Spinal Surgery*, Springer-Verlag (1983;66A:637)

Crock HV, Yoshizawa H: *The Blood Supply of the Vertebral Column and Spinal Cord in Man*, Springer-Verlag (1977;61B:523)

Crock HV, Yamagishi M, Crock MC (eds): *An Atlas of the Arteries and Veins of the Spinal Cord*, Springer-Verlag (1986;69B:172)

° Cruess RL (ed): *The Musculoskeletal System: Embryology, Biochemistry and Physiology*, Churchill Livingstone (New York) (1982;65A:286; 65B:681)

Cruess RL, Rennie WRJ (eds): *Adult Orthopaedics*, Churchill Livingstone (New York) (1984;66A:1503; 67B:512)

° Curry J: *Mechanical Adaptations of Bone*, Princeton University Press (1984;67A:510)

Dahlin DC: *Bone Tumors*, 3rd ed., Charles C Thomas (1978;60A:1160)

Dalinka MK (ed): *Arthrography*, Springer-Verlag (1980;63A:509; 64B:267)

D'Ambrosia R (ed): *Musculoskeletal Disorders: Regional Examination and Differential Diagnosis*, 2nd ed., CB Slack (1986;69A:637)

D'Ambrosia R, Drez D Jr: *Prevention and Treatment of Running Injuries*, JB Lippincott (1982;64A:637)

Dandy DJ: *Arthroscopic Surgery of the Knee*, Churchill Livingstone (Edinburgh) (1981; 64A:478; 64B:267)

Dandy DJ: *Arthroscopy of the Knee: A Diagnostic Color Atlas*, Butterworth (Publishers) (1984;67A:1150; 67B:687)

D'Angio GJ, Evans AE (eds): *Bone Tumours and Soft-Tissue Sarcomas*, Edward Arnold Publishers (1985;68B:170)

Daniel RK, Terzis J: *Reconstructive Microsurgery*, JB Lippincott (1977;60A:573)

Das Gupta TK: *Tumors of the Soft Tissues*, Appleton-Century-Crofts (1983;67A:989)

Dawson DM: *Entrapment Neuropathies*, JB Lippincott (1983;66A:1326)

Debrunner HU: *Orthopaedic Diagnosis*, 2nd ed., Thieme (1982;66B:155)

DePalma's Management of Fractures and Dislocations, 3rd ed., JB Lippincott (1981;64A:158; 64B:389)

DePalma AF: *Surgery of the Shoulder*, 3rd ed., WB Saunders (1983;65A:1361; 66B:309)

Department of Health and Social Security, Training Council for Orthotists: *Classification of Orthoses*, Her Majesties Stationery Office (1980; 63B:311)

Dequeker JV, Johnston CC Jr: *Non-invasive Bone Measurements: Methodological Problems — Radiogrammetry, Single and Dual Photon Absorptiometry and C-T Densitometry*, I.R.L.Press (1983; 65A:1360; 65B:682)

DeSmet AA: *Radiology of Spinal Curvature*, CV Mosby (1985;67A:1149)

Detrisac DA, Johnson LL: *Arthroscopic Shoulder Anatomy: Pathologic and Surgical Implications*, CB Slack (1986;68A:958)

Devas M (ed): *Geriatric Orthopaedics*, Academic Press (1977;60B:449)

Dibos PE, Wagner HN Jr: *Atlas of Nuclear Medicine, Vol 4: Bone*, WB Saunders (1978;61A:798)

Dickson RA, Bradford DS (eds): *Management of Spinal Deformities*, Butterworth (Publishers) (1984;67B:852)

°° Dickson RA, Wright V (eds): *Musculoskeletal Disease* Heinemann (London) (1984;67B:165)

° Dieppe P, Calvert P: *Crystals and Joint Disease*, Chapman and Hall (1983;65A:1037)

Dieppe PA, et al: *Atlas of Clinical Rheumatology*, Lea & Febiger (1986;68A:1309)

Dihlmann W: *Radiologic Atlas of Rheumatic Diseases*, Thieme (1986;69A:158; 69B:859)

Dirheimer Y: *The Craniovertebral Region in Chronic Inflammatory Rheumatoid Disease*, Sprnger-Verlag (1977;61B:263)

°° Dixon AD, Sarnat BG (eds): *Normal and Abnormal Bone Growth: Basic and Clinical Research*, Alan R Liss (1985;68B:344)

Dorr LD (ed): *Techniques in Orthopaedics: Revision of Total Hip and Knee*, Edward Arnold Publishers (1984;67B:341)

Dowling JJ: *Musculoskeletal Disease: Staged for Rapid Comprehension*, Yearbook Medical Publishers (1985;68B:172)

°° Drennan JC: *Orthopaedic Management of Neuromuscular Disorders, Grune & Stratton (1983;65A:1038)

Ducheyne P, van der Perre G, Aubert AE (eds): Biomaterials and Biomechanics 1983: Proceedings of the Fourth European Conference on Biomaterials, Elsevier (1984;67B:344)

Duckworth T: Lecture Notes on Orthopaedics and Fractures, Blackwell Scientific Publishers (1980;63B:311)

Dunsker SB, et al (eds): The Unstable Spine (Thoracic, Lumbar and Sacral Regions), Grune & Stratton (1986;68A:798; 69B:515)

°° Duthie RB, Bentley G (eds): Mercer's Orthopaedic Surgery, 2nd ed., Edward Arnold Publishers (1983;66B:152)

Edeiken J: Roentgen Diagnosis of Diseases of Bone, 3rd ed., Williams & Wilkins (1981;64B:512)

Eftekhar NS (ed): Infection in Joint Replacement Surgery: Prevention and Management, CV Mosby (1984;67A:1149; 67B:851)

Eftekhar NS: Principles of total hip arthroplasty, CV Mosby (1978;62A:493; 63B:306)

Egloff DV: Surgery of the Hand: Free Tissue Transfers by Nerve and Vascular Microanastomoses, Editions Medicine et Hygiene (1984;68B:343)

Engel J, Kessler I (eds): The War Injuries of the Upper Extremity, S Karger (1979;61B:525)

Engh CA, Bobyn JD: Biological Fixation in Total Hip Arthroplasty, CB Slack (1985;68B:342)

Enneking WF: Clinical Musculoskeletal Pathology, Slorter Printing Company (1978;60A:869)

Enneking WF: Musculoskeletal Tumor Surgery, Vols. 1 and 2, Churchill Livingstone (New York) (1983;65A:1361; 66B:620)

° Epps CH Jr (ed): Complications in Orthopaedic Surgery, JB Lippincott (1978;61A:478)

Epstein BS: The Vertebral Column (Atlas of Tumor Radiology), Yearbook Medical Publishers (1974;60B:448)

Epstein HC: Traumatic Dislocation of the Hip, Williams & Wilkins (1980;63B:145)

Evans P (ed): The Knee Joint: A Clinical Guide, Churchill Livingstone (Edinburgh) (1986;69B:515)

°° Evarts CM (ed): Surgery of the Musculoskeletal System, Churchill Livingstone (New York) (1983;66A:973; 67B:164)

Fairbank's Atlas of General Affections of the Skeleton, 2nd ed., Churchill Livingstone (Edinburgh) (1976;60B:300)

Farrell J: Illustrated Guide to Orthopedic Nursing, JB Lippincott (1977;60B:449)

° Feldman F (ed): Radiology, Pathology and Immunol-

ogy of Bones and Joints, Appleton-Century-Crofts (1978;63B:309)

Felson B (ed): Roentgenology of Fractures and Dislocations, Grune & Stratton (1978;61A:317)

Ferguson AB Jr: Orthopaedic Surgery in Infancy and Childhood, 5th ed., Williams & Wilkins (1981;64B:652)

Fess EE, Gettle KS, Strickland JW: Hand Splinting, CV Mosby (1981;63A:861; 64B:148)

Ficat RP, Arlet J: Ischemia and Necrosis of Bone, Williams & Wilkins (1980;63A:685; 64B:147)

° Ficat RP, Hungerford DS: Disorders of the Patello-femoral Joint, Williams & Wilkins (1977;60A:1159; 61B:389)

Finlay DBL, Allen MJ: Radiological Diagnosis of Fractures, Bailliére Timbatt (1984;68B:170)

Flatt AE: Care of the Arthritic Hand, 4th ed., CV Mosby (1983;65A:718; 65B:683)

°° Flatt AE: The Care of Congenital Hand Anomalies, Springer-Verlag (1977;60A:278; 61B:131)

Flatt AE: The Care of Minor Hand Injuries, 4th ed., CV Mosby (1979;62A:156; 62B:413)

Flynn JE (ed): Hand Surgery, 3rd ed., Williams & Wilkins (1982;64A:637; 64B:650)

Fogelman I (ed): Bone Scanning in Clinical Practice, Springer-Verlag (1987;69A:637; 69B:859)

°° Forrester DM, Brown JC (eds): Clinics in Rheumatic Diseases, Vol. 9, No. 2: Radiological Investigation in Rheumatology, WB Saunders (1984; 66B: 312)

Forrester DM, Brown JC, Nesson JW: Radiology of Joint Disease, 2nd ed., WB Saunders (1978;61A:637)

Fowles JV: Skeletal Trauma Notes, Williams & Wilkins (1985;68B:514)

Fowles JV: Surgical Anatomy and Pathology for Orthopaedic Surgeons, Williams & Wilkins (1983;66B:156)

Frankel VH, Nordin M (eds): Basic Biomechanics of the Skeletal System, Lea & Febiger (1980;64A:1118)

Freeland AE, Jabaley ME, Hughes JL: Stable Fixation of the Hand and Wrist, Springer-Verlag (1986;69A:1309)

°° Freeman MAR (ed): Adult Articular Cartilage, 2nd ed., Pitman Medical (1979;61B:525)

Freeman MAR (ed): Arthritis of the Knee: Clinical Features and Surgical Management, Sprnger-Verlag (1980;63A:509; 63B:647)

Freiberger RH, Kaye JJ, Spiller J: Arthrography, Appleton-Century-Crofts (1979;63B:146)

Friedlaender GE, Mankin HJ, Sell KW (eds): Osteochondral Allografts: Biology, Banking, and Clini-

cal Applications, JB Lippincott (1984;66A:317; 67B:515)

Galasko CSB: *Skeletal Metastases*, Butterworth (Publishers) (1986;69A:797)

°° Galasko CSB, Weber DA (eds): *Radionuclide Scintigraphy in Orthopaedics*, Churchill Livingstone (Edinburgh) (1984;67A:509; 67B:688)

Galasko CSB (ed): *Principles of Fracture Management*, Churchill Livingstone (Edinburgh) (1984;68B:169)

Gale RP (ed): *Recent Advances in Bone Marrow Transplantation*, Alan R Liss (1983;66B:624)

Gartland JJ: *Fundamentals of Orthopaedics*, 3rd ed., WB Saunders (1979;63A:861)

Gatter R: *A Practical Handbook of Joint Fluid Analysis*, Lea & Febiger (1984;66A:814)

Gehweiler JA Jr, Osborne RE Jr, Becker RF: *Radiology of Vertebral Trauma*, WB Saunders (1980;63A:861)

Gerhardt JJ, King PS, Zettl JH: *Amputations: Immediate and Early Prosthetic Management*, JK Burgess (1982;65A:141; 65B:230)

Gerhart JJ, et al (eds): *Interdisciplinary Rehabilitation in Trauma*, Williams & Wilkins (1987;69A:798)

Gershwin ME, Robbins DL (eds): *Musculoskeletal Diseases of Children*, Grune & · Stratton (1983;67B:164)

Ghadially FN: *Fine Structure of Synovial Joints: A Text and Atlas of the Ultrastructure of Normal and Pathological Articular Tissues*, Butterworth (Publishers) (1983;66B:311)

° Ghista DN (ed): *Osteoarthro-mechanics*, Charles C Thomas (1981;64A:477)

Ghista DN: *Spinal Cord Injury Medical Engineering*, Charles C Thomas (1986;69A:797)

Ghista DN, Roaf R (eds): *Orthopaedic Mechanics*, Academic Press (1978;61B:390)

Ghista DN, Roaf R (eds): *Orthopaedic Mechanics: Procedures and Devices*, Vols. 2 and 3, Academic Press (1981;65B:108)

Goldberg MJ: *The Dysmorphic Child*, Raven Press (1987;69A:1309)

° Golding DN: *Synopsis of Rheumatic Diseases*, 3rd ed., Yearbook Medical Publishers (1979;62A:157)

Goldman AB, Dines D, Warren RF: *Shoulder Arthrography: Technique, Diagnosis, and Clinical Correlations*, JB Lippincott (1982;65A:717)

Goldstein LA, Dickerson RC: *Atlas of Orthopaedic Surgery*, 2nd ed., CV Mosby (1981;64B:388)

Gossling HR, Pillsbury SL (eds): *Complications of Fracture Management*, JB Lippincott (1984;66A:1502)

° Gozna ER, Harrington IJ: *Biomechanics of Musculoskeletal Injury*, Williams & Wilkins (1982;64A:798)

Grana WA (ed): *Update in Arthroscopic Techniques*, Edward Arnold Publishers (1984;67B:343)

Grech P: *Casualty Radiology*, Chapman & Hall (1981;64B:150)

Grech P: *Hip Arthrography*, Chapman & Hall (1977;60B:300)

Green DP (ed): *Operative Hand Surgery*, Vols. 1 and 2, Churchill Livingstone (New York) (1982;65A:142; 65B:527)

Green SA: *Complications of External Skeletal Fixation: Causes, Prevention and Treatment*, Charles C Thomas (1981;65B:528; 64A:797)

Greenfield GB: *Radiology of Bone Diseases*, 3rd ed., JB Lippincott (1980;63A:861)

Grieve GP: *Common Vertebral Joint Problems*, Churchill Livingstone (Edinburgh) (1981; 64B:389)

Gruebel Lee DM: *Disorders of the Hip*, JB Lippincott (1983;65A:1214)

Gustilo RB: *Management of Open Fractures and Their Complications*, WB Saunders (1982;65B:230)

Guyot J: *Atlas of Human Limb Joints*, Sprnger-Verlag (1981;63A:861; 64B:512)

Hackenbroch M, Witt AN (eds): *Atlas of Orthopaedic Operations, Vol. 1: Surgery of the Spine*, WB Saunders (1979;64B:266)

Hajdu SI: *Differential Diagnosis of Soft Tissue and Bone Tumors*, Lea & Febiger (1986;68A:797)

Hajdu SI: *Pathology of Soft Tissue Tumors*, Lea & Febiger (1980;62A:684)

Halford AE (ed): *Clinical Podogeriatrics*, WB Saunders (1981;64A:157)

Hall AJ, Stenner RW: *Manual of Fracture Bracing*, Churchill Livingstone (Edinburgh) (1985;68B:343)

°° Ham AW, Cormack DH: *Histophysiology of Cartilage, Bone, and Joints*, JB Lippincott (1979;62B:415)

Hamdy RC: *Paget's Disease of Bone*, Prager Scientific (1981;64B:147)

Hamilton WC (ed): *Traumatic Disorders of the Ankle*, Springer-Verlag (1984;66A:1150)

Hardy RW (ed): *Seminars in Neurological Surgery: Lumbar Disc Disease*, Raven Press (1982;65B:371)

Harris JD, Copeland K (eds): *Orthopaedic Engineering (Proceedings of the Conference, Oxford, 1977)*, Biological Engineering Society (1978;61B:523)

Harris JH, Harris WH: *The Radiology of Emergency Medicine*, Williams & Wilkins (1981;65B:230)

Harris NH (ed): *Postgraduate Textbook of Clinical*

Orthopaedics, PSG Publishers (**1983;66A:1150; 66B:620**)

Harris WH (ed): *Advanced Concepts in Total Hip Replacement*, CB Slack (**1985;68B:166**)

Hartman JT: *Fracture Management*, Lea & Febiger (**1978;60A:1159**)

Hastings DE: *The Hand: Diagnosis and Indications*, 2nd ed., Churchill Livingstone (New York) (**1984;67A:174**)

Haughton VM, Williams AL: *Computed Tomography of the Spine*, (**1982;64A:958; 65B:371; 66B:793**)

Heim U, Pfeiffer KM: *Small Fragment Set Manual*, Springer-Verlag (**1982;65B:680**)

Helfet AJ: *Disorders of the Knee*, 2nd ed., JB Lippincott (**1982;65A:286; 65B:106**)

Helfet AJ, Lee DMG: *Disorders of the Foot*, JB Lippincott (**1980;62A:1393; 63B:483**)

Helfet AJ, Lee DMG: *Disorders of the Lumbar Spine*, JB Lippincott (**1978;61B:131**)

Hempel D, Fischer S: *Intramedullary Nailing*, Thieme (**1982;65B:680**)

Henche HR: *Arthroscopy of the Knee Joint*, Springer-Verlag (**1980;63B:484**)

Hensinger RN (ed): *Standards in Pediatric Orthopaedics*, Raven Press (**1986;69B:170**)

Heppenstall RB (ed): *Fracture Treatment and Healing*, WB Saunders (**1980;62A:494; 63B:149**)

Hierholzer G, Müller KH (eds): *Corrective Osteotomies of the Lower Extremity after Trauma*, Springer-Verlag (**1985;68A:638; 68B:859**)

Hierholzer G, Rüedi Th, Allgöwer M, Schatzker J: *Manual on the AO/ASIF Tubular External Fixator*, Springer-Verlag (**1985;67B:852**)

Hirohata K, Morimoto K, Kimura H: *Ultrastructure of Bone and Joint Diseases*, 2nd ed., Igaku-Shoin (**1981;64A:478**)

Hollingsworth JW: *Management of Rheumatoid Arthritis and Its Complications*, Year Book Medical Publishers (**1978;60A:1014**)

Holt PJL (ed): *Clinics in rheumatic diseases, Vol. 7, No. 3: Endocrine and Metabolic Aspects of Rheumatic Disease*, WB Saunders (**1981;65B:231**)

Hooper G: *A Colour Atlas of Minor Operations on the Hand*, Wolfe Medical Publications (**1985;68B:171**)

Hoppenfield S, deBoer P: *Surgical Exposures in Orthopaedics: The Anatomic Approach*, JB Lippincott (**1984;66A:1502; 67B:513**)

Horan F, Beighton P: *Orthopaedic Problems in Inherited Skeletal Disorders*, Springer-Verlag (**1982;64B:651**)

Houghton GR, Thompson GH (eds): *Problematic Musculoskeletal Injuries in Children*, Butterworth (Publishers) (**1983;66B:465**)

Howorth B, Bender F: *A Doctor's Answer to Tennis Elbow — How to Cure It — How to Prevent It*, Chelsea House (**1977;60A:869**)

Huckstep RL: *A Simple Guide to Trauma*, 2nd ed., Churchill Livingstone (Edinburgh) (**1978;61B:264; 65B:372**)

Hueston JT, Tubiana R (eds): *Dupuytren's Disease*, 2nd ed., Churchill Livingstone (Edinburgh) (**1986;69B:514**)

° Hughes S (ed): *The Basis and Practice of Traumatology*, William Heinemann (**1983;65B:681**)

° Hughes S, Sweetnam R (eds): *The Basis and Practice of Orthopaedics*, William Heinemann (**1980;63B:649**)

Hughes SPF, Fitzgerald RH Jr (eds): *Musculoskeletal Infections*, Year Book Medical Publishers (**1986;69B:514**)

Hughes SPF (ed): *Current Operative Surgery: Orthopaedics and Trauma*, WB Saunders (**1985;68A:1134; 68B:514**)

Hughston JC, Walsh WM, Puddu G: *Patellar Subluxation and Dislocation (Saunders Monographs in Clinical Orthopaedics, Vol. 5)*, WB Saunders (**1984;66A:974; 67B:168**)

Hungerford DS, Krackow KA, Kenna RV (eds): *Total Knee Arthroplasty: A Comprehensive Approach*, Williams & Wilkins (**1984;66A:973, 1495**, correspondence; **67B:343**)

Hunter JM, et al (eds): *Tendon Surgery in the Hand*, CV Mosby (**1987;69A:798**)

Hunter JM, Schneider LH, Mackin EJ, Callahan AD (eds): *Rehabilitation of the Hand*, 2nd ed., CV Mosby (**1984;67B:342**)

Hunter LY, Funk FJ (eds): *Rehabilitation of the Injured Knee*, CV Mosby (**1984;67A:669; 68B:167**)

Huvos AG: *Bone Tumors*, WB Saunders (**1979;62A:157**)

Imhauser G: *The Idiopathic Clubfoot and Its Treatment*, Thieme (**1986;69A:158**)

°° Inman VT: *The Joints of the Ankle*, Williams & Wilkins (**1976;60A:141**)

°° Inman VT, Ralston HJ, Todd F: *Human Walking*, Williams & Wilkins (**1981;63A:1038; 64B:148**)

Insall JN (ed): *Surgery of the Knee*, Churchill Livingstone (New York) (**1984;66A:812; 67B:169**)

Institution of Mechanical Engineers and British Orthopaedic Association: *Engineering Aspects of the Spine* (papers read at the conference, 1980), Mechanical Engineering Publications (**1980; 63B:311**)

Jackson DW, Drez D Jr (eds): *The Anterior Cruciate Deficient Knee: New Concepts in Ligament Repair*, CV Mosby (**1987;69A:1118**)

Jackson JP, Waugh W (eds): *Surgery of the Knee Joint*, Chapman & Hall (**1984;66B:796; 67A:174**)

Jaffe N (ed): *Bone Tumors in Children*, PSG Publishing (**1979;62A:685**)

Jahss MH: *Disorders of the Foot*, Vols. 1 and 2, WB Saunders (**1982;65B:106**)

James CCM, Lassman LP: *Spina Bifida Occulta*, Grune & Stratton (**1981;64A:478; 64B:513**)

Jayson MIV (ed): *The Lumbar Spine and Back Pain*, 2nd ed., Pitman Medical (**1980;63B:310**)

Jeffreys E: *Disorders of the Cervical Spine*, Butterworth (Publishers) (**1980;62B:538**)

Jenkins DHR (ed): *Ligament Injuries and Their Treatment*, Chapman & Hall (**1985;68B:688**)

Jenkins DAR et al: *Manual of Spinal Surgery*, Butterworth (Publishers) (**1981;64A:798**)

° Jewett DL, McCarroll HR Jr (eds): *Nerve Repair and Regeneration*, CV Mosby (**1980;62A:1230**)

Johnson LL: *Comprehensive Arthroscopic Examination of the Knee*, CV Mosby (**1977;60A:869; 61B:262**)

Johnson LL: *Diagnostic and Surgical Arthroscopy*, 2nd ed., CV Mosby (**1981;64A:1118; 64B:147**)

Johnson RM (ed): *Advances in External Fixation*, Yearbook Medical Publishers (**1980;63B:651**)

°° Jowsey J: *Metabolic Disease of Bone*, WB Saunders (**1977;61B:262**)

Kane WJ (ed): *Current Orthopaedic Management*, Churchill Livingstone (New York) (**1981;64B:149**)

Kassity KJ, McKittrick JE, Preston FW (eds): *Manual of Ambulatory Surgery*, Springer-Verlag (**1982;66B:153**)

Katz JF: *Common Orthopedic Problems in Children*, Raven Press (**1981;64B:515**)

Katz JF: *Legg-Calvé-Perthes Disease*, Prager Scientific (**1984;67B:516**)

Katz JF, Siffert RS (eds): *Management of Hip Disorders in Children*, JB Lippincott (**1984;66B:795**)

Katznelson A, Nerubay J (eds): *Progress in Clinical and Biological Research, Vol. 99: Osteosarcoma, New Trends in Diagnosis and Treatment*, Alan R Liss (**1982;65B:682**)

Kay NRM: *Complications of Total Joint Replacement*, Springer-Verlag (**1985;68B:859**)

Keats TE: *Atlas of Normal Roentgen Variants that May Simulate Disease*, 3rd ed., Year Book Medical Publishers (**1984;66A:1502**)

Keim HA: *The Adolescent Spine*, 2nd ed., Springer-Verlag (**1982;65B:679**)

Kelikian H, Kelikian AS: *Disorders of the Ankle*, WB Saunders (**1985;68B:168**)

°° Kelley WN, Harris ED Jr, Ruddy S, Sledge CB (eds): *Textbook of Rheumatology*, 2nd ed., WB Saunders (**1985;68B:513**)

Kelsey JL: *Epidemiology of Musculoskeletal Disorders*, Oxford University Press (**1982;65A:717**)

Kennedy JC (ed): *The Injured Adolescent Knee*, Williams & Wilkins (**1979;61A:956; 62B:138**)

Kessel L: *Clinical Disorders of the Shoulder*, Churchill Livingstone (Edinburgh) (**1982; 64B:514; 65A:286**)

Kessel L, Boundy U: *Colour Atlas of Clinical Orthopaedics*, Wolfe Medical Publications (**1980;63B:307**)

Kieffer SA, Heitzman ER (eds): *Atlas of Cross-sectional Anatomy*, Harper & Row (Hagerstown MD) (**1979;61A:958**)

Kiene RH, Johnson KA (eds): *Symposium on the Foot and Ankle*, CV Mosby (**1983;65A:1036**)

Kilgore ES Jr, Graham WP III (eds): *The Hand: Surgical and Non-surgical Management*, Lea & Febiger (**1977;60A:573; 60B:590**

Kirby NG, Blackburn G (eds): *Field Surgery Pocket Book*, Her Majesties Stationery Office (**1981;64B:268**)

Kirkaldy-Willis WH: *Managing Low Back Pain*, Churchill Livingstone (New York) (**1983; 66A:318; 66B:624**)

Klenerman L (ed): *The Foot and Its Disorders*. 2nd ed., Butterworth (Publishers) (**1982;65A:1360; 66B:311**)

Kostuik JP, Gillespie R (eds): *Amputation Surgery and Rehabilitation: The Toronto Experience*, Churchill Livingstone (New York) (**1981; 64B:651**)

Kozak GP, Hoar CS Jr, Rowbotham JL, et al (eds): *Management of Diabetic Foot Problems*, WB Saunders (**1984;67B:514**)

Krakauer LJ, et al (eds): *1985 Year Book of Sports Medicine*, Blackwell Scientific Publishers (**1986;68B:516**)

Kricun R, Kricun ME: *Computed Tomography of the Spine: Diagnostic Exercises*, Aspen Publishers (**1987;69A:797**)

Kulund DN: *The Injured Athlete*, JB Lippincott (**1982;65A:718**)

Lamb DW: *A Colour Atlas of the Surgery of Flexor Tendon Injuries of the Hand*, Wolfe Medical Publications (**1984;67B:688**)

Lamb DW (ed): *The Paralysed Hand*, Churchill Livingstone (Edinburgh) (**1987;69A:958**)

Lamb DW, Kuczynski K (eds): *The Practice of Hand Surgery*, Blackwell Scientific Publishers (**1981;64A:797; 64B:390**)

Laskin RS, Denham RA, Apley AG: *Replacement of the Knee*, Springer-Verlag (**1984;67A:350; 67B:686**)

Leach RE, Hoaglund FT, Riseborough EJ: *Controversies in Orthopaedic Surgery, WB Saunders (1982;64A:1407)

Lee AJC, et al (eds): Advances in Biomaterials, Vol. 4: Clinical Applications of Biomaterials, J Wiley & Sons (1982;65B:370)

Lee DMG, Hirsch DM: Disorders of the Hip, Lea & Febiger (1983;66B:795)

Leffert RD: Brachial Plexus Injuries, Churchill Livingstone (New York) (1985;68A:1310; 68B:859)

Letournel E, Judet R: Fractures of the Acetabulum, Springer-Verlag (1981;64A:1406; 64B:648)

Levin ME, O'Neal LW (eds): The Diabetic Foot, CV Mosby (1977;60A:277)

Levy SW: Skin Problems of the Amputee, Warren H Green (1983;66A:638)

Lewis RC Jr: Handbook of Traction, Casting and Splinting Techniques, JB Lippincott (1977;60A:422)

Lichtenstein L: Bone Tumors, 5th ed., CV Mosby (1977;60A:574; 60B:448)

Ling RSM (ed): Complications of Total Hip Replacement, Churchill Livingstone (Edinburgh) (1984;67B:687)

Lippert FG III, Farmer JA (eds): Psychomotor Skills in Orthopaedic Surgery, Williams & Wilkins (1984;67A:669; 67B:513)

Lister G: The Hand: Diagnosis and Indications, 2nd ed., Churchill Livingstone (Edinburgh) (1984;67B:169)

Lloyd-Roberts GC, Ratliff AHC: Hip Disorders in Children, Butterworth (Publishers) (1978;60A:1158; 61B:264)

Loach A: Anaesthesia for Orthopaedic Patients, Edward Arnold Publishers (1983;66B:464)

Louis R: Surgery of the Spine: Surgical Anatomy and Operative Approaches, Springer-Verlag (1983;65A:1360)

Lovell W, Winter RB (eds): Pediatric Orthopaedics, 2nd ed. Vols. 1 and 2, JB Lippincott (1986;68A:1133)

Lusted LB, Keats TE: Atlas of Roentgenographic Measurement, 4th ed., Year Book Medical Publishers (1978;61A:317)

Maatz R, et al (eds): Intramedullary Nailing and Other Intramedullary Osteosyntheses, WB Saunders (1986;69A:317; 69B:515)

Machleder HI (ed): Vascular Disorders of the Upper Extremity, Futura (1983;66B:468)

Macnab I: Backache, Williams & Wilkins (1977;60A:422; 60B:299)

Macnicol MF: Aids to Orthopaedics, Churchill Livingstone (Edinburgh) (1984;67B:688)

Macnicol MF, Lamb DW: Basic Care of the Injured Hand, Churchill Livingstone (Edinburgh) (1984;67B:515)

Maitland GD: Vertebral Manipulation, 4th ed., Butterworth (Publishers) (1977;60B:148)

Malluche HH, Faugere MC: Atlas of Mineralised Bone Histology, S Karger (1986;69A:317)

Mann RA (ed): Surgery of the Foot, 5th ed., CV Mosby (1986;69B:171)

Maquet PGJ: Biomechanics of the Hip: As Applied to Osteoarthritis and Related Conditions, Springer-Verlag (1985;68B:166)

Maquet PGJ: Biomechanics of the Knee: With Application to the Pathogenesis and the Surgical Treatment of Osteoarthritis, 2nd ed., Springer-Verlag (1984;66A:478)

Marcove RC: The Surgery of Tumors of Bone and Cartilage, 2nd ed., Grune & Stratton (1984;67A:829)

Marcus RE (ed): Trauma in Children, Aspen Publishers (1986;69A:638)

Marcus SA, Block BH (eds): Complications in Foot Surgery: Prevention and Management, 2nd ed., Williams & Wilkins (1984;67B:514)

°° Mason JK (ed): Pathology of Violent Injury, Yearbook Medical Publishers (1978;61A:318)

Matev IB: Reconstructive Surgery of the Thumb, Pilgrims Press (1983;66B:623)

Mathes SJ, Nahai F (eds): Clinical Applications for Muscle and Musculocutaneous Flaps, CV Mosby (1982;65A:430; 65B:682)

Matter P, Rittmann WW: The Open Fracture, Yearbook Medical Publishers (1978;62A:493)

Mattingly S (ed): Rehabilitation Today, Update Publishers Limited (1977;60B:450)

May HL (ed): Emergency Medicine, J Wiley & Sons (1984;67B:166)

°° McCarty DJ (ed): Arthritis and Allied Conditions, 9th ed., Lea & Febiger (1979;62A:157)

McCulloch JA, Macnab I: Sciatica and Chymopapain, Williams & Wilkins (1983;66A:156; 67B:168)

McDougall DJ: A Handbook of Experiences with the Application of Wrist, Hand and Finger Orthoses, Dundee Royal Infirmary (1986;68B:516)

McGraw JB, Arnold PG: McGraw and Arnold's Atlas of Muscle and Musculocutaneous Flaps, Hampton Press (1986;69A:477)

McGregor IA: Fundamental Techniques of Plastic Surgery and Their Surgical Applications, 7th ed., Churchill Livingstone (Edinburgh) (1980; 63B:149)

McKibbin B (ed): Recent Advances in Orthopaedics, No. 3 (1979;62B:538; 63A:174. No. 4, Churchill Livingstone (Edinburgh) (1983;66B:619)

McMaster JH: The ABC's of Sports Medicine, S Karger (1982;65A:142; 65B:372)

McMinn RMH: *A Colour Atlas of Applied Anatomy,* Wolfe Medical Publicatons (**1984;67B:341**)

McMinn RMH, Hutchings RT, Logan BM: *A Colour Atlas of Foot and Ankle Anatomy,* Wolfe Medical Publications (**1982;65B:232**)

McRae R: *Clinical Orthopaedic Examination,* 2nd ed., Churchill Livingstone (Edinburgh) (**1984;66B:155**)

McRae R: *Practical Fracture Treatment,* Churchill Livingstone (Edinburgh) (**1981;64B:514**)

Meals RA, Lesavoy MA: *Hand Surgery Review,* Williams & Wilkins (**1981;65A:717**)

Mears DC: *External Skeletal Fixation,* Williams & Wilkins (**1983;65A:1214; 66B:309**)

Mears DC, Rubash HE: *Pelvic and Acetabular Fractures,* CB Slack (**1986;68A:1310**)

Menelaus M: *The Orthopaedic Management of Spina Bifida Cystica,* 2nd ed., Churchill Livingstone (Edinburgh) (**1980;62B:539**)

Meisel AD, Bullough PG: *Atlas of Osteoarthritis,* Lea & Febiger (**1984;67A:989**)

Meyers MH: *Fractures of the Hip,* Yearbook Medical Publishers (**1985;68A:478; 68B:516**)

Meyers MH (ed): *The Multiply Injured Patient with Complex Fractures,* Lea & Febiger (**1984;66A:1325; 67B:166**)

Micheli LJ (ed): *Pediatric and Adolescent Sports Medicine,* JB Lippincott (**1984;66A:813; 67B:172**)

Milford L: *The Hand,* 2nd ed., CV Mosby (**1984;66B:156**)

Mills KLG: *Guide to Orthopaedics, Vol 1: Trauma,* Churchill Livingstone (Edinburgh (**1981;64B:149**)

Mirra JM: *Bone Tumors: Diagnosis and Treatment,* JB Lippincott (**1980;63A:685; 63B:308**)

Mittelbach HR: *The Injured Hand: A Clinical Handbook for General Surgeons,* Springer-Verlag (**1979;62A:684**)

Moberg E: *The Upper Limb in Tetraplegia,* Thieme (**1978;61B:525**)

Moberg E: *The Upper Limb in Tetraplegia,* Thieme (**1978; 61B:525**)

Moe JH et al: *Scoliosis and Other Spinal Deformities,* WB Saunders (**1978;60A:868; 61B:263**)

Moll JMH (ed): *Ankylosing Spondylitis,* Churchill Livingstone (Edinburgh) (**1980;63B:651**)

Moll JMH: *Management of Rheumatic Disorders,* Chapman & Hall (**1983;67B:170**)

Moore KL: *Clinically Oriented Anatomy,* Williams & Wilkins (**1980;64B:268**)

Morrey F: *The Elbow and Its Disorders,* WB Saunders (**1985;69A:318**)

Morscher E (ed): *Cementless Fixation of Hip Endoprostheses,* Springer-Verlag (**1984;66A:813**)

Motamed HA: *Anatomy, Radiology and Kinesiology of Hand-Unit,* 2nd ed., Motamed Medical Publishing (**1982;65B:372**)

Motamed HA: *Surgery of Hand-Unit in Adults and Children,* Privately Published (**1979;62A:684; 62B:539**)

Mubarak SJ, Hargens AR: *Compartment Syndromes and Volkmann's Contracture,* WB Saunders (**1981;64A:798; 64B:389**)

Muckle DS: *Injuries in Sport,* 2nd ed., PSG Publishers (**1982;64B:515**)

Muckle DS: *An Outline of Fractures and Dislocations* Churchill Livingstone (Edinburgh) (**1985;68B:343**)

Muckle DS (ed): *Femoral Neck Fractures and Hip Joint Injuries,* Chapman & Hall (**1977;60B:448**)

Müller ME, et al: *Manual of Internal Fixation,* 2nd ed., Springer-Verlag (**1979;62A:862**)

Müller W: *The Knee: Form, Function and Ligament Reconstruction,* Springer-Verlag (**1983;65A:1037; 66B:311**)

Nakano KK: *Neurology of Musculoskeletal and Rheumatic Disorders,* Houghton Mifflin (**1979;61A:637**)

Nance EP Jr, Heller RM, Kirchner SG, Kaye JJ: *Advanced Exercises in Diagnostic Radiology, Vol. 17: Emergency Radiology of the Pelvis and Lower Extremity,* WB Saunders (**1983;67B:344**)

Napier J: *Hands,* George Allen & Unwin (**1980;63B:307**)

Newton TH, Pitts DG (eds): *Computed Tomography of the Spine and Spinal Cord,* Clavadel (**1983;66A:478; 66B:793**)

°° Nickel VL (ed): *Orthopaedic Rehabilitation,* Churchill Livingstone (New York) (**1982;65A:572; 65B:683**)

Nicolle FV, Dickson RA: *Surgery of the Rheumatoid Hand,* William Heinemann (**1979;62B:413**)

Nixon HH, Waterston D, Wink CAS (eds): *Selected Writings of Sir Dennis Browne,* The Trustees of the Sir Dennis Browns Memorial Fund (**1983;66B:624**)

Nordin BEC (ed): *Metabolic Bone and Stone Disease,* 2nd ed. Churchill Livingstone (Edinburgh) (**1984;67B:171**)

Norkin CC, White DJ: *Measurement of Joint Motion: A Guide to Goniometry,* FA Davis Company (**1985;68B:172**)

Nursing Photobook Series: Working with Orthopaedic Patients, Intermed Communications (**1982;65A:142**)

O'Brien BMcC: *Microvascular Reconstructive Surgery,* Churchill Livingstone (Edinburgh) (**1977;60A:573; 60B:148**)

Oestrich AE, Crawford AH: *Atlas of Pediatric Orthopaedic Surgery*, Thieme (1985;68A:798)

Ogden J: *Pocket Guide to Pediatric Fractures*, Williams & Wilkins (1987;69A:1118)

Ogden JA: *Skeletal Injury in the Child*, Lea & Febiger (1982;64A:1407; 65B:525)

Ogilvie-Harris DJ, Lloyd GJ (eds): *Personal Injury* Churchill Livingstone (Edinburgh) (1986;69B: 688)

Omer GE Jr, Spinner M: *Management of Peripheral Nerve Problems*, WB Saunders (1980;63B:308)

Ortner DJ, Putschar WGJ: *Identification of Pathological Conditions in Human Skeletal Remains*, Smithsonian Institution Press (1981;65B:231)

Owen R, Goodfellow J, Bullough (eds): *Scientific Foundations of Orthopaedics and Traumatology*, William Heinemann (1980;63B:482)

Owen-Smith MS: *High Velocity Missile Wounds*, Edward Arnold Publishers (1981;63B:650)

Panayi GS, Johnson PM (eds): *Immunopathogenesis of Rheumatoid Arthritis*, Reed Books (1979;62B:288)

Pandey S: *Intra-articular & Allied Injections*, WB Saunders (1982;66B:468)

Panush RS (ed): *Principles of Rheumatic Diseases*, J Wiley & Sons (1981;65B:107)

Park JB: *Biomaterials: An Introduction*, Plenum Press (1979;61A:957)

Parsons V: *Colour Atlas of Bone Disease*, Wolfe Medical Publications (1980;63B:307)

Paterson CR, MacLennan WJ: *Bone Disease in the Elderly*, J Wiley & Sons (1984;67B:516)

Paterson JK, Burn L: *An Introduction to Medical Manipulation*, MTP Press (1985;68B:169)

Pauwels EKJ, Schütte HE, Taconis WK (eds): *Bone Scintigraphy*, Leiden University Press (1981;64B:512)

Pauwels F: *Biomechanics of the Locomotor Apparatus*, Springer-Verlag (1980;64B:392)

Pavlov H, Ghelman B, Vigorita VJ: *Atlas of Knee Menisci: An Arthrographic-Pathologic Correlation*, Appleton-Century-Crofts (1983;66B:795)

Pearce GH: *The Medical Report and Testimony*, Beacons Field Publications (1979;62B:539)

Pearson JR, Austin RT: *Accident Surgery and Orthopaedics for Students*, 2nd ed., Lloyd Luke Medical Books (1979;62B:414)

Perren SM, Schneider E (eds): *Biomechanics: Current Interdisciplinary Research*, Martinus Nijhoff (1985;68B:515)

Pettersson H, Gilbert MS: *Diagnostic Imaging in Haemophilia: Musculoskeletal and Other Hemorrhagic Complications*, Springer-Verlag (1985; 68B:172)

Pettersson H, Harwood-Nash DCF: *CT and Myelography of the Spine and Cord: Techniques, Anatomy and Pathology in Children*, Springer-Verlag (1982;65A:717)

Pickett JC, Radin EL (eds): *Chondromalacia of the Patella*, Williams & Wilkins (1983;67B: 687)

Pierre M (ed): *The Nail*, Churchill Livingstone (Edinburgh) (1981;64B:515)

Pope MH, Frymoyer JW, Andersson G (eds): *Occupational Low Back Pain*, Praeger (1984;67A:990; 68B:169)

Porter RW: *Management of Back Pain*, Churchill Livingstone (Edinburgh) (1986;69B:515)

Porter RW: *Understanding Back Pain*, Churchill Livingstone (Edinburgh) (1983;66B:467)

Post M: *Physical Examination of the Musculoskeletal System*, Churchill Livingstone (Edinburgh) (1987;69A:798)

Post M (ed): *The Shoulder*, Lea & Febiger (1978;61A:477; 62B:287)

Post MJD (ed): *Computed Tomography of the Spine*, Williams & Wilkins (1984;67B:341)

Powell M (ed): *Orthopaedic Nursing and Rehabilitation*, 9th ed., Churchill Livingstone (Edinburgh) (1986;69B:170)

Poznanski AK: *The Hand in Radiologic Diagnosis*, 2nd ed., WB Saunders (1984;66A:1326)

Proctor H, London PS: *Principles of First Aid for the Injured*, 3rd ed., Butterworth (Publishers) (1977;60B:148)

Rainniger K (ed): *Encyclopedia of Medical Radiology*, Vol. 5, Part 6: (Bone Tumors), Springer-Verlag (1977;60A:573)

Ranawat CS (ed): *Total-Condylar Knee Arthroplasty: Technique, Results, and Complications*, Springer-Verlag (1985;68A:957; 68B:687)

Rang M (ed): *Children's Fractures* 2nd ed., JB Lippincott (1982;65A:718; 66B:464)

Regazzoni P, Rüedi Th, Winquist R, Allgöwer M: *The Dynamic Hip Screw Implant System*, Springer-Verlag (1985;68B:172)

Regnauld B: *The Foot*, Springer-Verlag (1986; 69B:514)

Reid DAC, Gosset J (eds): *Mutilating Injuries of the Hand*, Butterworth (Publishers) (1979;61B: 524)

Reid DAC, McGrouther DA: *Surgery of the Thumb*, Butterworth(1986;68A:797)

Reid DAC, Tubiana R (eds): *Mutilating Injuries of the Hand*, 2nd ed., Churchill Livingstone (Edinburgh) (1984;67A:350; 67B:342)

Reid SE, Reid SE Jr: *Head and Neck Injuries in Sport*, Charles C Thomas (1984;67A:510)

Reilly T (ed): *Sports Fitness and Sports Injuries*, Faber & Faber (1981;63B:650)

Resnick D, Niwayama G (eds): *Diagnosis of Bone and Joint Disorders*, WB Saunders (1981;64A:157)

Revell PA: *Pathology of Bone*, Springer-Verlag (1986;68A:638; 68B:687)

Ritter MA, Gosling C: *The Knee: A Guide to the Examination and Diagnosis of Ligament Injuries*, Charles C Thomas (1979;61A:478)

° Roaf R: *Posture*, JB Lippincott (1977;60A:869; 60B:591)

Roaf R: *Spinal Deformities*, (1977;60A:278; 60B:147. 2nd ed., 1980;63B:484)

Roaf R, Hodkinson LJ: *The Paralysed Patient*, JB Lippincott (1977;60A:277)

Roaf R, Hodkinson LJ: *Textbook of Orthopaedic Nursing*, 3rd ed., Blackwell Scientific Publishers (1980;63B:148)

Rob C, Smith Sir R (gen eds): *Operative Surgery*, 3rd ed. *Accident Surgery*, Butterworth (Publishers) edited by PS London (1978;61B:389). *The Hand*, edited by RG Pulvertaft (1977; 60B:148). *Orthopaedics*, edited by G Bentley (1979;62A:318; 62B:288)

Robertson E: *Rehabilitation of Arm Amputees and Limb-Deficient Children*, Balliére Timball (1978;61B:391)

Robin GC, Makin M, Steinberg R (eds): *Osteoporosis*, J Wiley & Sons (1983;66A:156)

°°° Rockwood CA, et al (eds): *Fractures*, 2nd ed., JB Lippincott (1984;68A:158)

°° Rodrigo JP: *Orthopaedic Surgery: Basic Science and Clinical Science*, JB Lippincott (1985;68A:957; 69B:170)

Rogers LF (ed): *Radiology of Skeletal Trauma*, Vols. 1 and 2, Churchill Livingstone (New York) (1982;65A:430; 65B:681)

Roo T de, Schroder HJ: *Pocket Atlas of Skeletal Age*, Williams & Wilkins (1977;60A:142)

° Root MI, Orien WP, Weed JH: *Clinical Biomechanics, Vol. 2: Normal and Abnormal Function of the Foot*, Clinical Biomechanicals (1977;60A:868)

Rothman RH, Simeone FA (eds): *The Spine*, Vols. 1 and 2, 2nd ed., WB Saunders (1982;65B:526)

Rothschild BM: *Rheumatology: A Primary Care Approach*, Yorke Medical Books (1982;66B:621)

Rowe JW, Dyer L (eds): *Care of the Orthopaedic Patient*, Blackwell Scientific Publishers (1977;60B:449)

Rüedi T, von Hochstetter A, Schlumpf R: *Surgical Approaches for Internal Fixation*, Springer-Verlag (1984;66A:638)

Rütt A, Hackenbroch M, Witt AN (eds): *Atlas of Or-thopaedic Operations, Vol. 2: Surgery of the Lower Leg and Foot*, WB Saunders (1980;64A:477)

Rushton N, Greatorex RA, Broughton NS: *Colour Atlas of Surgical Exposures of the Limbs*, Edward Arnold Publishers (1985;68B:168)

Rutherford WH et al (eds): *Accident and Emergency Medicine*, Pitman Medical (1980;62B:538)

Ryan JR: *Orthopaedic Surgery*, Henry Kimpton (1977;61B:131)

Saha AK: *Recurrent Dislocation of the Shoulder: Physiopathology and Operative Corrections*, 2nd ed., Thieme (1981;66B:312)

Salter RB: *Textbook of Disorders and Injuries of the Musculoskeletal System*, 2nd ed., Williams & Wilkins (1983;66A:157; 66B:620)

Samilson RL (ed): *Orthopaedic Aspects of Cerebral Palsy*, JB Lippincott (1975;60B:147)

Sanders GT: *Lower Limb Amputations: A Guide to Rehabilitation*, FA Davis Company (1985;68A:958; 69B:171)

Sandzén SC Jr: *Atlas of Wrist and Hand Fractures*, 2nd ed., PSGB Publishing (1986;68A:1133; 69B:170)

Sandzén SC Jr (ed): *Current Management of Complications in Orthopaedics*, Williams & Wilkins (1985;68A:157)

Sandzén SC Jr (ed): *The Hand and Wrist*, Williams & Wilkins (1985;68B:515)

Sanerkin NG, Jeffree GM: *Cytology of Bone Tumours*, John Wright & Sons (1980;63B:652)

Sarmiento A, Latta LL: *Closed Functional Treatment of Fractures*, Springer-Verlag (1981;64B:388)

Sarrafian SK: *Anatomy of the Foot and Ankle: Descriptive, Topographic, Functional*, JB Lippincott (1983;65A:1361; 66B:796)

Savastano AA (ed): *Total Knee Replacement*, Appleton-Century-Crofts (1980;62A:1229; 63B:648)

Schafer MF, Dias LS: *Myelomeningocele: Orthopaedic Treatment*, Williams & Wilkins (1983;66B:794)

Schajowicz F: *Tumors and Tumorlike Lesions of Bones and Joints*, Springer-Verlag (1981;63A:1357; 64B:512)

Schatzker J (ed): *The Intertrochanteric Osteotomy*, Springer-Verlag (1984;67A:509; 68B:687)

Schauwecker F: *Practice of Osteosynthesis: Primary Care. An Accident Surgery Atlas — Ligaments, Joints, Bones*, 2nd ed., Thieme (1982;65A:572)

Schneider FR: *Orthopaedics in Emergency Care*, CV Mosby (1980;63A:174; 63B:650)

Schneider LH: *Flexor Tendon Injuries*, CV Mosby (1985;67A:1149)

Schneider RC, Kennedy JC, Plant ML (eds): *Sports Injuries*, Williams & Wilkins (1986;69B:171)

Schnitzlein HN, Murtagh FR: *Imaging Anatomy of*

the Head and Spine: A Photographic Color Atlas of MRI, CT, Gross and Microscopic Anatomy in Axial, Coronal, and Sagittal Planes, Urban & Schwarzenberg (1985;68A:157)

Schramm J, Jones SJ (eds): *Spinal Cord Monitoring*, Springer-Verlag (1985;68A:957)

Schultz KP, Krahl H, Stein WH (eds): *Late Reconstructions of Injured Ligaments of the Knee*, Springer-Verlag (1978;61A:958; 62B:138)

° Scoles PV: *Pediatric Orthopaedics in Clinical Practice*, Yearbook Medical Publishers (1982;65A:141)

°° Scott JT (ed): *Copeman's Textbook of the Rheumatic Diseases*, 6th ed., Churchill Livingstone (Edinburgh) (1986;69B:859)

Scott WN, Nisonson B, Nicholas JA (eds): *Principles of Sports Medicine*, Williams & Wilkins (1984;67A:829; 67B:851)

Sculco TP (ed): *Orthopaedic Care of the Geriatric Patient*, Williams & Wilkins (1985;67A:989)

Segal P, Jacob M: *The Knee*, Wolfe Medical Publishers (1984;68B:167)

Segelov PM (ed): *Manual of Emergency Orthopaedics*, Churchill Livingstone (Edinburgh) (1986;69B:688)

Seimon LP: *Low Back Pain: Clinical Diagnosis and Management*, Appleton-Century-Crofts (1983;66A:477, 1144 correspondence; 67B:168)

Selecki BR (ed): *Low Back Disability*, Australasian Medical Publishing (1978;60A:1159; 61B:523)

° Seligson D (ed): *Concepts in Intramedullary Nailing*, Grune & Stratton (1985;67A:1455)

° Seligson D, Pope M: *Concepts in External Fixation*, Grune & Stratton (1982;65B:108)

Semple C: *Primary Management of Hand Injuries*, Pitman Medical (1979;63B:308)

Serafin D, Buncke HJ Jr (eds): *Microsurgical Composite Tissue Transplantation*, CV Mosby (1979;61A:1263)

Sevastik J, Goldie I (eds): *The Young Patient with Degenerative Hip Disease*, Almquist & Wiksell (1985;68A:1309; 69B:171)

°° Sevitt S: *Bone Repair and Fracture Healing in Man*, Churchill Livingstone (New York) (1981;63B:483)

Shahriaree H (ed): *O'Connor's Textbook of Arthroscopic Surgery*, JB Lippincott (1983;66A:1326; 67B:169)

Shapiro R: *Myelography*, 4th ed., Yearbook Medical Publishers (1984;66A:974)

°° Sharnoff JG: *Prevention of Venous Thrombosis and Pulmonary Embolism*, MTP Press (1980;63B:309)

Sharrard WJW: *Paediatric Orthopaedics and Fractures*, 2nd ed., Blackwell Scientific Publishers (1979;62A:1230; 62B:287)

Sheon RP, Moskowitz RW, Goldberg VM: *Soft Tissue Rheumatic Pain*, Lea & Febiger (1982;64A:1118)

Shields CL Jr (ed): *Manual of Sports Surgery*, Springer-Verlag (1987;69A:958)

Shizhen Z, Yongjian H, Wenchum Y (eds): *Microsurgical Anatomy*, MTP Press (1985;68B:860)

Siegel IM: *Clinical Management of Muscle Disease*, CV Mosby (1977;60A:141)

Silber SJ (ed): *Microsurgery*, Williams & Wilkins (1979;63B:148; 68B:344)

Sim FH: *Diagnosis and Treatment of Bone Tumors: A Team Approach. A Mayo Clinic Monograph*, Charles C Thomas (1983;65A:878)

Simmons DJ, Kunin AS (eds): *Skeletal Research: An Experimental Approach*, Academic Press (1979;63B:145)

Simon WH (ed): *The Human Joint in Health and Disease*, Pendragon Press (1978;61B:390)

Sissons HA, Murray RO, Kemp HBS: *Orthopaedic Diagnosis: Clinical, Radiological, and Pathological Coordinates*, Springer-Verlag (1984;67A:989; 67B:512)

Smillie IS: *A Colour Atlas of Traditional Meniscectomy*, Wolfe Medical Publications (1983;66B:467)

Smillie IS: *Diseases of the Knee Joint*, 2nd ed., Churchill Livingstone (Edinburgh) (1980;63A:509)

Smillie IS: *Injuries of the Knee Joint*, 5th ed., Churchill Livingstone (Edinburgh) (1978;61A:956; 61B:526)

Smith NJ (ed): *Sports Medicine: Health Care for Young Athletes*, Butterworth (Publishers) (1983;66A:813)

Smith R: *Biochemical Disorders of the Skeleton*, Butterworth (Publishers) (1979;62B:137)

Smith R, Francis MJO, Houghton GR: *The Brittle Bone Syndrome: Osteogenesis Imperfecta*, Butterworth (Publishers) (1983;66A:156; 66B:465)

Soeur R: *Fractures of the Limbs: The Relationship Between Mechanism and Treatment*, Charles C Thomas (1981;64A:573; 64B:648)

Sokoloff L (ed): *Clinics in Rheumatic Diseases*, WB Saunders (1986;68B:688)

Sokoloff L (ed): *The Joints and Synovial Fluid*, Vol. 1, Academic Press (1978;63B:146). Vol. 2, Academic Press (1980;63B:310)

Somerville EW: *Displacement of the Hip in Childhood*, Springer-Verlag (1982;64A:1407; 65B:106)

Soren A: *Histodiagnosis and Clinical Correlation of Rheumatoid and Other Synovitis*, JB Lippincott (1978;60A:1160)

Spengler DM: *Low Back Pain: Assessment and Man-

agement, Grune & Stratton (1982;65A:572; 65B:526)

Sperryn PN: *Sport and Medicine*, Butterworth (Publishers) (1983;66B:312)

Spiegel PG (ed): *Topics in Orthopaedic Trauma*, Edward Arnold Publishers (1984;67B:165)

Spinner M: *Injuries to the Major Branches of the Peripheral Nerves of the Forearm*, 2nd ed., WB Saunders (1978;61A:477)

Spinner M (ed): *Kaplan's Functional and Surgical Anatomy of the Hand*, 3rd ed., JB Lippincott (1984;66A:1503)

Steinmetz ND: *MRI of the Lumbar Spine: A Practical Approach to Image Interpretation*, CV Slack (1986;69A:637)

Stewart JDM, Hallet JP: *Traction and Orthopaedic Appliances*, 2nd ed., CV Slack (1983;66B:794)

Stoker DJ: *Knee Arthrography*, Chapman & Hall (1980;63B:648)

° Stokes IAF (ed): *Mechanical Factors and the Skeleton*, John Lieby Company (1981;64B:515)

Stoll BA, Parbhoo S, (eds): *Bone Metastasis: Monitoring and Treatment*, Raven Press (1983;66A:477; 66B:465)

Strickland JW, Steichen JB (eds): *Difficult Problems in Hand Surgery*, CV Mosby (1982;65B:527)

Sugarbaker PH, Nicholson TH (eds): *Atlas of Extremity Sarcoma Surgery*, JB Lippincott (1984;67A:990)

Sumner-Smith G (ed): *Bone in Clinical Orthopaedics*, WB Saunders (1982;65B:107)

°° Sunderland Sir S: *Nerves and nerve injuries*, 2nd ed., Churchill Livingstone (Edinburgh) (1978;61B:524)

Sutherland DH: *Gait Disorders in Childhood and Adolescence*, Williams & Wilkins (1984;67B:516)

Sutton JC (ed): *Current Concepts in Chemonucleolysis: The Royal Society of Medicine International Congress and Symposium*, Series No. 72, Royal Society of Medicine (1985;68B:171)

Swanson SAV, Freeman MAR (eds): *The Scientific Basis of Joint Replacement*, Pitman Medical (1977;60B:591)

Swash M, Schwartz MS: *Neuromuscular Diseases*, Springer-Verlag (1981;64B:516)

Symmers WStC (ed): *Systemic Pathology, 2nd ed., Vol. 5: Nervous System, Muscle, Bone Joints*, Churchill Livingstone (Edinburgh) (1979; 62B:415)

Tachdjian MO (ed): *Congenital Dislocation of the Hip*, Churchill Livingstone (New York) (1982;65A:285; 65B:526)

Taleisnik J: *The Wrist*, Churchill Livingstone (New York) (1986;68B:859)

Tax HR: *Podopediatrics*, Williams & Wilkins (1980;63B:149)

Thijn CJP: *Arthrography of the Knee Joint*, Springer-Verlag (1979;62A:157)

Tile M: *Fractures of the pelvis and Acetabulum*, Williams & Wilkins (1984;66A:1325; 67B:167)

Tillman K: *The Rheumatoid Foot*, Thieme (1979;62A:685; 62B:413)

Torg JS: *Athletic Injuries to the Head, Neck and Face*, Lea & Febiger (1982;64A:1408)

Trickey EL, Hertel P (eds): *Surgery and Arthroscopy of the Knee*, Springer-Verlag (1986;69A:317)

Tronzo RG (ed): *Surgery of the Hip Joint*, 2nd ed., Springer-Verlag (1984;68B:513)

Troup IM, Wood MA: *Total Care of the Lower Limb Amputee*, Pitman Books Ltd (1982;64B:650)

Tscherne H, Gotzen L (eds): *Fractures with Soft Tissue Injuries*, Springer-Verlag (1984;67B:686)

Tubiana R (ed): *The Hand*, Vol. 1, WB Saunders (1981;67A:830; 64B:390)

Tubiana R (ed): *The Hand*, Vol. 2, WB Saunders (1985;68B:168)

Turco VJ: *Club Foot*, Churchill Livingstone (New York) (1981;64A:158; 64B:392)

° Turek SL: *Orthopaedics: Principles and Their Application*, 4th ed., JB Lippincott (1984;67B:512)

Turner RH, Scheller A (eds): *Revision Total Hip Arthroplasty*, Grune & Stratton (1982;64A:1406; 66B:152)

Uhthoff HK, Stahl E (eds): *Current Concepts of Diagnosis and Treatment of Bone and Soft Tissue Tumors*, Springer-Verlag (1984;66A:1325; 67B:515)

Uhthoff HK, Stahl E (eds): *Current Concepts of External Fixation of Fractures*, Springer-Verlag (1982;65A:877; 65B:370)

Uhthoff HK, Stahl E (eds): *Current Concepts of Infections in Orthopaedic Surgery*, Springer-Verlag (1985;68B:342)

Uhthoff HK (ed): *Current Concepts of Bone Fragility*, Springer-Verlag (1986;69A:477)

° Urist MR (ed): *Fundamental and Clinical Bone Physiology*, JB Lippincott (1981;63A:1198; 63B:483)

°° Vaughan J: *The Physiology of Bone*, 3rd ed., Clarendon Press (1981;64B:516)

Verdan C (ed): *Tendon Surgery of the Hand*, Churchill Livingstone (Edinburgh) (1979; 62B:288)

Vidić B, Suarez FR: *Photographic Atlas of the Human Body*, CV Mosby (1984;67B:166)

Vincenzini P: *Ceramics in Surgery*, Elsevier (1983;66B:624)

Vinken PJ, Bruyn GW (eds): *Handbook of Clinical Neurology, Vol. 32: Congenital Malformations of* the Spine and Spinal Cord, North Holland Publishing Company (1978;61B:132)

Vitali M, et al: Amputations and Prostheses, Balliére Timball (1978;61B:391)

Von Torklus D, Nicola T (eds): Atlas of Orthopaedic Exposures, 2nd ed., Urban & Schwarzenberg (1986;69A:158; 69B:515)

Wadsworth TG (ed): The Elbow, Churchill Livingstone (Edinburgh) (1982;64B:649)

Wainwright D: Arthritis and Rheumatism: What They Are — What You Can Do to Help Yourself, Elliot Right Way Books (1982;65B:371)

Walker PS: Human Joints and Their Artificial Replacements, Charles C Thomas (1977;60A:1014)

Watanabe M (ed): Arthroscopy of Small Joints, Igaku-Shoin (1985;68A:1134; 69B:860)

Watkins RG: Surgical Approaches to the Spine: An Atlas of Surgical Anatomy, Springer-Verlag (1983;65A:1213)

Watson M (ed): Practical Shoulder Surgery, Grune & Stratton (1985;68B:343)

Watson N: Practical Management of Musculo-skeletal Emergencies, Blackwell Scientific Publishers (1985;68B:344)

Watson N, Smith RJ: Methods and Concepts in Hand Surgery, Butterworth (Publishers) (1986;69A:317)

Watson N, Smith RJ (eds): Methods and Concepts in Hand Surgery, Butterworth (Publishers) (1986;69B:860)

Weber BG, Brunner C, Freuler F (eds): Treatment of Fractures in Children and Adolescents, Springer-Verlag (1980;62A:1392)

Weber BG, Magerl F: The External Fixator: AO/ASIF Threaded Rod System Spine Fixator, Springer-Verlag (1985;67A:1310; 68B:342)

Weeks PM, Wray RC: Management of Acute Hand Injuries, 2nd ed., CV Mosby (1978;61A:317)

Weir J, Abrahams P: Atlas of Radiological Anatomy, Springer-Verlag (1978;61A:638)

Weiss L, Gilbert HA (eds): Bone Metastasis, GK Hall (1981;64A:478)

Weissman SD (ed): Radiology of the Foot, Williams & Wilkins (1983;67B:514)

Welsh RP, Shephard RJ: Current Therapy in Sports Medicine 1985–86, CV Mosby (1985;69B:516)

White AA III, Panjabi MM: Clinical Biomechanics of the Spine, JB Lippincott (1978;61A:956)

White AH: Back School and Other Conservative Approaches to Low Back Pain, CV Mosby (1983; 65A:877)

White AH: Spine, Hanley & Belfus (1986;69B:860)

Whittle M, Harris D (eds): Biomechanical Measurement in Orthopaedic Practice, Oxford University Press (1985;69A:1118)

Whittle M (ed): Biomechanical Measurement in Orthopaedic Practice, Clarendon Press (1985; 68B:514)

Wiesel SW, Bernini P, Rothman RH: The Aging Lumbar Spine, WB Saunders (1982;65B:679)

Wilgis EFS: Vascular Injuries and Diseases of the Upper Limb, JB Lippincott (1983;66B:622)

Wilkinson JA: Congenital Displacement of the Hip Joint, Springer-Verlag (1985;68A:157; 68B:513)

Williams JGP: Colour Atlas of Injury in Sport, Wolfe Medical Publishers (1980;63B:485)

Williams JGP: Injury in Sport, Bayer UK Ltd (1978;61B:132)

Williams PF (ed): Orthopaedic Management in Childhood, Blackwell Scientific Publishers (1982;65A:1213; 65B:525)

Williams TF (ed): Rehabilitation in the Aging, Raven Press (1984;66B:796)

Wilner D: Radiology of Bone Tumors and Allied Disorders, WB Saunders (1982;64A:1406)

Wilson DH, Flowers MW: Accident and Emergency Handbook, Butterworth (Publishers) (1985; 68B:344)

Wilson DH, Hall MH: Casualty Officer's Handbook, 4th ed., Butterworth (Publishers) (1979;62B:414)

Wilson FC (ed): The Musculoskeletal System: Basic Processes and Disorders, 2nd ed., JB Lippincott (1982;65A:573)

Wilson JN (ed): Watson–Jones Fractures and Joint Injuries, 6th ed., Vols. 1 and 2, Churchill Livingstone (Edinburgh) (1982;65B:680)

Winter RB: Congenital Deformities of the Spine, Thieme (1983;66A:157)

Wiseman R: Of Wounds, of Gun-shot Wounds, of Fractures and Luxations (facsimile reprint from Several Chirurgicall Treatises, 1676), Kingsmead Press (1977;60B:447)

Wolfe RD: Knee Arthrography: A Practical Approach, WB Saunders (1984;67B:343)

Wolff J: The Law of Bone Remodelling, Springer-Verlag (1986;69A:478)

Wolfort FG (ed): Acute Hand Injuries, Little, Brown (1980;63B:484)

Wright V (ed): Bone and Joint Disease in the Elderly, Churchill Livingstone (Edinburgh) (1983; 66B:466)

Wright V (ed): Clinics in Rheumatic Diseases: Measurement of Joint Movement, Vol. 8, No. 3, WB Saunders (1982;66B:621)

Wu KK: Diagnosis and Treatment of Polyostotic Spinal Tumors, Charles C Thomas (1982;65A:285)

Wyke B (ed): A Back Pain Bibliography, Lloyd Luke Medical Books (1983;65B:679)

Wynn Parry CB (ed): Clinics in Rheumatic Diseases,

Vol. 10, No. 3: The Hand, WB Saunders (1984;68B:168)

Wynne-Davies R, Hall CM, Apley AG: *Atlas of Skeletal Dysplasia,* Churchill Livingstone (Edinburgh) (1986;69B:172)

Yablon IG, Segal D, Leach RE (eds): *Ankle Injuries,* Churchill Livingstone (New York) (1983;65A:877; 66B:154)

Yaghmai I: *Angiography of Bone and Soft Tissue Lesions,* Springer-Verlag (1979;62A:684)

Yashon D: *Spinal Injury,* Appleton-Century-Crofts (1978;61A:477)

Zancolli E: *Structural and Dynamic Bases of Hand Surgery,* 2nd ed., JB Lippincott (1979;62A:156)

Zarins B, Andrews JR, Carson WG Jr (eds): *Injuries to the Throwing Arm,* WB Saunders (1985;67A:1454)

Zauder HL (ed): *Anesthesia for Orthopedic Surgery,* FA Davis Company (1980;62A:1392)

Zuidema GD, Rutherford RB, Ballinger WF II (eds): *The Management of Trauma,* 3rd ed., WB Saunders (1979;63B:146)

ORTHOPEDIC JOURNALS*

Acta Orthopedica Belgica, [Acta Medica Belgica (Brussels)], 1945 (6)

Acta Orthopedica Scandinavica (with supplements), [Munksgaard (Copenhagen)], 1930 (6)

Advances in Orthopedic Surgery, Williams & Wilkins, 1977 (6)

Advances in Trauma, Year Book Medical Publishers, 1986 (1)

American Journal of Emergency Medicine, WB Saunders, 1983 (6)

Annals of Emergency Medicine, [Am. Coll. of Emerg. Physicians (Dallas)], 1972 (1)

Annual Advances in Bone and Mineral Research, [Elsevier (Amsterdam)], 1983 (1)

Archives of Orthopedic and Traumatic Surgery, [Springer (New York)], 1903 (6)

Arthroscopy, Raven Press, 1985 (4)

Clinical Orthopedics and Related Research, JB Lippincott, 1952 (12)

Emergency Medicine, [Cahmers (New York)], 1969 (21)

Emergency Medicine Clinics of North America, WB Saunders, 1983 (4)

Foot and Ankle, Williams & Wilkins, 1980 (6)

Hand, [Churchill Livingstone (Edinburgh)], 1968

Hand Clinics, WB Saunders, 1985 (4)

Injury, Butterworth (Publishers), 1969 (6)

Instructional Course Lectures AAOS, CV Mosby (1)

International Orthopedics, Springer-Verlag, 1977 (4)

Italian Journal of Orthopedics, [Gagg. Editore (Bologna)], 1975 (4)

Italian Journal of Sports Traumatology, [Editrice Kurtis (Milan)], 1979 (4)

Japanese Orthopedic Association Journal, [Nippon Seikei, Geka Gakkai Zasshi (Tokyo)], 1926 (12)

Journal of Arthroplasty, Churchill Livingstone (New York), 1986 (4)

Journal of Bone and Joint Surgery (American Volume), [JBJS (Boston)], 1903 (9)

Journal of Bone and Joint Surgery (British Volume), [Editorial Society of B & J Surgery (London)], 1903 (5)

Journal of Hand Surgery, [Churchill Livingstone (Edinburgh)], 1975

Journal of Orthopedic Trauma, Raven Press, 1987 (4)

Journal of Orthopedic Research, Raven Press, 1983 (4)

Journal of Pediatric Orthopedics, Raven Press, 1981 (26)

Journal of Trauma, Williams & Wilkins, 1961 (12)

Neuro-Orthopedics, Springer-Verlag, 1986 (4)

Orthopedic and Traumatic Surgery, [Kauphara (Tokyo)], 1958 (12)

Orthopedic Clinics of North America, WB Saunders, 1970 (9)

Orthopedics, CB Slack, 1978 (12)

Plastic and Reconstructive Surgery, Williams & Wilkins, 1946 (12)

Scandinavian Journal of Plastic and Reconstructive Surgery, [Almqvist & Wiksell Periodical Co. (Stockholm)], 1966 (12)

Seminars in Orthopedics, Grune & Stratton, 1986 (4)

Spine, JB Lippincott, 1976 (10)

Yearbook of Emergency Medicine, Year Book Medical Publishers, 1981 (1)

Yearbook of Orthopedics, Year Book Medical Publishers, 1940 (1)

SELECTED BIBLIOGRAPHY*

Interpretive Skills and Examination (Chapter 1)

D'Ambrosia RD: *Musculoskeletal Disorders— Regional Examination and Differential Diagnosis.* JB Lippincott, 1977.

---

* Year indicates date of first issue. Numbers in parentheses indicate number of issues per year.

* See pages 479–480 for the meaning of the asterisks that precede some of the references.

DeBrunner HU: *Orthopaedic Diagnosis*, 2nd ed., Thieme (Stuttgart), 1982.

DeGowin EL, DeGowin RI: *Bedside Diagnostic Examination*. MacMillan, 1976.

Hoppenfeld S: *Physical Examination of the Spine and Extremities*. Appleton-Century-Crofts, 1976.

McRae R: *Clinical Orthopedic Examination*. Churchill Livingstone, 1976.

Morgan WL, Engel L: *The Clinical Approach to the Patient*. WB Saunders, 1977.

Post M: *Physical Examination of the Musculoskeletal System*, Year Book Medical Publishers, 1987.

Ritter MA, Gosling C: *The Knee, Guide to Exam and Diagnosis of Ligament Injuries*. Charles C Thomas, 1977.

Infection and Inflammation (Chapter 2)

°°° Aegerter E, Kirkpatrick JD: *Orthopedic Diseases, Physiology, Pathology, and Radiology*, 4th ed. WB Saunders, 1975.

Burris C: *Post-Traumatic Osteomyelitis*. JB Lippincott, 1976.

° Jaffe HL: *Metabolic, Degenerative and Inflammatory Diseases of Bones and Joints*. Lea & Febiger, 1972.

Lichtenstein L: *Diseases of Bones and Joints*, 2nd ed. CV Mosby, 1975.

° Woods CG: *Diagnostic Orthopedics — Pathology*. Blackwell Scientific Publishers, 1972.

Injury and Repair: Fractures (Chapters 3 – 5)*

°°° Apley AG: *System of Orthopedics and Fractures*, 5th ed. Butterworth, 1972. (MS, NP)

°°°° Blount WP: *Fractures in Children*. Williams & Wilkins, 1955. (MS, RP)

°°° Cave EF, Burke JF, Boyd RJ: *Fracture Management Injuries*. Year Book Medical Publishers, 1983. (RP)

Chapchal G: *Pseudoarthroses and Their Treatment*. Thieme, 1979. (SF)

°°° Charnley J: *Closed Treatment of Common Fractures*, 3rd ed. Williams & Wilkins, 1976. (RP)

---

* The letters in parentheses at the end of some references indicate the intended readers: MS = medical student; NP = nurse practitioner; RP = residents, practioners; SF = special focus.

Clowes, *Trauma, Sepsis and Shock*. Dekker, 1983.

Connolly JF: *DePalma's The Management of Fractures and Dislocations: An Atlas*, 3rd ed. WB Saunders, 1981.

Devas M: *Stress Fractures*, Churchill Livingstone (Edinburgh), 1975. (SF)

Duckworth R: *Lecture Notes on Orthopedics and Fractures*. Blackwell Scientific Publications, 1980. (SF)

Fleson B: *Roentgenology of Fractures and Dislocation*. Grune & Stratton, 1978. (SF)

°°° Flatt AE: *The Care of Minor Hand Injuries*. CV Mosby, 1979. (SF)

Gehweiler JA Jr, Osborne RG, Becker RF: *Radiology of Vertebral Trauma*. WB Saunders, 1980. (SF)

°° Guttman L: *Spinal Cord Injuries*. Blackwell Scientific Publications, 1976. (SF)

Hardy AG, Rossier AB: *Spinal Cord Injuries*. Acton Pub Sci, 1975. (SF)

Hartman JT: *Fracture Management — A Practical Approach*. Lea & Febiger, 1978. (NP)

Heim, Pfeiffer: *Small Fragment Set Manual, ASIF Group Companion Volume to Manual of Internal Fixation*. Springer-Verlag, 1974. (RP)

Heppenstall RB: *Fracture Treatment and Healing*. WB Saunders, 1980. (RP)

James F: *AAOS — The Athlete's Knee — Surgical Repair and Reconstruction* (24 contributors). CV Mosby, 1980. (SF)

Johnson RM: *Advances in Internal Fixation*. Year Book Medical Publishers, 1980. (SF)

Kennedy JC: *The Injured Adolescent Knee*. Williams & Wilkins, 1979. (RP)

Kuntscher G: *The Callus Problem*. Altner, Peter, Warren H Green, 1974. (RP)

Mason JK: *The Pathology of Violent Injury*. Year Book Medical Publishers, 1978. (SF)

Matter P, Rittman WW: *The Open Fracture*. Year Book Medical Publishers, 1978. (SF)

Mittelbach HR: *The Injured Hand. A Clinical Handbook for General Surgeons*. Springer-Verlag, 1979. (SF)

Muckles DS: *Femoral Neck Fractures and Hip Joint Injuries*. Chapman-Hill, 1977. (SF)

° Müller ME, Allgower M, Schneider R, Willenegger H: *Manual of Internal Fixation (Fractures) Techniques Recommended by the AO Group*, 2nd ed. Springer-Verlag, 1977. (RP)

° O'Donohue DH: *Treatment of Injuries to Athletes*. WB Saunders, 1976. (RP)

Owen-Smith MS: *High Velocity Missile Wounds*. Edward Arnold, 1981. (SF)

Perren SM, Rittman WW: *Cortical Bone Healing*

After Internal Fixation and Infection. Springer-Verlag, 1974. (SF)

Pierce DS, Nickel VH: *The Total Care of Spinal Cord Injuries.* Little, Brown, 1977. (SF)

°°° Rang M: *Children's Fractures.* Blackwell Scientific Publications, 1983. (RP)

Reilly T: *Sports Fitness and Sports Injuries.* Faber & Faber, 1981. (SF)

°°°° Rockwood CA, Green DP: *Fractures,* 2nd ed. (3 vols.). JB Lippincott, 1984. (RP)

°°° Salter RB: *Textbook of Disorders and Injuries of the Musculoskeletal System.* Williams & Wilkins, 1970. (MS, NP)

°°° Schneider FR: *Orthopedics in Emergency Care.* CV Mosby, 1980. (RP)

Schultz KP, Krahl H, Steven WU: *Late Reconstruction of Injured Ligaments of the Knee.* Springer-Verlag, 1978. (SF).

Sevitt S: *Bone Repair and Fracture Healing in Man.* Churchill Livingstone (Edinburgh), 1981. (SF)

°°° Shires TG: *Care of the Trauma Patient,* 2nd ed. McGraw-Hill, 1979. (RP)

°° Smillie IS: *Injuries of the Knee Joint.* Churchill Livingstone (Edinburgh), 1978. (SF)

°°°° Walt AJ: *Early Care of the Injured Patient, Committee on Trauma, American College of Surgeons.* WB Saunders, 1982. (MS, NP)

Weber BG, Brunner C, Freuler F: *Treatment of Fractures in Children and Adolescents.* Springer-Verlag, 1980. (SF)

Weeks PM, Gilula LA, Manske PR, et al: *Acute Bone and Joint Injuries of the Hand and Wrist: A Clinical Guide to Management.* CV Mosby, 1981. (SF)

° Weeks PM, Wray RC: *Management of Acute Hand Injuries.* CV Mosby, 1978. (SF)

Williams JGP: *A Color Atlas of Injury in Sports.* Wolfe Medical Publishers, 1980. (SF)

°°° Wilson JN: *Watson-Jones Fractures and Joint Injuries.* Churchill Livingstone (Edinburgh), 1976. (RP)

Wolfort FG: *Acute Hand Injuries: A Multispecialty Approach.* Little, Brown, 1980. (SF)

Soft Tissue Injury and Wound Repair (Chapter 6)

Dunphy JE: *Wound Healing.* Medical Update Series. Medical Communication Press, 1974.

°° Glynn LE: *Tissue Repair and Regeneration.* Vol. 3. *Handbook of Inflammation.* Elsevier/North Holland Biomedical Press, 1981.

°°° Hunt TK, Dunphy JE: *Fundamentals of Wound Management.* Appleton-Century-Crofts, 1979.

Mencker L: *Biologic Basis of Wound Healing.* Harper & Row, 1975.

°°° Peacock EE, VanWinkle W Jr: *Wound Repair,* 2nd ed. WB Saunders, 1970.

Sevitt W: *Reactions to Injury and Burns and Their Clinical Importance.* William Heinneman, 1974.

Sports Medicine

James F: *AAOS — The Athlete's Knee — Surgical Repair and Reconstruction* (24 contributors). CV Mosby, 1980.

Kennedy JC: *The Injured Adolescent Knee.* Williams & Wilkins, 1979.

O'Donohue DH: *Treatment of Injuries to Athletes.* WB Saunders, 1976.

Reilly T: *Sports Fitness and Sports Injuries.* Faber & Faber, 1981.

Smillie IS: *Injuries of the Knee Joint.* Churchill Livingstone (Edinburgh), 1978.

Williams JGP: *A Color Atlas of Injury in Sports.* Medical Publishers, Wolfe, 1980.

Aseptic Necrosis of Bone (Chapter 7)

°°°° Davidson JK: *Aseptic Necrosis of Bone.* Excerpta Medica/America, 1976.

°°°° Catterall A: *Current Problems in Orthopaedics.* Churchill-Livingstone, 1982.

Jaffe HL: *Metabolic Degenerative and Inflammatory Diseases of Bones and Joints.* Lea & Febiger, 1972.

Proceedings of the Conference on Aseptic Necrosis of the Femoral Head: Surgery Study Sections, National Institutes of Health, United States Public Health Service, 1964.

Proceedings of a Symposium on Dysbaric Osteonecrosis. Beckman EL, Elliott DH (eds): Public Health Service National Institute for Occupations Safety and Health, Superintendent of Documents, U.S. Government Printing Office, 1974.

Zinn WM: *Idiopathic Ischemic Necrosis of the Femoral Head in Adults.* Thieme, 1971.

Arthritis (Chapter 8)

°°° Ansell BM: *Rheumatoid Disorders in Childhood.* Butterworth, 1980.

Andrews GP, Ansell BM: *Surgical Management of*

Juvenile Chronic Polyarthritis. Grune & Stratton, 1978.

Boyle JA, Buchanan WW: *Clinical Rheumatology*. Blackwell Scientific Publications, 1971.

Cruess RL, Mitchell NS: *Surgical Management of Degenerative Arthritis of the Lower Limb*. Lea & Febiger, 1975.

°°° Flatt AE: *Care of the Arthritic Hand*, 4th ed. CV Mosby, 1983.

Freeman MAR: *Arthritis of the Knee: Clinical Features and Surgical Management*. Springer-Verlag, 1981.

Goldie I: *Surgery in Rheumatoid Joints*. S Karger, 1981.

Golding DN: *A Synopsis of Rheumatoid Disease*. Year Book Medical Publishers, 1979.

Gschwend M: *Surgical Treatment of Rheumatoid Arthritis*. WB Saunders, 1981.

Katz W: *Rheumatoid Diseases: Diagnosis and Management*. JB Lippincott, 1977.

°°°° Kelley WN, Harris ED, Jr, Ruddy S, Sledge CB: *Textbook of Rheumatology*. WB Saunders, 1981.

Maroudas A, Holborow EJ: *Studies in Joint Disease*. Pitman, 1980.

Mason M, Curry HLF: *An Introduction to Clinical Rheumatology*. Pitman Medical, 1975.

°°°‡ McCarty DJ: *Arthritis and Allied Conditions*. Lea & Febiger, 1979.

Moll JMH: *Ankylosing Spondylitis*. Churchill-Livingstone, 1980.

Nicolle FV, Dickson RA: *Surgery of the Rheumatoid Hand*. William Heinemann, 1979.

Nuki G: *The Aetopathogenesis of Osteoarthritis*. Pitman Medical, 1980.

°°°° Rodman GP, Schmacher HR (eds): *Primer on the Rheumatic Diseases*. 8th ed. William Byrd Press, 1983.

Scott JT (ed): *Coperman's Textbook of the Rheumatism Diseases*. 6th ed. Churchill Livingstone (Edinburgh), 1986.

°°° Sokoloff L: *The Joints and Synovial Fluid*. Academic Press, 1978.

Tillerman K: *The Rheumatoid Foot*. Thieme, 1979.

Tumors and Tumor-like Lesions (Chapter 9)

°°°° Dahlin DC: *Bone Tumors — General Aspects and Data on 6221 Cases*. Charles C Thomas, 1978.

°°°° Enneking WF: *Musculoskeletal Tumor Surgery*. 2 Vols. Churchill-Livingstone, (New York, Edinburgh), 1983.

°°°° Enzinger F, Lattes R, Torloni H: *Histological Typing of Soft Tissue Tumors*. WHO (Geneva), 1969.

°°° Enzinger R, Weiss SW: *Soft Tissue Tumors*. CV Mosby, 1983.

Grundmann F: *Malignant Bone Tumors*. Springer-Verlag, 1976.

°°°° Hajdu S: *Pathology of Soft Tissue Tumors*. Lea & Febiger, 1980.

°°° Huvos AG: *Bone Tumors — Diagnosis, Treatment and Prognosis*. WB Saunders, 1979.

°°°° Jaffe HL: *Tumors and Tumor-like Lesions of Bone*. Lea & Febiger, 1956.

Jaffe N: *Bone Tumors in Children*. PSG Publications, 1979.

°° Lichtenstein L: *Bone Tumors*, 5th ed. CV Mosby, 1977.

Marcove RC: *The Surgery of Tumors of Bone and Cartilage*. Grune & Stratton, 1981.

°°° Mirra JA: *Bone Tumors — Diagnosis and Treatment*. JB Lippincott, 1980.

Price CHG, Ross FGM: *Bone — Certain Aspects of Neoplasia. Proceedings of the 24th Symposium of the Colston Research Society*. Butterworth, 1973.

° Sanerkin NF, Jeffree GM: *Cytology of Bone Tumors*. J Wright & Sons, 1980.

°°°° Schajowics F, Ackerman C, Sissons H: *Histological Typing of Bone Tumors*. WHO (Geneva), 1972.

°°°° Schajowicz F: *Tumors and Tumor-like Lesions of Bone and Joints*. Springer-Verlag, 1981.

°°°° Spjut H, Dorfman H, Fechner RE, Ackerman LV: *Tumors of Bone and Cartilage*. Armed Forces Institute of Pathology, 1971.

°°° The Netherlands Committee on Bone Tumors: *Radiological Atlas of Bone Tumors*. Norton & Co., 1975.

Emergency Room Trauma

Blount WP: *Fractures in Children*. Williams & Wilkins, 1955.

Cave EF, Burke JF, Boyd RJ: *Fracture Management Injuries*. Year Book Medical Publishers, 1983.

Charnley J: *Closed Treatment of Common Fractures*. 3rd ed. Williams & Wilkins, 1976.

Flatt AE: *The Care of Minor Hand Injuries*. CV Mosby, 1979.

Gehweiler JA Jr, Osborne RG, Becker RF: *Radiology of Vertebral Trauma*. WB Saunders, 1980.

Rockwood CA, Green DP: *Fractures*, 2nd ed., 3 Vols. JB Lippincott, 1984.

Rockwood CA: *Emergency Care and Transportation*

of the Sick and Injured. Committee on Injuries, American Academy of Orthopaedic Surgeons. George Banta, 1971.

Shires TG: Care of the Trauma Patient, 2nd ed. McGraw-Hill, 1979.

Walt AJ: Early Care of the Injured Patient. Committee on Trauma American College of Surgeons. WB Saunders, 1982.

Wilson JN: Watson-Jones Fractures and Joint Injuries. Churchill Livingstone (Edinburgh), 1976.

Index

Note: Page numbers followed by f designate figures and those followed by t designate tables.